Informatics and Nursing

Opportunities and Challenges

SEVENTH EDITION

Informatics and Nursing

Opportunities and Challenges

SEVENTH EDITION

Kristi Miller, PhD, CPPS, CNE, RN

Associate Professor, Mary Black College of Nursing
University of South Carolina Upstate, Spartanburg, SC

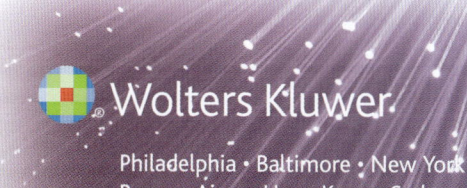

Philadelphia • Baltimore • New York • London
Buenos Aires • Hong Kong • Sydney • Tokyo

Vice President and Publisher: Julie K. Stegman
Director of Nursing Education and Practice Content: Jamie Blum
Acquisitions Editor: Joyce Berendes
Associate Director of Content Management: Staci Wolfson
Development Editor: Karen C. Turner
Editorial Coordinator: Varshaanaa Muralidharan
Marketing Manager: Wendy Mears
Editorial Assistant: Sara Thul
Design Coordinator: Stephen Druding
Art Director, Illustration: Jennifer Clements
Production Project Manager: Justin Wright
Manufacturing Coordinator: Margie Orzech-Zeranko
Prepress Vendor: TNQ Tech

Seventh Edition
Copyright © 2025 Wolters Kluwer

Copyright © 2019 Wolters Kluwer. Copyright © 2016 Wolters Kluwer. Copyright © 2013 and 2010 Wolters Kluwer Health | Lippincott Williams & Wilkins. Copyright © 2003, 1999 Lippincott Williams & Wilkins. All rights reserved. This book is protected by copyright. No part of this book may be reproduced or transmitted in any form or by any means, including as photocopies or scanned-in or other electronic copies, or utilized by any information storage and retrieval system without written permission from the copyright owner, except for brief quotations embodied in critical articles and reviews. Materials appearing in this book prepared by individuals as part of their official duties as U.S. government employees are not covered by the above-mentioned copyright. To request permission, please contact Wolters Kluwer at Two Commerce Square, 2001 Market Street, Philadelphia, PA 19103, via email at permissions@lww.com, or via our website at lww.com (products and services).

9 8 7 6 5 4 3 2 1

Printed in Mexico

Library of Congress Cataloging-in-Publication Data

ISBN-13: 978-1-975220-66-2

Cataloging in Publication data available on request from publisher.

This work is provided "as is," and the publisher disclaims any and all warranties, express or implied, including any warranties as to accuracy, comprehensiveness, or currency of the content of this work.

This work is no substitute for individual patient assessment based upon healthcare professionals' examination of each patient and consideration of, among other things, age, weight, gender, current or prior medical conditions, medication history, laboratory data and other factors unique to the patient. The publisher does not provide medical advice or guidance and this work is merely a reference tool. Healthcare professionals, and not the publisher, are solely responsible for the use of this work including all medical judgments and for any resulting diagnosis and treatments.

Given continuous, rapid advances in medical science and health information, independent professional verification of medical diagnoses, indications, appropriate pharmaceutical selections and dosages, and treatment options should be made, and healthcare professionals should consult a variety of sources. When prescribing medication, healthcare professionals are advised to consult the product information sheet (the manufacturer's package insert) accompanying each drug to verify, among other things, conditions of use, warnings and side effects and identify any changes in dosage schedule or contraindications, particularly if the medication to be administered is new, infrequently used or has a narrow therapeutic range. To the maximum extent permitted under applicable law, no responsibility is assumed by the publisher for any injury and/or damage to persons or property, as a matter of products liability, negligence law or otherwise, or from any reference to or use by any person of this work.

LWW.com

About the Author

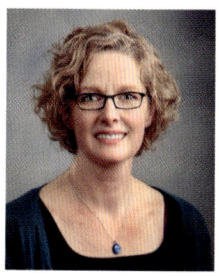

Dr. Kristi Miller is an associate professor of nursing at the Mary Black College of Nursing at the University of South Carolina Upstate and serves as the director of the graduate programs within the College of Nursing. She is board-certified as a patient safety specialist and is a certified nurse educator. Her nursing credentials include a PhD from East Tennessee State University where she focused on nursing education and patient safety; a Master of Science in Nursing Education and a Bachelor of Science in Nursing from Western Carolina University; and an associate degree in nursing from Asheville-Buncombe Community-Technical College. Before becoming a nurse, Kristi worked as a molecular biologist after obtaining a Master of Science in Biology from the Indiana University School of Medicine and a Bachelor of Science in Biology from Ball State University.

Kristi's expertise is in patient safety, nursing education, and the scholarship of teaching and learning. Her current research is focused on measuring nursing student informatics competencies and cultivating a just culture in schools of nursing. She is also passionate about diversity, equity, inclusivity, and civility. She has received several teaching awards, including a service learning and community engagement award for teaching excellence, a faculty/staff information literacy award, and an open educational resources award. She teaches traditional face-to-face classes as well as blended and online classes across the nursing curriculum in the following programs: baccalaureate in nursing, RN-BSN, Master of Science in Nursing, and Doctor of Nursing Practice. She has served as a consultant in nursing education and patient safety and as a speaker at local, regional, national, and international conferences.

Kristi has clinical nursing experience in a variety of settings, including oncology nursing, integrative health, cancer research, women's health, and home health, and she has functioned as a patient safety officer in clinical and nursing education settings. She has always been an active user of informatics and is an advocate for the use of data collection and analysis to support nursing education and patient safety.

Reviewers

Erica Alexander, PhD, RN, CNE
Professor, MSN Program Coordinator
Blessing-Rieman College of Nursing & Health Sciences
Quincy, Illinois

Chito Belchez, DNP, MSN, RN, NPD-BC
Clinical Assistant Professor
School of Nursing
University of Kansas
Kansas City, Kansas

Allison Divine, EdD, MSN, RN, CNE
Graduate Nursing Program Director
Henderson State University
Arkadelphia, Arkansas

Lyndsey Gates, MSN, RN
MSN Programs Coordinator
School of Nursing
Norwich University
Northfield, Vermont

Cynthia Hicks, DNP, RN, CMC
Cerner Surginet Clinical Analyst
Medasource – Indiana University Health
Indianapolis, Indiana

Sarita James, PhD, RN, CNE
Professor and Director
School of Nursing
Louisiana State University of Alexandria
Alexandria, Louisiana

Bonnie Kehm, PhD, RN
Faculty Program Director, Baccalaureate and Master of Science Programs
School of Nursing
Excelsior University
Albany, New York

Lilly Mathew, PhD, RN
Associate Professor of Nursing Informatics
CUNY School of Professional Studies
New York, New York

Teresa Niblett, DNP, MS, RN-BC
Chief Nursing Informatics Officer
TidalHealth System
Salisbury, Maryland

Ronda Order, APRN, PhD
Associate Teaching Professor
Pensacola Christian College
Pensacola, Florida

Shelly Randall, PhD
Associate Professor
Arkansas Tech University
Russellville, Arkansas

Ivy Razmus, RN, WOCN, PhD
Assistant Professor
University of Detroit Mercy
Detroit, Michigan

Jaime Rohr, MSN, RN-BC
Faculty Specialist
Bronson School of Nursing
Western Michigan University
Kalamazoo, Michigan

Debra Shelton, CNE
Adjunct Faculty
Northwestern State University
Shreveport, Louisiana

Jaime Sinutko, RHIA, PhD
Assistant Professor
University of Detroit Mercy
Detroit, Michigan

Daryle Wane, PhD
BSN Program Director
Pasco-Hernando State College
New Port Richey, Florida

Preface

The American Nurses Association (ANA) defines nursing informatics as "the specialty that transforms data into needed information and leverages technologies to improve health and health care equity, safety, quality, and outcomes." For many years, there has been a call for nurses to play a more central role in guiding the future of healthcare in the United States. An understanding of informatics is required for nurses to be full partners in redesigning healthcare in the United States. Nurses trained in informatics are needed to engage in effective workforce planning and policymaking. Informatics skills are needed to design, implement, utilize, and evaluate current and emerging technology in healthcare facilities.

The American Association of Colleges of Nursing (AACN) and the National League for Nursing (NLN) have identified informatics as an essential competency for all nurses, ranging from the beginning practitioner to the Doctor of Nursing Practice (DNP), Doctor of Philosophy (PhD), and Doctor of Nursing Science (DNSc). Domain 8 of the AACN Essentials outlines informatics and healthcare technology competencies for entry- and advanced-level education. A call for nursing education to adopt informatics competencies for all levels of education also came from the Technology Informatics Guiding Education Reform (TIGER) Initiative, aimed at using informatics for improving practice with evidence-based information.

The first edition of this textbook, *Computers in Nursing*, published in 1999 and was one of the first textbooks to address core informatics competencies for all nurses. Each edition, including this seventh edition, was designed to capture the innovative advancements in nursing informatics core competencies and applications and to teach students about integrating informatics into practice. This book has been redesigned to meet the challenges set forth by the National Academies of Sciences, Engineering, and Medicine and the competencies outlined in the AACN Essentials to incorporate concepts of diversity, equity, and social justice into all aspects of nursing care.

Audience

The information in this textbook is important for every nurse, from prelicensure to Doctor of Nursing practice. Besides providing introductory information about nursing informatics, the book can be used for a standalone course in nursing informatics or in a program in which informatics is threaded throughout the curriculum.

Updates

In this seventh edition, the original six units were rearranged into five units to improve the organization and flow of the content. Chapters were combined and streamlined for ease of use.

Content updates to the seventh edition include:

- Coverage of advances in healthcare information technology like artificial intelligence, telehealth, and home monitoring.
- How informatics can address social determinants of health including information literacy and access to high-speed internet.
- How informatics has been used to respond to the COVID-19 pandemic and how it can support efforts to deal with future global health crises.
- The AACN Essentials and the HIMSS TIGER competencies guide the content in each chapter.

- AACN Essentials Domain 8: Informatics and Healthcare Technologies Competencies and Subcompetencies for both entry level and advanced levels are included in this textbook.
- Applicable AACN Essentials entry- and advanced-level subcompetencies from all 10 domains are covered in this textbook.
- HIMSS TIGER Competencies are also covered in this textbook.
- Removal of the QSEN scenarios to reflect their adoption by the AACN Essentials.
- Addition of a case study at the beginning of each chapter linking key chapter concepts with thought-provoking questions throughout the chapters to encourage the development of clinical judgment.
- Ideas for discussion and activities as well as practice questions at the end of each chapter.
- Revision of chapter summaries into bulleted lists with bullet points for each of the major chapter headings.
- Removal of the chapter on legal and ethical issues and the weaving of these topics throughout the book with specific links to the ANA Code of Ethics provisions and interpretive statements.
- A new chapter on patient safety designed by a patient safety expert that links informatics concepts to concepts of civility, advocacy, communication, and just culture.
- Removal of hyperlinks to encourage the learner to find information using internet search skills.
- Increased focus on keeping the patient at the center of care.

Unit I, "What Is Informatics?", introduces readers to nursing informatics concepts including an introduction to nursing informatics; and the theoretical basis, educational preparation, and professional identity of informatics nurses.

Unit II, "Technology", provides an overview of healthcare information technology and includes essential computer concepts, computer networking and online communication, mobile healthcare technology, telehealth, and emerging technology.

Unit III, "Using Data to Improve Patient Outcomes", introduces the learner to basic nurse informatics skills needed to create knowledge from data. This unit includes how to find information, tools for collecting and analyzing data, and an overview of how to disseminate data.

Unit IV, "The Role of the Informatics Nurse", introduces the reader to informatics as a specialty including the role of the informatics nurse in supporting quality improvement projects and managing electronic health records. Students will be introduced to interoperability concepts in this unit.

Unit V, "Using Informatics to Improve Patient Outcomes", provides specific examples of how the informatics nurse can increase the quality of healthcare. Topics include information literacy, how to protect patient privacy and confidentiality, and patient safety concepts.

Key terms in each of the book's chapters are defined in the glossary. Because nursing students often identify information technology terminology as new and challenging, the glossary terms provide learning support.

In summary, the topics in this textbook address informatics competencies and applications needed by all nurses, now and in the future. Nurses with communication skills enhanced with the use of technology, computer fluency, information literacy skills, and knowledge of informatics terminology and clinical information systems can assist in shaping nursing practice to improve patient outcomes, contribute to the scholarship of nursing, and reduce health disparities.

TEACHING AND LEARNING RESOURCES

To facilitate mastery of this text's content, a comprehensive teaching and learning package has been developed to assist faculty and students.

Resources for Instructors

Tools to assist you with teaching your course are available upon adoption of this text at https://thePoint.lww.com/MillerInformatics7e.

- **PowerPoint Presentations** provide an easy way for you to integrate the textbook with your students' classroom experience, via either slide shows or handouts.

- A **Test Bank** lets you put together exclusive new tests from a bank containing hundreds of questions to help you in assessing your students' understanding of the material. Test questions link to chapter learning objectives.
- An **Image Bank** lets you use the photographs and illustrations from this textbook in your PowerPoint slides or as you see fit in your course.
- **Maps for the AACN Essentials, and HIMSS TIGER Competencies.**

  Lippincott CoursePoint is a rich learning environment that drives course and curriculum success to prepare students for practice. Lippincott CoursePoint is designed for the way students learn. The solution connects learning to real-life application by integrating content from *Informatics and Nursing: Opportunities and Challenges* with interactive modules. Ideal for active, case-based learning, this powerful solution helps students develop higher level cognitive skills and asks them to make decisions related to simple-to-complex scenarios.

  Lippincott CoursePoint for *Informatics and Nursing: Opportunities and Challenges* features the following:

- **Leading content in context:** Digital content from *Informatics and Nursing: Opportunities and Challenges* is embedded in our Powerful Tools, engaging students and encouraging interaction and learning on a deeper level.
  - The complete interactive eBook features annual content updates with the latest evidence-based practices and provides students with anytime, anywhere access on multiple devices.
  - Full online access to *Stedman's Medical Dictionary for the Health Professions and Nursing* ensures students can work with the best medical dictionary available.
- **Powerful tools to maximize class performance**: Additional course-specific tools provide case-based learning for every student:
  - **Interactive Modules** help students quickly identify what they do and do not understand, so they can study smartly. With exceptional instructional design that prompts students to discover, reflect, synthesize, and apply, students actively learn. Remediation links to the digital textbook are integrated throughout.
  - **Journal Articles** highlight how informatics is pivotal in improving clinical decision-making and patient outcomes. Collectively, the articles underscore the critical role of informatics in advancing nursing practices and shaping the future of healthcare.
- **Data to measure students' progress**: Student performance data provided in an intuitive display lets instructors quickly assess whether students have viewed interactive modules outside of class as well as see students' performance on related NCLEX-style quizzes, ensuring students are coming to the classroom ready and prepared to learn.

  To learn more about Lippincott CoursePoint, please visit: http://www.nursingeducationsucces.com/coursepoint

Acknowledgments

Several colleagues at USC Upstate contributed to this seventh textbook edition. Dr. Teri Harmon revised Chapter 2, and Dawn Henderson revised Chapter 3; both have a depth of knowledge about informatics. Andrew Kearns shared his library expertise for Chapter 7 edits on digital libraries.

I am also grateful for the help I received from the other contributors listed at the beginning of each chapter. Their input and perspective has been invaluable. In addition, the feedback from peer reviewers, faculty, and students who have used the textbook helped to guide the changes and updates.

Numerous others assisted in editing and rewriting, including Staci Wolfson, Associate Director of Content Management at Wolters Kluwer and Karen C. Turner, freelance editor.

Thank you to my husband Wes Miller and my four children, Brent, Nicole, Riley, and Trenton for allowing me the time and space to complete this much needed work. They missed me but understood my passion and drive to complete this and get it out into the world. I am grateful to my friends and colleagues as well; without their support, I would not have been able to accomplish this important undertaking. I dedicate this book to those who have experienced poor health outcomes and healthcare disparities due to racism, bias and social injustice and I pledge to do what I can to make a difference.

Contents

About the Author v
Reviewers vi
Preface viii
Acknowledgments xi

UNIT I: WHAT IS INFORMATICS?

1. Introduction to Nursing Informatics 3
Kristi Miller

What Is Informatics? 6
   Healthcare Informatics 6
   Nursing Informatics: A Historical Perspective 6
   The Informatics Nurse 7
   Benefits of Nursing Informatics 10

Federal Standards for Healthcare Informatics 11
   Office of the National Coordinator for Health Information Technology 11
   Federal Laws 11

Healthcare Informatics Professional Organizations 11
   Interdisciplinary Organizations 12
   Nursing Informatics Organizations 13

Nursing Informatics Competencies 13
   The TIGER International Competency Synthesis Project 13
   The AACN Essentials: Core Competencies for Professional Nursing Education 14

Ethics and Nursing Informatics 15
   ANA Code of Ethics for Nurses 17
   The International Council of Nurses Code of Ethics 17

Summary 18
Discussion Questions and Activities 18
Practice Questions 19

2. Professional Characteristics: Theories and Career Pathways 22
Teri Harmon and Kristi Miller

Theories That Support Informatics 24
   Data, Information, Knowledge, and Wisdom Model 24
   Sociotechnical Theory 26
   Change Theories 27
   General Systems Theory 29
   Chaos Theory 30
   Cognitive Science 31

Becoming an Informatics Nurse 31
   Bedside Experience 31
   Standards and Competencies for Informatics Education 31
   Informatics Education Programs 32
   Certification 32

Tips for Starting an Informatics Career *34*
Continuing Education *35*
Professional Informatics Organizations *35*
Nursing Informatics as a Specialty *35*
Summary 36
Discussion Questions and Activities 36
Practice Questions 38

UNIT II: TECHNOLOGY

3. Essential Computer Concepts 43

Dawn Henderson and Kristi Miller

What Is a Computer? 45
   Computer Components 45
Types of Computers 46
   Servers *46*
   Mainframes *47*
   Personal Computers *47*
   Mobile Devices *47*
Operating System 47
   Examples of Operating Systems *47*
   Graphical User Interface *48*
   Computer Programming *48*
Data Storage 49
   Hard Drive *49*
   Solid-State Drives *50*
   Other Storage Hardware *50*
   Backing Up Data *50*
Cloud Computing 50
   Cloud Storage and Encryption *52*
   Sharing Files in the Cloud *52*
   Advantages and Limitations of Using the Cloud *53*

Software Applications 53
   Commercial Software *54*
   Open-Source Software *54*
   Freeware *54*
   Public Domain Software *55*
Summary 55
Discussion Questions and Activities 55
Practice Questions 55

4. Computer Networks and Online Communication 57

Elizabeth Riley, Veneine Cunningkin, Larronda Rainey, Jaime Sinutko, and Kristi Miller

Computer Networks 60
   Architecture *60*
   Types of Computer Networks *61*
   Network Connections *61*
The Internet 64
   Internet Access as a Social Determinant of Health *64*
   Internet Components *65*
Issues With Network Security 66
   Cyber Criminals *67*
   Computer Malware *67*
   Prevalence of Breaches *70*
   Protecting Against Security Breaches *71*
Online Communication 73
   Importance of Professionalism *73*
Social Media in Healthcare 75
   Social Networking Sites *75*
   Image-Based Platforms *77*
   Video-Sharing and Streaming Platforms *77*
   Microblogging *78*
   Other Online Communication Platforms *78*

  Social Media Guidelines......................*79*
  Safe Networking................................. *80*
 Misinformation **81**
  Detecting Misinformation................ *81*
  Combating Misinformation............. *82*
 Summary... **82**
 Discussion Questions and Activities... **83**
 Practice Questions **84**
 Practice Question Answers With Rationales...**84**

5. Mobile Healthcare Technology............ 88
 Kristi Miller, Elizabeth Riley, Veneine Cunningkin, and Larronda Rainey
 Mobile Devices.......................................**90**
  Smartphones and Tablet Devices *91*
  Connecting Mobile Devices.............. *92*
 Examples of mHealth.......................... **97**
  Mobile Medical Devices......................*97*
  Wearables... *98*
  Barcode Medication Administration....................................... *99*
  eBooks... *99*
  Internet Telephone *100*
  Video Conferencing.......................... *100*
  mHealth Software for Mobile Devices...*101*
 Mobile Devices in Clinical Practice...**103**
  Advanced Practice: Nurse Practitioner Use of mHealth *103*
  Use of Mobile Devices in Nursing Research *104*
 Advantages and Disadvantages of Using mHealth............................. **104**
  Smartphone Malware......................*105*
  Cyber Attacks on Medical Devices...*106*

 Future Trends...................................... **106**
  Speech Recognition *106*
  Artificial Intelligence *107*
  Nanotechnology................................*107*
 Summary... **108**
 Discussion Questions and Activities...**109**
 Practice Questions **109**

6. Telehealth.. 112
 Kristi Miller, Olivia Boice, Neal Reeves, and Brittany Beasley
 Telehealth Concepts..........................**114**
  Types of Telehealth *115*
  Telenursing..*116*
  Standards for Telenursing and Telehealth *116*
  Telehealth and Education................ *117*
 Examples of Telehealth.....................**117**
  Telehomecare....................................*118*
  Portable Monitoring Devices *118*
  Primary Care.......................................*120*
  Telemental Health............................*120*
  e-Intensive Care Units......................*120*
  Teletrauma Care................................ *123*
  Telehealth for Chronic Illness Management....................................... *123*
  Disaster Healthcare *124*
 Issues With Telehealth **125**
  High-Speed Internet Access.......... *125*
  Reimbursement *126*
  Regulation *127*
  Fraud..*127*
 Summary... **129**
 Discussion Questions and Activities... **129**
 Practice Questions **130**

UNIT III: USING DATA TO IMPROVE PATIENT OUTCOMES

7. Finding Information 135

Andrew Kearns, Meredith MacKenzie, and Kristi Miller

Creating Nursing Knowledge 137
- The Cyclical Nature of EBP 137
- The PICOT Question 138

Library Advantages 139

Using Databases for Research 140
- Metadata and Records 141
- Reference Managers.......................... 141
- Avoiding Plagiarism........................... 141
- Bibliographic Databases Pertinent to Nursing.......................... 142

Using a Search Interface..................145
- Boolean Connectors.......................... 146
- Other Limiters 146
- Subject Headings 148
- Searching Using MeSH Terms 148
- Advantages of Search Interfaces.. 148

Sources of Nursing Knowledge........150
- Scholarly Nursing Journals.............. 150
- Online Journals 150
- Open-Access Journals....................... 151
- Magazine, Newsletter, Newspaper, and Website Articles 152
- Government and Not-for-Profit Specialty Organization Information.. 152
- Professional Nursing Organization Information 152
- Laws, Rules, and Regulations......... 153
- Online Evidence-Based Resources 153
- Levels of Evidence............................. 154

Example of Conducting a Literature Search 154
- Search for the Best Evidence......... 154
- Conduct a Critical Appraisal of the Studies 157

Summary..157

Discussion Questions and Activities... 158

Practice Questions 159

8. Collecting Data.................................161

Kristi Miller

Data Collection Guidelines...............163
- Setting Goals 164
- Identifying Opportunities for Collecting Data 164
- Capturing Diversity........................... 165
- Overcoming Obstacles..................... 165

Data Collection Tools 166
- Polls... 166
- Surveys... 167
- Observation 169
- Interviews 169
- Focus Groups 169
- Experimentation 170
- Data from Data 170

Databases...171
- Database Management System..... 172
- Database Models............................... 172
- Database Design 173
- Database Software 174

Summary.. 174

Discussion Questions and Activities.. 174

Practice Questions 174

9. Analyzing Data................................. 176

Meredith Mackenzie, Jean Mellum, and Kristi Miller

Data Analysis in Nursing...................179

Data Analysis in EBP and Research... 180

Types of Data 180
- Structured Data................................. 181

Unstructured Data *181*
Big Data *181*

Sources of Standard Data **184**
U.S. Government *185*
U.S. Census Bureau *185*
Agency for Healthcare Research and Quality *185*
Centers for Medicare & Medicaid Services *185*

Tools for Data Analysis **186**
Analyzing Structured Data *186*
Analyzing Unstructured Data *189*
Big Data Technology *190*

Current Trends in Data Analytics **191**
Health Information Technology *191*
Artificial Intelligence to Improve Healthcare *191*
Clinical Decision Support Systems *192*

Summary **192**

Discussion Questions and Activities **193**

Practice Questions **193**

10. Disseminating Data 196

Kristi Miller, Joni Tornwall, Meredith Mackenzie, and Sarah Rusnak

Data Dissemination **199**

Presenting Data **199**
Choosing a Venue *200*
Presentations *200*
Posters *205*
Assessment and Evaluation *207*

Publishing Data **207**
How Do Scholarly and Academic Writing Differ? *207*
Choosing a Journal for Publication *208*

Universal Design **209**
Accessibility *209*
Usability *211*
Inclusivity *211*

Summary **212**

Discussion Questions and Activities **213**

Practice Questions **213**

UNIT IV: THE ROLE OF THE INFORMATICS NURSE

11. Roles and Responsibilities of the Informatics Nurse 219

Kristi Miller, Neal Reeves, Marilyn Faye Hughes, and Heather Shirk

IN Job Titles **223**
IN Specialist and Clinical Informatics Specialist *223*
Clinical Analyst *224*
Director or Manager of Clinical Informatics *224*
Nurse Educator or Instructor *224*
Chief Nursing Informatics Officer *224*
EHR Implementation Manager *225*

System Responsibilities of the IN ... **225**
System Implementation *225*
System Optimization and Utilization *229*
System Development *230*
Change/Control Management *232*

Other Responsibilities of the IN **234**
Quality Improvement *234*
Project Management *240*
Leadership *245*

Summary **246**

Discussion Questions and Activities **246**

Practice Questions **247**

12. Interoperability at the National and the International Levels..............250

Sally M. Villaseñor and Kristi S. Miller

Interoperability and Standards......252
- Levels of Interoperability...............253
- Standards 254

U.S. Efforts for Promoting Interoperability.............................254
- The Centers for Medicare & Medicaid Services 255
- Office of the National Coordinator for Health Information Technology..256
- The Centers for Disease Control and Prevention...................................257
- Unified Medical Language System...257

International Standards Organizations..................................259
- International Organization for Standardization 260
- International Electrotechnical Commission 261
- Health Level Seven 261
- International Classification of Disease 261
- International Classification of Functioning, Disability, and Health...262
- Digital Imaging and Communications in Medicine 262
- Comité Européen de Normalisation.....................................263
- International Health Terminology Standards Development Organization...263
- Development of International Standards 263

Billing Terminology Standardization 263
- ICD for Billing.....................................264
- Medicare Severity Diagnosis-Related Groups.............264
- The Healthcare Common Procedure Coding System 264
- Outcome and Assessment Information Set..................................264

The Importance of Interoperability in the Future of Healthcare..........265

Summary..265

Discussion Questions and Activities..266

Practice Questions 266

13. Electronic Health Records and Standardized Nursing Terminology...269

Kristi Miller and Melissa McNeilly

History and Trends of Healthcare Records...272
- Using Paper Records........................272
- Transition to Electronic Records ...273
- Modern Adoption of EHRs 274

Types of Electronic Records...........275
- Electronic Medical Records........... 275
- Electronic Health Records.............276
- Personal Health Records................277

Nursing Engagement With EHR Development and Design.............277
- Complaints About EHRs.................278
- EHR Design Problems......................278
- Nursing Research on EHRs.............279
- EHR Solutions.....................................279
- Nursing Advocacy for EHRs..........279

Standardized Terminology in Nursing...280
- Minimum Data Sets..........................281
- Interface Terminologies 281
- Reference Terminologies................283
- Nursing Information and Data Set Evaluation Center...........283

Barriers to Implementing Standardized Nursing Terminology.. 284
Summary... 284
Discussion Questions and Activities.. 285
Practice Questions 285

UNIT V: USING INFORMATICS TO IMPROVE PATIENT OUTCOMES

14. Information Literacy: A Road to Improved Patient Outcomes.............. 291

Sally M. Villaseñor and Kristi S. Miller

Information Literacy in Healthcare.. 293
- Information Literacy Competencies for Nurses 294
- Nursing Organizations Promoting Literacy............................ 294

Health Literacy.................................... 294
- Health Literacy Movement 296
- Health Literacy and Numeracy Surveys.. 297
- Factors that Affect Health Literacy.. 298
- Assessing Health Literacy in Patients 299
- Addressing Health Literacy Issues 299
- Providing Patient Information on Healthcare Agency Websites 302

Empowered Consumer..................... 304
- Key Legislative Developments...... 305
- Rise of Consumer Informatics....... 305
- Empowering the Healthcare Consumer to Achieve Information Literacy......................... 305

Summary... 309
Discussion Questions and Activities.. 309
Practice Questions 310

15. Protecting Patient Privacy and Confidentiality 313

Kristi Miller, Janna Lock, and Allison Devine

Privacy and Confidentiality.............. 315
- Ensuring Patient Privacy 315
- Protecting Confidentiality 316

Health Insurance Portability and Accountability Act 319
- HIPAA Privacy Rule 319
- Universal Patient Identifier.............. 321
- HITECH Act and HIPAA Protection... 321
- HIPAA Violations 321
- Limitations of HIPAA Protection..... 324

Data Security 325
- Protecting Data Accuracy 325
- Protecting Data From Unauthorized Internal Access 325
- Protecting Data From Unauthorized External Access...... 325
- Protection From Data Loss........... 326
- Data Security Breaches................... 326

Summary...328
Discussion Questions and Activities..329
Practice Questions 329

16. Applying Nursing Informatics to Patient Safety 331

Kristi Miller

Medical Errors 334
- Types of Errors.................................. 334
- Causes of Medical Errors 335
- Cost of Medical Errors 336

Measuring Patient Safety................. 337
- Counting Medical Errors 337
- Voluntary Error Reporting.............. 337
- Other Ways to Measure Errors...... 341

Preventing Errors 342

Systems Approach............................ 342
Root Cause Analysis......................... 343
*Health Information Technology
for Medication Error Prevention... 348*

Culture of Safety................................350
Measuring Safety Culture 353
Patient Safety Organizations......... 354

Summary...356
**Discussion Questions and
Activities..**356
Practice Questions 357

*Appendix A Creating a Database
With Microsoft Access 361*
*Appendix B Mastering Spreadsheet
Software to Assess Quality Outcomes......375*
*Appendix C Authoring Scholarly
Slide Presentations 392*
*Appendix D Authoring Scholarly
Word Documents 406*
Glossary.. 427
Index.. 441

UNIT I

What is Informatics?

Chapter 1	Introduction to Nursing Informatics
Chapter 2	Professional Characteristics: Theories and Career Pathways

The American Nurses Association (ANA) Scope of Nursing Informatics Practice states that "Nursing informatics is the specialty that transforms data into needed information and leverages technologies to improve health and health care equity, safety, quality, and outcomes" (ANA, 2022, p. 3). In this unit, you will find the basic skills and competencies needed to fulfill the role of an informatics nurse, ethical codes to guide your study on nursing informatics, the foundational theories that support informatics, and the educational and professional path to becoming an informatics nurse. This unit is foundational material for understanding the rest of the textbook.

Chapter 1 (Introduction to Nursing Informatics) provides an overview and history of nursing informatics. The chapter includes the rationale for using the Healthcare Information and Management Systems Society (HIMSS) Technology Informatics Guiding Education Reform (TIGER) Competencies and the American Association of Colleges of Nursing (AACN) Essentials to guide the content of the book. The role of the informatics nurse, the need for computer and information literacy skills, federal informatics guidelines, and professional organizations are also covered. A discussion of ethics and how they are tied to informatics concepts is provided. The Chapter 1 case study is on the Office of the National

Coordinator for Health Information Technology (ONC) 2020-2025 Federal Health Information Technology (IT) Strategic Plan.

Chapter 2 (Professional Characteristics, Theories and Career Pathways) explores informatics as a nursing specialty, including theories supporting nursing informatics and the educational and career pathways to becoming an informatics nurse. The work of Florence Nightingale is also discussed. The case study is on how Rogers' diffusion of innovation theory can help with the process of implementing medical devices into a clinical setting. The ethical duty of the nurse to engage in lifelong learning is also discussed.

REFERENCE

American Nurses Association (ANA). (2022). *Nursing informatics: Scope and standards of practice* (3rd ed.). American Nurses Publishing.

CHAPTER 1

Introduction to Nursing Informatics

Kristi Miller

OBJECTIVES

After studying this chapter, you will be able to:

1. Define and discuss the evolution of nursing informatics as a specialty and its benefits.
2. Identify federal agencies and laws for healthcare informatics.
3. Identify healthcare informatics professional organizations and explain their purpose.
4. Discuss the sources of nursing informatics competencies and how they support national healthcare goals.
5. Explain the importance of using ethical principles in nursing informatics.

AACN Essentials for Entry-Level Professional Nursing Education

1.1d	Articulate nursing's distinct perspective to practice.
8.1f	Explain the importance of nursing engagement in the planning and selection of healthcare technologies.
8.3d	Examine how emerging technologies influence healthcare delivery and clinical decision making.
8.3e	Identify impact of information and communication technology on quality and safety of care.
9.1a	Apply principles of professional nursing ethics and human rights in patient care and professional situations.
9.3e	Engage in professional activities and/or organizations.
9.4b	Adhere to the registered nurse scope and standards of practice.
9.5a	Describe nursing's professional identity and contributions to the healthcare team.
10.2d	Expand personal knowledge to inform clinical judgment.
10.3i	Recognize the importance of nursing's contributions as leaders in practice and policy issues.

AACN Essentials for Advanced-Level Nursing Education

1.1g Integrate an understanding of nursing history in advancing nursing's influence in healthcare.

8.3i Appraise the role of information and communication technologies in engaging the patient and supporting the nurse–patient relationship.

8.3j Evaluate the potential uses and impact of emerging technologies in healthcare.

8.5l Analyze the impact of federal and state policies and regulation on health data and technology in care settings.

9.1h Analyze current policies and practices in the context of an ethical framework.

9.5f Articulate nursing's unique professional identity to other interprofessional team members and the public.

HIMSS TIGER Competencies

Ethics in health internet technology

Information and knowledge management in patient care

Principles of health informatics

Teaching, training, education

KEY TERMS

- Code of ethics
- Code of Ethics for Nurses
- Computer literacy
- Healthcare information technology (HIT)
- Healthcare informatics
- Informatics
- Informatics nurse (IN)
- Information literacy
- Information technology (IT)
- Interoperability
- Nursing informatics
- Quality and Safety Education for Nurses (QSEN)
- Technology Informatics Guiding Education Reform (TIGER)

CASE STUDY

In your daily activities, you routinely use information and technology to do things like order groceries, request a ride, adjust your thermostat, or check your bank account. The rate of progress since the invention of the first computer in 1942 or the internet in 1983 is astounding. Healthcare has not matched the progress of mainstream technology. Most healthcare providers now use electronic health record (EHR) systems to record a patient's health history, but the information is still difficult for patients, caregivers, and healthcare providers to access across the wide variety of healthcare settings. Imagine a patient receiving care at a primary care office, an urgent care clinic, and an emergency department. Although it is a single patient, they may have multiple EHRs across these different systems.

To ensure healthcare technology is meeting the needs of consumers and providers, the Office of the National Coordinator for Health Information Technology (ONC) created a strategic plan in 2008 that is updated every 5 years. You can see the 2020-2025 Federal Health Information

Technology (IT) Strategic Plan in Figure 1-1. The plan outlines how to use IT to improve the connections among patients, caregivers, providers, and healthcare systems.

As you explore Figure 1-1, think about how the ONC strategic plan will impact nursing, and about how nursing, specifically nursing informatics, can impact the plan. Consider how the plan and a nurse with informatics skills could improve this patient's EHR scenario. As you read this chapter, think about how nursing informatics supports the vision of the ONC strategic plan to create "a health system that uses information to engage individuals, lower costs, deliver high-quality care, and improve individual and population health" (ONC, 2020, p. 3).

GOAL 1: Promote Health and Wellness

- **Objective 1a:** Improve individual access to usable health information
- **Objective 1b:** Advance healthy and safe practices through health IT
- **Objective 1c:** Integrate health and human services information

GOAL 2: Enhance the Delivery and Experience of Care

- **Objective 2a:** Leverage health IT to improve clinical practice and promote safe, high-quality care
- **Objective 2b:** Use health IT to expand access and connect patients to care
- **Objective 2c:** Foster competition, transparency, and affordability in healthcare
- **Objective 2d:** Reduce regulatory and administrative burden on providers
- **Objective 2e:** Enable efficient management of health IT resources and a nationwide workforce confidently using health IT

GOAL 3: Build a Secure, Data-Driven Ecosystem to Accelerate Research and Innovation

- **Objective 3a:** Advance individual- and population-level transfer of health data
- **Objective 3b:** Support research and analysis using health IT and data at the individual and population levels

GOAL 4: Connect Healthcare with Health Data

- **Objective 4a:** Advance the development and use of health IT capabilities
- **Objective 4b:** Establish expectations for data sharing
- **Objective 4c:** Enhance technology and communications infrastructure
- **Objective 4d:** Promote secure health information practices that protect individual privacy

Figure 1-1. The 2020-2025 Federal Health Information Technology Strategic Plan. (From Office of the National Coordinator for Health Information Technology (ONC). (2020, October). *2020-2025 Federal Health IT Strategic Plan*. HealthIT.gov. https://www.healthit.gov/topic/2020-2025-federal-health-it-strategic-plan)

"In attempting to arrive at the truth, I have applied everywhere for information, but in scarcely an instance have I been able to obtain hospital records fit for any purposes of comparison. If they could be obtained, they would enable us to decide many other questions besides the ones alluded to. They would show subscribers how their money was being spent, what amount of good was really being done with it, or whether the money was not doing mischief rather than good ..."

(Nightingale, 1863, p. 176)

Florence Nightingale is considered by many to be the first informatics nurse (IN), and her quote demonstrates some of the most important reasons for nurses to engage in informatics (you will learn more about her role in Chapter 2). This chapter will provide you with an overview of informatics, including the evolution of nursing informatics and the federal agencies and professional organizations that guide the use of informatics in nursing. You will also learn about the ethical principles, skills, and competencies needed to perform the role of the IN. All nurses need informatics knowledge to support the best possible patient outcomes; however, in future chapters, you will learn about career opportunities for nurses who want to specialize in informatics.

WHAT IS INFORMATICS?

The term "informatics" was first used in 1957 by a German computer scientist (Steinbuch, 1957). In the 1960s with increasing use of computers, the term became more widely accepted and was used to refer specifically to the use of computers (Sackett & Erdley, 2002). We can think of **information technology (IT)** as the use of electronic systems like computers or telecommunications for processing, storing, retrieving, and sending information. But **informatics** itself is the *application* of IT to the arts and sciences. Informatics encompasses library science as well as data science. It is the study of information, and the ways information is used by and impacts human beings and social systems. **Computer literacy** is the ability to perform various tasks or skills with a computer efficiently, whereas **information literacy** is the ability to know when information is needed and how to locate, evaluate, and effectively use it. This is a vital skill in informatics.

Informatics is used in a wide range of fields including technology development, business, cybersecurity, product management, government, and healthcare.

Healthcare Informatics

Healthcare informatics is the integration of computer and information science to manage healthcare information and technology. It applies to the generation, handling, communication, storage, retrieval, management, analysis, discovery, and synthesis of information and knowledge in all aspects of healthcare. Healthcare informatics is an interdisciplinary field that includes all branches of healthcare, including medicine, dentistry, and pharmacy. The duties of a healthcare informaticist include gathering and analyzing data and information; managing and implementing healthcare IT; and educating and training end users. **Healthcare information technology (HIT)** is IT used specifically for healthcare. It involves the processing, storage, and exchange of health information in an electronic environment.

Nursing Informatics: A Historical Perspective

Nursing informatics is a specialty of healthcare informatics. The original definition of nursing informatics was the use of computer technology in all nursing endeavors: nursing services, education, and research (Scholes & Barber, 1980). In the mid-1980s, there was a shift from a technology-oriented definition to an information-oriented definition when Schwirian (1986) created a framework model for nursing informatics investigators (Fig. 1-2). The base of this pyramid model uses "raw materials" (the information), with "technology" as only a supporting level in the framework.

The first widely circulated definition of nursing informatics that transitioned from technology to concepts was from Graves and Corcoran (1989) who defined nursing informatics as "a combination of computer science, information science and nursing science designed to assist in the management and processing of nursing data, information and knowledge to support the practice of nursing and the delivery of nursing care" (p. 227). The definition secured the position of nursing informatics within the practice of nursing and placed the emphasis on data, information, and knowledge (Staggers et al., 2001).

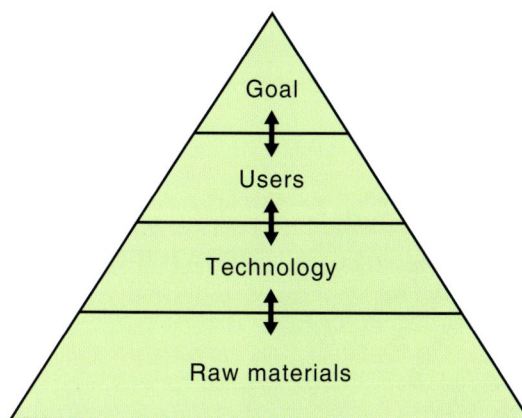

Figure 1-2. Schwirian's model of informatics. (Adapted from Schwirian P. (1986). The NI pyramid—A model for research in nursing informatics. *Computers in Nursing: CIN, 4*(3), 134-136. Retrieved from http://journals.lww.com/cinjournal/pages/default.aspx)

In 1992, the American Nurses Association (ANA) recognized nursing informatics as a subspecialty of nursing that combines nursing, information, and computer sciences for the purpose of managing and communicating data, information, and knowledge to support nurses and healthcare providers in decision making (Bickford, 2017). In 1993, the National Center for Nursing Research released the seminal report, *Nursing Informatics: Enhancing Patient Care* (Pillar & Golumbic, 1993), which set six program goals for nursing informatics research:

1. Establish a nursing language (useful in computerized documentation).
2. Develop methods to build clinical information databases.
3. Determine how nurses give patient care using data, information, and knowledge.
4. Develop and test patient care decision support systems.
5. Develop workstations that provide nurses with needed information.
6. Develop appropriate methods to evaluate nursing information systems.

These six goals are still pertinent, though today, the third goal would include "wisdom," because in 2008, the term was added to the data, information, and knowledge continuum (ANA, 2008).

The first administration of the informatics certification examination was in the fall of 1995 (Newbold, 1996). In 1997, the Division of Nursing of the Health Resources and Services Administration convened the National Advisory Council on Nurse Education and Practice. The council produced *A National Informatics Agenda for Nursing Education and Practice*, which made five recommendations (National Advisory Council on Nurse Education and Practice, 1997, p. 8):

1. Educate nursing students and practicing nurses in core informatics content.
2. Prepare nurses with specialized skills in informatics.
3. Enhance nursing practice and education through informatics projects.
4. Prepare nursing faculty in informatics.
5. Increase collaborative efforts in nursing informatics.

The National League for Nursing (NLN) published a position paper outlining recommendations for preparing nurses to work in an environment that uses technology (NLN, 2008). The paper outlined recommendations for nursing faculty, deans/directors/chairs, and the NLN. Examples of recommendations included the need for faculty to achieve informatics competencies and incorporate informatics into the nursing curriculum. In 2021, the ANA's *Nursing Informatics: Scope and Standards of Practice* stated that "Nursing informatics is the specialty that transforms data into needed information and leverages technologies to improve health and health care equity, safety, quality, and outcomes" (ANA, 2022, p. 3). This is the generally accepted definition of nursing informatics today.

The Informatics Nurse

In this textbook, you will learn nursing informatics competencies and skills that will support patient, provider, and organizational use of HIT. All nurses need informatics competencies and skills, but not all nurses will choose to become informatics nurses (INs). An **informatics nurse (IN)** is a nurse who enters the nursing informatics field because of interest or experience. They work to optimize information management and communication to improve the health of individuals, families, populations, and communities. Figure 1-3 shows

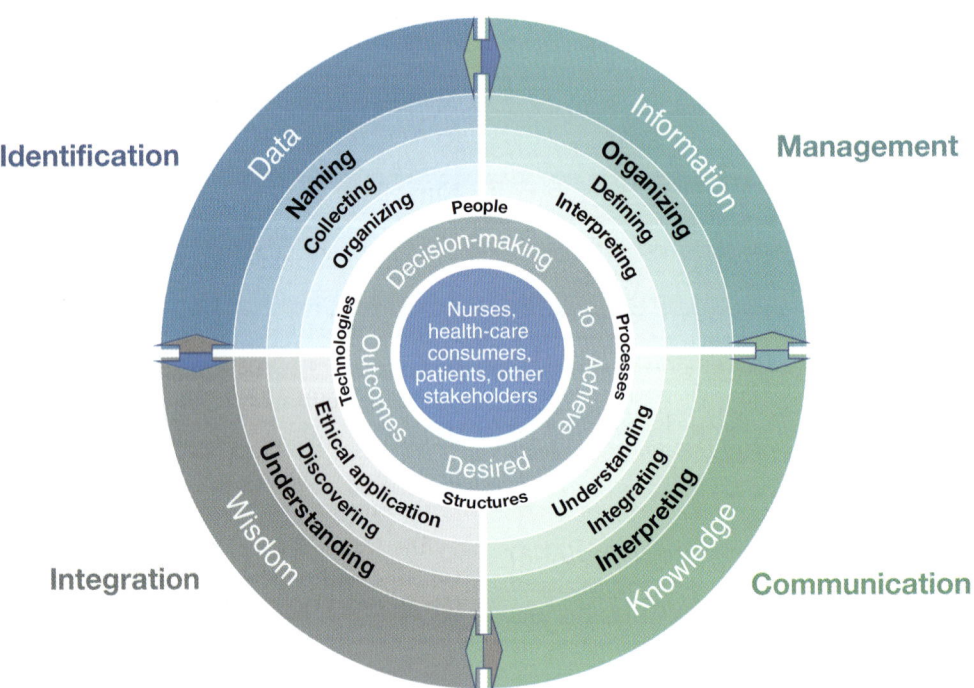

Figure 1-3. Nursing informatics specialty components and relationships. (From American Nurses Association (ANA). (2022). *Nursing informatics: Scope and standards of practice* (3rd ed.). Washington, DC: American Nurses Publishing.)

the nursing informatics specialty components and relationships. Each circle contains actions that can be taken by the IN to support the concepts of data, information, wisdom, and knowledge.

To guide the role of the IN, the ANA publishes *Nursing Informatics: Scope and Standards of Practice*. This book describes competencies for nursing informatics including national standards of practice and performance. It covers topics such as quality improvement, certification and credentialing, positions descriptions and performance appraisals, classroom teaching and in-service programs, and regulatory guidelines. It also presents concepts to be familiar with, including clinical decision support, big data, data analytics, and artificial intelligence (ANA, 2022). The ANA describes the following professional practice areas for the IN:

- Management, administration, and leadership
- Clinical informatics
- Data management and analytics
- Patient safety and quality
- Research and evaluation
- Compliance and integrity management
- Coordination, consultation, facilitation, and integration

All these concepts and practice areas will be covered in this textbook.

Some of the job titles you will find for nurses with informatics experience include:

- Nurse informaticist
- Nursing informatics specialist
- Nursing informatics clinician
- Clinical nurse informatics specialist
- Chief nursing informatics officer
- Perioperative IN

Box 1-1 describes a sample day in the life of an IN (additional coverage of this topic is found in Chapter 11). As you read through the tasks and

Box 1-1 A Day in the Life of an Informatics Nurse

My name is Teresa Niblett, and I am an informatics nurse specialist. I work for a healthcare system comprising a tertiary care regional medical center serving a large rural community, a broad network of primary and specialty ambulatory practices, and several joint ventures including home health, long-term care, medical equipment, outpatient surgery, urgent care, and outpatient diagnostics. We are 9 months post implementation of a new EHR system. Serving as a bedside nurse in the intensive care unit and a procedural nurse in the medical imaging department laid a solid foundation for a career in nursing informatics. My experience helps me connect to end users and address needs or concerns, which enable improved patient care. Many of the skills acquired through these clinical experiences such as the nursing process, critical thinking, prioritization, collaboration, conflict management, and multitasking, are applied daily.

These are the various activities I perform on a given day.

Rounding on clinical users with analysts: The days of the week, times of day, and area visited vary. My goals include finding out what's going well, identifying what can be improved, providing on-the-spot education, reporting issues that are difficult to detect, and strengthening the relationship between the user and analyst. In addition, I support end users during planned and unplanned system downtimes to support continuity of care and recovery.

Attend daily safety huddle: Each morning, department leads report out on any safety concerns occurring in the last 24 hours. If any involve the EHR, I support investigative follow-up and correction efforts. Recently, it was reported that a medication error occurred because a nurse failed to utilize barcode medication administration.

Facilitate decision making councils: Requests to create or change electronic order sets, documentation flow sheets, decision support rules, or reports and dashboards are made daily. Utilizing various informatics theories and a defined change control process, our organization empowers frontline staff to participate in decisions affecting system changes. Changes can be as simple as updating drop-down selections for wound care products. Other requests can be more complicated, such as adding new orders that flow to a nurse's task list. As a facilitator, I assist the teams in maintaining a charter, setting the agenda, engaging participants, following through on decisions, and communicating changes to affected stakeholders.

Support or sponsor optimization workgroup teams: Customizing care plan templates, standardizing bedside shift report handoff, and updating required documentation on admission and discharge are just a few examples of work that has been completed since we went live with our system. Currently, a team of nurses, providers, pharmacists, leaders, and analysts are collaborating to improve care for patients at risk for alcohol withdrawal. The goal is to detect patients at risk and intervene sooner, preventing negative health complications, stress, and avoidable resource utilization. Objective and subjective assessment findings have been researched. Assessment screening elements will be updated. Clinical decision support rules to alert users that a patient is scoring positively for withdrawal and what actions are needed will be created. Order sets will be updated to prescribe additional assessment tools and pharmacologic interventions to treat symptoms and prevent escalation. Reports to evaluate the effects of the changes will be created and utilized by the team.

(Continued)

> **Box 1-1** A Day in the Life of an Informatics Nurse *(Continued)*
>
> **Participate in weekly health information systems (HIS) and clinical operational leadership planning meetings:** Through participation at the various meetings, I gather information on new and ongoing projects and provide updates from other leadership teams. I help influence decisions and prioritize actions and resources. At the weekly leadership meeting, I hear about progress on the latest system update, lab instrument interface mapping, and document scanning improvement progress and vendor delays in receiving hardware for a new outpatient clinical. I can share details about workflow or throughput improvement efforts that depend upon system release deadlines, influence messaging details and communication channels to the organization about the planned system update, and advocate for resources to support validation of reports showing the organization is not meeting meaningful use requirements to send summaries of care for patients transferred or referred on discharge.
>
> **Networking and continuing education:** At least once a week, I participate in virtual calls or meetings with colleagues from other facilities in the state or region. We share successes, collaborate on challenges, and refer to other colleagues when able. I am involved with professional organizations such as ANIA, HIMSS, and AMIA at the local, state, and national level. This helps me to stay informed on new evidence or contribute feedback to proposed rulings. It also allows me to share about work our hospital has performed via presentations, posters, and webinars.
>
> My role as an informatics nurse specialist is exciting and rewarding. Every day we learn and apply knowledge to improve knowledge, process, and system design. We support clinicians in utilizing technology to deliver better care.
>
> *Teresa A. Niblett, RN-BC, MS,*
> *Chief Nursing Informatics Officer*

duties of the IN, make note of the concepts and terms with which you are not familiar. By the end of this textbook, you will have greater understanding of all the concepts and terms..

Benefits of Nursing Informatics

Danielle Siarri, a global nursing expert, said "healthcare and technology were separate entities that have now fused into one language which evolves daily" and "nursing informatics specialists are the translators" (HIMSS, 2019).

INs provide remarkable gifts to healthcare. They inform and influence IT systems. They spend a great deal of time developing, implementing, and optimizing HIT. The blend of clinical and technical knowledge and experience gives the IN a unique perspective. EHR vendors often hire INs to help design and build systems because they can recommend the best processes and most practical layouts. In addition, they can predict how staff will react to EHR features and prevent redundant or difficult workflow. The IN ensures evidence-based best clinical practice. They can influence the design of clinical systems to promote the use of evidence-based practices as well as train other nurses to use clinical IT systems.

The IN is involved in the development of new options for healthcare delivery, such as the use of smartphones, as well as in the design and implementation of telehealth systems, ensuring optimal usability. Once telehealth systems are implemented, the IN can educate patients using patient medical data and can support communication with their providers from across town or from the opposite side of the planet.

In summary, the IN supports more efficient EHRs, better HIT systems, research and application of clinical best practice, training of nurses, analysis of data to improve patient outcomes, and new ways to educate patients. Patients benefit from nursing informatics with fewer medical errors, more informed clinical decision making, shorter lengths of stay in hospitals, lower readmission and admission rates, and better patient self-management.

FEDERAL STANDARDS FOR HEALTHCARE INFORMATICS

The federal government plays an important role in the advancement of HIT. Federal agencies purchase, develop, and regulate HIT. They also fund and contribute to HIT research, development, and deployment at local, tribal, state, and national levels. In addition, federal agencies coordinate the alignment of standards between public and private entities and encourage innovation, best practice, and competition (ONC, 2020).

Office of the National Coordinator for Health Information Technology

In 2004, President George W. Bush called for adoption of interoperable EHRs for most Americans by 2014. **Interoperability**, covered in detail in Chapter 12, refers to the ability of two or more systems to pass information between each other and to use the exchanged information. The President also established the ONC to create and implement strategic plans to improve health and healthcare for all Americans through information and technology.

The 2008 *ONC-Coordinated Federal Health Information Technology Strategic Plan* focused on two goals—patient-focused healthcare and population health. The common themes for the goals included privacy and security, interoperability, adoption, and collaborative governance (ONC, 2008). The nation's shift toward interoperable EHRs has expanded and now incorporates patient-centered values so that all individuals, caregivers, and providers can expect reliable and timely access to electronic health information, a respect for individual preferences, and continuous learning and improvement.

The 2015–2020 ONC strategic plan was released with a vision of high-quality care, lower costs, healthy populations, engaged individuals, and a mission to "improve the health and well-being of individuals and communities through the use of technology and health information that is accessible when and where it matters most" (ONC, 2015). Around this time, the ONC created the Health IT Playbook to serve as a guide for successfully implementing an electronic health information program (HealthIT.gov, n.d.). The ONC has also created playbooks for health information exchange, certified health IT, privacy and security, and value-based care.

The 2020–2025 plan (see Fig. 1-1) is discussed in the case study. In this textbook, you will find many case studies that focus on healthcare challenges identified in the plan. The new plan focuses on decreasing healthcare spending, improving health outcomes, addressing the increasing rates of mental illness and substance use disorders, and increasing access to care, technology, and electronic health information (ONC, 2020).

Federal Laws

In 2009, the Health Information Technology for Economic and Clinical Health (HITECH) Act provided incentives for healthcare organizations and providers to implement HIT, including the use of EHRs. The 2010 Affordable Care Act (ACA) made improvements in healthcare coverage, lowered costs, and increased access to care (HHS.gov/HealthCare, 2017). The 21st Century Cures Act was signed into law in 2016 to promote research innovation and medical product development. The law works with the U.S. Food and Drug Administration's (FDA) research to incorporate patient perspectives into the development of new treatments, products, and devices (USFDA, n.d.).

The IN is responsible for knowing about federal regulations and laws that impact HIT to ensure that healthcare organizations are meeting requirements and guidelines and to provide the best possible care for patients.

HEALTHCARE INFORMATICS PROFESSIONAL ORGANIZATIONS

Informatics organizations focused on healthcare have been around since 1928. At the international, national, and local levels, they serve to promote the use of informatics for improved patient outcomes, reduced healthcare costs, and the generation of knowledge. These organizations connect informatics professionals from all areas of healthcare with conferences, meetings, membership directories, and discussion forums. They provide advocacy for informatics, continuing education, opportunities for career advancement, updates in the field of informatics, and venues for scholarly publications.

Interdisciplinary Organizations

Given the interdisciplinary nature of informatics, many of the formal organizations involve practitioners from all areas of healthcare. Some of these organizations have workgroups that are just for nurses.

Healthcare Information and Management Systems Society

The Healthcare Information and Management Systems Society (HIMSS) is a global organization that has offices across the United States and Europe, including Chicago, Washington, D.C., and Brussels (HIMSS, 2018). Founded in 1961, HIMSS is a not-for-profit organization dedicated to promoting a better understanding of healthcare information and management systems. HIMSS meets annually and publishes several guides to the field. They offer accreditation as a Certified Professional in Healthcare Information and Management Systems. HIMSS supports free access to the *Online Journal of Nursing Informatics*, which is published three times yearly. You will learn more about how HIMSS has been involved in developing nursing informatics competencies later in this chapter.

European Federation for Medical Informatics

The European Federation for Medical Informatics (EFMI) was founded in 1976 to advance international cooperation and dissemination in medical informatics. All European countries can be represented in EFMI by a suitable medical informatics society. EFMI's nursing working group was formed to support European nurses and nursing informatics as well as to build informatics contact networks (EFMI, 2018).

International Medical Informatics Association

The International Medical Informatics Association (IMIA) was established in 1967 as TC4, a Technical Committee within the International Federation for Information Processing. IMIA is a nonpolitical, international, scientific organization whose goals include promoting informatics in healthcare, promoting biomedical research, advancing international cooperation, stimulating informatics research and education, and exchanging information.

Many countries belong to IMIA through national organizations such as the American Medical Informatics Association (AMIA), which represents the United States, and EFMI (EFMI, 2018). The members have national meetings to focus on issues pertaining to their nations, allowing them to establish a national network where ideas can be shared and provide a place to gain information for specific national problems. These organizations also provide journals and are a source of up-to-date information for their country. The members of IMIA also take part in the World Congress on Medical and Health Informatics, or MedInfo, an international event that is held every 2 years.

The IMIA Nursing Working Group sponsors an international nursing informatics conference every 4 years. The themes of these conferences provide a perspective on how the concerns of nursing informatics have broadened from concerns with computers in nursing in the earliest years, through integrating caring and technology in nursing, to a realization of the impact of informatics on nursing knowledge, to the recognition of the importance of the consumer or human in healthcare.

American Health Information Management Association

The American College of Surgeons formed the American Health Information Management Association (AHIMA) in 1928 to improve clinical records and empower people to impact health (AHIMA, 2017). The name reflects the expansion of clinical information collected by single hospitals or providers to an evolving, integrated system that allows information to be shared between providers and organizations. AHIMA offers credentialing programs in health information management, coding, and healthcare privacy and security.

American Medical Informatics Association

The AMIA was formed in 1988 to support the development and application of medical informatics to support patient care, education, research, and administration (AMIA, n.d.). AMIA has over

5,600 members from fields like nursing, medicine, dentistry, and pharmacy who are experts in the science and practice of informatics. AMIA offers continuing education, annual conferences, a clinical informatics board review course for physicians, and a distance learning program called "AMIA 10×10" designed to train the next generation of informatics leaders. You can sign up for a daily newsletter without being a member. Membership includes digital access to the *Journal of the American Medical Informatics Association (JAMIA)*.

Nursing Informatics Organizations
American Nursing Informatics Association
In the United States, the largest nursing informatics professional association is the American Nursing Informatics Association (ANIA). Founded in 1982, the mission of ANIA is to advance nursing informatics through education, research, and practice in all roles and settings. ANIA has an annual conference, continuing education opportunities, networking, and career-building resources (ANIA, 2018). ANIA members have access to the *Journal of Informatics in Nursing* as well as reduced rates for the ANIA Nursing Informatics Certification course. AMIA's Nursing Informatics Working Group (NIWG) is responsible for promoting the integration of nursing informatics into the broader context of healthcare. NIWG also works to influence U.S. policymakers regarding the use of nursing information.

Alliance for Nursing Informatics
In 2004, the Alliance for Nursing Informatics (ANI) united many small local nursing informatics groups. The organization is sponsored by AMIA and HIMSS (Alliance for Nursing Informatics, n.d.). Membership is through affiliation with a nursing-focused informatics group, a nursing working group, or a local or national group. These groups retain their dues, programs, publications, and organizational structures but are united through ANI to create one voice for nursing informatics. Representatives of each of the organizational groups make up the governing director's group that guides the strategic goals and activities of ANI (n.d.). Their website features links to all the member groups. ANI membership includes access to the nursing working groups of AMIA, HIMSS, and ANIA.

British Computer Society Nursing Specialist Group
The British Computer Society (BCS) Nursing Specialist Group aims to disseminate information about current nursing informatics applications and to encourage the publication of research and development material in this area (BCS, 2018). This is accomplished by interacting with other groups such as the Royal College of Nursing, the Clinical Professions and Health Visitors' Association (CPHVA/Amicus), and the National Health Service (NHS) Connecting for Health Agency.

NURSING INFORMATICS COMPETENCIES
Nursing competencies include the skills, abilities, or knowledge necessary to achieve a specific goal and include emotional, social, and cognitive aspects (Thye, n.d.). There are several methods for measuring competence in nursing informatics. Staggers et al. (2001) conducted a study to determine informatics competencies for nurses and subsequently created a Nursing Informatics Competencies Questionnaire (Chung & Staggers, 2014). Three domains of competency have been identified, including computer skills, informatics knowledge, and informatics skills (Staggers et al., 2001). Additional competencies have been defined by informatics and nursing organizations. The author of this textbook has developed a nursing informatics competency self-assessment that aligns with the AACN Essentials. Take the assessment now (https://redcap.link/ydujb52g), and again after you have finished your informatics course of study to see what informatics competencies to focus on as you continue your nursing career.

The TIGER International Competency Synthesis Project
The **Technology Informatics Guiding Education Reform (TIGER)** initiative from HIMSS began in 2009 in response to the increased use of HIT in healthcare (Gugerty & Delaney, 2009). The TIGER initiative aims to provide the global health workforce with innovative informatics tools and resources and to integrate informatics into healthcare education, certification, practice, and research through an equitable, inclusive, interdisciplinary, and intergenerational approach (HIMSS, n.d.).

> **Box 1-2** TIGER International Competency Synthesis Project's *Recommendation Framework 2.0*: Summary of Health Informatics Core Competencies
>
> | | |
> |---|---|
> | Applied computer science | Information and knowledge management in patient care |
> | Assistive technology | Interoperability and integration |
> | Change/stakeholder management | IT risk management |
> | Clinical decision support by IT | Leadership |
> | Communication | Learning techniques |
> | Consumer health informatics | Legal issues in health IT |
> | Data analytics | Medical technology |
> | Data protection and security | Principles of health informatics |
> | Documentation | Process management |
> | e/mHealth, telematics, telehealth | Project management |
> | Ethics in health IT | Public health informatics |
> | Financial management | Quality and safety management |
> | Care processes and IT integration | Resource planning and management |
> | ICT/systems (applications) | Strategic management |
> | ICT/systems (architectures) | System lifecycle management |
> | Information management research | Teaching, training, education |
>
> Reprinted from Hübner, U., Thye, J., Shaw, T., Elias, B., Egbert, N., Saranto, K., Babitsch, B., Procter, P., & Ball, M. J. (2019). Towards the TIGER International framework for recommendations of core competencies in health informatics 2.0: extending the scope and the roles. *Studies in Health Technology and Informatics, 264*, 1218–1222.

TIGER was formed to develop informatics competencies that all practicing and graduating nursing students should have to provide safe, quality, competent care.

The TIGER International Competency Synthesis Project's (ICSP) *Recommendation Framework 2.0* (Box 1-2) is a set of competencies that are global in nature and inclusive of other disciplines (Hübner et al., 2019). The international informatics competencies were created by compiling national case studies submitted by HIMSS global community members and responses to a survey that asked about informatics and clinical nursing, nursing management, quality management, IT management, and coordination of interprofessional care (HIMSS, 2021). These new competencies include communication and leadership to address the interprofessional nature of informatics.

> **CASE STUDY**
>
> How can the HIMSS TIGER competencies be used to achieve objectives from the ONC Federal Health IT Strategic Plan (see Fig. 1-1)? (Hint: Think about ONC Objective 4d.)

The AACN Essentials: Core Competencies for Professional Nursing Education

In 1986, the American Association of Colleges of Nursing (AACN) published its first list of essentials for education for professional nursing to provide an educational framework for the preparation of nurses at 4-year colleges and universities. The *AACN Essentials: Core Competencies for Professional Nursing Education* provides a framework for nurses at all levels of nursing education, including those who are already working at the bedside and those in advanced practice nursing programs.

The AACN developed the newest version of nursing essentials based on the **Quality and Safety Education for Nurses (QSEN)** initiative. The QSEN project aimed to improve nurses' education to deliver safe and quality care (Curcio, 2021). The nursing role in achieving quality and safety standards is crucial, and nurses are often considered the last defense between the patient and potential errors (Altmiller & Hopkins-Pepe, 2019). You will learn more about the role of nursing informatics and patient safety in Chapter 16.

The AACN Essentials have been used to guide the content of this book. As of April 2021, the 10 domains of the Essentials are:

1. Knowledge for nursing practice
2. Person-centered care
3. Population health
4. Scholarship for the nursing discipline
5. Quality and safety
6. Interprofessional partnerships
7. Systems-based practice
8. Informatics and healthcare technologies
9. Professionalism
10. Personal, professional, and leadership development

Each domain includes competencies and subcompetencies that represent nursing as a unique profession. Box 1-3 shows an example of one of the competencies and its subcompetencies under the "Informatics and Healthcare Technologies" domain.

The competencies are applicable across four spheres of care during the lifespan: disease prevention/promotion of health and well-being; chronic disease care; regenerative or restorative care; and hospice/palliative/supportive care (AACN, 2021). The domains and competencies are the same for entry and advanced levels of education, but the subcompetencies are geared toward each level (see Box 1-3). You will find all these discussed throughout this textbook.

> **CASE STUDY**
>
> How are the AACN Essentials used to achieve the goals of the ONC Federal Health IT Strategic Plan (see Fig. 1-1)? (Hint: Think about ONC Objective 1a and Subcompetencies 8.2b and 8.2c.)

ETHICS AND NURSING INFORMATICS

Professionals are bound by their pertinent **codes of ethics**, which are made up of statements of the professionals' values and beliefs. These are based on ethical principles like those found in Table 1-1. According to a seminal article by Curtin (2005), ethical choices have three characteristics. First, choices always involve conflict of values that are extremely important. Second, scientific inquiry can influence the choice made in a value conflict, but it cannot provide an answer. Finally, the process involves deciding which value is most important. Curtin (2005) suggests that any decision made about conflicts of fundamental values will have lasting and unexpected consequences on human concern areas. For the public good and protection, professionals who are involved with the use of

---

> **Box 1-3** Competency 8.2 of the AACN Essentials
>
> **8.2 Use information and communication technology to gather data, create information, and generate knowledge**
>
> *Entry-Level Professional Nursing Education*
> 8.2a Enter accurate data when chronicling care.
> 8.2b Explain how data entered on one patient impacts public and population health data.
> 8.2c Use appropriate data when planning care.
> 8.2d Demonstrate the appropriate use of health information literacy assessments and improvement strategies.
> 8.2e Describe the importance of standardized nursing data to reflect the unique contribution of nursing practice.
>
> *Advanced-Level Nursing Education*
> 8.2f Generate information and knowledge from health information technology databases.
> 8.2g Evaluate the use of communication technology to improve consumer health information literacy.
> 8.2h Use standardized data to evaluate decision making and outcomes across all systems levels.
> 8.2i Clarify how the collection of standardized data advances the practice, understanding, and value of nursing and supports care.
> 8.2j Interpret primary and secondary data and other information to support care.
>
> From American Association of Colleges of Nursing (AACN). (2021). The essentials: Core competencies for professional nursing education. https://www.aacnnursing.org/Portals/42/AcademicNursing/pdf/Essentials-2021.pdf

TABLE 1-1 Ethical Principles

Autonomy	Self-rule/determination
Beneficence	Doing what is best for the individual
Nonmaleficence	Doing no harm
Veracity	Truth telling
Fidelity	Honesty
Paternalism	Making decisions on behalf of others
Justice	Being fair
Respect for others	Appreciation for human dignity

Box 1-4 AACN Essentials Subcompetencies Related to Ethics

Entry-Level Professional Nursing Education Competencies
- 1.2e Demonstrate ethical decision making.
- 3.1i Identify ethical principles to protect the health and safety of diverse populations.
- 4.3a Explain the rationale for ethical research guidelines, including institutional review board (IRB) guidelines.
- 4.3b Demonstrate ethical behaviors in scholarly projects including quality improvement and EBP initiatives.
- 8.5b Demonstrate ethical use of social networking applications.
- 9.1a Apply principles of professional nursing ethics and human rights in patient care and professional situations.
- 9.1c Demonstrate ethical behaviors in practice.
- 9.1e Report unethical behaviors when observed.
- 9.5d Demonstrate ethical comportment and moral courage in decision making and actions.

Advanced-Level Nursing Education
- 1.2h Employ ethical decision making to assess, intervene, and evaluate nursing care.
- 3.3f Incorporate ethical principles in resource allocation in achieving equitable health.
- 3.6g Participate in ethical decision making that includes diversity, equity, and inclusion in advanced preparedness to protect populations.
- 4.3e Identify and mitigate potential risks and areas of ethical concern in the conduct of scholarly activities.
- 4.3h Implement processes that support ethical conduct in practice and scholarship.
- 4.3i Apply ethical principles to the dissemination of nursing scholarship.
- 7.2l Evaluate health policies based on an ethical framework considering cost-effectiveness, health equity, and care outcomes.
- 8.4f Employ electronic health, mobile health, and telehealth systems to enable quality, ethical, and efficient patient care.

healthcare informatics "must be bound by ethical, moral, and legal responsibilities" (p. 352).

The concept of conflicting values is central to informatics. As an example, the ethical principles of autonomy and beneficence are often in conflict when discussing the use of radiofrequency identification devices (RFIDs) to track the location of nursing staff or patients or to monitor patients in their homes to assess changes in symptoms. Nurses must be knowledgeable about ethical principles, the professional code of ethics for nurses, pertinent laws, and conflict resolution skills. Even without a universal structured curriculum in ethics, nurses abide by ethical principles while caring for patients and families. In fact, according to the Gallup Poll, nursing has been considered the most ethical profession since 1999, except for in 2001, the year of the September 11 terrorist attacks, when firefighters topped the list (Brenan, 2023).

Ethics in health internet technology is a HIMSS TIGER competency. The AACN Essentials mentions ethics in nine of the entry-level subcompetencies and 13 of the advanced-level subcompetencies (Box 1-4).

> **Box 1-4** AACN Essentials Subcompetencies Related to Ethics (*Continued*)
>
> - 8.5h Assess potential ethical and legal issues associated with the use of information and communication technology.
> - 9.1h Analyze current policies and practices in the context of an ethical framework.
> - 9.1i Model ethical behaviors in practice and leadership roles.
> - 9.1j Suggest solutions when unethical behaviors are observed.
> - 9.1k Assume accountability for working to resolve ethical dilemmas.

ANA Code of Ethics for Nurses

The ANA **Code of Ethics for Nurses** (2015) addresses issues that concern acting on behalf of the patient's interests, privacy, and confidentiality. In relation to nursing informatics, it provides general statements that could be useful when addressing conflicts or dilemmas in interactions with others (within and outside the agency) resulting from the creation of, access to, and/or disposition of electronic health information data. In this textbook, you will find a discussion of ethical principles in many chapters. Box 1-5 lists the nine provisions and the chapters in which they are discussed. The ANA has written interpretive statements for each of the provisions, which can be found on the ANA Code of Ethics website. The interpretive statements are included in the Code of Ethics to explain the application of each provision and are related to informatics concepts in this textbook when applicable.

The International Council of Nurses Code of Ethics

The International Council of Nurses (ICN) Code of Ethics for Nurses has four elements, each with a list of related standards. The elements are:

1. Nurses and patients or other people requiring care or services
2. Nurses and practice
3. Nurses and the profession
4. Nurses and global health

> **Box 1-5** ANA Code of Ethics for Nurses
>
> - **Provision 1** The nurse practices with compassion and respect for the inherent dignity, worth, and unique attributes of every person (Chapters 4, 14, and 16).
> - **Provision 2** The nurse's primary commitment is to the patient, whether an individual, family, group, community, or population (Chapters 3 and 5).
> - **Provision 3** The nurse promotes, advocates for, and protects the rights, health, and safety of the patient (Chapters 3, 4, 15, and 16).
> - **Provision 4** The nurse has authority, accountability, and responsibility for nursing practice; makes decisions; and takes action consistent with the obligation to promote health and to provide optimal care (Chapters 3 and 16).
> - **Provision 5** The nurse owes the same duties to self as to others, including the responsibility to promote health and safety, preserve wholeness of character and integrity, maintain competence, and continue personal and professional growth (Chapters 2 and 3).
> - **Provision 6** The nurse, through individual and collective effort, establishes, maintains, and improves the ethical environment of the work setting and conditions of employment that are conducive to safe, quality healthcare (Chapters 3 and 16).
> - **Provision 7** The nurse, in all roles and settings, advances the profession through research and scholarly inquiry, professional standards development, and the generation of both nursing and health policy (Chapter 13).
> - **Provision 8** The nurse collaborates with other health professionals and the public to protect human rights, promote health diplomacy, and reduce health disparities (Chapters 5, 8, 12, and 14).
> - **Provision 9** The profession of nursing, collectively through its professional organizations, must articulate nursing values, maintain the integrity of the profession, and integrate principles of social justice into nursing and health policy (Chapters 4, 11, 12, and 13).

The full ICN Code of Ethics for Nurses is available online (ICN, 2021). Most countries with professional nurses have codes of ethics. The ICN website also has links to codes of ethics for nurses in other countries, including France, Italy, Germany, Japan, Sweden, and Brazil.

SUMMARY

- **What is informatics?** Informatics is the application of IT to the arts and sciences. Healthcare informatics is the integration of computer and information science to manage healthcare information and technology. Nursing informatics is the specialty that transforms data into needed information and leverages technologies to improve health and healthcare equity, safety, quality, and outcomes. An IN works to optimize information management and communication to improve the health of individuals, families, populations, and communities. The ANA provides professional practice areas of informatics nursing. Benefits of nursing informatics include more efficient technology development, research and application of clinical best practice, training of nurses, analysis of data to improve patient outcomes, and new ways to educate patients. Patients benefit from nursing informatics with fewer medical errors, better informed clinical decision making, and better patient self-management.
- **Federal standards for healthcare informatics.** Federal agencies and laws contribute to development and standardization of healthcare informatics. The ONC creates and implements strategic plans to improve health and healthcare for all Americans through information and technology. The HITECH Act provided incentives for healthcare organizations and providers to implement HIT. The 21st Century Cures Act promotes research innovation and medical product development.
- **Healthcare informatics professional organizations.** Interdisciplinary and nursing informatics-specific organizations connect informatics professionals from all areas of healthcare with conferences, meetings, and membership directories. They provide advocacy for informatics, continuing education, opportunities for career advancement, updates in the field of informatics, and venues for scholarly publications.
- **Nursing informatics competencies.** Competencies are skills, abilities, and/or knowledge necessary to achieve a specific goal and include emotional, social, and cognitive aspects. Competencies arise through research and from organizations like the HIMSS TIGER initiative and the AACN Essentials. Competencies include computer and information literacy, communication, leadership, and advocacy.
- **Ethics and nursing informatics.** Nurses must be knowledgeable about ethical principles, the professional code of ethics for nurses, pertinent laws, and conflict resolution skills. The ANA Code of Ethics for Nurses and the ICN Code of Ethics for Nurses support nursing competency in this area.

DISCUSSION QUESTIONS AND ACTIVITIES

1. Before you continue reading this book, take the Pretest for Attitudes Toward Computers in Healthcare (P.A.T.C.H. Scale), which can be found by searching online. The 50-item test is a valid and reliable self-report measure of attitudes toward computers in healthcare (Kaminski, 2011). You can download a certificate and the results will be emailed to you. How did your score compare with the scale interpretation chart? Take the test again at the end of your course of study to see if your attitudes have changed.
2. Locate the 2020-2025 Federal Health IT Strategic Plan and discuss how knowledge of informatics can support one of the objectives. Give examples.
3. Compare informatics, healthcare informatics, and nursing informatics. Consider definitions, goals, and team members.
4. You are a nurse working for a small primary care office that has recently begun using an EHR. How could informatics nursing skills support the office staff with utilizing the EHR effectively?
5. Look up the HITECH Act or the 21st Century Cures Act and discuss any recent news articles

about either of them and how they might impact nursing care.
6. Choose an informatics professional organization and discuss how to become a member, the benefits of membership, and how this organization supports nursing informatics.
7. Explore Box 1-1, "A Day in the Life of an Informatics Nurse." Choose a task or job discussed and learn more about it. Does this look like a job you would enjoy? Try to find a job listing for this role, the qualifications, and how much you might be paid.
8. List three informatics competencies you feel confident about and three you want to improve. Explain your choices.
9. Look up the ANA Code of Ethics for Nurses. Choose a provision that interests you and discuss one of the interpretive statements and how it applies to nursing informatics.
10. Search the internet for recent news about nursing informatics. What did you find to support the statement, "Informatics nurses provide remarkable gifts to healthcare"?

PRACTICE QUESTIONS

1. Which statement by the nurse indicates an understanding of nursing informatics?
    a. "Florence Nightingale provided the first definition of nursing informatics."
    b. "Healthcare informatics is the application of information technology to the arts and sciences."
    c. "In the 1980s, the ANA recognized nursing informatics as a subspecialty of nursing."
    d. "In 2008, the ANA added wisdom to the definition of nursing informatics."
2. Match the nursing informatics specialty components (data, information, wisdom, knowledge) with supporting actions. Each of the four terms can be used more than once.
    _____ a. Naming
    _____ b. Organizing
    _____ c. Understanding
    _____ d. Collecting
    _____ e. Ethical application
    _____ f. Integrating
3. Which statement by the nurse demonstrates an understanding of the function of the federal government in supporting informatics in healthcare?
    a. "The first ONC strategic plan focused on increasing rates of mental illness."
    b. "The HITECH Act provides incentives for healthcare organizations to implement HIT."
    c. "The 21st Century Cures Act guides the implementation of electronic health information programs."
    d. "The Centers for Medicare & Medicaid Services incorporates patient perspectives into the development of new treatments."
4. Which statement about a healthcare informatics professional organization is accurate?
    a. The Alliance for Nursing Informatics (ANI) united many local, smaller, nursing informatics groups.
    b. The American Nursing Informatics Association (ANIA) publishes the *Online Journal of Nursing Informatics*.
    c. The Healthcare Information and Management Systems Society (HIMSS) is the largest nursing informatics organization in America.
    d. The American College of Surgeons formed the American Medical Informatics Association (AMIA).
5. Which of these competencies are HIMSS TIGER competencies for nursing informatics? (Select all that apply.)
    a. Communication
    b. Quality and safety management
    c. Effectively use electronic communication tools
    d. Promote patient engagement with health data
    e. Computer skills
    f. Ethics in health IT

REFERENCES

Alliance for Nursing Informatics (ANI). (n.d.). *About us: Alliance for nursing informatics*. http://www.allianceni.org/about-us

Altmiller, G., & Hopkins-Pepe, L. (2019). Why quality and safety education for nurses (QSEN) matters in practice. *Journal of Continuing Education in Nursing, 50*(5), 199–200. https://doi.org/10.3928/00220124-20190416-04

American Association of Colleges of Nursing (AACN). (2021). *The essentials: Core competencies for professional nursing education*. https://www.aacnnursing.org/Portals/42/AcademicNursing/pdf/Essentials-2021.pdf

American Health Information Management Association (AHIMA). (2017). *AHIMA facts*. http://www.ahima.org/about

American Medical Informatics Association (AMIA). (n.d.). About AMIA. Retrieved April 25, 2023 from https://amia.org/about-amia

American Nurses Association (ANA). (2008). *Nursing informatics: Scope and standards of practice*. American Nurses Publishing.

American Nurses Association (ANA). (2015). *Code of ethics for nurses with interpretive statements*. Silver Spring. https://www.nursingworld.org/practicepolicy/nursing-excellence/ethics/code-of-ethics-for-nurses/

American Nurses Association (ANA). (2022). *Nursing informatics: Scope and standards of practice* (3rd ed.). American Nurses Publishing.

American Nursing Informatics Association (ANIA). (2018). *American Nursing Informatics Association main menu*. https://www.ania.org/

Bickford, C. J. (2017). The professional association's perspective on nursing informatics and competencies in the US. *Studies in Health Technology and Informatics, 232*, 62–68.

Brenan, M. (2023, January 10). *Nurses retain top ethics rating in U.S., but below 2020 high*. Gallup News. https://news.gallup.com/poll/467804/nurses-retain-top-ethics-rating-below-2020-high.aspx

British Computer Society (BCS). (2018). About us | The Chartered Institute for IT. http://www.bcs.org/category/5651

Chung, S. Y., & Staggers, N. (2014). Measuring nursing informatics competencies of practicing nurses in Korea: Nursing informatics competencies questionnaire. *Computers Informatics Nursing, 32* (12), 596–605. https://doi.org.10.1097/CIN.0000000000000114

Curcio, D. (2021). Engaging students in a QI/QM presentation to enhance QSEN concept learning. *Teaching and Learning in Nursing, 16*(3), 269–272. https://doi.org/10.1016/j.teln.2021.01.006

Curtin, L. L. (2005). Ethics in informatics: The intersection of nursing, ethics, and information technology. *Nursing Administration Quaterly, 29*(4), 349–352.

European Federation for Medical Informatics (EFMI). (2018). *NURSIE - nursing informatics in Europe*. https://www.efmi.org/workinggroups/nursie-nursing-informatics-in-europe

Graves, J. R., & Corcoran, S. (1989). The study of nursing informatics. *Image—Journal of Nursing Scholarship, 21*(4), 227–231.

Gugerty, B., & Delaney, C. W. (2009). TIGER Informatics Competencies Collaborative (TICC) final report. http://tigercompetencies.pbworks.com/f/TICC_Final.pdf

Healthcare Information and Management Systems Society (HIMSS). (2018). About HIMSS. http://www.himss.org/about-himss

Healthcare Information and Management Systems Society (HIMSS). (2019, May 14). https://www.himss.org/resources/what-nursing-informatics

Healthcare Information and Management Systems Society (HIMSS). (2021, January 29). *TIGER international competency synthesis project*. https://www.himss.org/sites/hde/files/media/file/2021/01/29/tiger-icsp-recommendations.pdf

Healthcare Information and Management Systems Society (HIMSS). (n.d.). *Technology Informatics Guiding Education Reform (TIGER) interprofessional community*. Retrieved April 27, 2023 from https://www.himss.org/membership-participation/technology-informatics-guiding-education-reform-tiger-interprofessional-community

HealthIT.gov. (n.d.). *The ONC HealthIT playbook*. Retrieved April 26, 2023 from https://www.healthit.gov/playbook/

HHS.gov/HealthCare. (2017, March 16). *About affordable care Act*. http://www.hhs.gov/healthcare/rights/

Hübner, U., Thye, J., Shaw, T., Elias, B., Egbert, N., Saranto, K., Babitsch, B., Procter, P., & Ball, M. J. (2019). Towards the TIGER international framework for recommendations of core competencies in health informatics 2.0: Extending the scope and the roles. *Studies in Health Technology and Informatics, 264*, 1218–1222. https://doi.org/10.3233/SHTI190420

International Council of Nurses Code of Ethics (ICN). (2021). *The International Council Code of ethics for nurses*. https://www.icn.ch/sites/default/files/inline-files/ICN_Code-of-Ethics_EN_Web.pdf

Kaminski, J. (2011). *P.A.T.C.H. assessment scale v3*. Nursing Informatics Learning Center. https://nursing-informatics.com/niassess/plan.html

National Advisory Council on Nurse Education and Practice. (1997, December). *A national informatics agenda for nursing education and practice*. Retrieved from http://eric.ed.gov/?id=ED449700

National League for Nursing. (2008, May 9). Position statement: Preparing the next generation of nurses to practice in a technology-rich environment—An informatics agenda. Retrieved from http://www.nln.org/docs/default-source/professional-development-programs/preparing-the-next-generation-of-nurses.pdf?sfvrsn=6

Newbold, S. K. (1996). The informatics nurse and the certification process. *Computers in Nursing, 14*(2), 84–88, Retrieved from http://journals.lww.com/cinjournal/

Nightingale, F. (1863). *Notes on hospitals* (3rd ed.). Longman, Green, Longman, Roberts, & Green.

Office of the National Coordinator for Health Information Technology (ONC). (2008, July 3). *The ONC-coordinated federal health information technology strategic plan: 2008-2012*. https://www.healthit.gov/sites/default/files/hit-strategic-plan-summary-508-2.pdf

Office of the National Coordinator for Health Information Technology (ONC). (2015). *Federal health information technology strategic plan: 2015–2020*. https://www.healthit.gov/data/datasets/federal-health-it-strategic-plan-2015-2020-goals

Office of the National Coordinator for Health Information Technology (ONC). (2020, October). *2020-2025 federal health IT strategic plan*. HealthIT.gov. https://www.healthit.gov/topic/2020-2025-federal-health-it-strategic-plan

Pillar, B., & Golumbic, N. (1993). *Nursing informatics: Enhancing patient care*. National Center for Nursing Research, U.S. Department of Health and Human Services.

Sackett, K. M., & Erdley, W. S. (2002). The history of health care informatics. In Englebardt, S. & Nelson, R. (Eds.), *Healthcare informatics from an interdisciplinary approach* (pp. 453–477). Mosby.

Scholes, M., & Barber, B. (1980). Towards nursing informatics. In Lindberg, D. A. D. & Kaihara, S. (Eds.), *MEDINFO: 1980* (pp. 7–73). North Holland.

Schwirian, P. (1986). The NI pyramid-a model for research in nursing informatics. *Computers Informatics Nursing, 4*(3), 134–136. http://journals.lww.com/cinjournal/pages/default.aspx

Staggers, N., Gassert, C. A., & Curran, C. (2001). Informatics competencies for nurses at four levels of practice. *Journal of Nursing Education, 40*(7), 303–316. https://doi-org.uscupstate.idm.oclc.org/10.3928/0148-4834-20011001-05

Steinbuch, K. (1957). Informatik: Automatische Informationsverarbeitung (informatics—Automatic information processing). *Sel Nachr, 4*, 171.

Thye, J. (n.d.). *Understanding health informatics core competencies*. Retrieved April 27, 2023 from. https://www.himss.org/resources/health-informatics

U.S. Food and Drug Administration (FDA). (n.d.). *21st Century Cures Act*. Retrieved April 26, 2023 from https://www.fda.gov/regulatory-information/selected-amendments-fdc-act/21st-century-cures-act

CHAPTER 2

Professional Characteristics: Theories and Career Pathways

Teri Harmon and Kristi Miller

OBJECTIVES

After studying this chapter, you will be able to:

1. Describe the nursing theories that guide nursing informatics.
2. Explain how theories can guide the creation and implementation of systems.
3. Explain the process for becoming an informatics nurse and why certification in informatics is important.
4. Apply ethical principles to the duty of the informatics nurse to pursue lifelong learning.
5. Differentiate between the roles of informatics nurses and informatics nurse specialists.

AACN Essentials for Entry-Level Professional Nursing Education

- 1.1a   Identify concepts, derived from theories from nursing and other disciplines, which distinguish the practice of nursing.
- 1.2a   Apply or employ knowledge from nursing science as well as the natural, physical, and social sciences to build an understanding of the human experience and nursing practice.
- 1.2b   Demonstrate intellectual curiosity.
- 1.2d   Examine influence of personal values in decision making for nursing practice.
- 4.1c   Apply theoretical framework(s)/models in practice.
- 6.1a   Communicate the nurse's roles and responsibilities clearly.
- 9.1a   Apply principles of professional nursing ethics and human rights in patient care and professional situations.
- 9.3a   Engage in advocacy that promotes the best interest of the individual, community, and profession.
- 9.3e   Engage in professional activities and/or organizations.

AACN Essentials for Advanced-Level Nursing Education

1.2f Synthesize knowledge from nursing and other disciplines to inform education, practice, and research.1.2gApply a systematic and defendable approach to nursing practice decisions.1.2jTranslate theories from nursing and other disciplines to practice.4.1hApply and critically evaluate advanced knowledge in a defined area of nursing practice.9.3iAdvocate for nursing's professional responsibility for ensuring optimal care outcomes.9.1iModel ethical behaviors in practice and leadership roles.

HIMSS TIGER Competencies

Ethics in health internet technologyInformation and knowledge management in patient careLearning techniquesTeaching, training, educations associated the theory can increase the clinical implemen-factors with the tenets of Rogers's diffusion tation of medical technologies. The review of innovations theory (Warty et al., 2021). presents barriers to diffusion to better

As you read this chapter, think about how understand why only 7% of medical devices you could use the theories presented to that are invented make it to the bed-improve patient outcomes. For each theory, side. The factors they identified included try to imagine a specific application.

KEY TERMS

Chaos theory
Cognitive science
Data
Data, information, knowledge, and wisdom (DIKW) model
General systems theory
Informatics nurse specialist
Information
Knowledge
Lewin's field theory
Rogers's diffusion of innovations theory
Social informatics
Sociotechnical theory
Super user
Tacit knowledge
Wisdom

CASE STUDY

In the article *Barriers to the Diffusion of Medical Technologies Within Healthcare: A Systematic Review*, the authors demonstrate how Rogers's diffusion of innovations theory can increase the clinical implementation of medical technologies. The review presents barriers to diffusion to better understand why only 7% of medical devices that are invented make it to the bedside. The factors they identified included technology-specific challenges, clinical evidence/uncertainty, regulatory affairs, health technology assessment, reimbursement, and adoption. The authors associated the factors with the tenets of Rogers's diffusion of innovations theory (Warty et al., 2021).

As you read this chapter, think about how you could use the theories presented to improve patient outcomes. For each theory, try to imagine a specific application.

The characteristics of nursing as a profession include education, theory, service, autonomy, a code of ethics, and caring. Nursing theory helps distinguish nursing as a separate discipline from medicine and related sciences and assists nurses in understanding patients and their needs. There are many nursing theories that support the field of nursing informatics. Understanding the theory behind nursing informatics is important for understanding what makes this career path unique from other branches of nursing. This chapter presents how theories support the profession of nursing informatics, and the educational and professional pathways that will lead to practicing informatics.

THEORIES THAT SUPPORT INFORMATICS

In addition to being the founder of modern nursing, Florence Nightingale was a well-known and respected statistician. She was so respected that in 1858, she became the first female member of the Royal Statistical Society (The National Archives, n.d.). Before the term "informatics" was ever spoken, she collected and analyzed data on mortality and sanitation. She used these data to make improvements in patient care and reduce casualties in the Crimean War. After the war, she used data collection and analysis to support reformation of public healthcare by championing better, cleaner, healthier living conditions (The National Archives, n.d.).

Since the time of Florence Nightingale, multiple theories have been proposed to increase nursing knowledge surrounding informatics. These include the data, information, knowledge, and wisdom model; sociotechnical theory; change theories from Rogers and Lewin; general systems theory; chaos theory; and cognitive science. See Table 2-1 for a summary of what these theories contribute to informatics.

Data, Information, Knowledge, and Wisdom Model

In their seminal article on nursing informatics, Graves and Corcoran (1989) devised a model for nursing informatics based on Bloom's taxonomy. This model identified data, information, and knowledge as the key components of nursing informatics. The concept of wisdom was first added to this structure by Nelson and Joos (as cited in Joos et al., 1992), but was officially incorporated in the 2008 American Nurses Association's (ANA) *Nursing Informatics: Scope and Standards of Practice*. Wisdom is an important addition to nursing informatics because the practice of nursing should always consider the wisdom of the human being and not leave everything solely to technology. The **data, information, knowledge, and wisdom (DIKW) model** is concerned with facilitating the management and communication of nursing information within the field of healthcare. It focuses on nursing actions and interventions. This theory provides a nursing perspective, clarifies nursing values and beliefs, produces new knowledge, and develops standardized nursing terminology for use in electronic records.

Data

Data are discrete, objective facts that have not been interpreted (Clark, 2010) or placed in context; data are the most basic level of information. The DIKW model states that data are presented as the building blocks of meaning. However, without context, data are meaningless. An example is four body temperature measurements of 98.5°F, 98.7°F, 99.0°F, and 102.5°F.

Information

Information is made up of data that have some type of interpretation or structure; that is, they have context. Information is derived from combining different pieces of data (Clark, 2010). Using the body temperature example, information would include the understanding that these readings are body temperature measurements from a patient after surgery every 4 hours.

Knowledge

Knowledge is the combination of what one learns and skills one develops over time (Asiedu et al., 2022). How one manages and uses knowledge is also vital. If knowledge is not applied appropriately,

TABLE 2-1 Contributions of Theories to Informatics

Theory	Contributions to Informatics
Data, information, knowledge, and wisdom	Shows the relationship among data, information, knowledge, and wisdom and how they can facilitate management and communication
Sociotechnical and social informatics	Improves the interaction between an information system and the organizational culture
Change	Increases the chance of success in implementing a system by accounting for the reactions to the change
Rogers's diffusion of innovations	Demonstrates the pattern of acceptance of change and the process of decision making
Lewin's field	Demonstrates how a positive outcome is achieved in relation to a change
General systems	Directs the focus to the interaction of the parts of a system instead of to each individual part
Chaos	Shows that minor differences in the beginning of a system can yield big differences later and aids in nonlinear thinking
Cognitive science	Improves the design of screens

It limits its effectiveness of it. Again, using the temperature example, knowledge might involve recalling from nurse training that a temperature above 101.0°F in a patient following surgery could indicate the presence of an infection.

Wisdom

Wisdom involves knowing when and how to apply knowledge to a situation (Nation & Wangia-Anderson, 2019). For example, wisdom is demonstrated when you interpret an elevated postsurgical temperature of 102.5°F as a sign of an infection, prompting a call to the healthcare provider to obtain an order for blood cultures. Wisdom might also include confirming the elevated temperature by obtaining another reading to ensure that there was not an error in data collection.

The Continuum

The simplified example of interpreting an elevated temperature is used to make the process of converting data into wisdom easier to understand. In the DIKW model, informatics concepts fall on a continuum that depends on the person making decisions or on variables in the situation. A nurse with 10 years of experience may possess a great deal of **tacit knowledge**. This is knowledge that has been earned with experience and reflection and is so ingrained that it is difficult for the nurse to verbalize or acknowledge. This tacit knowledge provides a higher level of wisdom than that of a new nursing graduate.

The general idea of the DIKW model is that the move from data to wisdom is a progressive process that follows a given path. As one moves up the continuum, each level becomes more complex and requires intellect that is more developed. In practice, the lines between each of these entities are blurred and the process is repetitive and cyclical. The process of converting data into wisdom includes capturing, sorting, organizing, storing, retrieving, and presenting data to give it meaning and produce information.

Figure 2-1 is an illustration of this continuum that might apply to a nursing student or a new graduate. In this figure, data are combined to produce information, and information is combined to produce knowledge. Knowledge combined with experience then leads to wisdom.

Sociotechnical Theory

Introducing new technology is a social process that deeply affects an organization. Researchers have found that the new age of digital healthcare has the potential to increase or decrease stress levels in healthcare workers depending on how it is implemented (Lovell, 2021). In the middle of the last century, it became evident that not all implementations of technology were increasing productivity. This was when sociotechnical theory originated. **Sociotechnical theory** focuses on the interactions between social systems and technical systems when designing an organizational system. Social systems have to do with a person's knowledge, skill set, attitudes, and culture. Technical systems include hardware, software, equipment, and the systems within an organization (Feldthouse et al., 2022).

Research based on sociotechnical theory is aimed at maximizing performance by designing or redesigning systems that fit the organizational system into which they are implemented. The sociotechnical point of view, which is the basis of **social informatics**, holds that a good design is based on an understanding of how people work and the context of the work, not just technologic considerations (Feldthouse et al., 2022). The importance of social informatics can be seen by looking at the failures of implemented information systems. For example, in 2003, there was a much publicized shutdown by Cedars-Sinai Medical Center in Los Angeles of their new multimillion-dollar computerized provider order entry (CPOE). Physicians felt the CPOE represented a change that was too radical and that their interests were not sufficiently represented, that the system forced more work on them, and that it was poorly designed (Bass, 2003).

CASE STUDY

The case study presented barriers to the clinical implementation of medical technologies. How could the application of the sociotechnical theory increase the implementation of new technologies?

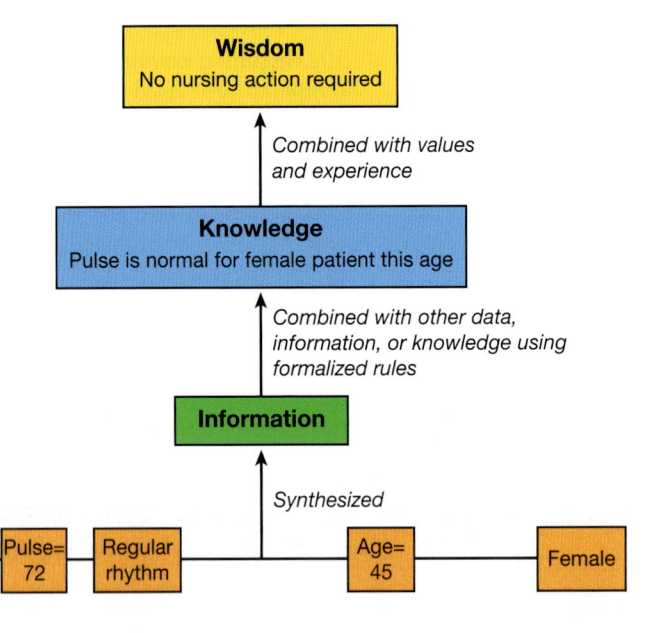

Figure 2-1. Progression of data to wisdom.

Change Theories

Change theories recognize that instituting a change, whether a minor one, such as a simple system upgrade, or a major one, such as moving from a paper record to an electronic system, can provoke discomfort. "What will this mean to me?" is often the first thought of a person faced with change. Ignoring the psychosocial nature of change often leads to the failure of a system. Everett Rogers and Kurt Lewin developed two theories that address the effects of change on people and organizations.

Rogers's Diffusion of Innovations Theory

Rogers's diffusion of innovations theory was first published in his 1962 book of the same name. This theory examines the pattern of acceptance that innovations follow as they spread across the population and the process of decision making that occurs in individuals when deciding whether to adopt an innovation. Although the theory was based on Depression-era rural research that studied how Midwestern farmers adopted hardier corn (Rogers, 2003), this theory is still widely applicable. Healthcare has undergone many changes in recent years, and as illustrated in the case study, Rogers's theory can help informatics nurses manage and implement change more effectively.

Categories of Change Adopters

Rogers classifies people into five categories (Fig. 2-2) and offers insight on how innovations are accepted by the general population (Rogers, 2003). Innovators, the first category, readily adopt innovations but constitute a small percentage (about 2.5%) of the population. These people are often seen as disruptive by those who are averse to risk taking, so innovators are usually unable to persuade others to adopt innovations. This job of persuasion is left to the next category, early adopters, who compose 13.5% of the population. They are respectable opinion leaders who function as promoters of an innovation. The next group, the early majority (34%), is averse to risks but will make safe investments. The late majority, who make up another 34% of the adopters, need to be sure that the innovation is beneficial. They may adopt the innovation not because they see a use for it, but because of peer pressure. The last group of 16% are termed laggards. They are suspicious of innovations and change and are quite resistant to adopt. Laggards must be certain that the innovation will not fail before they will adopt it. Instead of discounting this group, however, it is important to listen to them as they may grasp weaknesses that others fail to see. Since most adapters will be in the early or late majority, leaders should focus adoption efforts on them (Barrow et al., 2022).

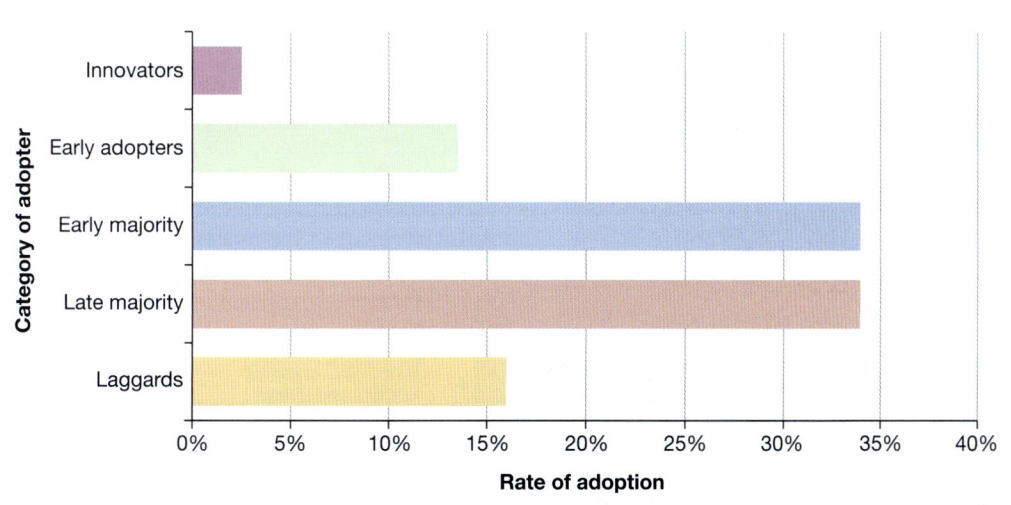

Figure 2-2. How individuals adopt innovation: innovators to laggards. (Data from Rogers' Diffusion of Innovations Theory, 1995. Reprinted from Melnyk B. M., & Fineout-Overholt E. (2015). *Evidence-based practice in nursing and healthcare: A guide to best practice* (5th ed.). Philadelphia, PA: Wolters Kluwer, with permission. Figure 17.1.)

Stages of Decision Making

In Rogers's theory, individuals go through five stages in deciding to adopt an innovation (Fig. 2-3). Like all stage theories, progress is not uniform, and adopters can show behaviors from more than one stage at a time or revert completely to an earlier stage. In the first stage, knowledge of an innovation, the potential adopter gains an understanding of how the innovation operates (Rogers, 2003). This can occur passively, through either education or advertisements, or actively in response to a felt need or incentives. The second stage, persuasion, is based on the perception of the relative advantage of the innovation, compatibility with existing norms, and its observability. At this stage, an individual forms an opinion about the innovation—negative, neutral, or positive. The third stage is called decision because the individual uses personal opinions to decide. A potential adopter may try the innovation or base an opinion on the experience and opinion of a respected peer who has tried the innovation. The individual then decides to either accept (adopt) or reject the innovation. If the decision is positive, the fourth stage, implementation, follows. At this stage, the adopter wants knowledge, such as how to use the innovation and how to overcome problems with its use. Confirmation, the fifth stage, may occur when reinforcement of the decision is sought. Conflicting information about the innovation may cause the adopter to reverse a decision.

CASE STUDY

The case study presented barriers to decision making associated with the factors of Rogers's theory. How might you use the five decision-making stages to convince a nursing administrator to adopt a new medical technology?

Lewin's Field Theory

Whereas Rogers's theory identifies the stages that individuals go through in making a change, **Lewin's field theory** provides a guide to helping individuals achieve a positive decision in relation to an innovation. This theory holds that human behavior is related to both personal characteristics and the individual's social environment (Smith, 2001). It focuses on the variables that need to be recognized during change and uses these variables to create a model of the stages that occur during change. Lewin divides change into three stages (or force fields): unfreezing, moving, and refreezing (Fig. 2-4). Ways of moving a group from the first to the last stage of change need to be part of the plan for implementing a system.

A real-world example of Lewin's theory occurred when the military health system transitioned to a new electronic medical record (EMR). This rollout involved many critical success factors like change champions, hands-on training, and helpful feedback. There were also critical barriers to implementation including technophobia, resistance to change, and problems with communication (Woody, 2020). Taking these success factors and critical barriers into account in future rollouts of the EMR increased efficiency in the process.

Unfreezing

The unfreezing stage is based on the idea that human behavior is supported by a balance of driving and restraining forces that create equilibrium. To institute change, the driving and restraining forces in the organizational culture and individual have to be changed. To unfreeze, one must identify and change the balance so that the driving forces are stronger than the restraining forces. Driving forces can be involvement in the process, respect of one's opinion, and continuous communication during the process. Unfortunately, restraining forces are harder

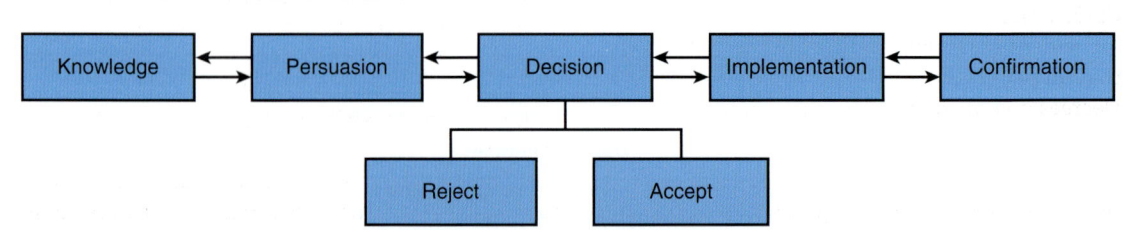

Figure 2-3. The five stages of Rogers's diffusion of innovations theory. (Adapted from Comscholar. Public domain.)

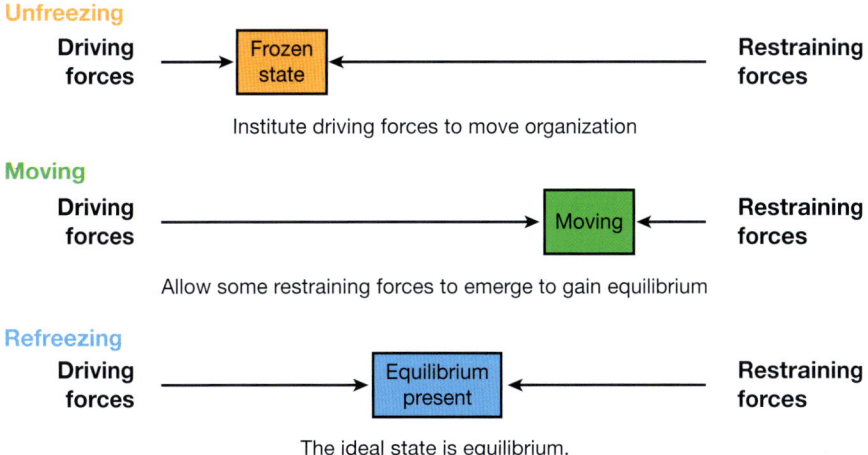

Unfreezing

Driving forces → Frozen state ← Restraining forces

Institute driving forces to move organization

Moving

Driving forces → Moving ← Restraining forces

Allow some restraining forces to emerge to gain equilibrium

Refreezing

Driving forces → Equilibrium present ← Restraining forces

The ideal state is equilibrium.
The more the restraining forces, the more difficult the change

Figure 2-4. The three stages of Lewin's field theory.

to identify and treat because they are often personal psychological defenses or group norms embedded in the organizational or community culture.

Moving

In the moving stage, the planned change is implemented. Its success depends on how situations were handled in the first stage. *This is not a comfortable period.* Anxieties are high, and if they are not successfully addressed, the change may be unsuccessful. Additionally, it is important to recognize that in this stage, movement may occur in the wrong direction. This is especially likely to happen if the new system has problems, if it is not supported by administration, or if it has had no end user involvement. Thus, it is important to thoroughly test the system before implementation for both bugs and usability, have the support of administration in the planning process, involve users so that the system serves them instead of creating more work, provide adequate training, and deal with any implementation problems immediately. In the Cedars-Sinai case, the new CPOE system created more work and resulted in a movement in the wrong direction despite a decree that all people must use the system (Bass, 2003). Decrees do not "move" people.

Refreezing

In the refreezing stage, equilibrium returns as the planned change becomes the norm and it is surrounded by the usual driving and restraining forces. For this state to occur, individuals need to feel confident with the change and feel in control of the procedures involved in the new methods. One way to assist this process would be to provide a well-designed help system that can provide solutions for frequently used procedures as well as those that a user may use only occasionally. Another approach that ensures equilibrium will occur is to have the organization recognize new skills. If the change is too strongly reinforced, it might be difficult to enact subsequent changes.

General Systems Theory

General systems theory is a method of thinking about complex structures such as an information system or an organization. A simplified description of systems theory holds that any change in one part of a system will be reflected in other parts of the system (von Bertalanffy, 1973). In systems theory, the focus is on the interaction among the various parts of the system instead of regarding each individual part as standing alone. It is based on the premise that the whole is greater than the sum of its parts, which is also the basis for holistic nursing.

Systems are open or closed. An open system continually exchanges information with the environment outside the system, while a closed system receives no input from the outside. Healthcare works better with open systems because they allow for free flow between information technology (IT), the environment, and the complexity of the healthcare team (Brown et al., 2019).

The objective of any system is to be in equilibrium, which is maintained by the correction forces from a feedback loop. Negative feedback results when there is a lack of something. The action it produces adds the missing item. Positive feedback results when there is too much of something. The action it produces takes away the excess. Both types of feedback restore a state of equilibrium. Whether feedback is positive or negative is based on what the system finds, not its action.

Feedback loops operate using input, process, and output (Fig. 2-5). Input involves adding information to a system, whether the information is an addition of an item (from negative feedback) or the removal of excess items (from positive feedback). Process is the throughput, or evaluation of the input, that the system performs using the input information. Output is the information or action that results from what the processing finds. This output may produce no action or the action needed from either negative or positive feedback.

Feedback loops may sound similar to the nursing process. A simple example is a patient with a high temperature. A nurse will *input* that temperature into a computer system. The computer will *process* that data by combining it with the order that if this patient's temperature is higher than a certain number, a specific medication should be given. The computer will *output* the instruction to provide the medication. This is positive feedback—there was too much of something (body heat). The action it produced was to tell the nurse to administer a medication.

Chaos Theory

Chaos theory has a mathematical basis and was first mentioned by a meteorologist in 1963 when attempting to predict the weather with a set of 12 equations (Dizikes, 2011). This theory suggests that minor changes in the beginning of a system can yield big differences later (Demir et al., 2019). This theory is often associated with the concept of the butterfly effect, or the idea that worldwide atmospheric conditions can be caused by the flapping of one butterfly's wings. The analogy comes from the small differences in the starting points (like a butterfly flapping its wings) that produce different effects that produce changes over time.

Chaos theory, like general systems theory, addresses an entire structure without reducing it to the elemental parts. This makes it useful with complex systems like information systems. The idea behind this theory is that what may appear to be chaotic has an order. It is based on the recognized fact that events and phenomena depend on initial conditions. For example, the conditions in which an information system is first envisioned will affect the overall design.

Chaos theory is nonlinear, allowing one to question assumptions one might normally reach using linear thought. For example, imagine a single pendulum. A weight attached to the end of a string will follow a predictable path. This is a linear system. Now imagine a double pendulum, or a pendulum with a second pendulum attached at the end. A double pendulum is highly sensitive to changes in initial conditions, like the weight of the item at the end of the string or the starting position of the pendulum arm. Small changes will lead to larger outcomes. Predicting the pattern the arms will trace is extremely difficult. This is a nonlinear system. Seeing things reframed in this nonlinear way can stimulate new thinking and new approaches.

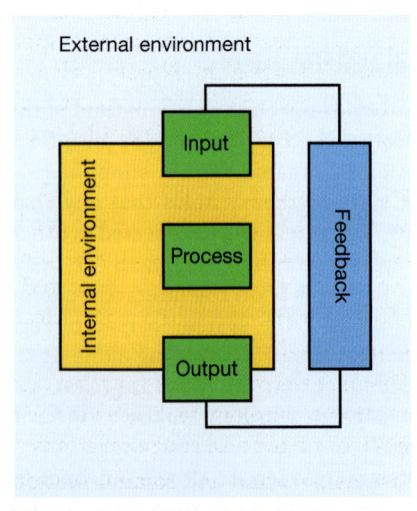

Figure 2-5. General systems theory.

(Search YouTube for "double pendulum chaos demonstration" to see the double pendulum in action.)

Cognitive Science

Cognitive science is the study of the mind and intelligence (Thagard, 2014) and how this information can be applied. It is interdisciplinary, including philosophy, psychology, neuroscience, linguistics, anthropology, and artificial intelligence, and it is a part of social informatics. It adds to informatics concepts that focus on how the brain perceives and interprets screens (Turley, 1996). This is important in all aspects of information systems. For example, when designing data input screens, the screen must be organized to facilitate data entry. Understanding cognitive theory when designing an electronic health record system could result in less stress for the end user.

BECOMING AN INFORMATICS NURSE

As discussed, understanding the theory behind the subject of informatics is vital to understanding the path that leads to practice. The path to becoming an informatics nurse is similar to the path of any other specialty nursing practice. You will first need to obtain your license as a registered nurse (RN). Employers typically prefer nurses with Bachelor of Science in Nursing (BSN) degrees for specialty practices such as informatics. Gaining experience at the bedside, pursuing an advanced degree, certification, gaining informatics skills, and membership in professional organizations will further support this career goal.

Bedside Experience

Bedside experience is essential for informatics nurses because it provides firsthand experience with the equipment and an understanding of how it is used within the organization. Furthermore, it allows the nurse to become familiar with the EMR system and the processes involved.

Today, many nurses practicing in the field of nursing informatics gained their knowledge through self-learning and continuing education. However, there is a move toward requiring advanced formal academic preparation in the field, especially for higher level jobs. Nevertheless, before beginning a career in informatics, it is helpful to have a thorough understanding of clinical practice in one's discipline, which can be gained through at least 5 years of experience in the field (ANA, 2015). Computer competency alone, though helpful, is insufficient for a career in informatics. Computers are only a tool in informatics; information management is the focus. This knowledge requires clinical experience.

Standards and Competencies for Informatics Education

Basic informatics knowledge is essential for safe and effective nursing practice at the generalist level and all advanced practice levels. Understanding the possibilities and limitations of information management and technology assists the nurse in having realistic expectations of information systems. In Chapter 1, the Healthcare Information and Management Systems Society (HIMSS) health informatics core competencies and the American Association of Colleges of Nursing (AACN) Essentials were discussed. Other organizations have published standards for informatics nursing education. *Nursing Informatics: Scope and Standards of Practice*, 3rd Edition (2022) "describes a competent level of nursing care at each level of nursing informatics practice and provides comprehensive overviews of the dynamic and complex practice of the nursing informatics specialty." The National League for Nursing also has an informatics toolkit designed to assist faculty in teaching informatics, which is available on their website.

The AACN developed the new Essentials in 2021 that clearly specify the competencies for healthcare professionals in informatics at the entry and advanced levels of nursing. Domain 8 of the AACN Essentials is "Informatics and Healthcare Technologies" and includes:

- 8.1 Describe the various information and communication technology tools used in the care of patients, communities, and populations.
- 8.2 Use information and communication technology to gather data, create information, and generate knowledge.

- 8.3 Use information and communication technologies and informatics processes to deliver safe nursing care to diverse populations in a variety of settings.
- 8.4 Use information and communication technology to support documentation of care and communication among providers, patients, and all system levels.
- 8.5 Use information and communication technologies in accordance with ethical, legal, professional, and regulatory standards, and workplace policies in the delivery of care.

You can view all the Essentials domains, competencies, and subcompetencies in the AACN Essentials (AACN, 2021).

> **CASE STUDY**
>
> Box 2-1 shows the results of a survey of nurse leaders about the competencies required of informatics nurses (Collins et al., 2017). Recall that in the case study, Rogers's theory was applied to difficulties with the implementation of new healthcare technology. Which of the competencies in Box 2-1 might be useful for removing barriers to technology implementation, such as technology-specific challenges, clinical evidence/uncertainty, regulatory affairs, health technology assessment, reimbursement, and adoption?

Informatics Education Programs

While some employers will hire tech-savvy BSN-prepared nurses for informaticist jobs, there is an increasing demand for nurse informaticists to have master's degrees, and some will advance their education even further by earning doctoral degrees (Nurse.org, n.d.) (Fig. 2-6).

The four categories for nursing informatics education are:

1. Graduate programs with a specialty in nursing informatics
2. Graduate and undergraduate programs with minors or majors in nursing informatics
3. Individual courses in nursing informatics within graduate/undergraduate programs
4. Online courses

Online courses may be standalone continuing education courses, part of a program that leads to a certificate in nursing informatics, or part of a formal degree-granting program that may or may not be 100% online.

Many educational institutions have informatics programs. The overall discipline of informatics has a core curriculum supplemented by informatics principles and knowledge specific to each healthcare discipline. Every educational program will have a different focus. Some concentrate on applied informatics, others on informatics research. A course at the master's level should include content on integrating technology in practice, improving healthcare delivery, and analyzing strategies for using information communication technologies to reduce risk. Formal educational programs provide an excellent foundation for jobs in informatics, but as with all healthcare disciplines, there must be a commitment to lifelong learning.

At present, there is no accrediting body that examines informatics education as there is for nurse practitioner education programs. Prospective students need to ask many questions when examining programs. Questions to ask about an informatics program are listed in Box 2-2.

Certification

A nurse may choose to obtain specialized certification to work as an informatics nurse or as an informatics nurse specialist. Certification is offered by the American Nurses Credentialing Center (ANCC). The certification is valid for 5 years and nurses must meet the following specific requirements to be eligible to sit for the exam (ANCC, n.d.):

- Hold a current, active RN license in a state or territory of the United States or hold the professional, legally recognized equivalent in another country.
- Hold a bachelor's or higher degree in nursing or a bachelor's degree in a relevant field.
- Have practiced the equivalent of 2 years full-time as an RN.

Box 2-1 Competencies Expected of Informatics Nurses, Ranked by Priority

1. Ability to ensure that nursing values and requirements are represented in healthcare information technology (HIT) selection and evaluation
2. Including nursing information within HIT system
3. Budgeting using technology
4. Data-based planning and decision making through the utilization and synthesis of HIT system data
5. Ability to collaborate with other departments regarding project management and resource allocation for HIT system implementation
6. Ability to collaborate with chief medical officer peers related to HIT and needs of nurses and physicians
7. Ability to collaborate with interprofessional team in HIT selection process
8. Ability to advocate for the development (or purchase) and use of integrated, cost-effective HIT systems within the organization
9. Communicating a system and nursing vision about the benefits of HIT
10. Ability to involve frontline staff in the evaluation of HIT systems related to their practice
11. Ability to involve frontline staff in the development of HIT system requirements
12. Ability to involve frontline staff in appropriate aspects of HIT design, implementation, and testing related to their practice
13. Ability to see HIT as a top priority and strategic decision
14. Recognition of value of clinicians' involvement in all appropriate phases of HIT
15. Quality assurance using technology

Adapted from Collins, S., Yen, P., Phillips, A., Kennedy, M. K. (2017). Nursing informatics competency assessment for the nurse leader: The Delphi study. *The Journal of Nursing Administration*, 47(4), 212–218. https://doi.org/10.1097/NNA.0000000000000467

- Have completed 30 hours of continuing education in informatics nursing within the last 3 years.
- Meet one of the following practice hour requirements:
  - Have practiced a minimum of 2,000 hours in informatics nursing within the last 3 years
  - Have practiced a minimum of 1,000 hours in informatics nursing in the last 3 years and completed a minimum of 12 semester hours of academic credit in informatics courses that are part of a graduate-level informatics nursing program
  - Have completed a graduate program in informatics nursing containing a minimum of 200 hours of faculty-supervised practicum in informatics nursing

Box 2-2 Questions Prospective Students Should Ask of an Informatics Program

These questions are in addition to those normally asked of any educational program.
1. What is the focus of the informatics program? For example:
   a. Clinical systems
   b. Knowledge generation/research
   c. Decision support
   d. Healthcare specialty
2. What types of jobs do graduates of the program obtain?
3. Who are the faculty in informatics?
   a. What is their informatics experience?
   b. What are their qualifications to teach informatics?
   c. What are their interests in informatics?
4. Is there a preceptorship or internship?
   a. If so, for how long?
   b. How are these assignments found?
5. How long has the program been operating?
6. What courses are currently available and what courses are being planned but are not yet offered?
7. If the program is online, how much on-campus time is required?

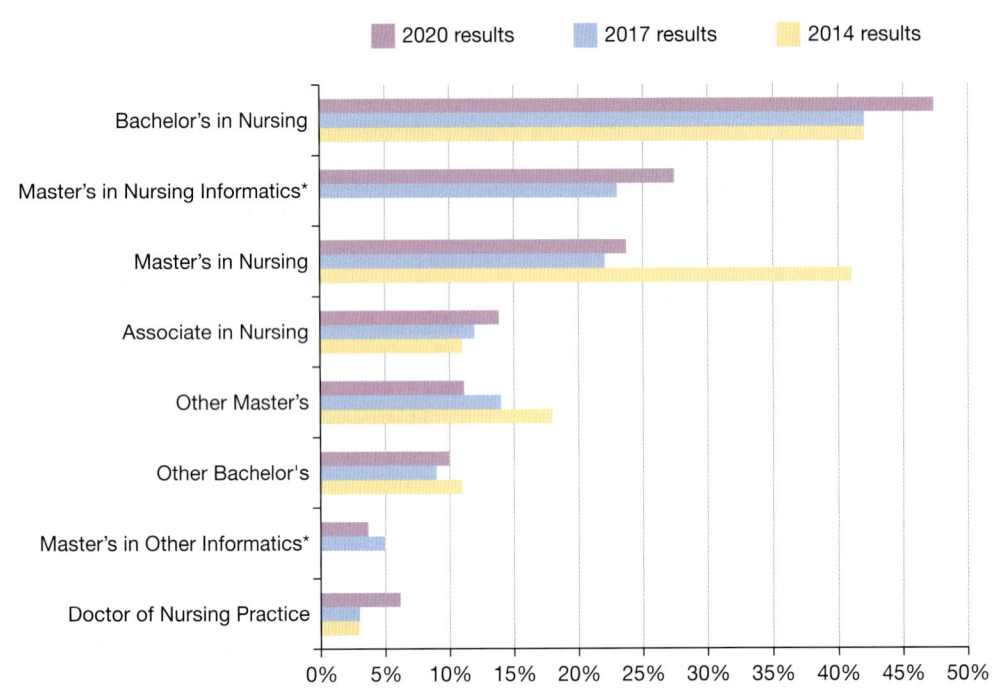

Figure 2-6. Advanced degrees of nursing education for informatics nursing are increasing. *New options in 2017. (Adapted from HIMSS. (2022). *2020 nursing informatics workforce survey*. https://www.himss.org/sites/hde/files/media/file/2020/05/15/himss_nursinginformaticssurvey2020_v4.pdf)

Once an RN completes the requirements and passes the exam, they will earn a credential of Informatics Nursing Certification (NI-BC).

Nursing informatics is evolving and growing quickly. According to a recent survey, certification in informatics took a significant jump from 49% in 2017 to 58% in 2020 (HIMSS, 2022). Certification is also helpful for compensation: 56% of informatics nurses who hold a certification in informatics have a salary of more than $100,000 compared with 39% of those pursuing certification and 40% of those not pursuing certification (HIMSS, 2022).

Check the ANCC website to stay up to date with any changes in requirements for certification (ANA, 2022). The American Nursing Informatics Association (ANIA) is in partnership with ANCC, so there are special discounts available for certification and certification review courses (Janetti, Inc., ANIA, n.d.).

Tips for Starting an Informatics Career

Though preparation for a career as an informatics nurse typically involves getting an advanced degree, there are other ways to get started. One possibility is becoming a super user. A **super user** achieves expertise with a new system (such as an EMR) and then trains and mentors other nurses to become proficient. Another opportunity is to volunteer for committees that work with the informatics department, as well as take part in studies, training, and research with exposure to expert knowledge and skills. Networking is also useful. By networking with experts who work in informatics, the nurse can gain a better understanding of the role. Consider setting up an interview with a practicing informatics nurse to learn about the certifications, degree programs, best practices, and ways to improve a resume and marketability (Gaines, 2022).

Continuing Education

All informatics careers require continuing education that is often obtained at professional conferences. The American Medical Informatics Association (AMIA), HIMSS, and the American Health Information Management Association (AHIMA) have large educational and research meetings including tutorials for novice practitioners. Additionally, some universities sponsor 1- or 2-week intensive informatics courses. Three annual conferences, one sponsored by Rutgers College of Nursing, a second one by the University of Maryland School of Nursing, and a third by ANIA, are all excellent places for continuing education. Read the Ethical Considerations box to learn about how continuing education supports the ANA Code of Ethics.

ETHICAL CONSIDERATIONS FOR PROFESSIONAL GROWTH

The ANA Code of Ethics Provision 5 states that the nurse owes the same duties to themselves as to others, including the responsibility to promote health and safety, preserve wholeness of character and integrity, maintain competence, and continue personal and professional growth. Principle 5.5 focuses on the role of the nurse in the maintenance of competence and continuation of professional growth. Professional growth requires a commitment to lifelong learning. This learning can include continuing education, self-study, networking with other professionals, achieving specialty certification, or obtaining an advanced degree. Think about what you have learned in this chapter and apply it to Principle 5.5 (ANA, 2015). What would you consider minimum evidence of an informatics nurse maintaining competence and continuing professional growth? Identify one opportunity from this chapter that you would consider to meet this principle, and justify your response.

Professional Informatics Organizations

Joining a professional informatics organization will help in the process of becoming a successful informatics nurse because of the opportunities for networking and professional growth and development. In Chapter 1, you learned that these organizations provide opportunities for advocacy, continuing education, and knowledge sharing at conferences at the local, regional, national, and international levels. Multidisciplinary organizations to consider include the European Federation for Medical Informatics (EFMI), the International Medical Informatics Association (IMIA), HIMSS, and AHIMA. Informatics organizations specific to nursing include the ANIA, the Alliance for Nursing Informatics (ANI), and the British Computer Society (BCS) Health Nursing Group. Consider asking a practicing informatics nurse about what organizations they participate in.

Nursing Informatics as a Specialty

Nursing is a subspecialty in informatics with roles and tasks in both disciplines. It is important to differentiate between an informatics nurse and an informatics nurse specialist. An informatics nurse is someone who enters the nursing informatics field because of an interest or experience (ANA, 2022). An **informatics nurse specialist** (INS) is an RN with a graduate-level degree in informatics or a closely related field (Houston et al., 2019). Both nurses can also get special certification to work in this area. Nurses working in this area may focus on some or all of these areas:

- Administration, leadership, and management
- Systems analysis and design
- Compliance and integrity management
- Consultation
- Coordination, facilitation, and integration
- Development
- Educational and professional development
- Genetics and genomics
- Information management/operational architecture

- Quality and performance improvement
- Research and evaluation
- Safety and security

Practice in each of these areas requires different knowledge and skills on the part of the informatics nurse. Some of the roles and responsibilities in these areas are summarized in Table 2-2.

The basic role of the informatics nurse is to improve care, improve the health of patients and the public, and improve cost-effectiveness (Houston et al., 2019). Whereas some informatics nurses have only on-the-job training, certified INSs work in settings where there is increased complexity and expectations for systems. Keep in mind that although the roles of informatics nurses and INSs may differ, there is often much overlap, and job descriptions vary from agency to agency. Understanding the roles of informatics nurses and INSs assists clinical nurses in working with them to improve clinical systems. Chapter 11 covers the role of the informatics nurse in more detail.

SUMMARY

- **Theories that support informatics.** Understanding the theories behind nursing informatics allows the nurse to better understand what makes nursing informatics unique. Notable theories in the field of nursing informatics include the DIKW model, sociotechnical theory, change theories from Rogers and Lewin, general systems theory, chaos theory, and cognitive science. Each of these theories can be used to increase patient outcomes by guiding the creation and implementation of systems.
- **Becoming an informatics nurse.** To become an informatics nurse, the nurse needs a nursing license and bedside experience as well as competencies in informatics. The AACN has developed standards for informatics education and other nursing organizations have published standards for the profession. Informatics education includes online, graduate, and certification programs, and continuing education helps practicing informatics nurses stay current in the field. Professional informatics organizations provide opportunities for advocacy, continuing education, and knowledge sharing. Note that there is a difference between an informatics nurse (someone who enters the field because of interest or experience) and an INS (someone with a graduate degree in an informatics field).

DISCUSSION QUESTIONS AND ACTIVITIES

1. Why is it important to learn about informatics nursing theories?
2. Consider the case study article (Warty et al., 2021). What changes to Rogers's diffusion of innovations model did the authors recommend? Do you agree or disagree with their conclusions? Defend your answer.
3. Choose one informatics theory and find an article in which that theory has been used to improve patient outcomes. Discuss whether you agree or disagree with the author's conclusions.
4. Search the internet for two formal educational programs in nursing informatics that would most interest you. Identify three factors about the programs that are the most interesting to you and explain why.
5. Investigate the activities of an informatics professional organization. Some methods for accomplishing this include checking the home page, attending a meeting, or interviewing a member or officer in one of the groups. Which organization would you consider joining and why?
6. Explore the ANIA website.
    - What resources are available on the website?
    - Describe the purpose of the ANIA professional organization.
    - Were you able to identify any continuing education resources? If so, provide an example.

TABLE 2-2 Roles and Responsibilities of Informatics Nurses and Informatics Nurse Specialists

Roles	Responsibilities
Informatics Nurse	
Systems educator	Plans, coordinates, and facilitates education for all computer applications and computer software for all user groups. Develops and trains all user groups on clinical computer applications and online documentation processes. If employed by a vendor, may be responsible for documenting a new system and providing "train the trainer" education to healthcare agency personnel.
Information technology nursing advocate	Assesses the needs and opportunities for nurses with the technology. Looks at both the functional and operational needs of clinical users when using the system and translates these needs into information technology–specific solutions
Super user	Supports the system for a specified unit. Assists users with functionality, procedural issues, and basic troubleshooting. Often holds a clinical position in the assigned unit
System specialist	May work at many different levels from the unit to the full agency. Acts as a link between nursing and information services and is both a nursing resource and a representative
Clinical systems coordinator/analyst	Responsible for coordinating aspects of planning, design, development, implementation, maintenance, and evaluation of the clinical information system. Troubleshoots issues with systems. Supports a clinical system
Informatics Nurse Specialist	
Project manager	Plans and implements an informatics project. Must be able to communicate effectively with all levels of management, users, and system developers. Must also be cognizant of all factors involved in the project including, but not limited to, managing change, assessing the need for the new project, and planning for its implementation
Consultant	Provides expert advice, opinions, and recommendations from consultant's area of expertise. Must be able to analyze what the client wants, as well as what is needed, and integrate these to create what is possible, technologically and politically. May be employed within an organization, by a vendor, or be self-employed

(Continued)

TABLE 2-2 Roles and Responsibilities of Informatics Nurses and Informatics Nurse Specialists (Continued)

Roles	Responsibilities
Director of clinical informatics	Facilitates the development, implementation, and integration for an agency information system. Assists in developing the strategic and tactical plans of the system. Develops plans for implementation and gaining acceptance of systems
Researcher	Uses informatics to create new knowledge. Encompasses research in any area of nursing informatics. May be involved in basic research on the symbolic representation of nursing phenomena, clinical decision making, or applied research of information systems. Could be involved in developing decision support tools for nursing or models of representation for nursing phenomena
Product developer	Participates in the development of new information systems including designing, developing, and marketing of informatics solutions for nursing problems. Must understand the needs of both business and nursing
Policy developer	Contributes to health policy development by identifying nursing data, its availability, structure, and content, which are used to determine health policy. These policies encompass not only information management but also health infrastructure development and economics
Entrepreneur	Analyzes nursing information needs in clinical areas, education, administration, and research. Develops and markets solutions

PRACTICE QUESTIONS

1. Which term from the DIKW model involves knowing when and how to apply knowledge to a situation?
   a. Data
   b. Information
   c. Wisdom
   d. Knowledge

2. The theories supporting informatics come from many different areas. A nurse exploring knowledge, people, and technologic systems is focusing on which theory?
   a. Lewin's field theory
   b. Chaos theory
   c. Sociotechnical theory
   d. Rogers's diffusion of innovations theory

3. Which is true of the educational preparation for nursing informatics?
   a. HIMSS is an accrediting body that examines informatics education.
   b. The ANIA sponsors an annual conference that provides continuing education credits.
   c. The ANA recommends at least 10 years of experience in nursing before beginning a career as an informatics nurse.
   d. The AACN only defines informatics knowledge at an advanced practice level.

REFERENCES

American Association of Colleges of Nursing (AACN). (2008, October 20). *The essentials of baccalaureate education for professional nursing practice*. http://www.aacnnursing.org/Education-Resources/AACN-Essentials

American Association of Colleges of Nursing (AACN). (2021). *The essentials: Core competencies for professional nursing education* https://www.aacnnursing.org/Portals/42/AcademicNursing/pdf/Essentials-2021.pdf

American Nurses Association (ANA). (2015). *Code of ethics for nurses with interpretive statements*. Silver Spring. https://www.nursingworld.org/practice-policy/nursing-excellence/ethics/code-of-ethics-for-nurses/

American Nurses Association (ANA). (2022). *Nursing informatics: Scope and standards of practice* (3rd ed.). American Nurses Publishing.

American Nurses Credentialing Center (ANCC). (n.d.). *Informatics nursing certification*. https://www.nursingworld.org/our-certifications/informatics-nurse/

Asiedu, N. K., Abah, M., De-Graft Johnson, D., Wright, L. T. (Reviewing editor). (2022). Understanding knowledge management strategies in institutions of higher learning and the corporate world: A systematic review, *Cogent Business & Management, 9*, 1. https://doi.org/10.1080/23311975.2022.2108218

Barrow, J. M., Annamaraju, P., & Toney-Butler, T. J. (2022). *Change management*. In *StatPearls*. StatPearls Publishing.

Bass, A. (2003, June 1). *Health-care IT: A big rollout bust*. CIO Magazine ([serial on the internet]).

Brown, G. D., Pasupathy, K. S., & Patrick, T. B. (2019). *Health informatics: A systems perspective (second)*. Health Administration Press ; Association of University Programs in Health Administration. https://public.ebookcentral.proquest.com/choice/FullRecord.aspx?p=5520238

Clark, D. (2010, November 15). *Understanding and performance*. http://www.nwlink.com/~donclark/performance/understanding.html

Collins, S., Yen, P., Phillips, A., & Kennedy, M. K. (2017). Nursing informatics competency assessment for the nurse leader: The Delphi study. *Journal of Nursing Administration, 47*(4), 212–218. https://doi.org/10.1097/NNA.0000000000000467

Demir, M. S., Karaman, A., & Oztekin, S.D. (2019). Chaos theory and nursing. *International Journal of Caring Sciences, 12*(2), 1223–1227.

Dizikes, P. (2011, February 22). *When the butterfly effect took flight*. MIT News Magazine. http://www.technologyreview.com/article/422809/when-the-butterfly-effect-took-flight/

Feldthouse, D. M., Jacques, D. P., Fenelon, L., Robertiello, G., Pasklinsky, N., Fletcher, J., Groom, L. L., Doty, G. R., & Squires, A. P. (2022). Implementing an academic electronic health record in nursing education. *Journal of Informatics Nursing, 7*(2), 37–42.

Gaines, K. (2022, July 18). *Nursing informatics*. Nurse.org Career Guide Series. https://nurse.org/resources/nursing-informatics/

Graves, J. R., & Corcoran, S. (1989). The study of nursing informatics: *Image—Journal of Nursing Scholarship, 21*(4), 227–231.

Healthcare Information and Management Systems Society (HIMSS). (2022). *2020 nursing informatics workforce survey*. https://www.himss.org/sites/hde/files/media/file/2020/05/15/himss_nursinginformaticssurvey2020_v4.pdf

Houston, S. M., Dieckhaus, T., Kircher, B., & Lardner, M., (Eds.). (2019). *An introduction to nursing informatics, evolution, and innovation* (2nd ed.). CRC Press. https://doi.org/10.4324/9780429425974

Janetti Inc., A., & ANIA. (n.d.). *Nursing informatics certification review course*. Nursing Informatics Certification Review Course. American Nursing Informatics Association. Retrieved November 30, 2022, from https://www.ania.org/nursing-informatics-certification-review-course

Joos, I., Whitman, N. I., Smith, M. J. (1992). *Computer in small bytes*. National League for Nursing Press.

Lovell, T. (2021, May 19). *Technology must meet clinician needs to manage burnout HealthcareITNews*. https://www.healthcareitnews.com/news/emea/technology-must-meet-clinician-needs-manage-burnout

Nation, J., & Wangia-Anderson, V. (2019). Applying the data-knowledge-information-wisdom framework to a usability evaluation of electronic health record system for nursing professionals. *Online Journal of Nursing Informatics, 23*, 1.

Nurse.org. (n.d.). *What is nursing informatics?* Retrieved November 30, 2022, from https://nurse.org/resources/nursing-informatics/#how-do-you-become-an-informatics-nurse

Rogers, E. M. (2003). *Diffusion of innovations* (5th ed.). Free Press.

Smith, M. K. (2001). *Kurt Lewin: Groups, experiential learning and action research*. http://infed.org/mobi/kurt-lewin-groups-experiential-learning-and-action-research

Thagard, P. (2014, July 11). *Cognitive science—the Stanford encyclopedia of philosophy*. http://plato.stanford.edu/entries/cognitive-science/

The National Archives. (n.d.). *Florence Nightingale: Why do we remember her?* https://www.nationalarchives.gov.uk/education/resources/florence-nightingale/

Turley, J. (1996). Toward a model for nursing informatics: *Image—Journal of Nursing Scholarship, 28*(4), 309–313. https://doi.org/10.1111/j.1547-5069.1996.tb00379.x

von Bertalanffy, L. (1973). *General system theory: Foundations, development, applications*. Harmondsworth. Penguin.

Warty, R. R., Smith, V., Salih, M., Fox, D., Mcarthur, S. L., & Mol, B. W. (2021, October 15). Barriers to the diffusion of medical technologies within healthcare: A systematic review. *IEEE Access, 9*, 139043–139058. https://doi.org/0.1109/ACCESS.2021.3118554. https://ieeexplore.ieee.org/document/9562554

Woody, E. W. II (2020). MHS Genesis implementation: Strategies in support of successful EHR conversion. *Military Medicine, 185*(9–10), e1520–e1527. https://doi.org/10.1093/milmed/usaa184

UNIT II

Technology

Chapter 3	Essential Computer Concepts
Chapter 4	Computer Networks and Online Communication
Chapter 5	Mobile Healthcare Technology
Chapter 6	Telehealth

This unit will provide you with an overview of healthcare information technology. As an informatics nurse, you need to be familiar with computers, networking, online communication, mobile healthcare technology, and telehealth to provide the best care for your patients. Technology is evolving at a rapid pace, and it is not possible to know everything about every innovation. Instead, focus on what these concepts have in common.

As you read these chapters, try to link what you are learning to what you already know about technology and patient care. Look for opportunities to apply what you are learning to the technology you use at work and in your life. Explore how you can contribute to the technology evolution you are seeing around you. Note situations in which technology might be helpful or useful. Is there a problem on your unit that technology could solve? Is there a patient outcome that could be positively affected by technology? Reach out to your information technology team and explore ways to engage in creating and developing new technology for patient care. When nurses are involved in the development of technology, patients are served better.

Chapter 3 (Essential Computer Concepts) includes a case study on using cloud computing for a nursing information platform. It covers basic concepts of computers and operating systems, as well as storage and software.

Chapter 4 (Computer Networks and Online Communication) begins with a case study about how online communication was used to scam a hospital, and includes stories demonstrating the pitfalls of social media in the healthcare field. The first half of the chapter covers computer networks, the internet, malware, and protecting computers from cyber criminals. The second half of the chapter explores the importance of professionalism and civility for safe nursing practice, the pros and cons of social media in healthcare, and misinformation.

Chapter 5 (Mobile Healthcare Technology) begins with a case study demonstrating how mobile healthcare technology can improve patient outcomes in underserved communities. The chapter covers the basics of mobile devices with examples of how they are used for patient care, software for mHealth, and how mHealth is used in clinical practice. Advantages and disadvantages and future trends are also discussed as well as ethical considerations of the primacy of the patient's interests.

Chapter 6 (Telehealth) covers all aspects of telehealth including the wide array of uses in the healthcare field and the barriers to its use, including limited internet access and reimbursement issues. The case study is on project ECHO, which provided funds for telehealth and home-based telemonitoring for the Navajo Nation during the COVID-19 pandemic.

CHAPTER 3

Essential Computer Concepts

Dawn Henderson and Kristi Miller

OBJECTIVES

After studying this chapter, you will be able to:
1. Identify the components of a computer.
2. Discuss the characteristics and uses of various types of computers.
3. Discuss differences in operating systems.
4. Explain best practices for storage and retrieval of data.
5. Describe cloud computing and identify its uses.
6. Give examples of different software applications.

AACN Essentials for Entry-Level Professional Nursing Education

8.1a Identify the variety of information and communication technologies used in care settings.
8.1b Identify the basic concepts of electronic health, mobile health, and telehealth systems for enabling patient care.
8.1d Describe the appropriate use of multimedia applications in healthcare.
8.3a Demonstrate appropriate use of information and communication technologies.
8.5c Comply with legal and regulatory requirements while using communication and information technologies.
9.1a Apply principles of professional nursing ethics and human rights in patient care and professional situations.

AACN Essentials for Advanced-Level Nursing Education

8.1g Identify best evidence and practices for the application of information and communication technologies to support care.
8.3j Evaluate the potential uses and impact of emerging technologies in healthcare.
8.5h Assess potential ethical and legal issues associated with the use of information and communication technology.

HIMSS TIGER Competencies

Applied computer science

Assistive technology

Data protection and security

Ethics in health internet technology

Information and communications technology systems applications

Legal issues in health internet technology

KEY TERMS

Applications	Flash drive	Server
Backup	Freeware	Shareware
Bugs	Graphical user interface (GUI)	Smartphone
Central processing unit (CPU)	Hard disk drives (HDDs)	Software
Cloud computing	Mainframe computer	Solid-state drive (SSD)
Code	Motherboard	Storage drive
Computer	Open-source software	Supercomputer
Computer programming (coding)	Operating system (OS)	Tablet
Data encryption	Public domain software	Universal serial bus (USB) port
Debugging	Random access memory (RAM)	Workstation

CASE STUDY

Chen et al. (2022) described building a nursing information platform (NIP) for patients of a general surgery (GS) unit using cloud computing technology. The goal of the author team was to construct a well-rounded hospital information system (HIS) to improve service quality and patient satisfaction. An HIS is designed to manage a hospital's operations and is composed of software components, data storage, security, and internal and external communication among providers and computer networks.

The authors describe the GS unit as complex and challenging with complications often occurring after surgery. Nurses on GS units must provide support, information, and guidance to patients as they recover, making GS an excellent unit to target with more efficient NIPs. The NIP would serve as a resource to improve nursing efficiency, reduce errors, and give nurses more time to care for patients directly. Cloud computing enables users to obtain required services on demand within the network. It has unique advantages of large-scale resource sharing, security, and reliability. The authors advocate for the construction of NIPs for complex units that need quick and reliable access to information supporting patient care (Chen et al., 2022).

How familiar are you with cloud computing and HISs? What skills would you need to be a contributing member of an NIP implementation team? As you read this chapter, think about how increased knowledge of computer concepts can support improved patient care.

Computers have become an integral part of patient care; it is now difficult to imagine healthcare without them. Beginning in the 1970s, nurse pioneers contributed to the use of computers in patient care activities. Examples include the development of the first computerized nursing unit, the Problem-Oriented Medical Information System (PROMIS) (Gordon, 1978), and the development and implementation of a computerized physician ordering system called *Eclipsys* (BaytechIT, 2018). New uses for computers are emerging daily; the use of telehealth has increased by over 50% since 2020, and drones can be used to transport blood samples from those living in remote areas (Smith, 2022). It is crucial that nurses not only be knowledgeable about emerging technology but also have the skills to innovate with the use of computers in patient care.

This chapter will discuss essential computer concepts, including types of computers and how they operate and how to access and use software applications. This chapter will also discuss cloud computing—the delivery of computing services over the internet. Knowing basic computer concepts will help you support optimal patient outcomes. The Ethical Considerations box discusses knowledge of computer concepts that support the American Nurses Association (ANA) Code of Ethics.

ETHICAL CONSIDERATIONS FOR COMPUTER CONCEPTS

Several provisions from the ANA Code of Ethics can relate to computers (2015):

- Interpretive Statement 2.3: Collaboration: Knowledge of computers and how they work meets this interpretive statement when you collaborate with patients using information, resources, and courage to participate in mutual decision making. Collaboration with computer programmers and information technology specialists is also needed when working with computers.
- Interpretive Statement 3.3: Performance Standards and Review Mechanisms: As a nurse, you need to demonstrate ongoing knowledge, skills, dispositions, and integrity for competence in practice. This relates specifically to knowledge of computers, which are an integral part of healthcare in today's world.
- Interpretive Statement 4.1: Authority, Accountability, and Responsibility: Nurses are accountable for maintaining their competence to ensure safe practice. This means nurses have a duty to learn about technologic advancements, evidence-informed practice mandates, and shifting patterns of healthcare delivery.
- Interpretive Statement 5.3: Preservation of Wholeness of Character: Nurses not only embrace the values of the profession but also display them in their communication and actions. Nurses must be careful in exerting undue influence on patients as they make decisions about using healthcare information technology.
- According to Interpretive Statement 6.3, you have a responsibility for the healthcare environment. This means participating in professional development about computer concepts and advocating for fair use of software.

WHAT IS A COMPUTER?

A **computer** is an electronic device that manipulates information (data) based on a program, software, or instructions. It can store, retrieve, and process data. In the world of healthcare, computers play an integral role in daily operations. They are used to record and store patient information, schedule medical appointments, monitor vital signs, keep track of medical inventory, track the spread of disease, facilitate research, and allow patients to care for themselves in their homes.

Computer Components

A computer is made up of multiple parts in two basic categories: hardware and software. Hardware are the physical structures housing the central processing unit, memory storage, and communication ports as well as peripheral devices like

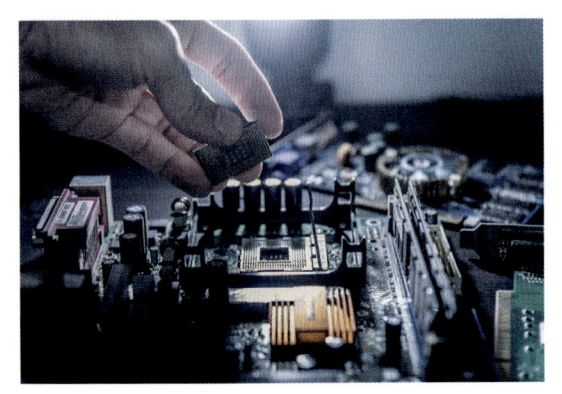

Figure 3-1. Computer components: putting a CPU onto the motherboard. (Shutterstock/TimeStopper69.)

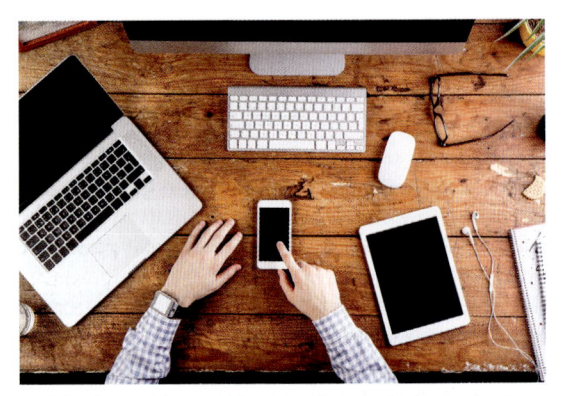

Figure 3-2. Types of computers: desktop, laptop, tablet, smartphone, and smartwatch. (Shutterstock/Ground Picture.)

printers, mouses, and keyboards. The minimum hardware needed for an electronic device to be considered a computer includes (Fig. 3-1):

- **Motherboard:** Primary circuit board holding the hardware in place, providing a connection between hardware components and devices
- **Central processing unit (CPU):** Processes and executes inputs from hardware and software. CPU speed is an important element to consider when purchasing a computer.
- **Random access memory (RAM):** Temporary data storage space holding information the CPU is actively using; when a program is open on a desktop, it is using RAM.
- **Storage drive:** Where data are stored on a permanent basis. Retrieving information from a storage drive takes more time than retrieving it from RAM, but data stored here are less likely to be lost, for example, in a power surge or if a computer is accidentally shut down while programs are open.

Software are the parts of a computer that are not physical. This includes data, programs, applications, and protocols. **Applications** are types of computer programs designed to assist the user in accomplishing tasks, such as word processing software or web browsers like Google Chrome.

You will learn more about hardware and software later in the chapter, but a computer science course includes even more details about these computer components. Nurses proficient in computer science are needed in informatics.

TYPES OF COMPUTERS

Computers have evolved into many different types over the last few decades (Fig. 3-2). Nurses have a responsibility to understand basic types of computers because they are so widely used in healthcare.

Servers

A **server** is a computer that provides information or services to other computers on a network. For example, an internet search yields results that are stored on a server. A server provides services to multiple clients. A single client can use multiple servers, and a single server can serve multiple clients. Examples of servers are database servers, file servers, mail servers, print servers, web servers, and application servers. Many healthcare organizations use file servers to store and share files internally. Application servers allow users in their networks to run and use applications without having to download and install them on their own computers. Mail servers make email communications possible in the same way a post office makes postal mail communication possible. Print servers allow one or more printers to be shared among many users. Web servers make connection to the internet possible. Most of the internet is based on the client–server model. Virtual servers also exist. They help healthcare organizations use and administer server resources more efficiently. Healthcare facilities can expand server capacity without having to find new space, increase power use, add staff, or turn to outsourcers for help.

Mainframes

A **mainframe computer** is a large, high-speed computer that supports peripheral computers or workstations. A **workstation** is a desktop computer in a network with many others and is more powerful than a personal computer due to the connection with the mainframe. A **supercomputer** is a large and powerful mainframe computer. The FRONTIER, the world's fastest computer, contains roughly 9.2 petabytes (9.2 million gigabytes) of storage or memory (BasuMallick, 2022). An example of the use of a supercomputer in healthcare is the MDGRAPE-3, a computer developed in Japan that is used to predict the structures of proteins. This supercomputer has been used to investigate mutations in protein folding in patients with epilepsy and leukemia and for accelerating COVID-19 research (Padhi et al., 2021).

Personal Computers

Developed in the late 1970s, personal computers are less expensive than mainframe computers and can be purchased and used by individuals. In 2000, more than 50% of all households in the United States owned a personal computer. However, sales have declined since 2012 as consumers have shifted their computer use to mobile smartphones and tablets. With the COVID-19 pandemic in 2020, personal computer sales increased as people began to work from home or attend virtual school (Encyclopedia Britannica, 2022).

Personal computers can be desktops, designed to be in a stationary location where all the components fit on or under a desk or table. They may also be laptops, which are sometimes viewed as mobile devices since they can be carried to different locations. Laptops tend to have less powerful CPUs than desktop computers, though this is changing as technology improves. A 1.3-gigahertz (GHz) processor and 2 to 4 GB of RAM are sufficient for using the internet and watching movies on any device, but faster processors and more memory may be needed for more complex tasks. Laptops and desktops may or may not have touch screens. A touch screen is a display device that allows the user to interact with a computer by tapping areas on the screen.

Mobile Devices

A mobile or handheld device is a computer small enough to be carried by hand. It wirelessly communicates and has capacity for general computing functions. Examples include tablets, smartphones, e-readers, and wearable technology.

- A **tablet** is a thin, lightweight, mobile computer with a touch screen. An example of a tablet is an Apple iPad. They are even more portable than laptops.
- **Smartphones** are phones that can also browse the internet, allow the user to play games, track health and fitness goals, and perform other functions wirelessly.
- An e-reader is an electronic device designed for reading books, such as the Amazon Kindle. Some e-readers use a special kind of display called *e-paper* that has less glare and is easier to read than traditional computer screens.
- Wearable technology includes fitness trackers and smartwatches. They are designed to be worn throughout the day. Fitness trackers track metrics like heart rate, activity, stress levels, sleep quality, and more. Some smartwatches also have smartphone capabilities.

OPERATING SYSTEM

Despite all its parts, the computer will do nothing unless it is told what to do. The **operating system (OS)** manages computer hardware and software, coordinates input from the keyboard with output on the screen, responds to the mouse and touch pad clicks, follows commands to save and retrieve files, and transmits commands to printers and other peripheral devices (GCFLearnFree, n.d.). An OS can boot, or turn on, the computer, manage memory, and load and start programs and data security.

Examples of Operating Systems

There are three main OSs for personal computers: Microsoft Windows, Apple macOS, and Linux. The Chromebook runs on Chrome OS. Additional OSs exist for smartphones and tablets like the Android OS and Apple iOS for the iPhone.

Windows has the most users at around 75%, followed by macOS and Linux (Statista Research Department, 2022). Though an Apple Macintosh computer is a personal computer, the term "PC" is often used to describe computers that operate using the Microsoft Windows OS, which has been around since 1985 (Microsoft, n.d.). Examples of computer brands that run on the Windows OS include Lenovo, Dell, Microsoft, Asus, and Acer. Benefits of using the Windows OS are that it is easily upgraded and has more options for different components such as motherboards, processors, storage drives, and video and graphics cards. In addition, PCs are less expensive than Apple computers and offer more features, software, and games and a wider variety of choices.

Apple released the first version of an OS for the Mac in 1984 (Gallagher, 2022). Macs are known for being user-friendly and are typically more intuitive to use. In addition, iPhones sync with Macs to download and save files among the phone, computer, and iCloud. Some also consider fewer choices to be another benefit. There are hundreds of PCs to choose from but fewer than 10 Apple computers. Macs have also been shown to be more secure; because there are fewer users, they are less vulnerable to viruses because hackers have a smaller pool of potential victims. However, they are generally more expensive than PCs and are more difficult to upgrade.

Linux was released as a free and open-source OS in the mid-1990s (The Linux Foundation, 2016). Linux is mostly used on servers, especially web servers, and it can also run supercomputers. Because Linux is free, it is also used to repurpose older computers.

Google released the Chrome OS in 2011 for Chromebooks (Bacchus, 2021). Chrome OS, which is an open-source project, represents a paradigm shift for operating systems because it is a combination of a web browser and OS.

Graphical User Interface

A **graphical user interface** (**GUI**, pronounced "gooey") is a graphics-based OS interface that uses icons, menus, and a mouse for the user to choose what they want the computer to do. Prior to the GUI, first used in the 1980s by Apple, computers used a disk operating system (DOS). DOS was text-based and required the user to remember a set of commands, such as "Delete," "Run," "Copy," and "Rename." The device screens were black and generally only displayed text and numbers. Unlike GUI, DOS allowed for only one program at a time to run, programs could not share information, and the user could not point and click to enter commands (Fig. 3-3).

Computer Programming

Computer programming (coding) is the process of writing code to facilitate computer actions. **Code** is text written by a computer programmer using a programming language. Examples of programming languages include C, C#, C++, Java,

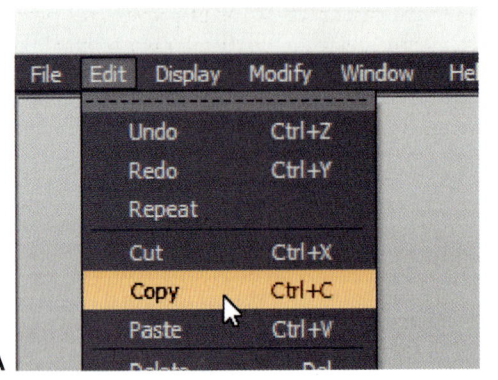

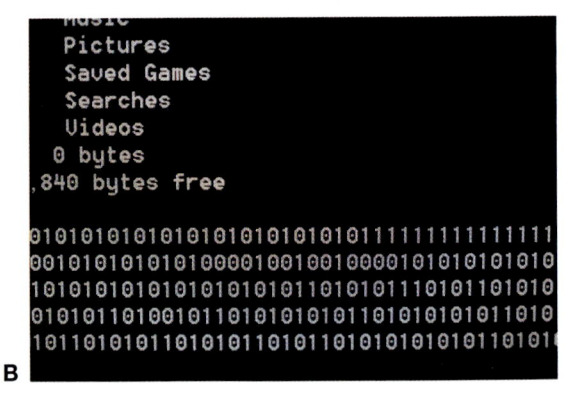

Figure 3-3. Comparing graphical user interface **(A)** to disk operating system **(B)**. (**A.** Shutterstock/eranicle; **B.** Shutterstock/Gullatawat Putchagarn.)

Linux, Perl, and Python. For example, on a PC, the computer code of a web page is visible by right-clicking on the page and selecting "View page source." A new window will appear, showing the computer code for the page. Programmers write code for OSs, applications, and other software programs.

Common tasks for computer programmers in healthcare include modifying electronic health record software to improve performance and resolving problems, such as when a software application crashes or becomes nonresponsive. Programmers often deal with **bugs**—a term that refers to computer system errors and issues. **Debugging** is the process of correcting computer system errors. Informatics nurses with computer programming skills are invaluable members of healthcare teams due to the unique perspective they can provide into how to build programs that will best facilitate quality patient care.

DATA STORAGE

One of the components of a computer is data storage, meaning information in the form of files, documents, and images that is recorded digitally and stored for future use. Storage systems can be electromagnetic, optical, or other media. A basic understanding of data storage is necessary to ensure information is stored in a way that allows quick and easy retrieval and protects patient privacy.

A storage drive houses the OS, applications, and data files. A computer needs at least one storage drive to function. Usually, this is an internal drive located inside the computer. Drive capacity is measured in bytes. A byte is a unit of data made of eight binary digits (i.e., zeros and ones), or enough data to represent a number, letter, or symbol. A gigabyte (GB) is 1 billion bytes, and a terabyte (TB) is 1 trillion bytes. Data storage in healthcare ensures that if a computer stops functioning, important medical records are not lost. Data storage needs to be reliable, cost-effective, secure, and compatible with an organization's infrastructure (Research Hub, 2022). Data storage can occur on a physical hard drive, solid-state drive, disk drive, digitally, or on the internet (in the cloud). Figure 3-4 shows different types of data storage.

Hard Drive

Hard disk drives (HDDs) are more common in older devices. An HDD contains moving parts—a motor-driven spindle that holds one or more flat, circular disks, coated with a thin layer of magnetic material. Advantages of HDDs are that they can hold a large amount of data (500 GB to 1 TB are common) and they are inexpensive (roughly 3 cents per gigabyte). For additional space, an external drive can be attached to the computer, usually through a universal serial bus (USB) port. External drives are also inexpensive and portable, making it easier to share files.

Disadvantages of HDDs are that they have slow operating speeds, especially with larger software applications. This is due to nonsequential storage of data, resulting in fragmentation, which causes small amounts of empty space to slowly take up storage space on the computer. If a computer is running slowly, the hard drive may need to be defragmented. This will free up storage space and help the computer run more efficiently. In addition, hard drives use a lot of power and produce heat, sometimes causing problems in small computers. Computers have internal fans or cooling devices, but overheating can lead to slow speeds

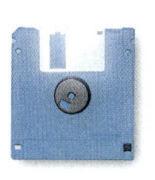

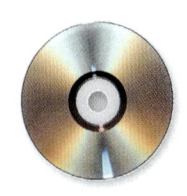

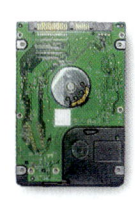

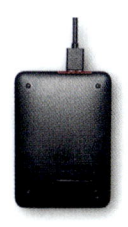

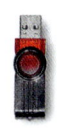

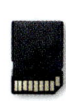

Figure 3-4. Storage devices. From left to right, floppy disc, CD, internal hard drive, external hard drive, flash drive, SD card, and microSD card. (Shutterstock/Kirin Phanithi.)

and crashes. An inexpensive external stand that contains a fan can help prevent overheating. At a minimum, avoid using laptops on surfaces that do not allow for good air flow.

Solid-State Drives

A **solid-state drive (SSD)** is the most common storage drive currently in use. An SSD is a memory chip using integrated circuits instead of a rotating disk. SSDs are a type of NAND flash memory (NAND stands for "NOT AND"). NAND is a type of nonvolatile storage technology, meaning it does not require power to retain data.

SSDs are more expensive and offer less storage than HDDs (64 to 256 GB); however, they are smaller and faster than HDDs, supporting more input and output operations per second. Other advantages include that they are noiseless and allow personal computers to be thinner and weigh less. They generate less heat and use less power than HDDs as well. Performance is not impacted by fragmentation, so defragmentation is not necessary. Finally, they have no moving parts.

Other Storage Hardware

In 1951, one of the first computers used magnetic tapes as storage devices. Floppy disks were used from 1971 until 1999 and could hold 240 MB of data (see Fig. 3-4). Compact disks (CDs) are optical storage devices that feature microscopic pits and bumps that disk drives read as binary data. They are prone to scratches and the storage capacity is limited to 700 MB, but they are inexpensive and take up little physical space. Digital video disks (DVDs) look like CDs and feature spiral tracks with more data capacity than CDs. A DVD uses an even finer laser than CDs due to the higher density and can hold up to 4.7 GB of data. They are also affordable and portable. However, newer computers are not made with CD/DVD drives, so use is limited to externally purchased disk drives.

Instead of CD/DVD drives, most computers and many other devices now have a **universal serial bus (USB) port** that serves as a connection for other devices. A **flash drive** plugs into a computer's USB port and relies on NAND flash memory just like SSDs. Flash drives feature fast read and write speeds with a capacity up to 256 GB. They are small, inexpensive, and designed to be portable storage solutions (see Fig. 3-4). Secure digital (SD) cards rely on flash memory as well and are designed for portable devices like smartphones and digital cameras. Most laptops have SD card readers. They are sold as full, miniSD, and microSD sizes with various capacities (Andrea, n.d.).

Backing Up Data

A **backup** is a copy of the data that can be used for recovery in case the original data are lost or corrupted. It is recommended that users back up data with three copies. Two should be local (e.g., on an external hard drive or the computer's hard drive) and the third should be on a cloud backup service. With this system, it is unlikely all data will be lost, even if a laptop is stolen, a hard drive crashes, or the internet goes down. The *New York Times* Wirecutter recommends a USB desktop hard drive as the most cost-effective external storage option. Though it has a smaller capacity and is more expensive, it does not require a power cord (Klosowski, 2021).

Windows has a tool that is included with the computer for backing up files called *File History*. This stores versions of computer files on an external hard drive. Once it is set up, backups happen automatically. On Macs, backups can be created using "Time Machine" (Fig. 3-5). Encrypting the backup ensures security. It is important to create a unique password that will not be forgotten because access to the backed-up files will not be possible without it.

CLOUD COMPUTING

Cloud computing refers to the ability to access software and file storage on remote devices using the internet (Fig. 3-6). This contrasts with the traditional method of establishing an onsite data center with servers or hosting the data on a personal computer. There are benefits

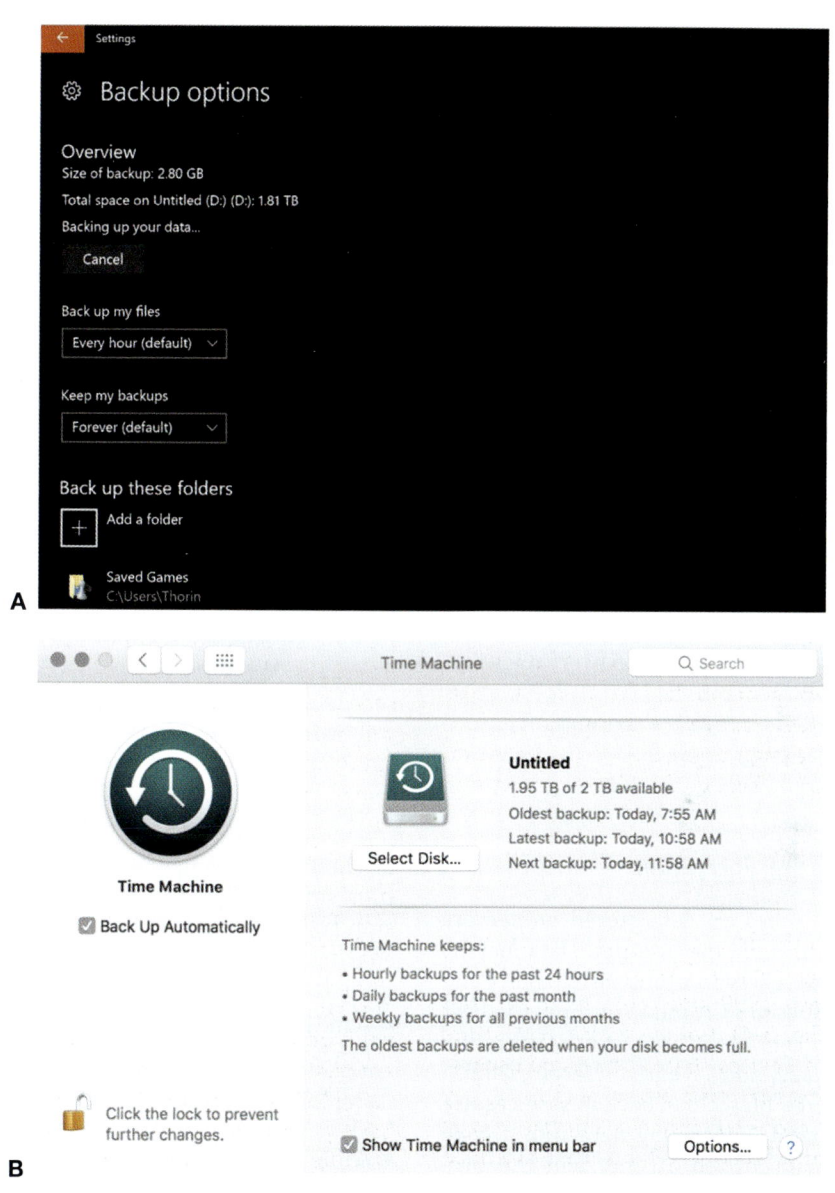

Figure 3-5. Backing up files with "File History" **(A)** and "Time Machine" **(B)**.

to using cloud computing in healthcare, including reduced costs, security, collaboration, and interoperability (the ability of two systems or organizations to exchange healthcare information). According to a survey of 500 information technology (IT) professionals at U.S. healthcare organizations, 70% say their organization has moved to the cloud and 20% say they hope to make the move in the next few years (DuploCloud, 2023). To access the cloud, a computer needs internet access and a cloud provider like Amazon, Google, Microsoft OneDrive, or Dropbox. Backing up an entire computer requires a large amount of storage, which may come with a cost. For example, Google charges $10 per month for 1 TB.

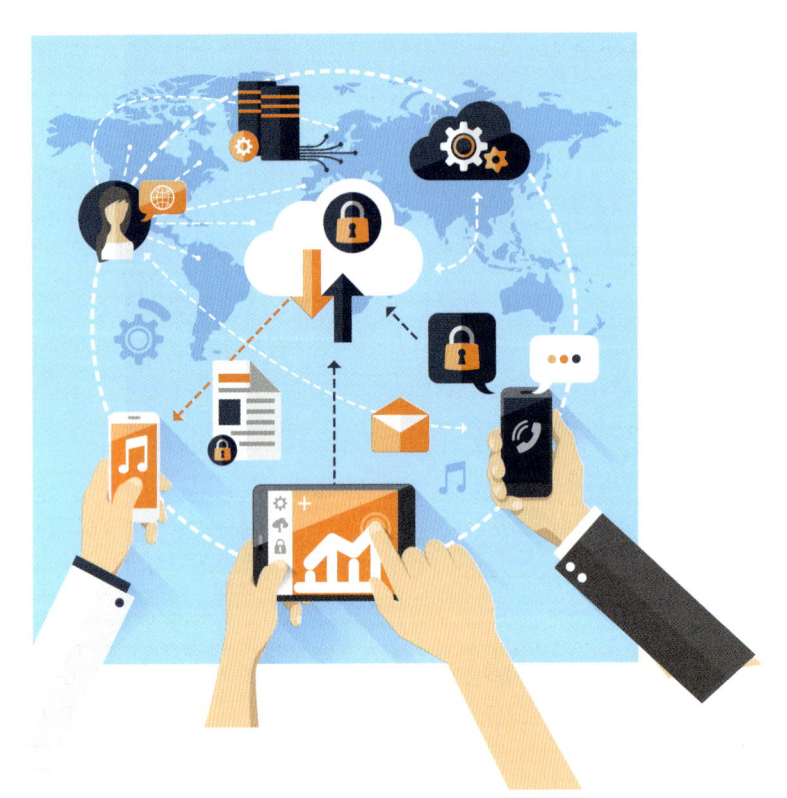

Figure 3-6. Cloud computing. (Shutterstock/Jiri Perina.)

Cloud Storage and Encryption

Cloud storage relies on data stored on servers that are accessible via the internet. Data may be stored on multiple servers to ensure reliability and access. According to *PCWorld* magazine, the best online backup services in 2022 were Carbonite, iDrive, Backblaze, and Livedrive (Jacobi, 2022). To protect stored files, cloud backup services use **data encryption** (converting data into a code to prevent unauthorized access), and the provider does not have a key to decrypt them. The Advanced Encryption Standard (AES) is a symmetric block cipher that the U.S. government selects to protect classified data. Most current cloud suppliers use 256-cycle AES encryption to secure information.

Sharing Files in the Cloud

The ability to create and edit files using cloud computing applications is another advantage of the cloud because users can share and edit files simultaneously, reducing the risk of version control issues. Common cloud computing sharing features include the ability to determine if:

- A file is publicly visible on the web where anyone can search and view it.
- A file is visible to anyone who has the link without a sign-in.
- A file is private and a sign-in is necessary to access the file.
- Shared users can view the file.
- Shared users can edit the file.
- Shared users can collaborate and edit files at the same time.
- Shared users can make comments on the file.

File sharing is used in many ways, for example, on group projects, meeting documents, petitions, surveys, and more. Access is dependent on the needs of the file owner who, with a click of a button, can change the status of who has access (Griffith, 2022).

Advantages and Limitations of Using the Cloud

There are many advantages of using the cloud (Griffith, 2022):
- Many cloud computing providers offer 1 to 200 GB of free file storage.
- The cloud offers universal access.
- Hard drives fail, and flash drives and SD cards are small and easy to lose while the cloud cannot be lost.
- Because computers crash and accidents happen, it is best to regularly back up files and have the backups located somewhere other than where the original document is stored. This is particularly important for files difficult to recreate.
- The ability to share and edit files with others simultaneously makes organizing files and their changes more efficient. The ability to access and edit files from any device connected to the internet that has the appropriate software makes files more accessible.

Limitations include (Griffith, 2022):
- Recurring fees
- Slower transfer speeds
- Capped capacity
- Since the user is not the owner of the site, they have no control over its availability. The site could be unavailable due to maintenance.
- Without internet access, the user cannot access the online applications or files.
- Popular cloud computing sites may be targets for cyber criminals.

Generally, files with patient information should not be located on the cloud without encryption. Some cloud computing sites offer site encryption, but for a fee, and users cannot view encrypted data without a code. Some fee-based storage solutions, such as Microsoft OneDrive for Business and Dropbox Business, provide additional file security.

> **CASE STUDY**
>
> The authors from the case study at the beginning of this chapter advocate for the use of cloud computing to construct NIPs for complex units that need quick and reliable access to patient care information. How might you advocate for cloud computing in a nursing unit if management is resistant to using the cloud?

SOFTWARE APPLICATIONS

Earlier in the chapter, hardware was defined as the physical parts of a computer. Software is not as easy to define. System software controls the internal functioning of a computer through the OS, and controls the peripherals like monitors, storage devices, printers, and speakers. Application software is a class of computer applications that allows the user to perform required tasks like word processing, data analysis and management, inventory, and payroll. Network software coordinates the communication between computers on a network. Driver software is used to support external devices like printers and wireless mice.

Think about the case study at the beginning of the chapter. The authors created an NIP for their GS unit (Chen et al., 2022). There are many similar health management system software applications in healthcare for providing billing and invoicing, care plan management, mobile access, patient records management, scheduling, and time tracking. Alora Home Health, MatrixCare Home Health, and Hummingbird are a few examples. Other types of healthcare-related software include (Paterska, 2022):
- Telemedicine software with in-app video conferencing, file transfer, and security
- Remote patient monitoring that can collect patient data outside traditional healthcare settings to gain more thorough information on a patient's health or conduct remote diagnosis
- Prescription software that allows providers to write and keep track of prescriptions

- Health tracking applications that track physical activity, movement, dieting, weight loss, and mental health and well-being.

Software is usually stored on an external memory device like a hard drive. When the program is being used, the computer puts the instruction in the RAM. This process of storing and executing instructions is called *running* or *executing* a program (Encyclopedia Britannica, 2022, August 24).

Certain application software works with a specific OS, which may play a role in which software or which OS to choose. When choosing software for healthcare organizations, the source and governing its use should be considered. Though most software is commercial and proprietary (owned by a company or individual and available for purchase), you may also consider open-source, shareware, freeware, and public domain software. It is important to know, understand, and abide by the software copyright policies for programs you use. When users accept software through any channel other than a reputable seller, they should be certain that they know what type of software it is. Unless obtained from a well-known vendor, the user should run a virus checker to verify that the file is safe to install.

Commercial Software

Commercial software is proprietary, meaning it has copyright protection, and you must purchase it. Examples include Microsoft Office and Adobe Photoshop. The terms of use display when you install the software and users must accept these terms to complete installation. Installation of proprietary software requires the user to register the software, a process that generally needs an internet connection. A key card for the software that includes the installation number may also be purchased. During installation, the user will be prompted to enter a number or code, such as the serial number, product key, or some other designation. Once this code is entered, the program checks to see if the code was previously registered before allowing installation. Although software is still available for purchase from a CD, it is more common now to purchase and download software from a website. If the software is installing from a CD, the location of the information is on the installation disks or the envelope in which the software disk came.

Shareware

Shareware is commercial software that is initially free to users but eventually requires a payment for the use of the software. As an example, many commercial software applications have a free trial period that allows you to try out the application before you purchase it. Some shareware has a paywall that blocks advanced features or only offers the full package for a limited time. Some shareware is fully functional and backed solely by voluntary donations.

Open-Source Software

Open-source software allows users to change the coding and share it with other users. The idea behind this is that by making source code available, many programmers who are not concerned with financial gain will find and eliminate bugs and make improvements to the code, producing a more useful, bug-free product. This peer review process is something that is absent in proprietary programs. Open source grew in the technologic community as a response to proprietary software owned by corporations. Examples include Firefox and LibreOffice.

Freeware

Freeware is an application the programmer has decided to make freely available to anyone who wishes to use it. Usually, it is closed-source with some restricted usage rights. Although it is free, the author usually maintains the copyright. Unless the program is open-source, a user cannot do anything with the program other than what the author specifies. Freeware has copyright protection. Examples include Instagram, Facebook, Adobe Reader, and Skype.

Free Cloud Office Applications

Many of the cloud computing office applications and file storage resources provide the ability to share files and folders with others. Examples of cloud computing software include office applications such as word processors, spreadsheets, notes, and media players. Some examples of free cloud-based office applications include Google

Drive and Apple iWork for iCloud. Both office suites include the ability to share and collaborate with others and access free storage solutions. With these cloud-based applications, users no longer need to download office software to their devices.

Public Domain Software

Public domain software is software with no copyright restrictions. Because there is no ownership, you can use the software without restrictions. Some freeware programs available on the internet are in the public domain, and they can be used any way the user desires, including making changes. Major examples of public domain software are the Linux OS, Apache web server, and JBoss application server.

SUMMARY

- **What is a computer?** A computer is an electronic device that stores, retrieves, and processes information. Nurses have a responsibility to understand basic computer technology, including hardware like the motherboard, CPU, RAM, and storage.
- **Types of computers.** Due to the widespread use of computers in healthcare, it is important for nurses to have a basic understanding of the types of computers in use, including servers, mainframes, PCs, tablets, and mobile devices.
- **Operating systems.** The OS manages all the hardware and software on a computer. Though there are several OSs to choose from, the best option is the one that fits the individual needs or the needs of an organization. Computer programmers write code to create OSs.
- **Data storage.** Knowing the basics of data storage will prevent unnecessary data loss. Most computers have SSDs for internal storage with enough memory to meet all the data storage needs, but there are many options, including SD cards, external hard drives, and DVD drives. It is good to have a plan for backing up data so that if a computer crashes, data will be protected.
- **Cloud computing.** Cloud computing is the ability to access software and store files using the internet. With more than 70% of healthcare organizations using the cloud, nurses need to understand the pros and cons of this technology.
- **Software applications.** Software is made up of programs that computers use to complete tasks or fill needs like managing complex healthcare information. Knowing the differences among commercial software, open-source, freeware, and shareware can inform decisions about which software is best.

DISCUSSION QUESTIONS AND ACTIVITIES

1. What should you consider when purchasing a computer for personal use? What would you purchase and why?
2. Identify the current OS on the computer you are using. Is it the most recent version? How many versions have there been of the OS you are using?
3. Are you using cloud technology on a desktop/laptop, phone, or tablet? If so, which cloud computing application are you using? Do an internet search to identify cloud computing resources that may help you or others. Summarize your findings.
4. A nursing classmate needs advice on backing up their computer. What storage resources could you suggest? What are the pros and cons of cloud computing? Would the type of computer in use be important? Explain your answer.
5. A friend sends you a web link to a program for you to install. What should you consider before doing so?
6. You wish to install a program that you have at home on another computer. What things should you consider?

PRACTICE QUESTIONS

1. A nurse has purchased proprietary software for their computer. To install it properly, what action is required?
    a. Call the vendor to set up service.
    b. Register the product.
    c. Be sure the software has a serial number.
    d. Skip the initial sign-in process.

2. The nurse is using software without copyright restrictions. What type of software is the nurse using?

   a. Freeware
   b. Open-source
   c. Public domain
   d. Shareware

3. The nurse is instructed to store patient information files in the cloud. What is the most important step to follow in the process?

   a. Accepting the terms of use
   b. Checking the site for viruses
   c. Checking the software copyright
   d. Encrypting the files

REFERENCES

American Nurses Association. (2015). *Code of ethics for nurses*. American Nurses Publishing. https://www.nursingworld.org/practice-policy/nursing-excellence/ethics/code-of-ethics-for-nurses/

Andrea, H. (n. d.). *13 different types of storage devices and disk drives used in computer systems*. Tech 21 Century. Retrieved January 21, 2023 from https://www.tech21century.com/different-types-of-storage-devices/

Bacchus, A. (2021, June 15). Chrome OS was born 10 years ago. Here are the highlights in its rise to power. https://www.digitaltrends.com/computing/chrome-os-turns-10-here-is-how-it-evolved/

BasuMallick, C. (2022, December 1). What is a supercomputer? Features, importance, and examples. https://www.spiceworks.com/tech/tech-101/articles/what-is-supercomputer/

BaytechIT. (2018, March 11). The history of healthcare technology and the evolution of EHR. https://www.baytechit.com/history-healthcare-technology/

Chen, Y., Wang, J., Gao, W., Yu, D., & Shou, X. (2022). Construction and clinical application effect of general surgery patient-oriented nursing information platform using cloud computing. *Journal of Healthcare Engineering, 2022*, 1–10.

DuploCloud. (2023, February 22). 70% of healthcare businesses have adopted cloud computing: DuploCloud report. https://www.globenewswire.com/news-release/2023/02/22/2613339/0/en/70-of-Healthcare-Businesses-Have-Adopted-Cloud-Computing-DuploCloud-Report.html

Encyclopedia Britannica. (2022, August 24). *Software*. In *Encyclopedia Britannica*. https://www.britannica.com/technology/software

Encyclopedia Britannica. (2022, September 20). *Personal computer*. In *Encyclopedia Britannica*. https://www.britannica.com/technology/personal-computer

Gallagher, W. (2022, January 24). Apple launched Macintosh on January 24, 1984 and changed the world—eventually. https://appleinsider.com/articles/19/01/24/apple-launched-macintosh-on-january-24-1984-and-changed-the-world----eventually

GCFLearnFree. (n.d.). What is an operating system? The operating system's job. https://edu.gcfglobal.org/en/computerbasics/understanding-operating-systems/1/

Gordon, C. A (1978). *Medical revolution that could...: The work of the PROMIS laboratory and Lawrence L. Weed, M.D*. US Department of Health, Education Welfare National Institute of Education. http://eric.ed.gov/ERICDocs/data/ericdocs2sql/content_storage_01/0000019b/80/3f/1a/15.pdf

Griffith, E. (2022, February, 15). *What is cloud computing? PC Magazine*. https://www.pcmag.com/how-to/what-is-cloud-computing

Jacobi, J. L. (2022, December 20). *Best online backup: We test the best services—Carbonite, iDrive, Backblaze, Livedrive*. PCWorld. https://www.pcworld.com/article/407149/online-cloud-backup-services-carbonite-idrive-backblaze-livedrive.html

Klosowski, T. (2021, September 29). *How to back up your computer*. Wirecutter. *New York Times*. https://www.nytimes.com/wirecutter/guides/how-to-back-up-your-computer/

Microsoft. (n.d.). The history of Microsoft. Retrieved June 17, 2022 from https://docs.microsoft.com/en-us/shows/history/history-of-microsoft-1985

Padhi, A., Rath, S. L. & Tripathi, T. (2021). Accelerating COVID-19 research using molecular dynamics simulation. *Journal of Physical Chemistry, 125*(32), 9078–9091. https://www.ncbi.nlm.nih.gov/pmc/articles/PMC8340580/

Paterska, P. (2022, December 6). See 16 types of emerging medical software that revolutionize the healthcare industry as we know it. https://www.elpassion.com/blog/most-popular-types-of-healthcare-software

Research Hub. (2022, September 6). What is data storage? Data storage types & attributes. https://www.cdw.com/content/cdw/en/articles/datacenter/what-is-data-storage.html#:~:text=Types%20of%20Data%20Storage,-There%20are%20two&text=this%20category%20include%3A,Hard%20Drives,Flash%20Drives

Smith, A. (2022, August 30). 16 jaw-dropping medical technology statistics of 2022. https://resources.10to8.com/blog/medical-technology-statistics/

Statista Research Department. (2022, May 23). Global market share held by computer operating systems 2012-2021, by month. https://www.statista.com/statistics/268237/global-market-share-held-by-operating-systems-since-2009/

The Linux Foundation. (2016). What is Linux? https://www.linux.com/what-is-linux

CHAPTER 4

Computer Networks and Online Communication

Elizabeth Riley, Veneine Cunningkin, Larronda Rainey, Jaime Sinutko, and Kristi Miller

OBJECTIVES

After studying this chapter, you will be able to:
1. Explain the importance of computer networks to patient care.
2. Provide examples of computer networks.
3. Analyze the different methods of connecting to the internet.
4. Discuss how the internet is used in healthcare.
5. Discuss computer network security threats.
6. Identify ways to protect computer networks from security breaches.
7. Explain what online communication is.
8. Identify the importance of professionalism and civility in online communication.
9. Examine the ethical and legal implications for unprofessional communication.
10. Discuss the use of social media in healthcare.
11. Compare the guidelines for use of social media.
12. Identify misinformation and fake news.

AACN Essentials for Entry-Level Professional Nursing Education

6.1e Communicate individual information in a professional, accurate, and timely manner.

7.2b Recognize the impact of health disparities and social determinants of health on care outcomes.

8.1a Identify the variety of information and communication technologies used in care settings.

8.1e Demonstrate the best practice use of social networking applications.

8.3a Demonstrate appropriate use of information and communication technologies.

8.4b Describe how information and communication technology tools support patient and team communications.

8.5a Identify common risks associated with using information and communication technology.

8.5b Demonstrate ethical use of social networking applications.

9.1a Apply principles of professional nursing ethics and human rights in patient care and professional situations.

AACN Essentials for Advanced-Level Nursing Education

8.1h Evaluate the unintended consequences of information and communication technologies on care processes, communications, and information flow across care settings.

8.1k Identify the impact of information and communication technologies on workflow processes and healthcare outcomes.

8.5h Assess potential ethical and legal issues associated with the use of information and communication technology.

8.5i Recommend strategies to protect health information when using communication and information technology.

HIMSS TIGER Competencies

Communication

Data protection and security

Ethics in health internet technology

Information and communications technology systems (applications)

Information and communications technology systems (architectures)

Information and knowledge management in patient care

Internet technology risk management

Legal issues in health internet technology

Quality and safety management

KEY TERMS

5G	Client	Extranet
Adware	Collective intelligence	Fake news
Algorithm	Computer virus	Firewall
Backdoor	Cyber criminal	Folksonomy
Bandwidth	Digital subscriber line (DSL)	Hacked
Blog	Disinformation	Hacker
Botnet	Distributed denial of service (DDoS)	Hardwired
Broadband		Hashtag
Chat	Domain name	Hoax
Civility	Drive-by-download	Hypertext transfer protocol (HTTP)
Click fraud	Ethernet	

Infodemic
Information disorder
Internet
Internet of medical things (IoMT)
Internet service provider (ISP)
Intranet
IP address
Keylogger
Listserv
Local area network (LAN)
Malware
Medjacking
Microblogs
Misinformation
Modem
Netiquette
Network

Network authentication
Nodes
Pharming
Phishing
Plain old telephone service (POTS)
Professional networking
Protocol
Ransomware
Router
Satellite
Search engines
Server
Social bookmarking
Social determinants of health (SDoH)
Social engineering
Social media
Social networking

Spam
Spyware
Topology
Trojan horse
Trolls
Universal resource locator (URL)
Virtual private network (VPN)
Warez
Web browser
Wide area network (WAN)
WiFi-protected access (WPA)
Wiki
Wireless (WiFi)
World Wide Web
Worm

CASE STUDY

- An employee at a Utah-based health system clicked on a link in an email that allowed hackers to gain access to the employee's login credentials. The health system's representatives believed the hacker was using phishing to gather usernames and passwords for financial fraud (McKeon, 2021).
- Two nurses in Tennessee were fired after posting a TikTok video mocking a pediatric patient who had a gunshot wound (Brusie, 2023).
- Misinformation on social media is linked to vaccine hesitancy. Sharing false information, even when later debunked, correlates with people either delaying vaccination or refusing a vaccine outright (Pierri et al., 2022).
- Cultural values may influence the ways in which people who identify as Latino or Latina engage with and act on cancer prevention and screening information on Facebook, which may lead individuals to bypass important procedures. Efforts are needed to leverage social media to empower this population to partake in prevention and screening actions that effectively reduce cancer health disparities (Rivera et al., 2022).

What do all these reports have in common? They highlight the explosive growth of the internet and online communication in conjunction with a lack of understanding about its effect on health outcomes. As you read this chapter, think about tools you can use in your workplace to ensure the safety of your peers, family, community, and patients as they engage with information found on the internet. In addition, consider how knowledge of computer networking can help keep the healthcare information of your patients safe and how social media can promote the goals of nursing.

Imagine you encounter a patient with a disease you cannot immediately recognize. Within seconds of typing the symptoms into the internet, you locate relevant information about the disease from an international healthcare organization. Healthcare professionals no longer have to wait for information to become available in a paper version of a medical journal. Rather, they can network with colleagues all over the world using computers and other devices to communicate and share information and ideas, often in real time. This is an example of how the ability to exchange information on a global scale is changing the healthcare profession.

Healthcare depends on communication—between the nurse and the patient, among healthcare professionals, and with the public. Since the first computers were able to communicate with each other in the late 1960s, communication about patient care has progressed to the point at which computers in an organization are connected not only to each other, but also to a worldwide network. However, society in general and healthcare professionals in particular are struggling to keep pace with the rapid evolution of online communication. With a multitude of interactive websites, instant news, and personal opinions not regulated by traditional media, it is important to discern evidence-based information from misinformation.

This chapter discusses computer networking, introducing pertinent terminology to use when talking about a problem with an information technology (IT) specialist, working on a committee related to networking technology, or advocating for equal access to high-speed internet. There is information about online security, security threats, and methods to protect computer devices. Finally, this chapter explores online communication in the healthcare setting, including applications and tools for online communication, use of social media, and how to deal with misinformation.

COMPUTER NETWORKS

A computer **network** consists of two or more computers that can exchange data and share resources with each other. A network system allows a variety of devices to share information seamlessly. Computer networks are made up of **nodes**, the connection points among network devices such as computers, routers, printers, or switches that can receive and send data from one endpoint to the other. Devices are connected by cables (wires), fiberoptics, or wireless signals, and the network is built with hardware (routers, switches, access points, and cables) and software (operating systems or applications). Devices can communicate because networks follow **protocols**, standardized sets of rules for formatting and processing data (IBM, n.d.). A network can range in size from a connection between a smartphone and a personal computer (PC) to the worldwide, multiuser computer connection known as the internet (Al-Fedaghi & Behbehani, 2020). The internet, social media, online searches, email, and modern healthcare exist because of computer networks.

Architecture

Computer network architecture refers to the physical and logical framework of a computer network. Architecture includes hardware, software, transmission media (wired or wireless), protocols, and topology. There are two types of computer networks, peer-to-peer (P2P) and client-server, that define how computers are organized and what tasks they will complete. Figure 4-1 illustrates these two types of networks.

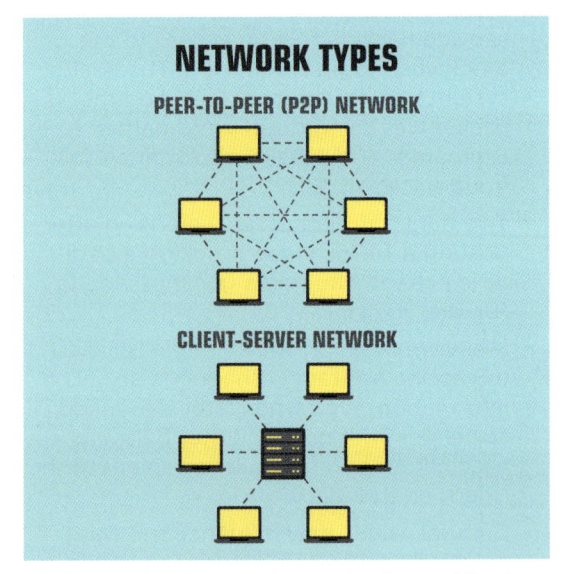

Figure 4-1. Computer network architecture. (Shutterstock/ShadeDesign.)

Peer-to-Peer

In P2P architecture, two or more computers are connected as "peers," giving them equal power and privileges on the network. A central server is not required for a P2P network. Each computer acts as both a **client** (a computer needing access to services) and a **server** (a computer serving the client accessing a service). Each peer makes resources available to the network, sharing memory, storage, processing power, and bandwidth (IBM, n.d.).

Client-Server

A client-server network uses a central server (or group of servers) to manage resources and deliver services to clients (devices) in the network. The clients in the network communicate with each other through the server via the internet. Unlike the P2P model, clients in a client-server architecture do not share resources. This architecture type is sometimes called a tiered model because it is designed with multiple levels or tiers.

Topology

Topology refers to how nodes in a network are arranged. The most common are bus, ring, star, and mesh (IBM, n.d.). Figure 4-2 shows common topologies.
- Bus: Every node is directly connected to a main cable.
- Ring: Nodes are connected in a loop, meaning each device has exactly two neighbors. Adjacent pairs are connected directly, and nonadjacent pairs are connected indirectly through multiple nodes.
- Star: All nodes are connected to a single hub and each node is indirectly connected through that hub.

- Mesh: The connections between nodes overlap. Full mesh means every node in the network is connected to every other node. Partial mesh means some nodes are connected to nodes with which they exchange the most data. Full mesh topology can be expensive and time-consuming to execute. Partial mesh provides less redundancy but is more cost-effective and simpler to execute. Mesh network topology is considered the most reliable and is the most used in the healthcare industry.

Types of Computer Networks

Geographic location can define a computer network. For example, a **local area network (LAN)** connects computers in a defined space such as a hospital or primary care office. A **wide area network (WAN)** can connect computers across continents. The internet is the largest example of a WAN. Table 4-1 outlines types of networks and the number and locations of connected computers.

The terms intranet and extranet are also ways to categorize network connections. An **intranet** is analogous to a LAN. It is a private network within an organization allowing users to share information. It may include features such as email, mailing lists, and user groups. Intranets are used in healthcare to keep patient information secure while still allowing healthcare workers to communicate about patient care. An **extranet** is more analogous to a WAN. It is defined as an extension of an intranet with added security features. It provides accessibility to the intranet to a specific group of outsiders, often business partners. Access requires a valid username and password (IntegralChoice, 2020).

Network Connections

Networks can be **hardwired**, connected physically with cables containing wires, or by using a **wireless (WiFi)** signal. Most healthcare agency networks, even those that use WiFi, are hardwired to some extent. Computers connected by cables are often referred to as LANs. These connections use Ethernet to connect computers in a physical space. **Ethernet** cables are designed to work with Ethernet ports, which can be found on routers, computers, televisions, and most

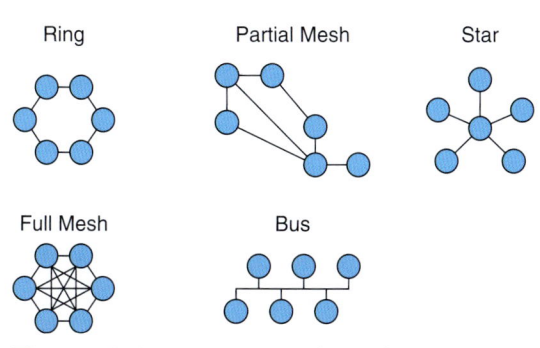

Figure 4-2. Computer network topology.

TABLE 4-1	Types of Networks
Personal area network (PAN)	Serves one person. An example is sharing and syncing content such as photos, email, and text between a smartphone and computer.
Local area network (LAN)	Confined to a small area within a short distance, such as a building or groups of buildings. Can be wireless (WLAN). Usually privately owned and managed.
Wide area network (WAN)	Encompasses a large geographic area. Might be two or more LANs. Ownership is collective or distributed.
Campus area network (CAN)	Encompasses a defined geographic area, such as a college campus. Smaller than a WAN and larger than a LAN.
Metropolitan area network (MAN)	Encompasses a city or town. Larger than a LAN and smaller than a WAN. Cities and governments own and manage MANs.
Virtual private network (VPN)	A secure, point-to-point connection between two nodes, a VPN establishes an encrypted channel to keep the user's identity and data inaccessible to hackers.

internet- and network-enabled devices. The benefits of hardwiring include faster internet and more reliable connectivity. The downside is that computers that are hardwired are not mobile (Ellis, 2023).

Wireless Connections

WiFi transmissions are limited in distance so they do not compete with other radio traffic. During the wireless system installation, nodes, which consist of a tiny router with a few wireless cards and antennas, are placed at strategic locations throughout the building or premises. Successful wireless communication depends on an adequate number of nodes and their placements. The distance of a device from a node affects the speed of transmission and whether one can use the network. The number of users per node also affects the speed of transmission.

Connection to a WiFi network requires the use of a modem and a router. The **modem**, a device that transmits digital information, connects with the **internet service provider (ISP)**, an organization that provides access to the internet. Examples of ISPs include AT&T, Verizon, Xfinity, and Spectrum. The **router**, which connects multiple computers to the same network, transmits the WiFi signal with the help of attached or internal antennas (Omboni et al., 2020). Sometimes, one device contains the router and modem.

A **digital subscriber line (DSL)** is a home network that connects a router to the internet with a regular phone line as opposed to Ethernet, which uses a television cable for the connection. In some rural areas, internet users may connect using a dial-up modem through a regular telephone line, called **plain old telephone service (POTS)**. **Satellite** connections are another type often found in areas with less developed infrastructure due to an inability to install and maintain nodes or communication towers. Connections are instead provided through communication satellites.

WiFi is less secure than hardwired transmission because it operates on a spectrum that can be used by anyone in range and on any device—the opposite of cellular networks (Chatzoglou et al., 2022).

WiFi-protected access (WPA) is a security standard for computing devices equipped with wireless internet connections. WPA was developed by the Wi-Fi Alliance to provide more sophisticated data encryption and better user authentication than wired equivalent privacy, the original WiFi security standard. WPA was replaced by WPA2 due to security issues (Vanhoef & Ronen, 2020). As of July 2020, any newly released device that is certified by the Wi-Fi Alliance must support WPA3 (Chatzoglou et al., 2022).

Network authentication is a standard for computer networks at home and at work. In the home setting, all users must enter the authentication code to access a secure WiFi network. Without the code, no new devices can connect to the network.

Network Connection Speed

Today, most internet connections use **broadband**, which refers to how much data the connection can transmit at once. The size, or **bandwidth**, of the broadband connection determines the speed of the network connection. The greater the bandwidth, the greater the simultaneous information transmission, just as a six-lane highway permits more cars to travel at the same time than a single-lane road. POTS transmits only a single frequency at one time; hence, a broadband connection offers more speed. Table 4-2 outlines different broadband connections available for using the internet (GCFGlobal, n.d.).

5G

WiFi networks linked to a router at home, work, or places such as coffee shops can be used free

TABLE 4-2 Types of Internet Connections

Connection Type	Pros	Cons
Fiberoptic cable	Supports high-speed data transfer Excellent signal reliability	More fragile than wire Frequently expensive
Television cable	Faster than dial-up and DSL Uses a television cable connection (can use internet and television at the same time) Supports high-speed data transfer	Available only where there is cable television service
Satellite	Faster than dial-up and DSL Available worldwide Can be powered by generator or battery	Affected by weather (heavy cloud cover and storms) Frequently expensive Requires use of a satellite dish
Digital subscriber lines (DSLs)	Faster than dial-up and DSL Uses a regular phone line (can use the phone and internet connection at the same time) Easy to install	Available only where there is phone service Connection speed slowed by longer distances from the provider
Dial-up	Inexpensive Easily available anywhere there is a telephone jack Easy to install	Very slow Less reliable Requires manual connection Uses a regular phone line (cannot use the phone and internet connection at the same time)

of cost, but free WiFi networks exist outside the range of a router. This is facilitated by **5G**, a term for the fifth-generation cellular network technology first deployed in 2019. 5G refers to the speed of the connection and follows implementation of 1G (first introduced in 1979), 2G, 3G, and 4G. 4G was adopted in 2009, but with the rapid introduction of new technologies, faster networking speeds were needed (Galazzo, 2020). 5G has a higher bandwidth, meaning it can be used to connect multiple devices and improve the quality of the internet in crowded areas. It can facilitate download speeds between 1 Gbps and 10 Gbps and upload speeds of 1 millisecond. This means that 5G internet connections can compete with cable internet and other hardwired connections. The actual speed depends on many factors, such as what network the user is connected to, the device they are using, and how many other people are also using it (De Looper, 2022).

> **CASE STUDY**
>
> Consider the examples in the case study. How could you design a computer network to maximize security features and avoid the scenarios presented? Think about the architecture, topology, and how the computers will be connected to each other and to the internet.

THE INTERNET

The **internet** is a worldwide network of interconnected computers, tablets, and smartphones as well as other internet-enabled devices. More than 21 billion devices are connected to the internet (Kelly et al., 2020). The **World Wide Web**, now more commonly called the "web," comprises the sites you see when you are connected to the internet. The internet is the network of connected devices that the web works on, carrying emails and files among users and devices. Think of the internet as a road that connects cities together, and the museums and restaurants you visit in those cities make up the web.

The initial development of the internet was to serve as a means of undisrupted military and scientific communication during a nuclear war and to provide the most economic use of resources (Science+Media Museum, 2020). Since then, government, industries, and academia have been partners in developing and implementing the internet. By the early 1990s, the internet had become familiar to most Americans, quickly getting assimilated into daily use around the world. Since its invention, the internet has revolutionized how and with whom we communicate by crossing national boundaries and long-established international protocols. It is now hard to imagine a world in which we do not have instant access to global information, communication, and entertainment. The free and open access to basic documents, especially protocol specifications, was key to the rapid growth of the internet. The development of faster bandwidth speeds was another key factor.

The internet has had a significant effect on healthcare. Information that was once delayed for weeks or months is now readily available within minutes for use by healthcare providers. The **internet of medical things (IoMT)** is the network of medical devices, hardware infrastructure, and software applications used to connect healthcare information technology. Sometimes referred to as the internet of things (IoT) in healthcare, the IoMT allows data to be sent, received, and stored among uniquely identifiable devices, such as glucose sensors and heart monitors. This system has allowed patients with varying degrees of complex health conditions to become more engaged in the self-management of their healthcare, leading to improved health outcomes (Kelly et al., 2020). For example, glucose monitors allow for better glycemic control, preventing blood sugar imbalance and reducing damage to tissues and trips to the hospital. When a patient with congestive heart failure transmits daily weight data, the provider can modify prescriptions that manage fluid volume, saving the patient time and money and possibly preventing a cardiac event.

Internet Access as a Social Determinant of Health

Research demonstrates that access to the internet is a **social determinant of health (SDoH)**, or a nonmedical factor that influences health outcomes (Early & Hernandez, 2021; Graves et al., 2021; Kim et al., 2021). Over 25% of Americans do not have broadband (high-speed or wide-data transmission) access and individuals without broadband are more likely to have poorer health outcomes and health literacy (Early & Hernandez, 2021; Raths, 2020). The Affordable Connectivity Program was funded by the U.S. Congress in 2021 to help provide internet access to individuals in the United States with limited means and/or living in rural areas. Nursing and healthcare organizations can continue to foster improved health equity by including digital equity in strategic plans and vision, sponsoring community partnerships for digital literacy, and contributing to research agendas focused on the effect of high-speed internet access on health equity (Early & Hernandez, 2021).

Internet Components

To understand the internet, it is helpful to understand some of the components you will encounter, including internet protocol addresses, universal resource locators, domain names, web browsers, and search engines. With better knowledge of these, you will be able to use the internet more efficiently.

IP Addresses

A device connected to the internet shows an internet protocol address (**IP address**) that identifies the internet connection in use at that moment. The IP address tells the internet "where" to deliver information. It identifies only the connection, not the user, and it will be different for each device connected to the same connection. An IP address does not travel with the user. If you use the wireless network at a coffee shop, that IP address will be different from the one at home, even if you use the same device.

To facilitate each online device having its own IP address, each ISP has a given number of IP addresses. These are assigned to online computers as either static (stays the same each time the device connects) or dynamic (may change each time the device connects). Most IP addresses assigned today are dynamic because this is more cost-effective. An IP address consists of a string of four sets of numbers separated by periods or dots. Each set of numbers can range from 1 to 255. Each device also has an assigned name (ICANN, 2022a).

Universal Resource Locator

A **universal resource locator (URL)** is a complete web address used to find a particular web page. While the domain is the name of the website, a URL leads to any one of the pages within the website. All web documents have a URL. URLs contain a domain name and descriptors and may include a folder name, a file name, or both. Figure 4-3 shows the parts of a URL. Note a forward slash indicates a folder. If a URL does not open a page, try modifying the URL by deleting items to the far right beginning with the file name (which occurs after a period or dot) and then the folder(s) until the domain or website address is left. The website organization may have moved the folders or files to a new URL. From the homepage website address, the user may be able to search for the file. If these steps do not work, use a search engine to see if the page still exists (Google Domains, n.d.).

Domain Name System

In 1998, the Internet Corporation for Assigned Names and Numbers (ICANN) was established to keep the internet "secure, stable, and interoperable" (ICANN, 2022a). ICANN is a global

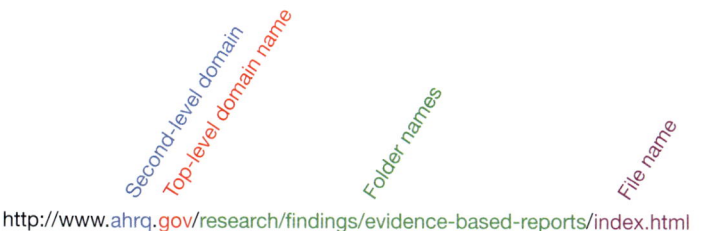

Figure 4-3. Anatomy of a URL.

http://www.ahrq.gov/research/findings/evidence-based-reports/index.html

nonprofit organization that works with individual government advisory organizations to determine domain names for website addresses. A **domain name** is a string of text that identifies an area of administrative autonomy, authority, or control within the internet. In general, a domain name identifies a network domain or an IP resource, such as a PC or server computer accessing the internet. Domain names are often used to identify services provided through the internet, such as websites and email services. As of the fourth quarter of 2023, there were 359.9 million domain name registrations (DNIB, 2024). The domain name text maps to a numeric IP address and is used to access a website from client software. In other words, a domain name is the text that a user types into a browser window to reach a particular website. For instance, the domain name for Google is "google.com". To obtain a domain name, users register the domain name with ICANN.

Domain names are typically broken up into two or three parts, each separated by a dot. When read right to left, the identifiers in domain names go from the most general to the most specific. The section to the right of the last dot in a domain name is the top-level domain (TLD). These include the "generic" TLDs such as ".com", ".net", and ".org" as well as country-specific TLDs, such as ".uk" (United Kingdom), ".cn" (China), and ".de" (Germany). Originally, there were five TLDs. Today, there are over 1,000 (ICANN, 2022b). To the left of the TLD is the second-level domain (2LD) and if there is anything to the left of the 2LD, it is called the third-level domain (3LD) (see Fig. 4-3).

Web Browsers

A **web browser**, or just "browser," is a tool enabling users to retrieve and display files from the internet. Web browsers use the client-server model of networking to retrieve web documents. The browser on the client computer requests a file from the server using a transmission protocol known as **hypertext transfer protocol (HTTP)**. The server has special software for using the protocol to receive the message, find the file, and send it back to the requesting computer (Fig. 4-4). A web address beginning with "https" indicates the protocol is encrypted and verified. HTTPS domain names are more secure than HTTP names.

There are many web browsers available, and having more than one installed on a device is useful when a page does not display correctly or an application does not run. Using a different web browser may correct the problem, and features vary among web browsers. Examples of popular web browsers include Google Chrome, Apple Safari, Microsoft Edge, and Mozilla Firefox.

Search Engines

Web browsers allow you to choose a **search engine**, a program that looks for and identifies items in a database that correspond to keywords or characters specified by the user. There are almost 300 different search engines. Common search engines include Google, Bing, Yahoo!, Ask.com, and DuckDuckGo. When searching for information, several engines may be necessary since they each use different **algorithms** (set of well-defined instructions to solve particular problems) to order the results. Classic search algorithms are evaluated on how fast they can find a solution and whether the solution is optimal. Although information retrieval algorithms must be fast, the quality of ranking and whether relevant results have been left out and irrelevant results included is more important.

ISSUES WITH NETWORK SECURITY

The phishing scam in the case study at the beginning of the chapter is just one example of a network security issue in the news. Many people

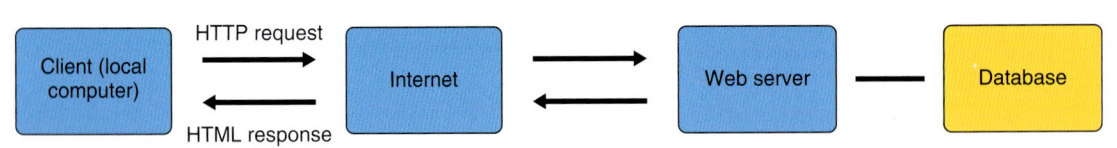

Figure 4-4. How a web browser works.

have received notifications that their names have been involved in a security breach, or perhaps they clicked on a link in an email only to discover that their computer no longer functioned properly. Any computer or device with internet access should be protected against cyber criminals.

Cyber Criminals

A **hacker** is anyone seeking to use a computer network to gain unauthorized access to data. Many hackers have gone on to be hired as IT experts or consultants to help test the limits of security of business networks. The term **hacked** means that data have been accessed by someone without permission. **Medjacking** refers to the practice of hacking a medical device with the intent to harm or threaten a patient (Cuningkin et al., 2021). A **cyber criminal** is a hacker who engages in criminal activity using computers or the internet.

Motives of cyber criminals include financial gain, espionage, access to information, personal glory, or influence. For example, Richard Pryce and Matthew Bevan hacked into military networks to try to prove the existence of aliens; Kevin Poulsen hacked into radio stations to win prize money (Cveticanin, 2022). Hacker groups have also been established; some well-known ones are the Legion of Doom, who published *The Hacker Manifesto*; Anonymous, known for politically motivated attacks; and the Masters of Deception, known for hacking phone companies (Cveticanin, 2022).

Computer Malware

Computer **malware** refers to software designed by cyber criminals to damage or disrupt a computer system. Several types of programs exist, all of which operate differently. Malware is designed to alter a device to suit the aims of the person deploying it (Petrosyan, 2022).

A **computer virus** is a type of malware limited to software, programs, or codes that self-replicates without the user's knowledge. Computer viruses may arrive in an email attachment, an electronic greeting card, or an audio or video file. They can corrupt or delete data on the computer or use email to send themselves to all the user's contacts. Like human viruses, computer viruses cause varying degrees of harm. Although a virus may exist on a computer, it cannot infect the computer until the user runs the program with the attached virus. If a computer is infected with a virus, the user may unknowingly share infected files and send emails with infected attachments, spreading the virus to others.

There are two methods cyber criminals use to get malware onto devices: social engineering and drive-by-download. **Social engineering** involves tricking computer users into downloading and installing malware (US-CERT Publications, 2020). This is the type of attack used in the Utah medical center example in the case study. For example, an email message that may look like it is from a legitimate sender could ask the reader to view a video or click a link. Clicking the link installs malware, often without the user's knowledge. The best practice is to never open files from an unknown sender. If a suspicious file comes from someone known to the user, they should check to ensure the sender meant to send it before opening it. Even a file created by a legitimate program, such as a word processor, might hide a virus.

Drive-by-download occurs when a web page design includes the malware (Rains, 2020). Opening the page automatically triggers the download and installation of the malware. It is also possible for malware to hide in advertisements of reputable, well-known websites (Rains, 2020). Once it is discovered, the owners of the website usually take immediate action to address the problem. Unfortunately, malware can make devices more susceptible to future complications and attacks, even after correcting the initial attack.

Phishing and Pharming

Phishing and pharming are older methods of cyber crime that attempt to get the user to reveal personal information such as a bank account number or a social security number. In **phishing**, the internet user receives an email message with a link and instructions to visit a website to perform some task that involves revealing personal information. Although the email message, link, or website look authentic, they are all designed by cyber criminals to extract personal information.

The example in Figure 4-5 is a phishing email. The sender is disguised as Automatic Data Processing (ADP), a company that provides

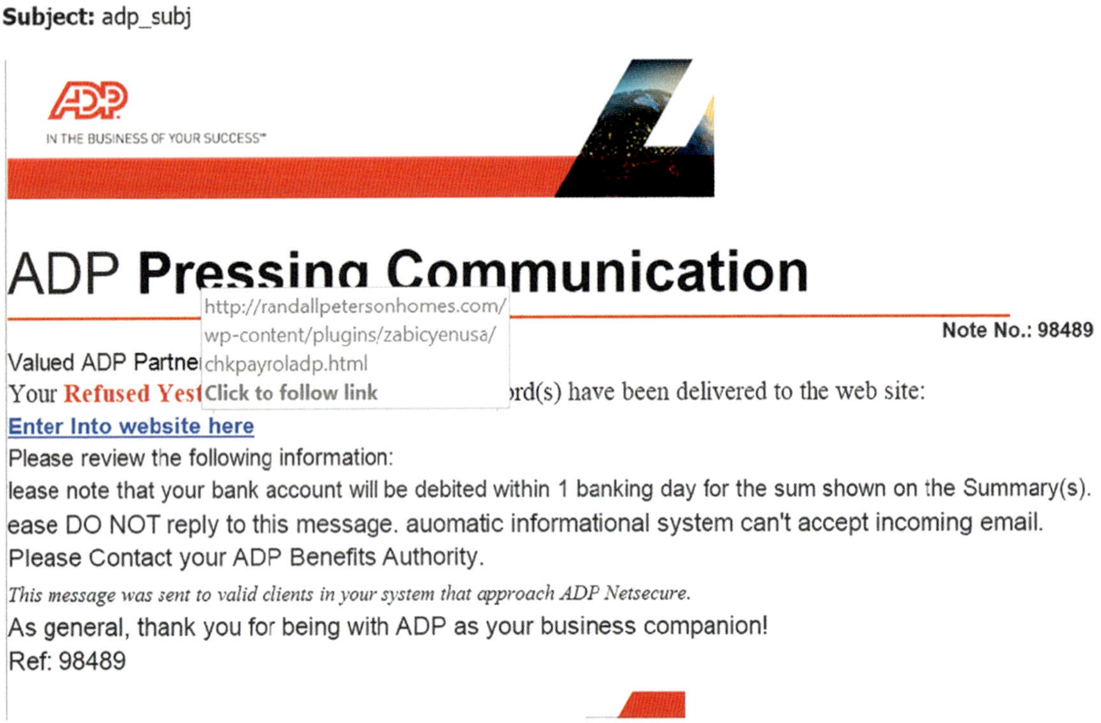

Figure 4-5

Subject: adp_subj

ADP Pressing Communication

Note No.: 98489

Valued ADP Partner
Your **Refused Yest**[...] rd(s) have been delivered to the web site:
Enter Into website here

[tooltip: http://randallpetersonhomes.com/wp-content/plugins/zabicyenusa/chkpayroladp.html — Click to follow link]

Please review the following information:
lease note that your bank account will be debited within 1 banking day for the sum shown on the Summary(s).
ease DO NOT reply to this message. auomatic informational system can't accept incoming email.
Please Contact your ADP Benefits Authority.
This message was sent to valid clients in your system that approach ADP Netsecure.
As general, thank you for being with ADP as your business companion!
Ref: 98489

Figure 4-5. Email scam with full weblink displayed.

---

payroll services. Note that some letters are missing from the left side of the email, and the text contains errors in grammar and spelling. Poor English usage and spelling errors should alert the user to potential phishing, scamming, virus, or other fraud schemes. However, email fraud is getting more sophisticated day-by-day, so that should not be the only thing to look out for with a potential phishing email. The user should also hover the cursor over the link to see the real URL, as shown in the figure. The real website the link connects to is not ADP, indicating the email is fraudulent.

Pharming results when an attacker infiltrates a domain name server and can route users to a different website. If you enter a domain name or URL for one of these sites, you are "pharmed" to a site designed by cyber criminals to extract personal information. Pharming is caused by inadequate security of the domain name server. Protection against this type of attack rests with those who maintain the domain name system servers.

Ransomware

Ransomware is malware that prevents the use of an affected computer. The two types of ransomware are lock screen and encryption (Microsoft, 2022). Lock screen ransomware displays a message demanding the user pay money to access the computer. Encryption ransomware encrypts files so they cannot be opened. Ransomware has been in the headlines over the last decade for its effect on healthcare facilities. In 2020 and 2021 alone, there were 168 ransomware attacks affecting 1,763 clinics, hospitals, and healthcare organizations (Bergal, 2022). Many attackers send phishing links or files to vulnerable employees to gain access to the computer network. When this happens, the healthcare organization must lock down the entire network (email, electronic healthcare record, management systems, etc.) and begin restoring system backup files. If backup files are not sufficient or the IT team is not able to mitigate the spread of the attack, then ransoms may be paid to the attackers to stop the spread and unlock the data.

In 2020, a patient experiencing an aortic aneurysm was being transported by ambulance for emergency care; however, when the ambulance arrived, it was turned away. The emergency room had been shut down due to the lockdown of services related to a ransomware attack. The ambulance was rerouted to a hospital that was an hour farther away; the patient died shortly after (Ralston, 2020). Although this is currently the only confirmed death due to ransomware attacks on healthcare facilities, it is a chilling example of what can happen if appropriate security measures are not taken.

Botnet

A **botnet** is a group of computers that are hijacked by cyber criminals without the knowledge of the users. A botnet owner is termed a "herder," and the infected computer is a "drone" or "zombie." Botnet herders use social networking websites, popular online financial institutions, advertisements, auction sites, and online stores to gain access to computers.

Botnets are used for click fraud, distributed denial of service, keylogger, warez, and spam. **Click fraud** occurs when a person or bot pretends to be a legitimate user on a web page, clicking on an ad, a button, or some other type of hyperlink. The goal is to trick a service into thinking a real user is interacting with the page, often to obtain recognition and awards for site visits. **Distributed denial of service (DDoS)** occurs when a herder directs all the computers in its botnet to send requests to the same site at the same time, overwhelming the site and preventing legitimate access to it. Cyber criminals may demand ransom money to release the hijacked website. Botnets can use malicious **keylogger** software that tracks keystrokes made by a user to trace and steal passwords and bank account numbers. Botnets can also steal, store, or gain access to software that should rightfully be purchased. Software that has been stolen and unlawfully redistributed is called **warez**. A herder may install software on a drone computer that forwards **spam**, which is unsolicited, usually in the form of commercial messages such as emails, text messages, or posts (Xing et al., 2021). Most spam is only irritating and time-consuming, but some spam is designed to trick the user into sharing personal information so that cyber criminals can steal money or identities.

Worms

A **worm** is a small piece of malware that uses security holes and computer networks to replicate itself. A worm is not completely a virus, in that it does not need to attach to an existing program and it can become active without a person running a program. To accomplish replication, the worm scans the network for another machine with the same security hole and copies itself to the new machine. The action is repeated, creating an ever-growing chain of infected computers. Worms may cause harm to a network by consuming bandwidth. Some worms include a "payload," or code that is designed to do more than just spread the worm. A payload may delete files on the host computer or encrypt files. The cyber criminal then demands a ransom to unencrypt the file. Payloads can also create a **backdoor**, or way into a theoretically secure system that bypasses security and is undetected (Li et al., 2021).

Trojan Horses

A **Trojan horse** is a program that appears to be something it is not. It may appear to be a program that performs a useful action or something fun, such as a game, but when the program runs, it places malicious software on the device or creates a backdoor for hackers. Trojan horses do not infect other files or self-replicate.

A keylogger Trojan is a malicious software that monitors keystrokes, places them in a file, and sends the file to a remote attacker (Singh et al., 2021). Some keyloggers record all keystrokes; others are sophisticated enough to log keys only on specific sites, such as online banking sites. Parents who monitor their children's online activities also may use this type of software. Some sites prevent keylogging by having a user use the mouse to point to a visual cue instead of using the keyboard.

Adware

Adware is a software that automatically displays or downloads advertising material (often unwanted) when a user is online. Adware includes pop-up advertisements; paying to register the software installation may remove these ads.

Adware is often a legitimate revenue source for companies that offer free software. Software programs, games, or utilities designed and distributed as freeware often provide their software in a sponsored mode (Prasad & Rohokale, 2020). In this mode, depending on the vendor, most or all the features are enabled, but pop-up advertisements appear when the program is in use. Paying to register the software removes the advertisements. This software is not malicious but randomly displays paid advertisements when the program is used. It does not track user habits or provide personal information to a third party.

Spyware

Spyware is software that obtains information about the user's computer activities by transmitting data covertly from the hard drive. In contrast to adware, spyware tracks a user's web activity to tailor advertisements to them. Some adware is also spyware (Prasad & Rohokale, 2020), giving legitimate adware a negative connotation. Spyware is like a Trojan horse because it appears to be something it is not. Downloading and installing P2P file-sharing products, such as music and movie files, is a common way computers are infected. Although spyware appears to operate like legitimate adware, it is usually a separate program that can monitor keystrokes, including passwords and credit card numbers, and transmit this information to a third party. It can also scan a hard drive, read cookies, and change default homepages on web browsers. Sometimes, a licensing agreement, which few people read before clicking "Accept," informs users of the spyware installation with the program, though this information is usually in obtuse, hard-to-read language with misleading statements.

Hoaxes

A **hoax** is a fake warning about a virus or other piece of malicious code. The user may receive a message asking to delete a specific file on their device because it is a virus that activates and damages the device or files. Elaborate instructions for locating and deleting the file are typically included. If the user believes the hoax and deletes the file, they may discover that it is part of the operating system or other application program on the computer. Deleting the file often causes a problem with the operating system and repairing the damage can be a lengthy chore.

Emails that warn of viruses are often hoaxes. Although they are usually not harmful, they are a waste of time and clutter the internet and internal networks with useless messages. Hoaxes appear credible, frequently citing sources such as an official from a well-known company. They may tell the recipient to forward the message to everyone they know. They may even contain the statement, "This is not a hoax." Discard these messages and do not forward them. When there is a real virus, it is likely to be newsworthy, especially if it is new and antivirus programs do not have any protection against it.

Emails should arouse suspicion if any of the following characteristics are present (Yuliani et al., 2018):

- The message says tragic consequences will occur if a given action is not taken.
- The message promises money or a gift certificate for performing an action.
- Instructions or attachments claim to provide protection from a virus that is undetectable by antivirus software.
- The message says it is not a hoax.
- The logic is contradictory.
- There are multiple spelling or grammatical errors.
- The message says it should be forwarded.
- The message has already been forwarded multiple times, evidenced by a trail of email headers in the body of the message.

Prevalence of Breaches

According to the Identify Theft Resource Center Data Breach Report (ITRC, 2024), there were 3,205 data compromises impacting an estimated 353,027,892 people. This is a 72% increase from 2021, the year in which the highest number of breaches were reported. Healthcare was the top industry affected between 2018 and 2023. In 2023, healthcare industries experienced 809 compromises, mainly from cyberattacks, phishing, and ransomware impacting over 56 million victims (ITRC, 2024). The ramifications of security breaches are potentially devastating if the private information is used maliciously for personal gain. These statistics underscore that more must be done to protect the private and confidential information of healthcare consumers.

Breaches can be the result of hacks, viruses, or unauthorized access to digital records. They often occur due to the loss or theft of laptops and portable storage devices (flash drives, backup drives, etc.); when data on the devices is not encrypted, criminals may be able to access it. It might seem like security breaches always happen digitally, but they can happen because of lost paper records, tampering of postal mail, or stolen paper files. Cyber criminals receive a larger amount of media attention because it is possible to digitally steal thousands of records containing private information relatively invisibly and quickly.

A data security breach is unlawful and can result in fines, imprisonment, or both. Data breaches are also expensive. The average per-incident cost in 2019 was $3.92 million with healthcare-associated breaches costing $6.45 million per incident. The United States had the highest cost per record and per breach with an average of $15 million compared to $8.19 million elsewhere (Seh et al., 2020).

Protecting Against Security Breaches

To prevent the loss of personal information, time, energy, and money, it is important to protect all internet-connected devices against malware with the following precautions (Cuningkin et al., 2021; Microsoft, 2022):

- Avoid reusing passwords.
- Change passwords frequently.
- Use strong and unique passwords.
- Use a password manager program to store all passwords in an encrypted vault (either on a device or in the cloud). Examples of the most popular password managers include Keeper, Zoho Vault, Bitwarden, LastPass, and 1Password.
- Use antivirus software and keep it updated.
- Scan any files you receive with an antivirus program before installing or executing the file.
- Avoid revealing personal information via social networking sites.
- Do not open email from strangers.

- Do not open unexpected email attachments.
- Download the latest operating system and software updates. Many updates fix security holes.
- Back up files on a regular schedule. Experts recommend saving backups to an external hard drive and to a cloud. If they are only saved in one place, they are more vulnerable.

Virtual Private Networks

A **virtual private network (VPN)** allows users in an organization to communicate confidentially by securing the connection between the computer and the internet. A file is transmitted using an encrypted tunnel blocking its view regardless of the device used to send it. The VPN is an intranet with an extra layer of security that operates as an extranet. A VPN can provide access to patient data such as a patient's electronic health record (EHR) to authorized users who are not physically present in the healthcare setting. VPNs can also be used for patient portals. These are places where patients can renew prescriptions, make appointments, and send messages to their providers. Free VPNs that are available for Android and Apple devices should be avoided due to potential security risks. In fact, some free VPNs have been set up by cyber criminals (Islam et al., 2021).

Firewalls

A **firewall** for computers is like a firewall in a building; it acts to block destructive forces. Computer firewalls work closely with router programs to filter the traffic coming into and going out of a network or a private computer. The difficulty comes with deciding what level of security to set. For networks such as those in healthcare agencies, the network administrator sets the limits.

For a private computer, the best method is to accept the firewall defaults. Windows and Mac computer software includes firewalls. Reputable antivirus software manages the computer firewall and alerts the user of a security risk if the firewall is turned off by a virus. Given that new viruses and methods of attack are frequently created, occasionally check to make sure that the firewall is turned on. In addition to the firewall on computers, most wireless routers for homes include built-in hardware firewalls.

Antivirus Software

Despite its name, antivirus software protects against other malware in addition to viruses. Depending on the version, most antivirus software detects and removes viruses, email and internet malware, and spyware and provides firewall-type protection. However, consider downloading a separate antimalware application in addition to the antivirus software because one product sometimes detects something that the other one missed (FraudWatch International, 2022).

PCs are targeted more often than Macs because the majority of computers are PCs (Muchmore, 2022). Macs are also more secure because Apple is in full control of both the hardware and software, while Windows must be adapted to many different brands and models (Muchmore, 2022). Antivirus software often comes loaded onto computers. There are many different vendors of antivirus software, including free versions, some of which are of high quality. Popular additional antivirus software programs are Bitdefender, Webroot, McAfee, ESET, G Data Antivirus, Malwarebytes, and Norton.

Details may differ among vendors, but antivirus software operates by scanning files and/or the computer's memory, looking for patterns based on the signatures or definitions of known viruses that may indicate an infection. Antivirus software performs three types of scans:

1. A custom scan is of a designated folder or file the user wants to check. It generally takes only a few minutes.
2. A quick scan finds any malware currently active on the computer and can take 15 to 30 minutes or less.
3. A deep or full scan detects anything missed by the quick scan. Depending on the number of files on the computer, it can take 2 to 4 hours and uses a lot of the computer's processing ability. Many people choose to set this scan for times when the computer will be on but not in use.

The response when an antivirus program finds a virus varies with the software. Some software packages present the user with a dialogue box asking for permission to remove the virus, and others remove the virus without asking. For many, a preference can be set.

Antivirus software should be continually updated because malware authors continually create new ways to attack computers. Most antivirus software offers a setting option to make updates automatic. Once antivirus software is installed and updated, a deep or full scan of the entire computer should be done. Thereafter, the software may be able to be configured to scan specific files or folders at automatic intervals (Cybersecurity and Infrastructure Security Agency, 2019). For example, scanning any email attachments of web downloads is an excellent way to protect a system from malware. Once initial scans are done, antivirus software can operate in the background and check all the incoming and outgoing data for malicious operations. Even with an antivirus software installed, the first step toward protecting data is to keep a backup of important files stored in another location.

Data Encryption

Because technologic devices are tools used to manage private and secure files that include patient information, online banking, social security numbers, passwords, and other unique identifiers, the data are targets of cyber thieves. Data encryption software can be used to conceal an entire hard drive or selected files.

Encryption software is also available via download. Examples include Axcrypt Premium, Folder Lock, and Advanced Encryption Package (Rubenking, 2022). It is also wise to search for reviews of encryption software to find a solution that works the best for specific needs.

Security Pitfalls

Antivirus software and firewalls are not 100% effective. Although combining these technologies with good security habits reduces risks, frequent software updates further mitigate risks. If a computer is not protected, it becomes vulnerable to cyber criminals. If a computer begins to run slowly or programs do not run correctly, these may be signs that there are other processes or programs running in the background without permission. If security software suggests a patch or an update, these should be installed as soon as possible. Nurses should advocate for patients by making sure computer networks are secure and mitigation strategies are in place to protect devices from malware.

ONLINE COMMUNICATION

Communication involves a sender, receiver, message, and channel (the way the message is passed or transmitted). The following sections discuss communication occurring via online channels using the internet. Online communication happens through social media, email, phone, video conferencing, instant messaging, websites, blogs, podcasts, discussion forums, and more.

Many of these forms of communication rely heavily on writing. The reliance on words means that nonverbal communication (everything we use to convey information, meaning, context, or emotion that does not rely on words) is not available to support online communication. In groundbreaking research, Dr. Albert Mehrabian found that the tone of voice and intonation accounted for 38% of communication and nonverbal cues made up 55% (Mehrabian, 1967). As you learn about professional online communication, remember that only 7% of meaning is conveyed using written words, so choose them carefully.

Importance of Professionalism

A lack of professionalism can result in poor patient outcomes. Professionalism is not just about appearance, showing up on time, and being prepared. Those are all important in the role of a professional nurse, but conducting oneself with responsibility, integrity, and accountability are also important. The American Association of Colleges of Nursing (AACN) Essentials define what it means to be a professional nurse. Competency 6.1 directs nurses to communicate in a manner that facilitates a partnership approach to quality care delivery, and includes subcompetency 6.1e, to communicate individual information in a professional, accurate, and timely manner (AACN, 2021). The National Council of State Boards of Nursing (NCSBN) and the American Nurses Association (ANA) also provide guidelines for the use of social media, which will be discussed in more detail later in the chapter.

Although online communication opens up a world of opportunities for sharing thoughts, opinions, and experiences, the case study provides examples of cause for caution. It is possible for anything shared on the internet to be viewed by others. Despite attempts to delete posts or use privacy settings, attorneys, law enforcement, journalists, and advocacy associations may be able to gain access, so it is important to follow ethical and legal guidelines for anything posted, emailed, or messaged. Read the Ethical Considerations box to learn about how knowledge of professional behavior supports the ANA Code of Ethics.

ETHICAL CONSIDERATIONS FOR PROFESSIONAL BEHAVIOR

Provision 1 of the ANA Code of Ethics for Nurses (2015) states that the nurse practices with compassion and respect for the inherent dignity, worth, and unique attributes of every person. Specifically, Provision 1.5 requires nurses to cultivate civility, collaboration, and collegiality to ensure safe, quality patient care and outcomes; compassionate, transparent, and effective health services; and a hospitable work environment. The code goes on to say, "…any form of bullying, harassment, intimidation, manipulation, threats or violence will not be tolerated" (ANA, 2015, p. 4).

Provision 3 states that the nurse promotes, advocates for, and protects the rights, health, and safety of the patient. Interpretive Statement 3.1 goes on to discuss the protection of the right of the patient to privacy and confidentiality. This means the nurse has an ethical duty to refrain from sharing patient information on the internet.

Following ethical principles is not just about avoiding harm to oneself or patients; it is also about promoting the profession of nursing. Provision 9 states the profession of nursing, collectively through its professional organizations, must articulate nursing values, maintain the integrity of the profession, and integrate principles of social justice into nursing and health policy. Online communication provides the profession of nursing with tools to articulate and assert the values of nursing (Interpretive Statement 9.1) to the public as well as promoting the integrity of the profession (Interpretive Statement 9.2).

> **CASE STUDY**
>
> The case study gave an example of nurses who were fired for poor online communication. Think about that example and others you may have heard about or experienced. What are some specific guidelines you would include in a nursing handbook at a hospital, nursing home, or other medical practice about how nurses should conduct themselves online?

> **BOX 4-1** Ground Rules for Civility in the Workplace
>
> - Assume good will and best intentions.
> - Be respectful in interactions.
> - Use direct communication.
> - Role model professionalism, civility, and ethical conduct.
> - Listen carefully and with intention to understand.
> - Honor and respect diversity.
> - Be open to others' points of view.
> - Hold oneself and each other accountable for abiding by workplace norms.
>
> Data from Clark, C. (2017). *Creating and sustaining civility in nursing education,* 2nd ed. Washington, DC: American Nurses Association. Indianapolis, IN: Sigma Theta Tau International Publishing.

Civility

Many have experienced online interactions that begin as a discussion and rapidly devolve into an argument. **Civility** is defined as formal politeness and courtesy in behavior or speech and has been linked to improved patient outcomes. It is an important concept when discussing online communication. Dr. Cynthia Clark, a nurse leader and expert on civility has researched the effect of incivility on patient outcomes and has found that "disrespectful and uncivil behaviors in healthcare settings can have detrimental effects on individuals, teams, organizations and patient safety" (Clark, 2019, para. 1). Incivility affects three different stages of the cognitive system: (1) how attentive people are; (2) how people process information; and (3) how people use information to problem solve (Porath, 2016).

Civility represents standards set by society on how to effectively communicate with others and sets up a positive work environment that supports patient-focused care. An annual survey of 22 countries conducted by Microsoft provides a digital civility index (DCI) score. The survey asks about exposure to online incivility. Higher DCI scores indicate an increase in incivility. The global DCI score was 65% in 2021, which is the best it had ever been (up by 2% since 2020). Close to 90% of respondents stated that improved education is the way to increase online safety and civility (Thomas, 2022). Use what you learn in this chapter to educate your patients, peers, family, and friends about how to engage in civil online communication. Box 4-1 lists ground rules for civil behavior.

Netiquette

A search of the internet for guidelines for effective communication yields multiple sets of principles or rules. For example, the "seven Cs" is a list of ideal descriptors for written and spoken communication: clear, correct, complete, concrete, concise, considered, and courteous (Microsoft, 2023). While etiquette is defined as the customary code of polite behavior in society or among members of a particular profession or group, **netiquette** is defined as the correct or acceptable way of communicating on the internet. The rules may vary by context (e.g., texting, video conference, phone), but there are a few guidelines for maintaining good etiquette in online communication (MasterClass, 2022):

1. Follow the same standards of etiquette that would be followed in person. Internet anonymity encourages some people to communicate in ways they never would in real life.
2. Check sources of information. Many people on the internet share content that contains incorrect information. It is easy to spread misinformation online so only share content verified as accurate.
3. Keep online communication brief. Respect other people's time and avoid writing long posts or comments.
4. Avoid sarcasm. Although sarcasm is common in face-to-face communications for many, it relies on nonverbal communication, which is not possible online.

5. The communication platform matters. Email messages or discussion board posts are typically more formal than text messages or chatting online. Explore each situation thoughtfully before using emoticons, text speak, abbreviations, or improper capitalization.
6. Respect privacy. Limit the use of personal information on public, username-based websites and forums and avoid requesting personal information to respect the privacy of others.
7. Beware of all caps. Using all capital letters can be interpreted as yelling, so avoid using all caps in most internet writing, especially in public or more formal settings.

Nurses should be familiar with employer policies and procedures for online communication and social media use by staff members. Policies often include directives to avoid negative references to healthcare agencies or other employers.

SOCIAL MEDIA IN HEALTHCARE

Social media is defined as any platform for sharing stories, pictures, videos, career goals, research, and thoughts with others online using the internet. In healthcare, social media can be used to promote a business, share reviews, and provide resources. Although older patients regularly visit doctors and primary care providers, only 7% of those born between 1981 and 1996 regularly schedule preventive healthcare appointments (Ohio University, 2020). This group is more likely to get information from online sources than see a doctor in person. The collaborative nature of social media allows providers to discuss care options including optimal medications and treatments, successful procedures, and patient needs and questions. Healthcare organizations can use social media as a marketing tool, increasing awareness of what a specific organization can offer patients, or about advances in medical technology. Social media also allows for **professional networking**, where interactions focus on finding jobs, finding employees, and building a business.

Over 5 billion people were reported to be using social media in 2024, a number predicted to increase to over 6 billion by 2028 (Dixon, 2024). Examples of social media include social networking sites such as Facebook and LinkedIn; image-based sites such as Instagram and Pinterest; video-sharing platforms such as YouTube and TikTok; discussion forums; community platforms; and **blogs** (websites written in an informal style) (Fig. 4-6). It is not possible to discuss all of them, but it is important to be knowledgeable about the most popular sites to know where best to target job searches, community outreach, and research questions.

Social media sites serve to connect millions of users worldwide. Every month 38.7% of the global population uses Facebook, with over 1 billion stories shared daily (Bagadiya, 2024). As of 2023, there were over 556 active monthly users of X (formerly Twitter), and as of April 2024, X receives about 6.1 billion visits per month (Duarte, 2024). These sites are free and only require users to create a login and password. All are available as separate apps for smartphones and tablets. Each site is slightly different, but all meet the needs of people who have a particular interest who want to connect and share content.

Social media is ever-changing. Applications gain popularity, but that can quickly change. Many social media applications that were popular when this edition was being written may no longer be used by the time the book is published.

Academia and corporate businesses initially shunned the use of social networking. Today, it is common for colleges, universities, hospitals, and professional organizations to have a presence on Facebook, X, and other sites. Social media can be used by healthcare organizations to raise public awareness, combat misinformation, communicate during a time of crisis, and promote citizen engagement (Beveridge, 2022). In embracing the use of social media to connect with the public, it allows them to act on a more personal level and with a sense of community. Box 4-2 includes a sample of nursing professional associations with social media presences.

Since much of social media is open to the public, be mindful of civility and netiquette with every share or post. Consider creating two different accounts for personal and professional presences online.

Social Networking Sites

Social networking sites allow users to interact with other users and find people or groups with similar interests. There are several social networking sites that are commonly used in healthcare for

Most popular social networks worldwide as of January 2023

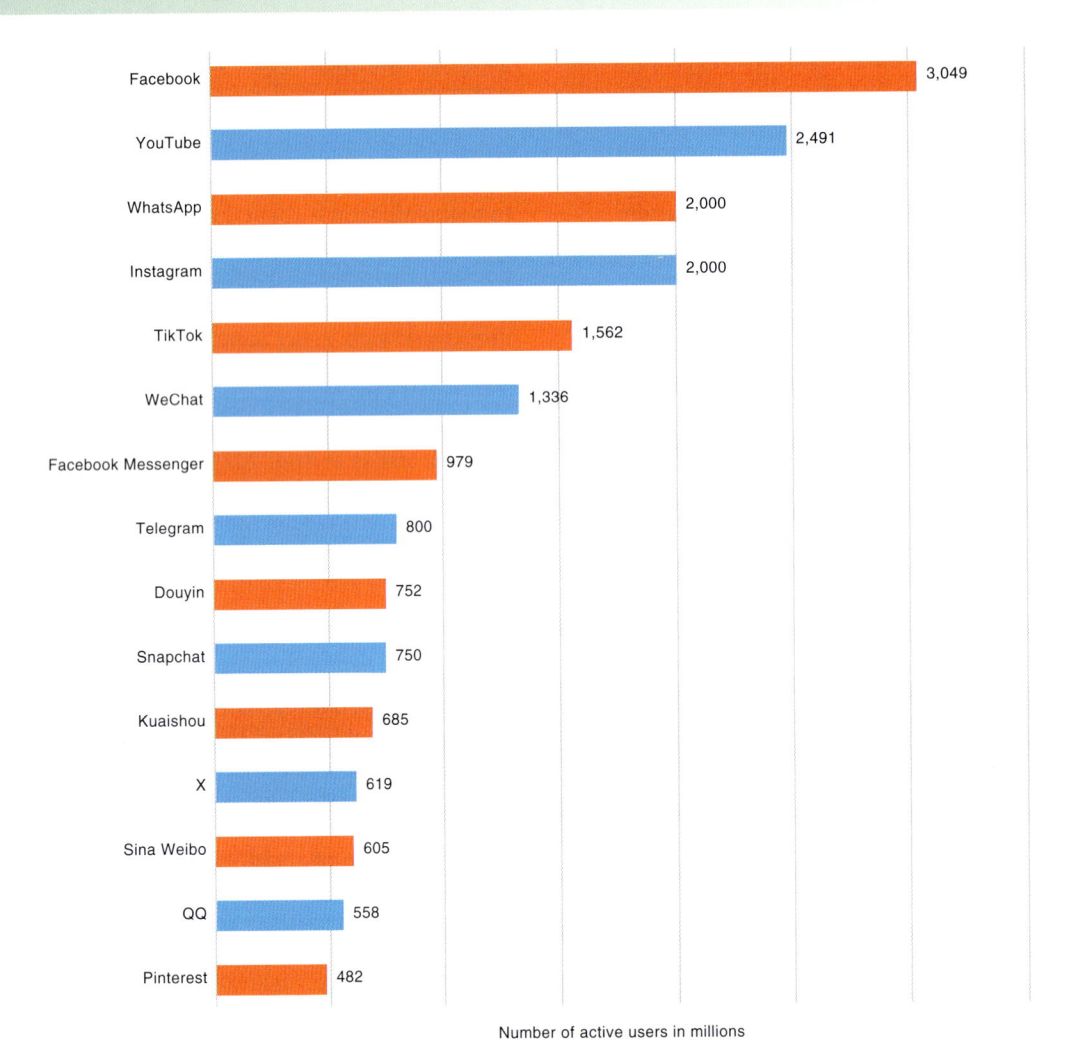

Platform	Number of active users (millions)
Facebook	3,049
YouTube	2,491
WhatsApp	2,000
Instagram	2,000
TikTok	1,562
WeChat	1,336
Facebook Messenger	979
Telegram	800
Douyin	752
Snapchat	750
Kuaishou	685
X	619
Sina Weibo	605
QQ	558
Pinterest	482

Number of active users in millions

Figure 4-6. Most popular social networks worldwide as of January 2023. (Data from *Statista: Social Media & User-Generated Content.* https://www.statista.com/statistics/272014/global-social-networks-ranked-by-number-of-users/)

professional networking, including Facebook, LinkedIn, and ResearchGate. To find any of these platforms online, just type the name into a search engine.

Facebook allows users to create personal pages and groups and post messages, photos, and videos. Users can also use the Messenger feature to talk to other members directly using text, photos, or video. Group Facebook pages run by organizations or businesses target specific audiences. Groups can be open to everyone, closed, or secret. Closed and secret groups require an invitation to participate.

Group administrators have access to several tools, such as the ability to create polls, promote events, and view analytics.

LinkedIn is a professional networking site. Like Facebook, users can choose individuals and groups with whom they want to connect. LinkedIn provides a way to connect with other business professionals, share information, or look for new career opportunities. LinkedIn is unique, in that users can build professional profiles, post resumes, and search for jobs. It also allows users to research and follow healthcare organizations, connect with

> **BOX 4-2** Examples of Professional Associations Using Social Networking Sites
>
> Look for the following groups on Facebook, LinkedIn, and X. Some are also available on Instagram and YouTube.
> - American Nurses Association (ANA)
> - American Association of Critical-Care Nurses (AACN)
> - National Council of State Boards of Nursing (NCSBN)
> - Healthcare Information and Management Systems Society (HIMSS)
> - Publisher Medline (PubMed)
> - Multimedia Educational Resources for Learning and Online Teaching (MERLOT)

peers, and stay up to date with industry news and trends. Medical professionals benefit from being on LinkedIn because of networking opportunities, the ability to demonstrate expertise, content sharing, and building a professional reputation (Sinclair-Brown, 2023).

ResearchGate is a professional networking site for researchers and scientists. It allows members to share research, post published papers, and collaborate with others. Like on LinkedIn, members can build a profile that includes education, work experience, and current position. Members can also use the site to post and find jobs. ResearchGate allows members to post peer-reviewed work and supplementary resources, such as data sets. Members can also post papers that have not been peer-reviewed to obtain feedback from others (ResearchGate, n.d.).

Image-Based Platforms

Content sharing is a component of social media and professional networking and photo sharing is a popular social media form. Examples of photo-sharing websites include Flickr, Google Photos, Instagram, Pinterest, and Shutterfly. These sites facilitate sharing photos with others as well as uploading files. Users must register and create a login and password to share photos.

Image sharing is a valuable tool for making public health resources available to the public. For example, the Centers for Disease Control and Prevention (CDC) has a public health image library available on their website at https://phil.cdc.gov/. This library offers an organized, universal, electronic gateway to the CDC's images.

Many healthcare organizations and professionals are turning to Instagram as a way of marketing themselves and reaching a wider audience. Instagram offers the ability to target an audience geographically and demographically. Getting followers from a target audience facilitates showcasing services, facilities, and success stories as well as fostering community engagement. Instagram is also a good resource for the latest trends in healthcare (Knott, 2023).

It is possible that an employer or patient can search online for photos or videos if they are accessible, which is why it is important to always consider civility and netiquette on these sites. Users must also adhere to the website terms of use and copyright law. There can be consequences for using an image on social media without the right permissions. Image copyright is the legal ownership of an image. If someone did not create an image, a permission to use it is needed unless it falls under fair use, images that can be used without permission if they are a benefit to the society. It is also possible to request written permission from the owner of the image, but that may require a fee. The safest option is to look for images that are in the public domain (Newberry, 2022).

Video-Sharing and Streaming Platforms

Video-sharing sites include the ability to search and find videos as well as post user-generated videos if they adhere to the terms of the website. To upload a video, the user must register with the service and create a login and password. For a fee, most video-sharing sites provide users with much larger uploading and storage capacities. These platforms also allow users to comment and interact with video creators, sometimes in real time. Copyright restrictions that apply to images also apply to videos.

Popular video-sharing platforms include YouTube and TikTok. YouTube is a free video-sharing website where users can create and watch videos as well as interact with other video creators using the comments feature. Created in 2005, it is the second most popular social media site (see Fig. 4-6) with users watching approximately 6 billion hours of video each month (Bump, 2022).

YouTube allows healthcare organizations and individuals to explain their brand and promote products and services. It allows medical professionals to provide timely information and patient education that can influence patient's behaviors and decisions. However, in a review by Osman et al. (2022), of 22,300 YouTube videos only 32% of videos appeared to be neutral, or not biased for or against, toward the health content being presented. The researchers state that YouTube is not a reliable source of medical and health-related information and that the popularity of a platform should not be considered a quality indicator. The authors recommend a system to promote higher-quality content that includes expert reviews and to include that assessment data in the ranking algorithm (the way YouTube and other social media platforms determine what videos come up in a search) (Osman et al., 2022).

TikTok is a social media app for smartphones and tablets that allow users to watch or share short video clips. The app allows for public and private content distribution. What began as a fun way to add effects, music, and split-screen duet videos can now be used by professional organizations and companies for awareness, promotion, or sales (Bump, 2022). It is also an effective way to target a younger audience.

Microblogging

Microblogs are concise blog posts (under 300 words) that may have images, GIFs, links, infographics, videos, or audio clips. Although the term microblogging is relatively new, the practice is not, having been made popular with the advent of Twitter, now X. A microblog could be as simple as a sentence fragment and as complex as a message advertising Nursing Informatics Day (May 12). X and Reddit are two popular platforms for microblogging, but microblogs can be posted on almost any platform.

On X, users can post messages of 280 characters or less, though paid users can tweet up to 25,000 words as of June 2023 (Mehta, 2023). X requires users to register and create a login and password, but the basic service is free. Users can post, report, or reply to other posts, allowing them to connect with others who share interests or might be interested in the topic. X also allows users to post photos and short videos. Posts are shared with other X users, and users can choose whom to follow to see their posts. The @ sign is a connector symbol for the user's name, for example, @HIMSS. The # sign or **hashtag** identifies the keyword or topic of the post, for example, #Nurses4HIT.

X can be useful for healthcare communication because it allows users to keep up with breaking news from professional organizations such as the Future of Nursing, Interdisciplinary Nursing Quality Research Initiative, HealthIT, and the CDC. During natural disasters, X users can send posts to inform the affected population about various situations.

Reddit is a social news platform and discussion website. After signing up for an account, users can search for and submit content to the site that includes links, texts, images, and videos. Topics are organized into communities or "subreddits." Users upvote posts, making them more likely to be seen. Subreddits of interest to informatics include medical news, health, health issues, and healthcare industry. Reddit is the fourth most visited site in the U.S. behind Facebook, Pinterest and Instagram (Dixon, 2024).

Other Online Communication Platforms

There are many other ways to collaborate and share information with other healthcare professionals. Users might use social bookmarking to share favorite websites, tag them with keywords, and share the sites with others. Group discussion forums, listservs, and wikis are other options that support collaboration. Cloud office suite software provides ways that one or more users can create word processing, spreadsheets, and presentations synchronously or asynchronously (discussed in more detail in Chapter 3).

Social Bookmarking

A bookmark is a term for identifying a favorite website. **Social bookmarking** allows the user to save bookmarks to the cloud where they are available on all your computers, smartphone, and other devices with an internet connection, and then share them with others. Reddit, Pinterest, and Diigo are examples of social bookmarking platforms where people share and tag their favorite websites and see tags from other users.

Social bookmarking sites use **folksonomy** taxonomies to organize tags into categories (Anissimov, 2022). Folksonomies are a form of **collective intelligence**, which emerges from the collaboration, collective efforts, and competition of many individuals. The tags are word descriptors, often achieved by collaborative group consensus.

Group Discussion Forums

Every topic imaginable can be found in group discussion forums such as listservs, wikis, and chats. Users can find them by searching terms such as "online nursing communities," "nursing discussion lists," or "nursing listserv." To find a specialty forum, include the name of the specialty in the search. An example of a nursing forum is National League for Nursing (NLN) Connect, a forum for members of the NLN that went live in 2023. The community allows nurse educators and scholars to directly engage with one another (NLN Connect, n.d.).

A **listserv** is a method of communicating with a group of people via a group email address. Those belonging to the list, called subscribers, receive all the messages. Users can reply to the original message if they have something to share on the same subject or start a new thread with a new message if they want to start a new topic. The archives of many listservs are organized by the subject line in the message.

A **wiki** is a piece of server software that allows users to freely create and edit content on a web page using any web browser; this is an example of collaborative knowledge sharing. Editing authority may be public or available only to those invited to participate in the wiki by the creator. Wikis can be private or public; for example, a wiki designed for committee work or nursing research would be private. The culture of the group is a factor that affects the effectiveness of wiki collaboration. Users must be willing to share knowledge, exchange ideas, and remain open-minded to create an updatable knowledge management repository. There are numerous free wiki sites available, including dooWikis, Wikidot, and Google sites.

Wikipedia is a popular, free, publicly edited, online encyclopedia, which began in 2001 and now has more than 6.6 million English-language articles (Wikipedia, n.d.). Users collaboratively create, improve, and discuss Wikipedia articles. There is a public history of changes (an audit trail), and contributors should note that their internet address will be publicly available in the history. To prevent vandalism of popular pages, some Wikipedia articles are "semi-protected," meaning only registered users can make changes to the articles. Wikipedia is addressing the quality of articles by designating "featured articles" and "good articles" that are reviewed by Wikipedia editors and meet certain quality criteria (Wikipedia Contributors, 2023). Wikipedia also flags questionable articles believed to be incomplete or inaccurate. The strength of Wikipedia is that it provides updated information on an ever-expanding number of topics. For technical information, Wikipedia is often one of the most up-to-date sources of information.

Chat is a type of interactive online communication. Both messaging and chat involve two or more individuals, but chatting takes place within an application. Chatting is a feature available in course learning management systems (LMSs) such as Blackboard, Moodle, or D2L. In an LMS, the computer screen shows a list of the participants as they enter the chat room. Some chat software allows users to use their real names or an alias (also known as a handle). Many social media apps such as Skype, Discord, TeamSpeak, and Slack offer chat capabilities.

Social Media Guidelines

The NCSBN and ANA collaborated on a set of guidelines for social media. The guidelines and video are accessible by searching for "NCSBN Social Media Guidelines for Nurses." Box 4-3 lists social media guidelines complied from a number of professional nursing organizations.

One of the biggest concerns with using social media in healthcare is the potential for breaching the Health Insurance Portability and Accountability Act (HIPAA) of 1996 or not adhering to a healthcare institution's policies (NCSBN, 2018). Online communication must never contain

BOX 4-3 Social Media Guidelines

1. Review your posts to ensure they are appropriate for your audience. For example, it would be inappropriate to post an image of yourself at a party with a drink in your hand on a page that is viewed by your employers.
2. Be aware of the privacy settings on each social media platform you use. What are you posting that is available to the public versus trusted friends? Can friends of friends see your posts and share them?
3. Follow your employer's social media policies even when you are not at work and avoid posting while you are at work. You can be held accountable for your behavior on social media in all settings.
4. Never share any patient care information. For example, if you post "I had a tough patient today," you may be violating patient privacy. Others may be able to infer who your patients are based on the date of the post. If you see a post that violates patient privacy, report it immediately.
5. Share credible information. Sharing misinformation can harm the health and well-being of the public. Use what you have learned about evaluating information to ensure that you are posting factual information that is supported by research.
6. Do not take photos at work. If you do, blur out your badge in any images and remove any visible logos identifying where you work.
7. Use a respectful, civil, and professional tone in your posts. Avoid negativity in posts about the nursing profession, your patients, coworkers, and employer.
8. Maintain professional boundaries with patients and their loved ones and avoid connecting with them on social media.

Data from American Nurses Association. (n.d.). *Social Media*. Accessed January 26, 2023. https://www.nursingworld.org/social/; Jeyaraman, M, Ramasubramanian, S, Kumar, S, Jeyaraman, N, Selvaraj, P, Nallakumarasamy, A, Bondili, SK, & Yadav, S. (2023, May 16). Multifaceted role of social media in healthcare: Opportunities, challenges, and the need for quality control. *Cureus*, 15(5):e39111. https://doi.org/10.7759/cureus.39111.; and Wells, S. (2024, February 19). *Do's and Don'ts of Social Media Use for Nursing Professionals*. American Association of Critical-Care Nurses. https://www.aacn.org/blog/dos-and-donts-of-social-media-use-for-nursing-professionals

---

names or identifiers of patients, families, or other staff members. Moreover, it should not contain any type of information that might even indirectly identify people in the clinical setting. Examples of inappropriate use of social and electronic media include the story from the case study in which nurses posted a TikTok mocking a patient and were fired (Brusie, 2023). In another case, a nurse was fired for posting a photo on social media of a baby with a birth defect (Acevedo, 2021). Even when no malice is intended, nurses and healthcare providers who indiscriminately share stories, photos, and videos related to practice face serious punishments. Examples of penalties include dismissal from a nursing program, termination from work as a nurse, revoking of a nursing license by the state board of nursing, lawsuits, fines, or jail time (NCSBN, 2018). Chapter 15 goes into more detail about protecting patient privacy and confidentiality.

Safe Networking

Social and professional networking privacy policies remain in constant flux. It is important that users read the privacy policies before selecting a networking site. Social media sites allow users to choose privacy settings, such as who can view the user's posts, share their photos, and connect with the user. Unless the user customizes the settings, the default setting is often for information to be public.

Social media can be hacked. A hacker may exploit a security flaw or a network security breach. For example, some high-profile X accounts were hacked in 2017 (Barrett, 2017). The hackers posted swastikas and references to Nazi Holland and Germany from the affected accounts. Hackers illegally access devices or websites to steal people's personal information, which they use to commit crimes such as theft. Many people shop, bank, and pay bills online; keep personal data in social media accounts; and keep credit card numbers stored on vendor websites. A hacker can do a lot of damage even if only one account or device is compromised, but damage can be extreme if a social media site is attacked. To make matters worse, hackers are difficult to stop because they may be located outside the United States and use cutting-edge technology to evade law enforcement and acquire large amounts of information. If you are hacked, have your devices inspected, change your passwords, monitor your financial accounts, notify others, and report hacking to the Federal Bureau of Investigation.

MISINFORMATION

With the rise in internet usage to share information, researchers have begun to discuss **information disorder**, which is the sharing or developing of false information with or without the intent of harm (Kandel, 2020). **Misinformation** is false or inaccurate information with or without intention. It can be spread in several ways. Microtargeting on social media platforms gears misinformation at a specific group of people. **Trolls** are people who use inflammatory, insincere, digressive, extraneous, or off-topic messages online to obscure and drown out opposing views and evidence-based content. **Disinformation** is intentional misinformation that includes misleading or biased information, manipulated narratives or facts, and propaganda. Disinformation can be spread by governments, extremist groups, and individuals seeking to sway public opinion. **Fake news** is also intentional and can be defined as a story or article that is verifiably false. It is meant to manipulate people's perceptions of real facts, events, and statements through a seemingly trustworthy source.

The COVID-19 pandemic and response were accompanied by an **infodemic** of information, or a large increase in the volume of information associated with a specific topic in a short period of time. This led to a manipulation of information that was amplified through social media (WHO, 2022).

In a systematic review of 31 studies that analyzed fake news related to health, X, Facebook, and YouTube were found to be critical in spreading misinformation related to the COVID-19 pandemic (Borges do Nascimento et al., 2022). The study reports that during major crises or disasters, "the overproduction of data from multiple sources, the quality of the information, and the speed at which new information is disseminated create social and health-related impacts" (Borges do Nascimento et al., 2022, para. 1). The authors found that poor-quality health-related information was propagated on social media, amplifying vaccine hesitancy and exploration of treatments unsupported by science. For example, 20% to 30% of videos on YouTube about emerging infectious diseases were found to contain inaccurate or misleading information (Borges do Nascimento et al., 2022). The negative effect of widespread misinformation includes polarized opinions, escalating fear and panic, and decreased access to healthcare. The vaccine example in the case study demonstrates the danger of misinformation in causing poor health outcomes.

In an infodemic, there is so much information that it can be hard for healthcare workers to find trustworthy sources and reliable guidance when it is needed. This can affect decision making, especially when immediate answers are expected and there is not enough time to analyze the evidence. There is no quality control over what is published. Anyone can write or publish anything on social media channels.

Detecting Misinformation

Although it might seem that students today are savvy when it comes to online or digital content, this is not always the case. A study of 1,060 first-year college students found that the students used the order of Google search results to determine trustworthiness of information. Additionally, after selecting a website, the students were unable to evaluate it for credibility. They rarely considered the source of the website or examined the author's credentials (Ziv & Bene, 2022). The International Federation of Library Associations and Institutions (IFLA) has recommendations for how to spot fake news. They include (IFLA, 2021):

- Consider the source. Check the credentials of the author.
- Read beyond. Read the entire content, not just the headline.
- Supporting sources? Check whether the references cited support the story.
- Do others agree? Search for other sites or authors who agree or disagree.
- Is it a joke? Research to make sure it is not satire.
- Check your biases. Make sure your own beliefs are not affecting your judgment.
- Ask the experts. Check with fact-checking sites or official sources.
- Look before you share. Do not share stories you have not checked out first.

Combating Misinformation

Strategies that can help with combating fake news include finding industry solutions, interfering with economic incentives, and creating products to interfere with the amplification of misinformation (Flostrand et al., 2019). Importantly for nursing students and practicing nurses, however, it is providing education to improve news literacy. For example, it is important to understand how to fact-check news stories. Fact-checking sites include Politifact, Snopes, NPR Fact-Check, and Hoax Slayer. However, studies have determined that many consumers doubt the ability of fact-checking tools to retrieve completely true information (Nieminen & Rapeli, 2019). The Stanford History Education Group (SHEG) has free lesson plans that address improved news literacy skills at the SHEG website. The site is free but requires users to create a login and password to access the learning materials. In addition to history lessons and assessments, the site has an assessment for civic online reasoning, which is the ability to judge the credibility of information online (Stanford History Education Group, n.d.).

Nurses have a responsibility to detect and deal with misinformation and disinformation to ensure patient safety. You can help patients identify misinformation and direct them to evidence-based information. Other ways to combat incorrect information include awareness campaigns for patients and healthcare providers, including scientific evidence in health-related content in mass media, and improving media and health literacy. Unit V of this book goes into detail on each of these topics. Social media platforms can also be used to counter false or misleading information, but further studies are needed to determine the best way to accomplish this.

CASE STUDY

The case study provides an example of misinformation related to vaccines. How could you plan to react to a patient who brings misinformation they found on the internet as evidence of why they will not get a lifesaving or health-promoting treatment?

SUMMARY

- **Computer networks.** In healthcare, a computer network connects two or more computers in multiple ways to provide improved patient care. Understanding the architecture and topology of networks can help improve network security and lead to more efficient functionality. Networks are often defined by geography and can be as small as a LAN in a primary care office to a WAN such as the World Wide Web. Computers can be hardwired together physically or can be connected using WiFi signals.
- **The internet.** The internet is a global network of interconnected computers, tablets, smartphones, and other internet-enabled devices. Access to the internet is an SDoH, and nurses have a responsibility to not only understand this aspect of computer networking, but to advocate for equity. Knowledge of IP addresses, URLs, domain names, web browsers, and search engines help people use the internet efficiently.
- **Issues with network security.** Network security is a concern for all healthcare providers due to its effect on patient care and privacy. Breaches are increasingly common and can cost organizations millions of dollars and result in delayed care that can lead to patient harm and even death. Cyber criminals have many tools for attacking computer

networks including social engineering such as phishing and pharming and drive-by-downloading that triggers malware downloads. Examples of malware include ransomware, botnets, worms, adware, and spyware. Protecting against security breaches involves being careful with passwords and emails. VPNs, firewalls, antivirus software, and data encryption are also useful for preventing data breaches.

- **Online communication.** Just like in-person communication, online communication involves a sender, receiver, message, and channel. There are many platforms for online communication. It is important to remember that nonverbal communication is often not available when communicating online. Communicating with professionalism and civility supports patient safety, improves patient outcomes, and results in employee satisfaction. The ANA, NCSBN, and AACN have guidelines for how to behave professionally.

- **Social media in healthcare.** Social media represents opportunities and challenges. Nurses have a responsibility to protect patient privacy and confidentiality but also to use social media to promote the profession of nursing. Social media platforms provide social networking, photo and video sharing, microblogging, discussion boards, social bookmarking, and group discussion capabilities.

- **Misinformation.** Misinformation is intentionally or unintentionally false information. Disinformation and fake news are terms referring to information and news that is verifiably and intentionally false. The COVID-19 pandemic and social media have led to an infodemic of information that makes it difficult to tell facts from fiction, which can lead to poor health outcomes and affect patient safety. The nurse can use tools for detecting and combating misinformation and educate patients to help them make more informed decisions about their healthcare.

DISCUSSION QUESTIONS AND ACTIVITIES

1. Classify the networking architecture used in a hospital nursing unit setting. Consider the equipment used to chart patient data, control intravenous infusions, access medications, and control blood sugar.

2. Analyze the methods you use to connect to the internet for work and personal use. What are the differences and similarities?

3. Search the internet for a graphic from the Agency for Healthcare Research and Quality called *Poverty and Access to Internet, by County* (AHRQ, 2021). Explore the graphic to better visualize the link between poverty and access to high-speed internet. What trends do you see in the United States? What is internet access like in your area? Do you know of any local initiatives to increase access to high-speed internet?

4. Do an internet search that extends your understanding of types of computer networks. Summarize your finding along with examples of their use.

5. Compare three types of malware. Explain how the malware might infect a computer.

6. Imagine you are a member of a professional practice committee. One of the items under discussion is the development of a policy for nurses' uses of social networking websites. What resources might you recommend as references for the policy? What are some possible policies that are important to consider?

7. Compare three social media platforms that are useful in healthcare.

8. Rewrite the following email that was sent from a nurse to their supervisor using what you have learned in this chapter about professional and civil online communication.

    "Hey Marcy, I know you must be exhausted from the long hours they make you work here. I AM SO TIRED of ths plaic! ☺ Can you please give me some extra time off? I really need a break after taking care of Mrs. Smith in room 306 with the number of times she had to go to the bathroom and how mean she was to all of us. Plus the CNAs are just not carrying their weight."

9. A fellow nursing student shows you a picture of a patient's wound they posted on Facebook. What should you do?

10. Conduct a literature search in a digital library to find an article that extends your understanding of safe social media use.
11. Search the internet for social media privacy breaches made by nurses and healthcare workers over the past 3 years. Discuss the ethical and legal implications for the practice breaches.
12. Compare the guidelines for the use of social media from the NCSBN and the ANA. Describe the use of the guidelines in your school and workplace settings.
13. A patient asks what you think about a video they saw on YouTube discussing the dangers of the COVID-19 vaccines. What is your best response?
14. You decided to use social networking to connect with other nurse professionals and to share your research interests.
    - What social media platform might you use? What is your rationale?
    - What, if any, information should you refrain from publishing on the site?
    - What would you do if a current patient contacted you using social media to ask questions about their care?

PRACTICE QUESTIONS

1. Email warnings should arouse suspicion if which characteristic is present?
   a. The message says that there is a virus hidden in a file on your computer.
   b. The message is from a known email address of a coworker.
   c. The information in the email is logical.
   d. There are no spelling or grammatical errors.
2. Which type of software tracks an individual's web browsing to tailor advertisements based on personal history and use?
   a. Adware
   b. Spyware
   c. Trojan horse
   d. Worm
3. Which type of network within an organization allows users to share information privately?
   a. Extranet
   b. VPN
   c. Intranet
   d. Mobile network
4. Which is an appropriate action for the nurse to take to maintain professionalism when using social media?
   a. Accepting a patient's friend request on Facebook
   b. Setting personal social media accounts to a private viewing mode
   c. Sharing a patient's conditions and details, but removing their name
   d. Having a conversation in a members-only social media work group about a patient
5. Which application would the nurse find most useful to share news updates on nursing informatics with other nurses interested in the same topic?
   a. X
   b. Social bookmarking
   c. YouTube
   d. Wiki

REFERENCES

Acevedo, N. (2021, October 2). Florida nurse fired after posting photos of baby born with birth defect on social media. https://www.nbcnews.com/news/us-news/florida-nurse-fired-after-posting-photos-baby-born-birth-defect-n1280627

Agency for Healthcare Research and Quality (AHRQ). (2021, June). Poverty and access to internet, by county. https://www.ahrq.gov/sdoh/data-analytics/sdoh-tech-poverty.html

Al-Fedaghi, S., & Behbehani, B. (2020). How to document computer networks. Journal of Computer Science, 16(6), 723–734. https://doi.org/10.3844/jcssp.2020.723.434

American Association of Colleges of Nursing (AACN). (2021, April 6). Core competencies for professional nursing education. https://www.aacnnursing.org/Essentials

American Nurses Association (ANA). (n.d.). Social media. Retrieved January 26, 2023. https://www.nursingworld.org/social/

Anissimov, M. (2022, December 26). What is a folksonomy? EasyTech Junkie. https://www.easytechjunkie.com/what-is-a-folksonomy.htm

Barrett, B. (2017, March 15). Hack brief: High-profile twitter accounts overrun with swastikas. https://www.wired.

com/2017/03/hack-brief-high-profile-twitter-accounts-overrun-swastikas/

Bagadiya, J. (2024, April 6). 38 facebook statistics and facts for every marketer in 2024. *SocialPilot*. https://www.socialpilot.co/facebook-marketing/facebook-statistics#:~:text=On%20average%2C%20350%20million%20photos,by%20Facebook%20users%20each%20day

Bergal, J. (2022). Ransomware attacks on hospitals put patients at risk. *PEW Research*. https://www.pewtrusts.org/en/research-and-analysis/blogs/stateline/2022/05/18/ransomware-attacks-on-hospitals-put-patients-at-risk#:~:text=In%202020%20and%202021%2C%20there,analyst%20for%20cybersecurity%20company%20Emsisoft

Beveridge, C. (2022, October 11). *How to use social media in healthcare: Examples + tips*. https://blog.hootsuite.com/social-media-health-care/

Borges do Nascimento, I. J., Pizarro, A. B., Almeida, J. M., Azzopardi-Muscat, N., Gonçalves, M. A., Björklund, M., & Novillo-Ortiz, D. (2022). Infodemics and health misinformation: A systematic review of reviews. *Bulletin of the World Health Organization, 100*(9), 544–561. https://doi.org/10.2471/BLT.21.287654

Brusie, C. (2023, January 6). *Nurses fired for mocking child with gunshot wound on TikTok*. https://nurse.org/articles/tiktok-nurses-fired-children-gunshot/

Bump, P. (2022, February 10). The best social media platforms for video content in 2022. *Hubspot*. https://blog.hubspot.com/marketing/go-to-social-media-video-platforms

Chatzoglou, E., Kambourakis, G., & Kolias, C. (2022). How is your Wi-Fi connection today? DoS attacks on WPA3-SAE. *Journal of Information Security and Applications, 64*, 103058.

Clark, C. (2019). Fostering a culture of civility and respect in nursing. *The Journal of Nursing Regulation, 10*(1), 44–54. https://doi.org/10.1016/S2155-8256(19)30082-1

Cuningkin, V., Riley, E., & Rainey, L. (2021). Preventing medjacking. *American Journal of Nursing, 121*(10), 46–50. https://doi.org/10.1097/01.NAJ.0000794252.99183.5e

Cveticanin, N. (2022, December 9). *Who are cybercriminals? A short guide*. DataProt. https://dataprot.net/articles/who-are-cybercriminals/

Cybersecurity and Infrastructure Security Agency. (2019). *Security tip (ST04-009) identifying hoaxes and urban legends*. http://www.us-cert.gov/ncas/tips/ST04-009

De Looper, C. (2022, April 20). 5G vs. Wi-Fi: How they're different and why you'll need both. *Digital Trends*. https://www.digitaltrends.com/mobile/5g-vs-wi-fi/

Dixon, S. J. (2024, May 17). Number of global social network users 2017-2028. *Statista*. https://www.statista.com/statistics/278414/number-of-worldwide-social-network-users/

Domain Name Industry Brief (DNIB). (2024, April 9). *Global domain name base trends*. https://dnib.com/dashboards/global-domain-name-base-trends

Duarte, F. (2024, April 25). X (formerly Twitter) user age, gender, & demographic stats for 2024. *ExplodingTopics*. https://explodingtopics.com/blog/x-user-stats

Early, J., & Hernandez, A. (2021). Digital disenfranchisement and COVID-19: Broadband internet access as a social determinant of health. *Health Promotion Practice, 22*(5), 605–610. https://doi.org/10.1177/15248399211014490

Ellis, J. (2023, January 4). What is an Ethernet cable and what does it do? *Comms Blog*. https://www.comms-express.com/blog/what-does-an-ethernet-cable-do/

Flostrand, A., Pitt, L., & Kietzmann, J. (2019). Fake news and brand management: A Delphi study of impact, vulnerability and mitigation. *Journal of Product & Brand Management*. http://www.emeraldinsight.com/1061-0421.htm

FraudWatch International (2022). *What is anti-malware?* https://fraudwatch.com/what-is-anti-malware-do-you-need-anti-malware-protection/

Galazzo, R. (2020, September 21). From 1G to 5G: The history of cell phones and their cellular generations. *CENGN*. https://www.cengn.ca/information-centre/innovation/timeline-from-1g-to-5g-a-brief-history-on-cell-phones/#:~:text=Launched%20by%20Nippon%20Telegraph%20and,1G%20to%20the%20United%20States

GCFGlobal. (n.d.). *How do I connect to the internet?* Retrieved January 23, 2023. https://edu.gcfglobal.org/en/computerbasics/connecting-to-the-internet/1/

Google Domains. (n.d.). *Web terms 101*. Retrieved January 24, 2023. https://domains.google/learn/web-terms-101/#:~:text=A%20URL%20(aka%20Universal%20Resource,the%20pages%20within%20the%20website

Graves, J. M., Abshire, D. A., Amiri, S., & Mackelprang, J. L. (2021). Disparities in technology and broadband internet access across rurality: Implications for health and education. *Family and Community Health, 44*(4), 257–265. https://doi.org/10.1097/FCH.0000000000000306

IBM. (n.d.). *What is a computer network?* Retrieved January 22, 2023. https://www.ibm.com/topics/networking

Identify Theft Resource Center (ITRC). (2024, January). *2023 data breach report*. https://www.idtheftcenter.org/publication/2023-data-breach-report/

IntegralChoice. (2020, November 5). *Intranet vs. Extranet*. https://www.integralchoice.com/intranet-vs-extranet-what-is-the-difference/

International Corporation for Assigned Names and Numbers (ICANN). (2022a). *What does ICANN do?* https://www.icann.org/resources/pages/what-2012-02-25-en

International Corporation for Assigned Names and Numbers (ICANN). (2022b). *List of top-level domains*. https://data.iana.org/TLD/tlds-alpha-by-domain.txt

International Federation of Library Associations and Institutions (IFLA). (2021, August 31). *How to spot fake news: COVID-19 edition*. https://repository.ifla.org/bitstream/123456789/1289/2/how-to-spot-fake-news-covid.pdf

Islam, M. Z., Khan, M. A. R., Hossain, M. I., & Hossain, R. (2021). Analysis: The importance of VPN for creating a safe connection over the world of internet. *International Journal of Advanced Research in Computer and Communication Engineering, 10*(10), 86–92. https://doi.org/10.17148/IJARCCE.2021.101017

Kandel, N. (2020). Information disorder syndrome and its management. *Journal of Nepal Medical Association, 58*(224), 280–285. https://doi.org/10.31729/jnma.4968

Kelly, J. T., Campbell, K. L., Gong, E., & Scuffham, P. (2020). The Internet of things: Impact and implications for health care delivery. *Journal of Medical Internet Research, 22*(11), e20135.

Kim, H., Mahmood, A., Goldsmith, J. V., Chang, H., Kedia, S., & Chang, C. F. (2021). Access to broadband internet and its utilization for health information seeking and health communication among informal caregivers in the United States. *Journal of Medical Systems, 45*(2), 24–29. https://doi.org/10.1007/s10916-021-01708-9

Knott, J. (2023, April 15). *Instagram marketing for doctors—tips to growing patient engagement*. https://intrepy.com/1000-instagram-followers-medical-practices/

Li, Y., Hua, J., Wang, H., Chen, C., & Liu, Y. (2021, May). DeepPayload: Black-box backdoor attack on deep learning models through neural payload injection. In *2021 IEEE/ACM 43rd international Conference on Software Engineering (ICSE)* (pp. 263–274). IEEE.

MasterClass. (2022, November 9). *Netiquette: 7 common netiquette rules*. https://www.masterclass.com/articles/netiquette

McKeon, J. (2021, August 25). *Healthcare phishing scam exposes PHI for 12K patients in UT. Health IT Security*. https://healthitsecurity.com/news/healthcare-phishing-scam-exposes-phi-for-12k-patients-in-ut

Mehrabian, A. (1967). Attitudes inferred from neutral verbal communications. *Journal of Consulting and Clinical Psychology, 31*(4), 414–417.

Mehta, I. (2023, June 27). *Twitter now allows subscribers to post 25,000-character-long tweets*. Tech Crunch. https://techcrunch.com/2023/06/27/twitter-now-allows-subscribers-to-post-25000-character-long-tweets/

Microsoft. (2022). *Ransomware*. https://www.microsoft.com/en-us/security/portal/mmpc/shared/ransomware.aspx

Microsoft. (2023, January 23). *The principles of communication*. https://learn.microsoft.com/en-us/microsoft-365/community/principles-of-communication

Muchmore, M. (2022, November 29). macOS vs. Windows: Which operating system is really better? *PCMag*. https://www.pcmag.com/news/macos-vs-windows-which-os-really-is-the-best#:~:text=Market%20share%20is%20another%20thing,Opens%20in%20a%20new%20window)

National Council of State Boards of Nursing (NCSBN). (2018). *A nurse's guide to the use of social media*. https://www.ncsbn.org/public-files/NCSBN_SocialMedia.pdf

National League for Nursing (NLN) Connect. (n.d.). *Welcome to NLN connect*. Retrieved January 25, 2023. https://nln.connectedcommunity.org/home

Newberry, C. (2022, July 19). Image copyright on social media: Everything you need to know. *Hootsuite*. https://blog.hootsuite.com/understanding-image-copyright/

Nieminen, S., & Rapeli, L. (2019). Fighting misperceptions and doubting journalists' objectivity: A review of fact-checking literature. *Political Studies Review, 17*(3), 296–309. https://journals.sagepub.com/doi/10.1177/1478929918786852

Ohio University. (2020, August 11). *The role of social media in health care: A public health perspective*. https://onlinemasters.ohio.edu/blog/social-media-in-healthcare/#:~:text=Individuals%20can%20share%20posts%20and,individuals%20with%20specific%20health%20problems

Omboni, S., Panzeri, E., & Campolo, L. (2020). E-Health in hypertension management: An insight into the current and future role of blood pressure telemonitoring. *Current Hypertension Reports, 22*(6), 42–13. https://link.springer.com/article/10.1007/s11906-020-01056-y

Osman, W., Mohamed, F., Elhassan, M., & Shoufan, A. (2022). Is YouTube a reliable source of health-related information? A systematic review. *BMC Medical Education, 22*(1), 382. https://doi.org/10.1186/s12909-022-03446-z

Petrosyan, A. (2022, July 7). *Distribution of windows malware 2019*. https://www.statista.com/statistics/221506/share-of-new-types-of-malware/

Pierri, F., Perry, B. L., DeVerna, M. R., Yang, K. C., Flammini, A., Menczer, F., & Bryden, J. (2022). Online misinformation is linked to early COVID-19 vaccination hesitancy and refusal. *Scientific Reports, 12*(1), 5966. https://doi.org/10.1038/s41598-022-10070-w

Porath, C. (2016). *Mastering incivility: A manifesto for the workplace*. Grand Central Publishing.

Prasad, R., Rohokale, V. (2020). Cyber threats and attack overview. In: *Cyber security: The lifeline of information and communication technology. Springer series in wireless technology*. Springer. https://doi.org/10.1007/978-3-030-31703-4_2

Rains, T. (2020). *Cybersecurity threats, malware trends, and strategies*. https://falksangdata.no/wp-content/uploads/2021/06/Tim.Rains-Cybersecurity.Threats.Malware.Trends.and_.Strategies.pdf

Ralston, W. (2020, November). The untold story of a cyberattack, a hospital and a dying woman. *Wired News*. https://www.wired.co.uk/article/ransomware-hospital-death-germany

Raths, D. (2020, June). Expanding internet access improves health outcomes. *Government Technology*. https://www.govtech.com/network/Expanding-Internet-Access-Improves-Health-Outcomes.Html

ResearchGate. (n.d.). *About us*. Retrieved January 25, 2023. https://www.researchgate.net/about

Rivera, Y. M., Moran, M. B., Thrul, J., Joshu, C., & Smith, K. C. (2022). When engagement leads to action: Understanding the impact of cancer (Mis)information among Latino/a Facebook users. *Health Communication, 37*(9), 1229–1241. https://doi.org/10.1080/10410236.2021.1950442

Rubenking, N. J. (2022, May 26). *The best encryption software for 2022*. https://www.pcmag.com/picks/the-best-encryption-software

Science+ Media Museum. (2020, December 3). *A short history of the internet*. https://www.scienceandmediamuseum.org.uk/objects-and-stories/short-history-internet

Seh, A. H., Zarour, M., Alenezi, M., Sarkar, A. K., Agrawal, A., Kumar, R., & Khan, R. A. (2020). Healthcare data breaches: Insights and implications. *Healthcare, 8*(2). 133, https://www.mdpi.com/2227-9032/8/2/133

Sinclair-Brown, J. (2023, January 12). *Four reasons why all doctors should be on LinkedIn*. https://www.bmj.com/careers/article/four-reasons-why-all-doctors-should-be-on-linkedin

Singh, A., Choudhary, P., Singh, A. K., & Tyag, iD. K., (2021, August). Keylogger detection and prevention. In *Journal of physics: Conference series* (Vol. 2007, No. 1, p. 12005). IOP Publishing. https://doi.org/10.1088/1742-6596/2007/1/012005

Stanford History Education Group. (n.d.). *Civic online reasoning*. https://sheg.stanford.edu/publications/research-articles

Thomas, L. (2022, February 7). Online civility improved in past year and is the best it's been since 2016, new Microsoft research shows. *Microsoft*. https://blogs.microsoft.com/on-the-issues/2022/02/07/safer-internet-day-online-civility-improves-2022-research/

US-CERT Publications. (2020). *Security tip (st04-014) avoiding social engineering and phishing attacks*. https://www.us-cert.gov/ncas/tips/ST04-014

Vanhoef, M., & Ronen, E. (2020, May). *Dragonblood: Analyzing the dragonfly handshake of WPA3 and EAP-pwd*. In *2020 IEEE Symposium on security and privacy (SP)* (pp. 517–533). IEEE. https://ieeexplore.ieee.org/abstract/document/9152782

Wikipedia Contributors. (2023, August 15). *Wikipedia: Featured articles*. https://en.wikipedia.org/wiki/Wikipedia:Featured_articles

Wikipedia (n.d.) *Main page*. https://en.wikipedia.org/wiki/Main_Page

World Health Organization (WHO). (2022, September 1). *Infodemics and misinformation negatively affect people's health behaviours, new WHO review finds*. https://www.who.int/europe/news/item/01-09-2022-infodemics-and-misinformation-negatively-affect-people-s-health-behaviours--new-who-review-finds

Xing, Y., Shu, H., Zhao, H., Li, D., & Guo, L. (2021). Survey on botnet detection techniques: Classification, methods, and evaluation. *Mathematical Problems in Engineering, 2021*, 1–24. https://doi.org/10.1155/2021/6640499

Yuliani, S. Y., Sahib, S., Abdollah, M. F., Al-Mhiqani, M. N., & Atmadja, A. R. (2018). Review study of hoax email characteristic. *International Journal of Engineering & Technology, 7*(3), 778–782.

Ziv, N. & Bene, E. (2022). Preparing college students for a digital age: A survey of instructional approaches to spotting misinformation. *Stanford History Education Group*. https://crl.acrl.org/index.php/crl/article/view/24799/33592

CHAPTER 5

Mobile Healthcare Technology

Kristi Miller, Elizabeth Riley, Veneine Cunningkin, and Larronda Rainey

OBJECTIVES

After studying this chapter, you will be able to:
1. Discuss the similarities and differences between computers and mobile devices and the components necessary for them to function.
2. Identify the ways mobile devices connect to each other and to the internet.
3. Describe the history and significance of different types of mHealth.
4. Explain what a mobile medical device is and give examples.
5. Discuss various software applications for mobile devices.
6. Explain how mobile devices are used in clinical practice.
7. Compare and contrast the advantages and disadvantages of using mHealth.
8. Discuss future trends in mHealth including nanotechnology and artificial intelligence.
9. Explore ethical issues related to mHealth.

AACN Essentials for Entry-Level Professional Nursing Education

3.3a Describe access and equity implications of proposed intervention(s).
7.2b Recognize the impact of health disparities and social determinants of health on care outcomes.
8.1b Identify the basic concepts of electronic health, mobile health, and telehealth systems for enabling patient care.
8.3c Use information and communication technology in a manner that supports the nurse–patient relationship.
8.3d Examine how emerging technologies influence healthcare delivery and clinical decision making.
8.4c Identify the basic concepts of electronic health, mobile health, and telehealth systems in enabling patient care.
8.5a Identify common risks associated with using information and communication technology.
9.1a Apply principles of professional nursing ethics and human rights in patient care and professional situations.

AACN Essentials for Advanced-Level Nursing Education

2.2g Demonstrate advanced communication skills and techniques using a variety of modalities with audiences.

8.1g Identify best evidence and practices for the application of information and communication technologies to support care.

8.3i Appraise the role of information and communication technologies in engaging the patient and supporting the nurse–patient relationship.

8.3j Evaluate the potential uses and impact of emerging technologies in healthcare.

8.3k Pose strategies to reduce inequities in digital access to data and information.

8.4f Employ electronic health, mobile health, and telehealth systems to enable quality, ethical, and efficient patient care.

8.5g Apply risk mitigation and security strategies to reduce misuse of information and communication technology.

8.5h Assess potential ethical and legal issues associated with the use of information and communication technology.

8.5k Advocate for policies and regulations that support the appropriate use of technologies impacting healthcare.

HIMSS TIGER Competencies

Data protection and security

Electronic/mobile health, telematics, telehealth

Ethics in health internet technology

Information and communications technology systems applications

Information and knowledge management in patient care

Internet technology risk management

Medical technology

KEY TERMS

Artificial intelligence (AI)
Barcode medication administration (BCMA)
Beaming
Bluetooth
Cell phone
Flash memory
Hotspot
Internet of medical things (IoMT)
Internet telephone
Medical device
Mobile device
Mobile healthcare technology (mHealth)
Mobile medical application
Mobile medical device
Mobile network
Nanotechnology
Near-field communication (NFC)
Password manager
Push notification
QWERTY keyboard
Random access memory (RAM)
Read-only memory (ROM)
Smartphone
Speech recognition software
Synchronization
Video conferencing
Voice over Internet Protocol (VoIP)
Wearable
Webcast
Webinar
Wireless (WiFi)

CASE STUDY

Gonzalez and colleagues (2021) conducted a scoping review of the use of mobile healthcare technology (mHealth) in Latinx communities, focusing on intervention studies to promote behavioral change and improve health outcomes. The Hispanic/Latinx demographic is the fastest growing demographic group in the United States, but this population has been disproportionately affected by health disparities and inequalities. Latinx individuals experience excess mortality from preventable diseases like diabetes, cervical cancer, and liver disease, and they were three times more likely to become infected with COVID-19 during the pandemic and nearly twice as likely to die from it as their non-Hispanic White counterparts. Since 35% of Latinx American adults rely on smartphones as their primary means of internet access at home (compared to 14% of White and 24% Black adults), there is great potential for developing mobile technologies for this population. The review found that text message reminders can improve patient adherence to medication regimens and access to care. Patients can be empowered to manage their health when feedback texts, personalized treatments, and two-way texting are included. Applications that combine texting with self-guided interactive content have the greatest potential to support mHealth use across cultures.

As you read this chapter, think about the role of the informatics nurse in supporting patient engagement. What can you do to increase access to mHealth? Are there opportunities to explore the use of mHealth with the goal of improving patient outcomes?

Healthcare services provided electronically via the internet are collectively known as eHealth. Under the broad umbrella of eHealth, **mobile healthcare technology (mHealth)** is defined as the use of wireless technologies, such as mobile phones, tablets, wearables, barcode readers, and others, to provide healthcare services and information. Fitness, diabetes management, depression, and sleep are just a few health factors that can be improved by the use of mHealth.

The use of mHealth has radically changed healthcare delivery on a global scale. Mobile devices are widely used today. According to the Pew Research Center (2021), 85% of American adults have a smartphone. Two-thirds of the largest U.S. hospitals offer applications for use on mobile devices. Approximately 62% of smartphone users have used a device to gather health-related information, making the use of mHealth more common than online banking, job searches, or accessing schoolwork or educational content (Pew Research Center, 2021).

mHealth encompasses everything from healthcare software applications (called apps) to electronic healthcare records (EHRs, covered in Chapter 13) to care given in the home using monitoring devices and telehealth (covered in Chapter 6). This chapter covers how mHealth is used to improve patient outcomes. You will read about the most used types of mHealth as well as advantages and disadvantages, clinical uses, ethical considerations, and how to protect your devices from cyber criminals.

MOBILE DEVICES

A **mobile device** can be a computer or other electronic device that is small enough to hold and operate in the hand; it is not hardwired to the internet. The most widely used mobile devices are smartphones and tablets. Because tablets are lightweight, portable, and easily cleaned, many nurses use tablets instead of laptops or desktop computers. Tablets and smartphones often include a microphone, audio recorder, and forward- and rear-facing cameras, meaning healthcare professionals must be careful not to take unauthorized photographs or recordings in the clinical setting.

Smartphones and Tablet Devices

The Psion Organiser was the first personal digital assistant (PDA) concept, developed in the early 1980s (Medindia, 2022). The first PDA design was primarily a personal information manager that included electronic telephone books and appointment calendars. The Newton MessagePad, developed by Apple in 1983, was the first popular PDA that featured a touch screen and handwriting capabilities. However, the PalmPilot, introduced by U.S. Robotics in 1996, was lightweight, fit in the palm of the hand, and had much better handwriting recognition than the Newton. As a result, it quickly dominated the market by 1999 (Medindia, 2022). PDAs ultimately paved the way for smartphones.

A **cell phone** is a short-wave wireless communication device that has a connection to a transmitter. The word "cell" refers to the area of transmission (cellular). Cell phones, like landline phones, require a paid subscription to the transmission service provider. **Smartphones** are cell phones with internet connectivity. IBM announced the first smartphone, known as Simon, in 1992 (Chantel, 2023). The smartphone combined features of the cellular telephone and personal information management software. It cost around $1,000 and weighed 1 kg (2.2 lb). In 1999, Qualcomm released the pdQ, which featured a cell phone and the Palm organizer.

The smartphone had not yet captured the attention of the market when Microsoft introduced the Pocket PC PDA in 2000, offering a compact version of the Windows operating system (OS). It gave users the ability to have more than one application open at the same time and the ability to view or edit Microsoft Office documents. In 2007, the first iPhone was released, and a year later, T-Mobile released the first Android phone (Chantel, 2023). Apple released the iPad tablet computer and iBookstore in 2010, triggering the start of a massive wave of consumer use of mobile devices by a variety of manufacturers. Other notable mobile device brands include the Microsoft Surface and various Android OS devices.

Mobile devices do not necessarily have the same OSs as computers (for a review of basic computer concepts, see Chapter 3). Although the OSs differ, the design of mobile-computing software is for interoperability (the devices work together). The OS determines the functions and software capabilities. Examples of these OSs include Apple iOS, Google Android, BlackBerry Research in Motion (RIM), Linux, Symbian, and Windows. The Google Android OS, released in 2008, is used by numerous mobile device manufacturers. Today, Android leads the market share, followed by Apple, for tablets and smartphones (Sharma et al., 2021).

By necessity, all mobile devices need to utilize battery power. Most mobile devices use rechargeable lithium-ion batteries, and innovations in mobile technology continue to improve battery life. Factors that shorten battery life are multitasking features, increased memory, audio, screen brightness, push-and-fetch email features, location services, and Bluetooth/wireless/cellular service connections. Always use the latest software updates, as they may improve battery life performance.

Mobile devices use three types of built-in memory: **read-only memory (ROM)**, which stores the operating and standard applications such as contacts, calendar, and notes; **random access memory (RAM)**, which stores all the add-on applications and data files and requires a small amount of continuous battery power; and built-in flash memory. Mobile devices use **flash memory** because it is nonvolatile, meaning that the applications and data will not disappear after the loss of battery power. Flash memory is also available as separate expansion cards. However, many healthcare organizations have limited the use of flash memory drives and cards due to their ability to transfer viruses.

Most mobile devices have a flat-screen liquid crystal display (LCD) and provide a touch screen for data input. **QWERTY keyboard** data entry (a keyboard layout common to the personal computer, PC) is available in all smartphones and tablets. It is called a QWERTY keyboard due to the layout of the top row of keys (Fig. 5-1). Unless there is a separate keyboard specifically designed for the mobile device, it is often easier to enter large amounts of data using a PC or paired keyboard, rather than the mobile device, and then synchronize the file with the mobile device.

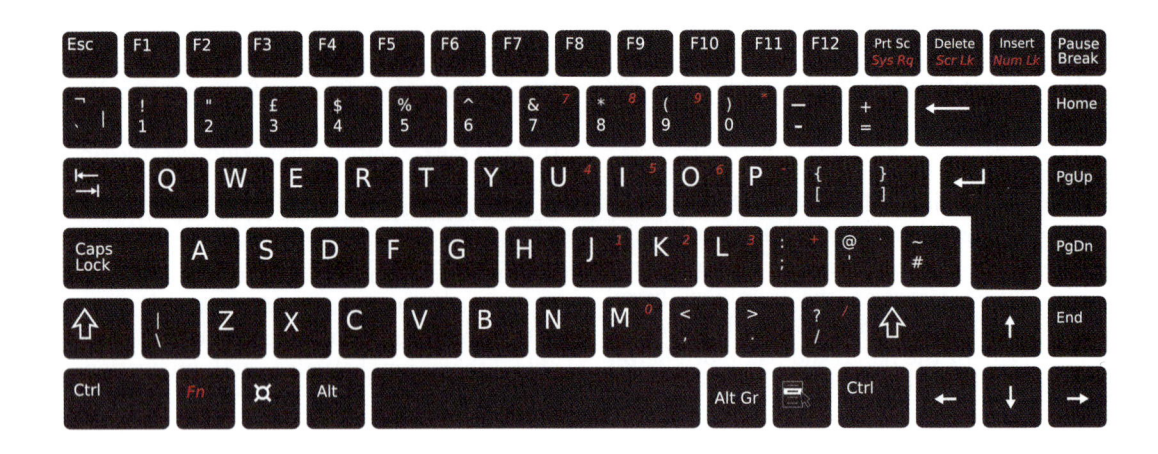

Figure 5-1. QWERTY keyboard. (Shutterstock/Uniquezen.)

Connecting Mobile Devices

Data transfer functions common to mobile devices include synchronization and connectivity using WiFi, cellular services, near-field communication (NFC), and Bluetooth. These allow for transfer of information among mobile devices and PCs, health information clinical systems, and other devices, such as headsets. A device that uses the internet to connect, share, and interact with others is considered "smart." Although usually small in size, smart devices typically have the computing power of a few gigabytes. Smartphones generally provide access to cellular services with a monthly fee. Most tablet devices have WiFi for internet access, while some also provide access to cellular services. Table 5-1 summarizes the primary ways mobile devices can communicate with each other.

Synchronization (sync) is when users share files between devices through a cloud-sharing application that facilitates copying changes back and forth. Most smartphones and tablets are not required to sync with a PC. Apps can automatically update when there is an internet connection and the ability to back up data to online cloud storage, such as OneDrive (Microsoft), G Cloud (Android), or iCloud (Apple devices). However, mobile devices can sync with desktops and laptops using proprietary software so that all the files on the two devices are the same.

The **internet of medical things (IoMT)** is the network of internet-connected medical devices, hardware infrastructure, and software applications used to connect healthcare information technology. The IoMT allows wireless and remote devices to securely communicate over the internet to allow rapid and flexible analysis of medical data.

WiFi

Wireless (WiFi) networking is a means of wireless device connectivity. WiFi is an industry standard (Deng et al., 2020). It uses a router that supports WiFi standard 802.11 to form a local area network. As new versions of standard 802.11 are approved, the speed of the wireless connection is improved and interference is reduced (Deng et al., 2020). WiFi networking is popular in people's homes because it allows multiple users to access the internet on multiple devices. WiFi networks are simple to set up using a software wizard that comes with the purchase of a wireless router.

Hotspot is a term used to identify a WiFi-enabled area where a person can use their WiFi-enabled mobile device to connect to the internet. Hotspots may be available at public libraries, colleges and universities, coffee shops, airport terminals, and hotels. Not all hotspots are public; many hotspots use encryption for security and require

TABLE 5-1 Wireless Connections

Connection Type	Description	Range	Security	Examples
WiFi	A radio signal sent from a wireless router to a nearby device, which translates the signal into data that can be seen and used. The device transmits a radio signal back to the router, which connects to the internet by wire or cable. The user sets up a router after purchasing a plan from an internet service provider. Internet access is possible anywhere a WiFi connection is present, such as in office buildings, shopping malls, restaurants, and other places.	WiFi routers operating on the 2.4-GHz band can reach up to 150 ft indoors and 300 ft outdoors.	Encryption must be enabled, and user must install updates.	Skyrunner, Spectrum, AT&T, EarthLink, Frontier, used to transfer large amounts of data at high speed
Cellular	Uses cellular signals from cell towers to connect to the internet as well as communicate with other cell phones. Allows the user to make phone calls and maintain internet access if there's a cellular tower nearby. Plans often come with data use limitations. Must have a cell phone plan to use. The speed at which the cellular network operates depends on the connection.	Users must be within 45 miles of a cell tower.	Encrypted by default	Verizon, Sprint, AT&T, T-Mobile

(Continued)

TABLE 5-1 Wireless Connections (Continued)

Connection Type	Description	Range	Security	Examples
Near-field communication (NFC)	A subset of radio frequency identity designed to be a secure form of data exchange; unique feature: device can be both an NFC reader and an NFC tag allowing devices to communicate peer-to-peer.	4 in or less	Not protected against eavesdropping; can be vulnerable to data modifications; may use higher-layer cryptographic protocols to establish secure channels	Contactless payment, tapping two phones, smart posters, beaming, connects smartphones and PCs to local printers
Bluetooth	Devices contain a Bluetooth radio computer chip and software for connectivity. Radio waves transmit information between devices directly.	Less than 32 ft, much weaker than WiFi or cellular signals	Can configure connections from "trusted devices;" passwords can be used to block cyber criminals	Headsets, speakers, battery-powered devices, AirDrop, beaming, in-home blood pressure monitoring
Radio frequency identification (RFID)	The process by which items are uniquely identified using radio waves comprises a tag, a reader, and an antenna. The reader sends an interrogating signal to the tag via the antenna, and the tag responds. Active RFID tags contain their own power source, but passive RFID tags do not. Three frequencies: low, high, and ultrahigh.	Active: read range of up to 330 ft Passive: read range from near contact up to 80 ft	Can send malicious data to systems that are susceptible to common attacks such as viruses, buffer overflows, and denial-of-service (DoS) assaults	Inventory, tool, staff and patient tracking, in place of product barcodes, employee identification badges

Connection Type	Description	Range	Security	Examples
Satellite	Radio waves are beamed down from satellites orbiting the earth. Data are sent and retrieved through a communication network that starts with your device and travels through the modem and satellite dish out to a satellite in space then back to ground stations on Earth known as network operations centers.	No limit, but problems with delays; 0.22 seconds for signal to transmit, limited only by the visibility of the satellite Using multiple satellites can allow for a signal to be transmitted to the other side of the world.	Encryption must be enabled, user must install updates	HughesNet and Viasat. Broadcasting, communication during natural disasters, transfer or large amounts of data, used in rural areas with no cell towers

Data from Laird Connect. (2019, June 28). *Connectivity Choices for your Medical Device and IoMT Application.* https://connectivity-staging.s3.us-east-2.amazonaws.com/2019-07/062019%20-%20White%20Paper%20-%20Medical.pdf; Peterson R. (2022, July 11). *Selecting a connectivity architecture for medical devices.* https://www.bench.com/setting-the-benchmark/selecting-a-connectivity-architecture-for-medical-devices.

the user to enter an access code or pay a fee for use. WiFi security is an important consideration. Hospitals that use WiFi have secure encrypted systems. Home routers include methods to address security issues in the setup information.

Smartphones and tablets with cellular capability can connect to the internet using regular cellular services. Cellular service users should be aware of their connection package agreement to avoid paying high fees for large data downloads. Users who need to access the internet using the cellular service as opposed to WiFi may consider having unlimited minutes as part of their cellular service agreement.

Mobile Networks

A **mobile network** is a communication network linking nodes, which are WiFi devices that receive signals and transmit them to the central server or rebroadcast them to another node. The first type of mobile network was known as 1G (first generation) and launched in the early 1980s in the United States. Mobile network technology has revolutionized over the decades. The newest and fastest mobile network is known as 5G (fifth generation) and has contributed to advancements in technology, business, and healthcare. Speed and accuracy are paramount since computers and mobile devices are tools designed to manage and manipulate data, provide social networking, and assist in various areas of healthcare. According to Dangi et al. (2021), 5G provides better speeds for internet usage due to greater bandwidths. This enhanced speed can allow users to stream high-definition videos, participate in virtual or augmented reality, and perform many other tasks while on the go. Many smartphones still use 4G technology, which provides sufficient speed for most everyday tasks.

Advancements are not without challenges. Security issues are still of concern regarding 5G networks, despite the use of security certificates, encryption, and user authentication. During the height of the COVID-19 pandemic, misinformation spread that 5G was responsible for the spread of the coronavirus. Some 5G cellular towers in populated areas of the United States were vandalized by people responding to this idea. Studies have also demonstrated the potential for electromagnetic interference from 5G related to aircraft in flight, as well as potential medical hazards due to radiation from 5G wireless devices (Kostoff et al., 2020; Solkin, 2021). The use of 5G has the potential to further widen the disparities in access to broadband internet due to the need to replace older technology to be able to use 5G networks.

Bluetooth

Bluetooth allows for a wireless, short-range (32 ft), low-power radio frequency connection to other Bluetooth-enabled devices (Todtenberg & Kraemer, 2019). When Bluetooth is enabled on a mobile device and paired with another Bluetooth device, it creates a personal area connection. Bluetooth can be used with external keyboards, to share files, to synchronize a mobile device with a PC, or for printing. Bluetooth headphones allow the user to wirelessly listen to music and have hands-free phone calls. Bluetooth-enabled devices can enhance efficiency and accuracy in healthcare settings by allowing patient information, such as vital signs, to be transmitted wirelessly to other Bluetooth devices (Fig. 5-2). Security is always a potential issue for wireless use, so it is a good idea to turn Bluetooth capabilities off when not in use.

Near-Field Communication

Mobile devices can communicate using a short-range (within a few centimeters) method called **near-field communication (NFC)**, a secure form of data exchange. A mobile device can be both an NFC reader and an NFC tag, allowing devices to

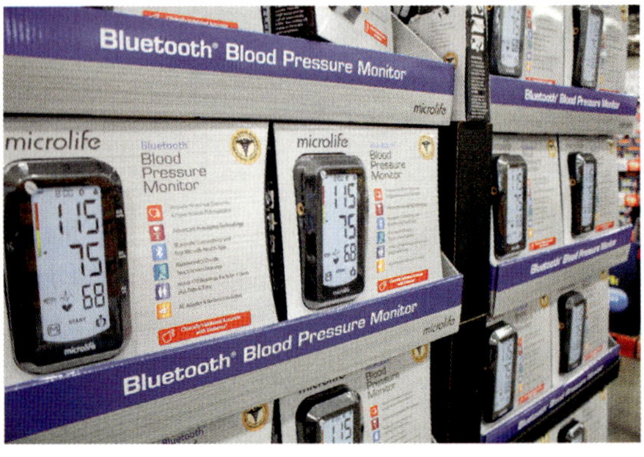

Figure 5-2. Bluetooth technology. (Shutterstock/The Image Party.)

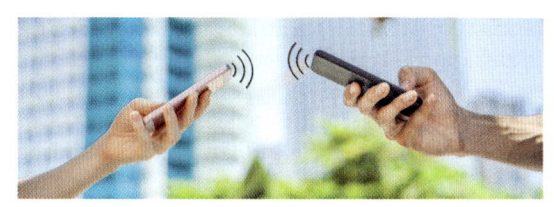

Figure 5-3. Beaming. (Shutterstock/Elizaveta Galitckaia.)

communicate peer-to-peer. Both Android Pay and Apple Pay use NFC. **Beaming**, a type of NFC, allows for wireless, short-range transmission of information to other beam-enabled devices with the same OS using infrared (IR) technology (Fig. 5-3). For example, Apple AirDrop provides beaming features for the Mac, iPad, and iPhone with iOS7+.

Since NFC is low-power, low-cost, easy to manufacture, and secure, it is a promising tool for health monitoring. Although NFC technology is not yet widely used in the healthcare field, it has great potential with wearable sensors. Research is being done on the use of NFC sensors for measuring vital signs, muscle stretching, and cholesterol levels, among other factors (Kang et al., 2021; Sun et al., 2022). This new technology could lead to more roles for informatics nurses in the future.

EXAMPLES OF mHEALTH

Beyond smartphones and tablets, the array of mHealth devices is vast. The discussion of mHealth examples here is not comprehensive. The goal is to provide an overview of the most widely used mHealth options to increase familiarity with its terminology and features. mHealth is growing so quickly, it is difficult to predict what will be relevant even in the near future.

Mobile Medical Devices

Box 5-1 provides the U.S. Food and Drug Administration (FDA) definition of medical devices. To summarize, a **medical device** is any device intended by the manufacturer to be used for a medical purpose. Examples of medical devices that are regulated by the FDA include stethoscopes, tongue depressors, anti-snoring devices, hearing aids, hospital gowns, and robotic surgical systems. The FDA also regulates medications, but these are chemical in nature; however, as nanotechnology (between 1 and 100 nm in diameter) advances, the line between medications and devices will become more difficult to discern. Nanotechnology is covered in more detail at the end of the chapter.

A **mobile medical device** is a medical device that can send or receive information via WiFi, Bluetooth, or cellular networks. Examples of mobile medical devices include smartphones, insulin pumps, pulse oximeters, and point-of-care

---

BOX 5-1 U.S. Food and Drug Administration Definition of a Medical Device

Per Section 201(h)(1) of the Food, Drug, and Cosmetic Act, a device is:

An instrument, apparatus, implement, machine, contrivance, implant, in vitro reagent, or other similar or related article, including a component part, or accessory which is:

- (A) recognized in the official National Formulary, or the United States Pharmacopoeia, or any supplement to them,
- (B) intended for use in the diagnosis of disease or other conditions, or in the cure, mitigation, treatment, or prevention of disease, in man or other animals, or
- (C) intended to affect the structure or any function of the body of man or other animals, and which does not achieve its primary intended purposes through chemical action within or on the body of man or other animals and which is not dependent upon being metabolized for the achievement of its primary intended purposes. The term "device" does not include software functions excluded pursuant to section 520(o).

From U.S. Food and Drug Administration (FDA). (2022 August 9). How to determine if your product is a medical device. https://www.fda.gov/medical-devices/classify-your-medical-device/how-determine-if-your-product-medical-device

devices for monitoring certain blood levels. In healthcare, these devices are used increasingly to improve patient safety, as in the case of smart card readers for identification, barcode readers for barcode medication administration, and smartphones for communication among members of the healthcare team. Figure 5-4 shows a variety of mobile medical devices.

Wearables

Wearables are smart devices that are worn on the body to obtain, analyze, and track patient data. The most prominent examples are smartwatches and fitness trackers, but other examples in healthcare include blood pressure monitors, glucose monitors, biosensors, and hearing aids (Fig. 5-5). These devices can obtain, analyze, and track patient data, such as heart rate, step count, and calories burned. Many consumers use these devices on their own to promote their health, tracking diet and exercise. While knowledge is still emerging on the benefits of wearables, studies suggest that there are many gaps in the research still to be investigated (Dian et al., 2020). Emerging literature is showing the potential for wearables in the use of patients with heart failure to help capture data on vital signs in conjunction with evidence-based heart failure care (DeVore et al., 2019). These are covered in more detail in Chapter 6.

Smartwatches

Smartwatch technology began in the early 1970s and has continued to evolve over the last five decades. Consumers did not purchase or use smartwatches in their early inception due to high costs, limited functionality, and appearance. In 2002, Fossil released a wearable digital wristwatch, the Fossil Palm Pilot. It displayed Palm

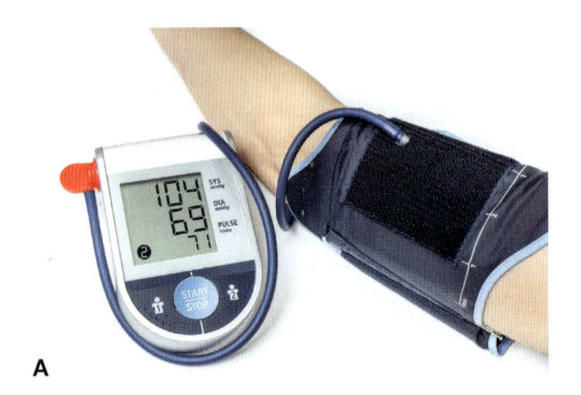

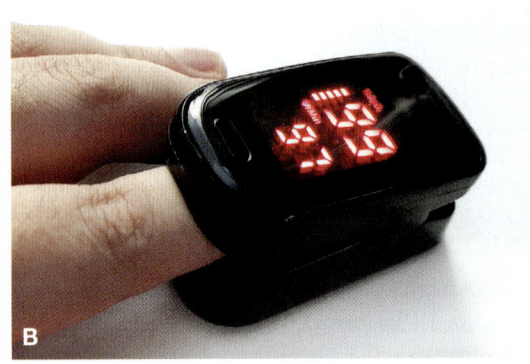

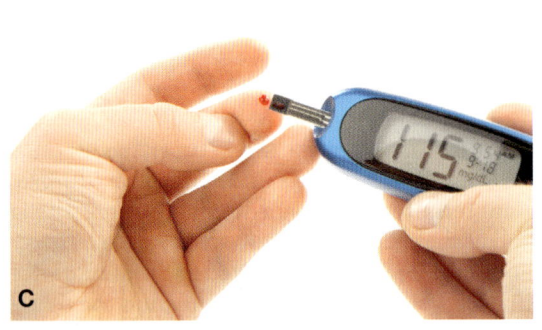

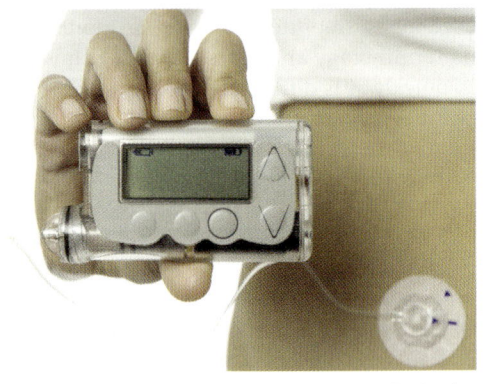

Figure 5-4. Examples of mobile medical devices. **A.** A blood pressure cuff. **B.** A pulse oximeter. **C.** A glucose monitor. **D.** An insulin pump. (**A.** Shutterstock/andriano.cz; **B.** Shutterstock/Blue Sky Pictures; **C.** Shutterstock/Dmitry Lobanov; **D.** Shutterstock/Click and Photo.)

Barcode Medication Administration

The use of **barcode medication administration (BCMA)** is an example of how the use of mobile technology can improve patient safety. BCMA is a point-of-care application for validation of medication administration that supports real-time recording of medications given to patients. BCMA interfaces with the electronic medication administration record to facilitate verification of patient identity as well as ensuring the patient receives the right medication, in the right dose, via the right route, at the right time (commonly known as "the five rights"). BCMA was designed to support patient safety in the administration of medication by providing checks and safeguards, but it is not a replacement for clinical judgment.

BCMA provides a familiar graphical interface that works with the EHR to both record medication administration and then make that information easily accessible to users of the EHR. Medication changes made by providers in the EHR are reflected in the BCMA as soon as the order is processed. Similarly, when a medication is administered using BCMA, the information is viewable in the EHR immediately (Fig. 5-6).

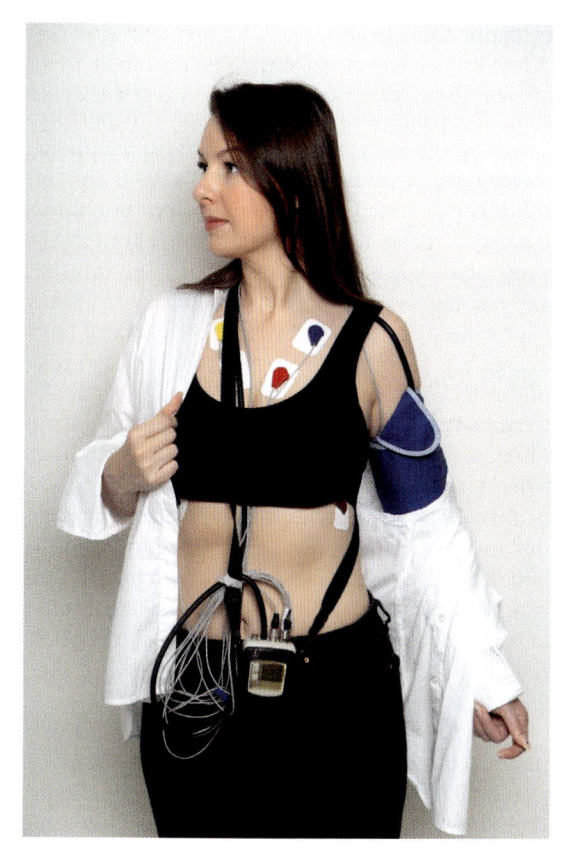

Figure 5-5. Example of a wearable device. (Shutterstock/vimpro.)

apps, such as an address book, calculator, and memo pad. There was also a stylus built into the wristband. Over the next 10 years, other iterations of smartwatches were released by companies such as Microsoft, Garmin, and Nike. The Sony SmartWatch was released in 2012. It most resembles the smartwatches that are popular today. It had a color display with apps, such as e-mail, music, and weather. The first Apple watch was released in 2015. Apple and Android smartwatches continue to be popular.

Most smartwatches are remotely controlled by the associated tethered phone. However, a few are long-term evolution (LTE)-enabled, which means that they have cellular service capabilities at an additional cost to the user's cellular plan. Current smartwatches function similarly to smartphones with capabilities for phone calls, text messages, email, and other apps.

eBooks

The popularity of eBooks is growing. In December 2013, eBooks outsold print books for the first time in history. Today, books, journals, and other publications can be easily accessed on mobile devices, giving users a digital library in the palms of their

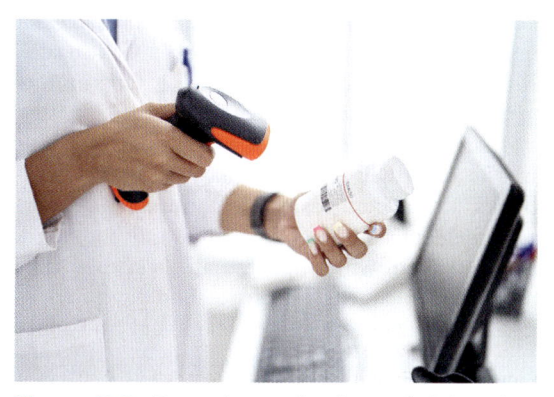

Figure 5-6. Barcode medication administration. (Shutterstock/Krakenimages.com)

hands. This is especially useful for nurses and other healthcare professionals because they can access knowledge easily and on the go. Clinical nurses commonly use references like nursing drug books, medical dictionaries, nursing procedures manuals, handbooks of diagnostic tests, and health assessment handbooks. The cost of an electronic references is usually comparable to the print version. Some printed nursing handbooks include app store information, so if the reader has a copy of the print book, they can download updates from an online store with resources for mobile devices.

Online bookstores that sell eBooks also sell eBook readers specific for the eBook file types in their stores. For example, Barnes & Noble sells the Nook, and Amazon sells the Kindle. Both eBook readers use WiFi to allow their users to purchase, download, and read eBooks sold in their stores. To read an eBook on a smartphone or tablet, the user may choose to have several eBook reader apps so they can access eBooks from different stores, libraries, and websites that provide access.

Most eBooks that can be purchased or borrowed from a library are protected by digital rights management (DRM), which provides copyright protection for eBooks, as well as commercial movies and music. DRM prevents the ability for users to make copies of eBooks. Because of DRM, users can read eBooks from the library app, and then they disappear from the user's app account when the loan expires. The Digital Millennium Copyright Act of 1998 made disabling DRM illegal in the United States.

However, not all eBooks are protected by copyright; some are free. Project Gutenberg (http://gutenberg.org) provides access to over 70,000 free eBooks without copyright protection. Examples of books for nursing include Florence Nightingale's *Notes on Nursing*, Clara Barton's *The Red Cross in Peace and War*, and Louisa May Alcott's *Hospital Sketches*.

Many publishers now offer nursing textbooks in eBook format as an alternative to print textbooks. The advantages of textbooks in eBook format include the ability to search and bookmark content. Also, when updates are available, they can be downloaded. Current technology provides opportunities for greater development and adoption of eBooks for nursing education. For example, eBooks can support embedded media, such as videos, embedded quizzes, and gaming.

Internet Telephone

Internet telephone, or telephony, refers to computer software and hardware that can perform functions usually associated with a telephone. **Voice over Internet Protocol (VoIP)** is the terminology for telephony products. VoIP provides a means to make a telephone call anywhere in the world with voice and video by using the internet and thereby bypassing the phone company. Many educational and healthcare institutions and businesses are switching from the conventional telephone to VoIP phones, which allow the user access to robust features similar to those on smartphones, such as conference and video calling. A benefit to using VoIP is that users can talk to people in other countries without paying any long-distance fees. In healthcare institutions, VoIP is beneficial because it allows improved communication with patients and providers on a global scale, and it reduces the cost and infrastructure needs required for dedicated phone lines (HBC Editors, 2022).

Free versions of VoIP software apps provide phone communication from computer to computer. Examples of free apps include Skype, FaceTime, FaceTime Audio, and WhatsApp. Skype allows free Skype-to-Skype voice and video calls, instant messaging, and file sharing. For an internet call, the user needs a microphone, speakers, and a sound card. If the device has a video camera, video calls are possible. The connection, computer processor, and software determine the number of people and quality of the connection. FaceTime and FaceTime Audio use the Apple iOS. FaceTime allows for video calls and FaceTime Audio allows audio calls on Apple computers, iPhones, and iPads using WiFi. WhatsApp is a messaging app that also allows users to make voice and video calls using WiFi on smartphones and tablets and on Apple or Windows OSs. The messaging and calls are encrypted. The messages can include images, videos, documents, user location, audio files, and more using a smartphone number.

Video Conferencing

Conference calls using the telephone used to be a way of life for those on teams or committees whose members lived in different geographical locations. Technology has advanced so that groups can meet using **video conferencing** (on screen). Video conferencing platforms, such as Microsoft Teams and Zoom, made remote work possible during the COVID-19 pandemic as people isolated to curb the spread of the virus. Much of the work that once took place in person, including visits to some healthcare settings, have moved online. The daily number of participants in Zoom meetings jumped from around 10 million at the end of December 2019 to more than 300 million 4 months later (Haddad, 2021).

Video conferencing allows participants to use a computer or a telephone connection. It is best practice to inform participants if the session is to be recorded and what the recording will be used for. Free teleconferencing applications are available. While they may not be as robust as the commercial applications, they offer affordable solutions. Examples include GoToMeeting, Google Hangouts, and Join.me.

Advantages of video conferencing include cost savings, increased employee productivity, transcription services that record and transcribe the spoken word into text, translation services for multilingual meetings, and file- and screen-sharing capabilities. Disadvantages include lack of more personal interactions, network connectivity issues, securing meetings (preventing unauthorized guests), complying with laws and regulations (especially in the healthcare field regarding privacy), organizing newly created data, and creating policies around new content types and sources.

A **webcast** is a one-way presentation, usually with video, to an audience who may be present either in a room or in a different geographical location. The webcast host often provides methods for the remote audience to ask questions, for instance, using chat functionality. Users can view the webcast "live" or later if recorded. The host can distribute the recording to others as a link on a web page or as an email file attachment.

A **webinar** is more like a live seminar. Users must log in to a website address. Although there is a speaker, the audience can ask questions during the presentation and the speaker can ask for feedback. Webinar software is available for enterprise and individual use. Faculty who teach courses online may use webinar software for office hours. Healthcare organizations use the software to conduct meetings and save employees inconvenience and travel costs. Professional organizations often offer free webinars to their members. Webinar software is available as a standalone or as embedded within a learning management system. It usually provides a means for video, audio, and chat. Zoom is an example of free webinar software.

mHealth Software for Mobile Devices

Healthcare software applications (apps) are abundant. At the peak, there were 53,979 mHealth apps available on the Apple Store alone (Statista, 2023a). In 2022, more than 86 million people in the United States (about 30% of adult smartphone owners) used a health or fitness app (Statista, 2023b). Smartphone and tablet owners can use apps to schedule hospital visits, communicate with physicians, follow recovery plans, track blood pressure, or achieve fitness goals (Fig. 5-7). Healthcare professionals use apps to access electronic health records, communicate with colleagues, look up medical references, and manage schedules.

A **mobile medical application** is designed to operate on a mobile platform and is intended either for use as an accessory to a regulated medical device or to transform a mobile platform into a regulated medical device (Hilliard, 2021). These applications are also regulated by the FDA to ensure their safety and effectiveness. The development and adoption of mobile medical apps has become widespread and is opening new and innovative ways to improve health and healthcare delivery.

Box 5-2 has a list of popular mHealth software categories and examples of apps. This is just a small example of the wide variety of healthcare apps for mobile devices.

CASE STUDY

Recall the case study at the beginning of this chapter. Are there mHealth applications that might be useful for patients from underserved communities? Think about how you would encourage patients to take advantage of mHealth applications.

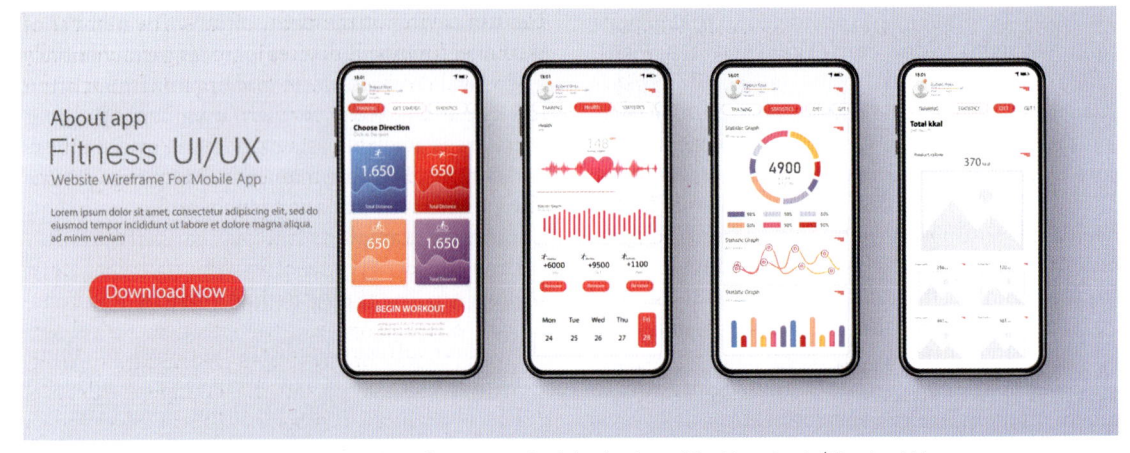

Figure 5-7. Fitness app collecting data from a wearable device. (Shutterstock/ZinetroN.)

BOX 5-2 mHealth Software Categories and Examples

Remote Monitoring
- Cardiio and Instant Heart Rate: Apps that allow the phone camera to measure pulse from a fingertip
- Diabetes:M: Calculates doses of insulin based on factors like exercise and stress and predicts blood sugar levels

Diagnostic
Sugar Sense: Analyzes glucose data from iHealth wearable glucometer

Condition Management
- Ovia Pregnancy and Baby Tracker: Tracks development of pregnancy, provides articles and tips, community, and Q&A
- Full Term: Labor contraction timer
- SmartBP: Blood pressure (BP) management app for recording, tracking, analyzing, and sharing BP; integrates with Bluetooth BP monitor

Online Consultations
MDLive and LiveHealth Online: Apps that host virtual appointments with doctors and therapists

Fitness Tracking
Fitbit: Health & Fitness: Allows users to track fitness progress, connect with friends, join communities, and start challenges; integrates with wearable Fitbit trackers

Nutrition and Weight Loss
MyFitnessPal: Exercise, calorie, and macronutrient tracker to support weight loss; includes meal scan feature that logs meals using smartphone camera

Reminders and Alerts
Medisafe Medication Management: Pill reminder and alarm, support for complex dosing schedules and management of healthcare appointments

Patient Health Records
Patient portal apps: Give patients access to personal health information from their various medical practitioners

Medical Compliance Applications
MyHealth: Allows patients to schedule healthcare appointments

Data from Ponomarov, S. (2022). What Types of Healthcare Apps Are Most Popular Among Consumers? https://digitalhealthbuzz.com/what-types-of-healthcare-apps-are-most-popular-among-consumers/

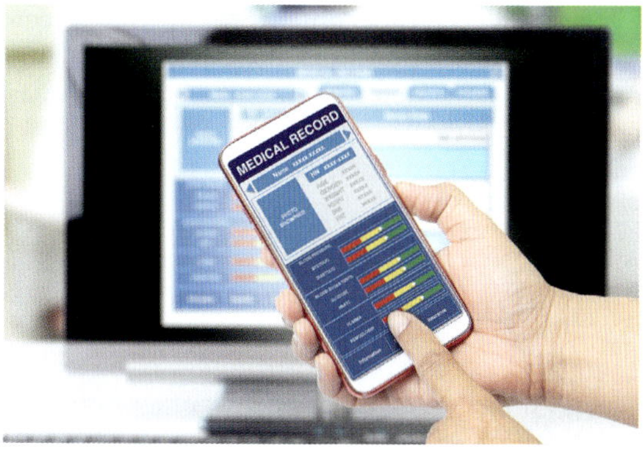

Figure 5-8. Patient portal software on a smartphone. (Shutterstock/panopstockool.)

Electronic Health Records and mHealth

Technologic advancements have enhanced the way healthcare providers manage electronic health records. Using mHealth software, patients and consumers are now able to interact with EHRs through patient portal software on mobile devices (Fig. 5-8). Most healthcare organizations have migrated from the use of paper records to completely electronic record keeping through clinical information systems. This provides for real-time charting of patient data (e.g., vital signs, intake/output, medication administration).

Many clinical information systems allow for syncing between EHRs and vital sign monitors and smart pumps, creating more ease and efficiency for healthcare providers when charting in the system. However, there are some disadvantages with the technology. Patients can read provider and nurse notes in real time as records are updated within the system, which means healthcare professionals need to be aware of charting sensitive information and using inclusive language. Healthcare providers must also continuously monitor for equipment malfunctions and be the last line of defense to prevent and mitigate security issues. EHR issues are discussed in more detail in Chapter 13.

MOBILE DEVICES IN CLINICAL PRACTICE

Mobile devices are used in clinical practice for a variety of reasons. Devices can free the nurse from looking for a reference book or finding a computer terminal to look up or enter data. Moreover, nurses can use devices at the point of care. The number of resources for mobile devices is growing exponentially every day. The best way to find apps and eBooks for clinical use is to search for them using the mobile app store or bookstore for the device. Potential buyers can also review user comments and ratings for the resources prior to making a purchase.

Ensuring nurses have access to updated information is a cornerstone of ensuring patient safety. Nurses find mobile devices affordable and indispensable in various nursing practice clinical settings including the medical–surgical nursing unit, the operating room, and the emergency department. A growing number of clinical information systems incorporate the use of mobile devices for point-of-need documentation. Wireless synchronization allows for real-time documentation in the electronic medical record (EMR).

Advanced Practice: Nurse Practitioner Use of mHealth

Nurse practitioners have quickly adopted the use of mobile devices into their practices. Two popular tools used in nursing are drug references and medical calculators. In addition to references used by the clinical nurse, nurse practitioners can monitor and evaluate patient progress. Patient Tracker is a program for patient care management. The free version allows users to enter up to 10 patients. For additional fees, users can access a pain assessment and blood sugar assessment and track an unlimited number of patients. Some EMR/EHR office systems, for example, eClinicalWorks, OneTouch EMR, and DrChrono EHR, have associated mobile device solutions for practitioners.

The practice setting for nurse practitioners can be busy. Prescription writing and coding for reimbursement of care can be automated with mobile device software. Prescription writing software such as Allscripts ePrescribe is available for mobile devices in addition to patient care management software. Although the mobile app is free, the user must have a paid subscription account for the software. There are also numerous software packages to identify International Classification of Diseases (ICD-10) and common procedural terminology (CPT) codes for billing of care. Search the mobile app stores using the terms "ICD" and "CPT."

> **CASE STUDY**
>
> Recall the finding by Gonzalez and colleagues (2021) in the case study that the Latinx community members they studied were more likely to engage with health information on their smartphones. Receiving a push notification through an app that a vaccination clinic is opening with Spanish-speaking providers could make a difference in health outcomes for Spanish-speaking people. Imagine also how important it is to have applications in both Spanish and English to improve health outcomes for this growing population. How can nurses advocate for using mHealth to reach underserved communities?

Use of Mobile Devices in Nursing Research

Mobile devices are useful for the research process. Users can administer and take web-based research surveys with a mobile device. The data from the surveys can be stored on the researcher's web server for aggregation and analysis. Researchers can use the audio recorder on a mobile device to record focus group interviews and then later download the recordings for data analysis. The camera on the mobile device can be used to take pictures to document changes that occurred because of a research treatment.

Mobile computers can assist in finding and storing literature citations used for library searches. For example, users can access their personal reference managers on mobile devices using apps such as EndNote or PaperShip for Mendeley and Zotero. The portability of the references saves time when visiting the library to search for journal articles and books or storing the call numbers for the book locations in the library. Libraries also lend more than books; they also lend CDs, DVDs, and computer equipment, such as laptops and iPods. Many college and health science libraries have extensive mobile device resources designed to assist healthcare students and professionals.

Most libraries also have websites, and a growing number of those websites are tablet- and smartphone-friendly. The design of mobile-friendly websites allows the content to fit the screen size without requiring horizontal scrolling. Additionally, the web address should be as short as possible to facilitate input, and the content should address what the mobile user needs.

ADVANTAGES AND DISADVANTAGES OF USING MHEALTH

There are benefits and shortcomings of mHealth, though many argue that the advantages far outweigh the disadvantages. Time management, improved communication and decision making, and access to information resources are often mentioned in the literature as positive outcomes of mobile devices in clinical settings (Sun et al., 2019). Instead of looking up information in multiple printed textbooks, nurses can query the mobile device, which can hold numerous textbooks. Patient safety and error reduction are also benefits. The ease of looking up reference information improves confidence and decreases errors in the clinical setting. Unlike the printed counterpart, you can update reference eBooks and renew subscriptions. Finally, the mobile device is easy for healthcare professionals to use when answering patient questions at the point of care.

Although mobile devices offer benefits, there are also shortcomings. While healthcare providers are using mobile devices in many areas, adoption may be slowed by a variety of factors (Sun et al., 2019). The culture of some settings does not support the use of mobile devices. Access to a mobile device and WiFi coverage may prove difficult. Rapid changes in technology can be problematic with no guarantees that the manufacturer of a given mobile device will continue to manufacture and offer support. The expense of the mobile devices is a common concern (Piuzzi et al., 2019). Some nursing programs require students to purchase devices, whereas others use grant money or incorporate the cost as a laboratory fee. The time involved with the selection and preparation of devices and education for users is another obstacle. There is a potential for misuse of mobile devices using the camera, scanner apps, and social media. Practicing nurses must be aware of the laws, policies, and procedures for use and never take unauthorized photos or make copies of any patient information with mobile devices. Doing so breaches patient privacy and confidentiality. There can be issues with faulty devices and short battery life. A final consideration is data security and the vulnerability of mHealth to attack by cyber criminals.

Smartphone Malware

The first cell phone virus, called Cabir, was detected in 2004. It impacted many models of phones. The virus installed itself automatically on the system when the user accepted a Bluetooth transmission from another user. When activated, it displayed a message on the screen with the text, "Caribe," and then started a continuous search for other devices to send itself to. Much like viruses that infect humans, Cabir was only able to transmit to phones within the 30-ft Bluetooth transmission radius.

Viruses that infect smartphones are not as common as PC viruses, but cyber criminals are aware of the increased use of phones and tablets, so they are rapidly switching their attention to these platforms. Smartphone viruses can potentially access all the contacts, apps, and stored information, such as credit cards or bank details, in the phone. They can also send texts on their own, and they can make phone calls to premium rate numbers or download other apps and run up a large bill. Android devices are the most commonly targeted by malware. Android users can install third-party apps directly from the internet without being vetted by the Google Play Store, and numerous manufacturers use the Android OS, each with a different level of security (McAfee, 2023).

The four most common ways to get a virus are to:
1. Download an infected app. There are many free apps for mobile devices, many of which come with malware.
2. Visit a compromised website. You may not know the site has been compromised.
3. Open attachments in emails or texts that contain malware.
4. Connect a device to a computer via a universal serial bus allowing viruses on the computer to transfer to the mobile device.

> **BOX 5-3** Using Passwords to Protect Data
>
> All mobile devices with any type of clinical data must be secure or encrypted using passwords or biometrics (such as fingerprint recognition). If passwords are used, they must be complex enough that they cannot be easily hacked. Tips for creating complex passwords include:
> - Use longer passwords of at least 10 to 12 characters.
> - Use words or characters that are easily remembered, but that are not personally identifiable, like the misspelled name of a fruit or flower, rather than the name of a family member or pet.
> - Use the first letter of each word in a familiar phrase.
> - Replace letters of the word with numbers or other keyboard characters. For example, the letter A might be replaced with the @ sign and the letter O with the number 0.
> - Do not reuse the same password for multiple accounts. Use a **password manager**, which will store unique passwords securely using encryption, so you can create many unique passwords.

Smartphone users should take the same precautions they do on for computers (there is more information about computer security in Chapter 3). For example, Box 5-3 includes tips for better password creation. Most important of all, if there is a need to store patient data, users must follow the policies and procedures outlined by their healthcare agency. Check with the agency's Health Insurance Portability and Accountability Act (HIPAA) officer for questions. Chapter 15 has more information about protecting patient privacy and confidentiality.

Cyber Attacks on Medical Devices

Take a moment to think about the many medical devices used in healthcare. Attacks on medical devices are a reality with the potential for severe consequences. Two models of Medtronic insulin pumps were recalled in June 2019 after a cybersecurity risk was identified related to the interconnectivity of the pump to other devices (FDA, 2019; Voelker, 2019). Similar vulnerabilities have been described in wireless implantable medical devices, such as implantable cardiac devices, insulin pumps, and infusion systems (Marin, 2018). In 2016, there was a disclosure that St. Jude Medical, a manufacturer of pacemakers and defibrillators, had security vulnerabilities. Dick Cheney, who was the U.S. Vice President at the time, had his implantable defibrillator wireless control disabled to avoid an attack by a cyber criminal with plans to disable the device. The WannaCry virus hit hospitals worldwide in 2016 and 2017, denying access to the hospital clinical information systems and demanding a ransom payment (Akbanov et al., 2019).

Cybersecurity of medical devices has become enough of a concern that in 2022, President Joe Biden added a section, "Ensuring Cybersecurity of Medical Devices," to the Federal Food, Drug, and Cosmetic Act. In 2023, the FDA began requiring new mobile medical device submissions to include documentation demonstrating that the device meets cybersecurity requirements (FDA, 2023).

FUTURE TRENDS

There is no way to completely predict the future of mHealth in education and clinical settings; however, there are trends that will likely continue. We can expect mobile devices to be easier to use with more intuitive software. Voice commands currently available to operate mobile devices can be expected to improve and become a primary method of data input. Mobile broadband for high-speed transfer of data will be an accessible and affordable feature for smartphones.

Medical devices are available and under development for integration with smartphones that can be used by both care providers and patients for monitoring and diagnostic purposes. Patients will be able to share medical information from the devices with their care providers electronically. Smartphones and tablets will likely continue to be appropriate for use in education, classroom, simulation clinical labs, and clinical settings. As the popularity of mobile devices increases, the pricing will continue to drop.

As the future unfolds, healthcare will harness the use of technology to improve patient care and save lives. In the event of a disaster, team notification will be done primarily using text messaging to smartphones. Clinical information systems will increase sending **push notifications**, mobile device messages, such as alerts for elevated lab values, poor air quality, or notification of an upcoming appointment.

It is possible that by publication, some concepts mentioned in this book will be outdated or no longer used. However, the following sections discuss trends on the rise.

Speech Recognition

Speech recognition software is designed to create text from speech. The user can speak to the device, and the program types the text so the user doesn't have to manually enter the text. Speech recognition is powered by artificial intelligence (AI). It enables computers and software applications to understand what people are saying to perform a task (Gordon, 2021). For example, the Alexa personal assistant speaker responds to commands after the user says "Alexa."

The healthcare industry first used speech recognition for medical reporting around 1994. Early versions of software required the user to learn how to talk to the computer rather than the computer learning to listen. Slow processing speeds and costs were a barrier (Parente et al., 2004).

In 2008, Google released Voice Search as an app in the iPhone's app store (Bhattacharya, n.d.). The popularity and convenience of the speech recognition feature triggered significant developments in accuracy of the software "understanding" speech. Apple also continued to improve the speech recognition feature with Siri, a "virtual personal assistant," that was integrated into iPhones in 2011 (Allen, 2021). Google and Apple use analytics from all their users to improve speech recognition.

Some apps also include voice recognition capabilities. The term for this feature is voice-to-text apps. For example, Facebook Messenger has voice recognition. Dragon Anywhere is a free app available for smartphones. Speech recognition, an add-on for the Chrome web browser, allows the user to dictate Google Docs files. Additionally, some commercially available programs allow dictation to the computer. One of the most popular for general work is Dragon NaturallySpeaking by Nuance Corporation. Nuance Corporation also has a version for medical documentation, which can translate spoken word to text, and it will read back the text (Nuance, n.d.).

Artificial Intelligence

Artificial intelligence (AI) is the ability of non-human machines to understand their surroundings and use information to achieve specific objectives (Rong et al., 2020). AI is transforming healthcare in multiple ways. It can be used in conjunction with mobile devices using sensors on the body to detect patterns and predict future occurrences of disease incidence. There are now mobile device apps that can help with skin cancer detection (Smak Gregoor et al., 2023). AI can collect patient data like vital signs or diagnostic results and use software to prioritize the information and help with decision support. AI can be used to visually analyze lab specimens and prioritize those that require a higher level of analysis by skilled providers (Siwicki, 2023). AI-based programs and chatbots can help pregnant people with advice during pregnancy (Rong et al., 2020).

AI is used to enhance communication. Chatbots use AI to answer frequently asked questions. Recognition of facial expressions as commands allows people with loss of autonomy to control wheelchairs and robot assistant vehicles without a joystick or sensors (Davis, 2023). AI can also be used to respond to patients in different languages and allow for real-time translation of medical information. AI-powered provider-to-patient translators can turn technical medical jargon into plain language using natural language processing. This use of AI allows complex medical notes to be translated into a fifth grade reading level, which can reduce health disparities influenced by lower healthcare literacy (Landi, 2023). Chapter 9 discusses how AI is used to analyze big data to predict diseases processes, such as seizures, strokes, and the spread of disease like COVID-19.

AI can streamline workflows, reduce administrative tasks, increase automation, improve quality and consistency, and reduce error rates (Bhattamisra et al., 2023). Advances in AI are allowing healthcare providers to spend more time on patient care and less time on administrative tasks. AI is useful for repetitive tasks and can be used for medication delivery, tracking input and output, and managing patient vital signs. Robots can be used to fill prescriptions, using computerized visualization to confirm the right dose and medication, and can then prepare the medications to be shipped to the patient's home (Siwicki, 2023).

An example of the use of AI to reduce administrative tasks includes monitoring for drug diversion or misuse, a time-intensive, traditionally manual task. Advanced analytics and machine learning allow software to identify suspicious behavior, automate management of controlled substances, and flag any issues that may need investigation (Siwicki, 2023). Federal healthcare agencies like the U.S. Department of Veterans Affairs (VA) process millions of paper and digital forms, applications, and images each year. AI can be used to extract data from documents to facilitate speedier healthcare decision making. The VA has been using AI to collect data to support insurance verification, referrals, scheduling, and patient care (Schroeder, 2023).

Nanotechnology

As previously stated, **nanotechnology** is work done at the nanoscale (1 to 100 nm in diameter; Nano.gov, n.d.). To provide a comparison, hemoglobin is 5.5 nm, and a strand of DNA is 2 nm in diameter.

Scientists envision many benefits from the use of nanotechnology in medicine (Nano.gov, n.d.), for example, using a nanoparticle to imitate high-density lipoprotein, the "good" cholesterol, to shrink plaque of atherosclerosis, or using nanoribbons to repair spinal cord injury. Researchers are working on nanotechnology that can allow for the administration of vaccines without needles. Read the Ethical Considerations box to learn about how knowledge of mHealth and nanotechnology supports the ANA Code of Ethics.

ETHICAL CONSIDERATIONS FOR MOBILE HEALTHCARE TECHNOLOGY

Provision 2 of the ANA Code of Ethics (2015) states that "The nurse's primary commitment is to the patient, whether an individual, family, group, community, or population." Interpretive Statement 2.1 challenges nurses to focus on the "primacy of the patient's interests" (ANA, 2015). Primacy means the patient is the most important part of care. It can be easy to lose sight of the patient when considering the wide variety of mHealth technology available. Nurses should try to involve patients in planning their care and ensure the patient finds the care plan acceptable and that they feel competent to use any proposed technology. The nurse should advocate for the patient's wishes when conflict arises. For example, if the patient wants to decline the use of a home monitoring device and instead come to the primary care office for monitoring, the nurse is obligated to find a reasonable solution that meets the needs of both the office and the patient.

Provision 8 of the ANA Code of Ethics states that "the nurse collaborates with other health professionals and the public to protect human rights, promote health diplomacy, and reduce health disparities" (ANA, 2015). When considering the use of emerging technology such as nanotechnology to treat patients, Salamanca-Buentello and Daar (2021) suggest that the risks may outweigh the benefits due to the ease with which nanoparticles could be unknowingly transmitted to anyone who may encounter them. The long-term effects of the use of nanotechnology in medicine are unknown, and analysis of literature published about nanotechnology reveals that the risks and benefits are not well understood. Therefore, nanotechnology can prompt concern for the health of the workers and the environment. Nanotechnology has the possibility of changing the ways we detect and treat disease. Does Provision 8 apply to this situation? If so, what is the responsibility of the nurse regarding the use of nanotechnology in patient care?

SUMMARY

- **Mobile devices.** The most common mobile devices are smartphones and tablets. Compared to traditional computers, mobile devices may have different OSs, displays, battery, memory, synchronization, data entry, and connectivity. Mobile devices can connect in many ways, including using WiFi mobile networks that include 5G as well as Bluetooth, cellular, and NFC.
- **Examples of mHealth.** Mobile medical devices are medical devices small enough to fit in your hand that can send or receive information wirelessly, such as smartphones, insulin pumps, pulse oximeters, and point-of-care monitoring devices. Uses of software for mobile devices include remote monitoring, diagnostics, condition management, online consultation, fitness and weight loss, reminders and alerts, patient health records, and medical compliance applications. Patient portal software can be accessed through smartphones, allowing patients instant access to their health records. Other examples of mHealth include wearables, smartwatches, BCMA, eBooks, internet telephones, and video conferencing.
- **Mobile devices in clinical practice.** Mobile devices allow nurses to access information in real time instead of having to rely on potentially outdated references, which is important for patient safety. Nurses also use mHealth for patient care management, for point-of-care testing, for blood glucose measurements, or when collecting vital signs. Mobile devices are used in nursing research for administering surveys, recording interviews, taking photos to document changes, or searching the literature.
- **Advantages and disadvantages of using mHealth.** Advantages of mHealth include saving time, time management, improved communication and decision making, and access to information resources. Disadvantages

include access to connectivity, the affordability of devices, keeping a device updated with rapid changes in technology, misuse of devices when interacting with patients, and data and security issues. Smartphone malware and cyber attacks on medical devices are both on the rise.

- **Future trends.** Trends in mHealth include increasing availability of mobile devices as costs continue to drop as well as increased access to the internet. Speech recognition will improve for easier use in healthcare settings. AI and nanotechnology are examples of cutting-edge trends on the rise.

DISCUSSION QUESTIONS AND ACTIVITIES

1. If you have access to a mobile device, discuss the connectivity of your device. Does the device have Bluetooth, NFC, beaming, or internet capabilities? Explain the advantages and disadvantages of each type of connection for accessing healthcare information.
2. Use the internet to preview an eBook that you might use on a mobile device. Discuss the similarities and differences between the printed book view and the electronic view.
3. Download a trial version of nursing reference software from the Internet. Use a search engine, such as Google, and enter the search term "nursing mobile software trial downloads." What do you discover?
4. Search for apps that are available in other languages. Explore healthcare apps for accessibility features like voice control or translation capabilities and discuss your findings.
5. Use a search engine to search for health science library mobile device websites.
6. Check with your local library to see if they lend mobile-computing devices such as laptops, iPads, and/or tablets.
7. Search for the national nanotechnology initiative and explore the website. List three new things you learned about nanotechnology. Did you learn anything that brings up ethical concerns for the potential for patient harm? Explain your answers.

PRACTICE QUESTIONS

1. Which type of networking would be useful for people living in an urban setting to search the internet?
   a. Bluetooth
   b. NFC
   c. WiFi
   d. Satellite
2. A patient you are educating uses a wireless insulin pump. Which would be an appropriate education topic to support the protection of patient information?
   a. How to connect the pump to public WiFi networks
   b. How to install security and software updates
   c. What to do if there is a power failure
   d. How to manage glucose and insulin levels
3. When educating patients regarding safe password creation, which statement is correct?
   a. Passwords should be of a personal nature.
   b. Passwords can be reused for multiple accounts.
   c. Passwords should be no more than eight unique characters.
   d. Passwords should replace letters of the word with numbers or other keyboard characters.
4. You have a patient with congestive heart failure who needs to monitor their vital signs daily. The patient lives in a remote area and cannot drive. Which mHealth option listed below is the best for this patient?
   a. A wearable device
   b. Video conferencing
   c. Access to a patient portal
   d. Use of BCMA

REFERENCES

Akbanov, M., Vassilakis, V., & Logothetis, M. D. (2019). Ransomware detection and mitigation using software defined networking: The case of WannaCry. *Computers & Electrical Engineering, 76,* 111-121. https://doi.org/10.1016/j.compeleceng.2019.03.012

Allen, J. (2021, October 4). 10 years of Siri: The history of Apple's voice assistant. Retrieved June 17, 2022, from https://www.techradar.com/news/siri-10-year-anniversary

American Nurses Association. (2015). *Code of ethics for nurses*. American Nurses Publishing. https://www.nursingworld.org/practice-policy/nursing-excellence/ethics/code-of-ethics-for-nurses/

Bhattacharya, J. (n.d.). Complete Google voice search history. Retrieved June 17, 2022, from https://seosandwitch.com/google-voice-search-history/#1-_When_Did_Google_Voice_Search_Start

Bhattamisra, S. K., Banerjee, P., Gupta, P., Mayuren, J., Patra, S., & Candasamy, M. (2023). Artificial intelligence in pharmaceutical and healthcare research. *Big Data and Cognitive Computing, 7*(1), 10. https://doi.org/10.3390/bdcc7010010

Chantel, J. (2023 April 25). Smartphone history: The timeline of a modern marvel. https://blog.textedly.com/smartphone-history-when-were-smartphones-invented#third

Dangi, R., Lalwani, P., Choudhary, G., You, I., & Pau, G. (2021). Study and investigation on 5G technology: A systematic review. *Sensors, 22*(1), 26. https://www.mdpi.com/1424-8220/22/1/26/htm

Davis, L. (2023, January 11). *Northwell releases AI-driven pregnancy chatbot*. Northwell Health. https://www.northwell.edu/news/the-latest/northwell-releases-ai-driven-pregnancy-chatbot

Deng, C., Fang, X., Han, X., Wang, X., Yan, L., He, R., Long, Y., & Guo, Y. (2020). IEEE 802.11 be WiFi 7: New challenges and opportunities. *IEEE Communications Surveys & Tutorials, 22*(4), 2136–2166. https://arxiv.org/pdf/2007.13401.pdf

DeVore, A. D., Wosik, J., & Hernandez, A. F. (2019). The future of wearables in heart failure patients. *JACC Heart Fail, 7*(11), 922–932. https://doi.org/10.1016/j.jchf.2019.08.008

Dian, F. J., Vahidnia, R., & Rahmati, A. (2020). Wearables and the Internet of Things (IoT), applications, opportunities, and challenges: A survey. *IEEE Access, 8*, 69200–69211. https://doi.org/10.1109/ACCESS.2020.2986329

Gonzalez, C., Early, J., Gordon-Dseagu, V., Mata, T., & Nieto, C. (2021). Promoting culturally tailored mHealth: A scoping review of mobile health interventions in Latinx communities. *Journal of Immigrant and Minor Health, 23*(5), 1065–1077. https://doi-org.uscupstate.idm.oclc.org/10.1007/s10903-021-01209-4

Gordon, C. (2021). *A market to harness: Speech recognition artificial intelligence (AI) innovations on the rise*. Forbes. https://www.forbes.com/sites/cindygordon/2021/12/23/a-market-to-harness-speech-recognition-artificial-intelligence-ai-innovations-on-the-rise/?sh=843a3ba134df

Haddad, M. (2021, April 10). *Love them or hate them, virtual meetings are here to stay*. The Economist. https://www.economist.com/international/2021/04/10/love-them-or-hate-them-virtual-meetings-are-here-to-stay

HBC Editors. (2022, March 29). Benefits & challenges of using VoIP technology in hospitals. https://healthcarebusinessclub.com/articles/healthcare-provider/technology/benefits_challenges-of-using-voip-technology-in-hospitals/#google_vignette

Hilliard, E. (2021, August 10). The proliferation of mobile medical devices—revolutionizing healthcare. https://sterlingmedicaldevices.com/thought-leadership/medical-device-design-industry-blog/proliferation-of-mobile-medical-devices/

Kang, S. -G., Song, M. -S., Kim, J. -W., Lee, J., & Kim, J. (2021). Near-field communication in biomedical applications. *Sensors (Basel), 21*(3), 703. https://www.mdpi.com/1424-8220/21/3/703

Kostoff, R. N., Heroux, P., Aschner, M., & Tsatsakis, A. (2020). Adverse health effects of 5G mobile networking technology under real-life conditions. *Toxicology Letters, 323*, 35–40. https://doi.org/10.1016/j.toxlet.2020.01.020

Landi, H. (2023, August 8). *Mint.com founder's health tech company launches AI tool to translate medical jargon for patients*. Fierce Healthcare. https://www.fiercehealthcare.com/health-tech/mintcom-founders-health-tech-company-launches-ai-tool-translate-medical-jargon#:~:text=Health%20tech%20company%20Vital%20launched,to%20the%20public%20in%20English

Marin, E. (2018). *Security and privacy of implantable medical devices* [Doctor of Engineering Science (PhD): Electrical Engineering]. Katholieke Universiteit Leuven.

McAfee. (2023, April 4). *How to remove viruses from your android phone*. https://www.mcafee.com/blogs/mobile-security/how-to-remove-viruses-from-your-android-phone

Medindia. (2022). History of PDA. http://www.medindia.net/pda/pda_history.htm

Nano.Gov. (n.d.). Nanotech 101. https://www.nano.gov/nanotech-101

Nuance. (n.d.). Medical speech recognition solutions. Retrieved June 26, 2022, from https://www.nuance.com/healthcare/provider-solutions/speech-recognition.html?_ga=2.111170116.1511985878.1656268118-690403584.1656268116&_gac=1.221991196.1656268574.5d830443aa741c4cd5e766fb0cda8dd4

Parente, R., Kock, N., & Sonsini, J. (2004). An analysis of the implementation and impact of speech-recognition technology in the healthcare sector. *Perspectives in Health Information Management, 1*, 5.

Pew Research Center. (2021, April 7). Mobile fact sheet. https://www.pewresearch.org/internet/fact-sheet/mobile/

Piuzzi, N., Strnad, G., Brooks, P., Hettrich, C. M., Higuera-Rueda, C., Iannotti, J., & Spindler, K. P., OME Cleveland Clinic Orthopaedics. (2019). Implementing a scientifically valid, cost-effective, and scalable data collection system at point of care: the Cleveland Clinic OME cohort. *The Journal of Bone & Joint Surgery, 101*(5), 458–464. https://doi.org/10.2106/JBJS.18.00767

Rong, G., Mendez, A., Assi, E. B., Zhao, B., & Sawan, M. (2020). Artificial intelligence in healthcare: Review and prediction case studies. *Engineering, 6*(3), 291–301. https://doi.org/10.1016/j.eng.2019.08.015

Salamanca-Buentello, F., & Daar, A. S. (2021). Nanotechnology, equity and global health. *Nature Nanotechnology, 16*(4), 358–361. https://doi.org/10.1038/s41565-021-00899-z

Schroeder, T. (2023, August 31). *AI-powered document understanding improves patient experiences and saves lives*. Federal News Network. https://federalnewsnetwork.com/commentary/2023/08/ai-powered-document-understanding-improves-patient-experiences-and-saves-lives/

Sharma, S., Kumar, R., & Rama Krishna, C. (2021). A survey on analysis and detection of Android ransomware. *Concurrency and Computation: Practice and Experience, 33*(16), e6272. https://doi.org/10.1002/cpe.6272

Siwicki, B. (2023, August 25). *Automation helps return time to patients, reduce clinician burnout*. Healthcare IT News. https://www.healthcareitnews.com/news/automation-helps-return-time-patients-reduce-clinician-burnout

Smak Gregoor, A. M., Sangers, T. E., Bakker, L. J. Hollestein, L., Uyl-de Groot, C. A., Nijsten, T., & Wakkee, M. (2023). An artificial intelligence-based app for skin cancer detection evaluated in a population-based setting. *NPJ Digital Medicine, 6*(1), 90. https://doi.org/10.1038/s41746-023-00831-w

Solkin, M. (2021). Electromagnetic interference hazards in flight and the 5G mobile phone: Review of critical issues in aviation security. *Transportation Research Procedia, 59*, 310–318. https://doi.org/10.1016/j.trpro.2021.11.123

Statista. (2023a). Number of mHealth apps available in the Apple App Store from 1st quarter 2015 to 3rd quarter 2022. https://www.statista.com/statistics/779910/health-apps-available-ios-worldwide/

Statista. (2023b). Number of health and fitness app users in the United States from 2018 to 2022. https://www.statista.com/statistics/1154994/number-us-fitness-health-app-users/

Sun, S. L., Hwang, H. G., Dutta, B., & Peng, M. H. (2019). Exploring critical factors influencing nurses' intention to use tablet PC in Patients' care using an integrated theoretical model. *Libyan Journal of Medicine, 14*(1), 1648963. https://www.tandfonline.com/action/showCitFormats?doi=10.1080/19932820.2019.1648963

Sun, X., Zhao, C., Li, H., Yu, H., Zhang, J., Qiu, H., Liang, J., Wu, J., Su, M., Shi, Y., & Pan, L. (2022). Wearable near-field communication sensors for healthcare: Materials, fabrication, and application. *Micromachines (Basel), 13*(5), 784. https://www.mdpi.com/2072-666X/13/5/784

Todtenberg, N., & Kraemer, R. (2019). A survey on Bluetooth multi-hop networks. *Ad Hoc Networks, 93*, 101922. https://doi.org/10.1016/j.adhoc.2019.101922

U.S. Food & Drug Administration (FDA). (2019, June 27). *FDA warns patients and health care providers about potential cybersecurity concerns with certain Medtronic insulin pumps* [press release]. https://www.fda.gov/news-events/press-announcements/fda-warns-patients-and-health-care-providers-about-potential-cybersecurity-concerns-certain

U.S. Food & Drug Administration (FDA). (2023, March 29). *Cybersecurity in medical devices frequently asked questions (FAQs)*. https://www.fda.gov/medical-devices/digital-health-center-excellence/cybersecurity-medical-devices-frequently-asked-questions-faqs

Voelker, R. (2019). Insulin pumps could be hacked. *Journal of the American Medical Association, 322*(5), 393. https://doi.org/10.1001/jama.2019.10645

CHAPTER 6

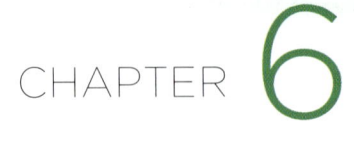

Telehealth

Kristi Miller, Olivia Boice, Neal Reeves, and Brittany Beasley

OBJECTIVES

After studying this chapter, you will be able to:
1. Discuss telehealth concepts and explain the difference between synchronous and asynchronous delivery as well as emerging uses of telehealth.
2. Identify the standards associated with telenursing and how telehealth can be used to deliver education to patients and providers.
3. Explain the various ways telehealth can be used to provide care to patients.
4. Discuss how telehealth can be used to treat patients with chronic diseases.
5. Explore how access to high-speed internet, reimbursement, federal and state regulation, and fraud impact telehealth delivery.

AACN Essentials for Entry-Level Professional Nursing Education

8.1b Identify the basic concepts of electronic health, mobile health, and telehealth systems for enabling patient care.

8.3c Use information and communication technology in a manner that supports the nurse–patient relationship.

8.4c Identify the basic concepts of electronic health, mobile health, and telehealth systems in enabling patient care.

8.5c Comply with legal and regulatory requirements while using communication and information technologies.

8.5f Deliver care using remote technology.

AACN Essentials for Advanced-Level Nursing Education

8.3i Appraise the role of information and communication technologies in engaging the patient and supporting the nurse–patient relationship.

8.3j Evaluate the potential uses and impact of emerging technologies in healthcare.

8.3k Pose strategies to reduce inequities in digital access to data and information.

8.4f Employ electronic health, mobile health, and telehealth systems to enable quality, ethical, and efficient patient care.

8.5h Assess potential ethical and legal issues associated with the use of information and communication technology.

HIMSS TIGER Competencies

Information technology risk management

Information and knowledge management in patient care

Teaching, training, education

KEY TERMS

Asynchronous telehealth	Robotics	Telemental health
E-intensive care	Store-and-forward (S&F)	Telemedicine
Holoportation	Synchronous telehealth	Telenursing
Portable monitoring devices	Telehealth	Telepresence
Remote patient monitoring	Telehomecare	Teletrauma

CASE STUDY

Lack of access to affordable, quality healthcare plays a role in the life expectancy of Native Americans in the United States; it is an average of 5.5 years fewer than that of people of all other U.S. demographic groups. For example, for the Navajo Nation, the COVID-19 pandemic drastically increased the number of patients but shut down many of the primary care and specialist practices available to them. In May of 2020, the Navajo Nation had the highest number of COVID-19 cases per capita in the United States. By August 2020, the disease had killed more Navajo people per capita than in any U.S. state (Begay et al., 2021).

To combat this inequity, Project Extension for Community Health Outcomes (ECHO) uses technology such as multipoint video conferencing and the internet to provide mentoring to the few providers caring for patients on tribal lands, using an interactive structured curriculum. Technology is also being used with home-based telemonitoring, in which smart thermometers (Fig. 6-1) are being used to predict disease hotspots by collecting data online whenever a user takes someone's temperature or interacts with the application (app) to self-report symptoms (Begay et al., 2021).

Another obstacle the Navajo Nation has experienced is issues with telecommunication infrastructure. Up to 30% of Navajo households lack electricity (Begay et al., 2021). Many have limited access to telephone services and reliable high-speed internet. In an area where lack of healthcare is prevalent, solid telecommunication options would help with patient education, emergency response, and critical services.

As you read this chapter, think about the role of the nurse in telehealth and how you can advocate for equitable health outcomes in your community using emerging technology.

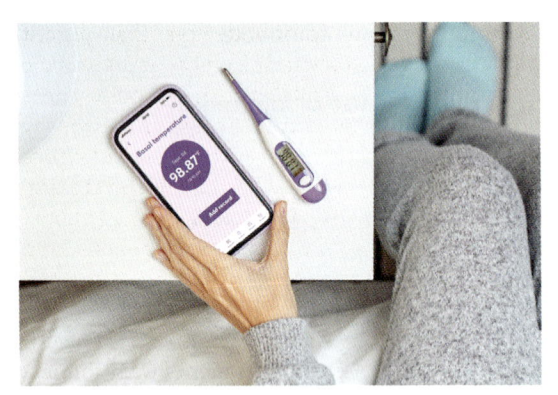

Figure 6-1. Smart thermometer. (Shutterstock/Hassel Stock.)

Telehealth is thought to have begun in 1879 when a mother phoned the family doctor in the middle of the night because she was afraid her baby had croup. The doctor asked that she put the phone close to the child so he could hear the cough (Genes, 2018). In the 1920s, the radio was used to give medical advice to clinics on ships. In the late 1950s, closed-circuit television links were established between the Nebraska Psychiatric Institute and Norfolk State Hospital for psychiatric consultations (NIHAN, 2022).

In the 1970s, the National Aeronautics and Space Administration (NASA) began the Space Technology Applied to Rural Papago Advanced Health Care (STARPAHC) program (Reifegerste et al., 2022). This program used the remote location of the Papago reservation and the less restrictive laws in Arizona to test the ability to monitor astronauts in space. Since then, NASA has been using telehealth to monitor biometrics of astronauts to learn how their bodies function in space. NASA is now using telemedicine for the International Space Station to monitor, diagnose, and treat astronauts if they become ill (Simpson et al., 2020). NASA is even using **holoportation** technology, which allows 3D models of healthcare providers to be transmitted live and in real time. Users can see, hear, and interact with remote participants in 3D as if they are present in the same space (Garcia, 2022). Not all telehealth applications are this dramatic, but this demonstrates the power of telehealth in the delivery of healthcare.

Today, home-based telemonitoring may include real-time audio and video messaging tools that connect providers with patients. Remote tools such as blood pressure monitors, Bluetooth-enabled digital scales, Fitbits, and other wearable devices can relay biometric information to providers. Data can be paired with individual symptom reports collected with smartphone apps or electronic health records. Technology-based apps can be used to monitor symptoms on a large scale, allowing the prediction of future pandemics. Computer concepts (Chapter 3), networking (Chapter 4), and mHealth (Chapter 5) are covered in other chapters and contain information important to understanding telehealth. This chapter will teach you about telehealth concepts, telenursing, how to use telehealth, and legal and ethical issues concerning the use of telehealth. Although much attention has been given to the aspect of telehealth that addresses the delivery of acute care or specialist consultations, telehealth is far more versatile.

TELEHEALTH CONCEPTS

Terms such as telehealth and telemedicine are often used interchangeably to refer to health services delivered using electronic technology to patients at a distance. According to the Health Resources and Services Administration (HRSA), **telemedicine** refers to the delivery of remote clinical services through the electronic exchange of patient information between two sites for improving the patient's health status. **Telehealth** is a broader term that extends beyond the delivery of clinical services to include provider training, such as continuing medical education, and administrative meetings in addition to clinical service offerings (HealthIT.gov, 2023; HRSA, 2023).

Telehealth is used for situations when the patient and the healthcare professional cannot meet in person. Reasons include being in different geographic locations, the inability of patients to leave their homes, or locales that are inaccessible, such as Antarctica or space (CCHP, 2022). The same reasons may lead two or more healthcare professionals to use telehealth to meet, consult, or teach. As seen in the case study, telehealth is useful when there are only a few providers available to treat patients who live in remote, inaccessible, or large geographic areas for both meeting with patients and for getting consultations from experts.

Types of Telehealth

Generally, telehealth visits are conducted in two ways to deliver healthcare: asynchronous and synchronous. **Asynchronous telehealth** happens in different time frames for the sender and receiver. This type of telehealth uses **store-and-forward (S&F)** technology in which a digital camera, scanner, or other technology (e.g., x-ray machine) is used to capture a still image or video electronically. The patient health information (image and/or data) is transmitted from the originating site (where the patient is) to another site for the healthcare professional to review and interpret at a later time (CCHP, 2022). Some examples of S&F include email or messaging in the electronic health record or other secured app, wound care using image evaluation, vital sign monitoring, and laboratory results evaluation. This method of telehealth communication is often used to gather data prior to an in-person or synchronous telehealth visit or with follow-up care.

Synchronous telehealth involves two-way interaction in real time, often using a microphone and camera and sometimes specialized monitoring devices. Synchronous telehealth requires the use of telecommunication devices that permit two-way communication. The oldest of these is the telephone, but current telehealth technology generally includes video conferencing using two-way video and audio. Using telehealth technology does not have to be complicated. Many telehealth services only require the patient to have a cell phone, tablet, or laptop with a camera, microphone, and speaker. Figure 6-2 summarizes synchronous and asynchronous telehealth.

Both asynchronous and synchronous telehealth may make use of other instruments with connectivity to a telehealth cart or with the ability to transmit data to a clinician at a different location. These assessment instruments can include but are not limited to an otoscope, a camera to capture skin observations, and a stethoscope. They can be used either in real time or in S&F mode. **Remote patient monitoring** is the measurement and/or transmitting of patient data to a monitoring center or healthcare professional (NCTRC, 2021). This can be done in a variety of situations to monitor health conditions such as chronic diseases in the home environment or in the hospital to monitor acute conditions (Fig. 6-3).

By using a combination of **robotics** (use of robots) and virtual reality, a surgeon can perform surgery by manipulating instruments remotely. This use of robotics is a form of **telepresence**,

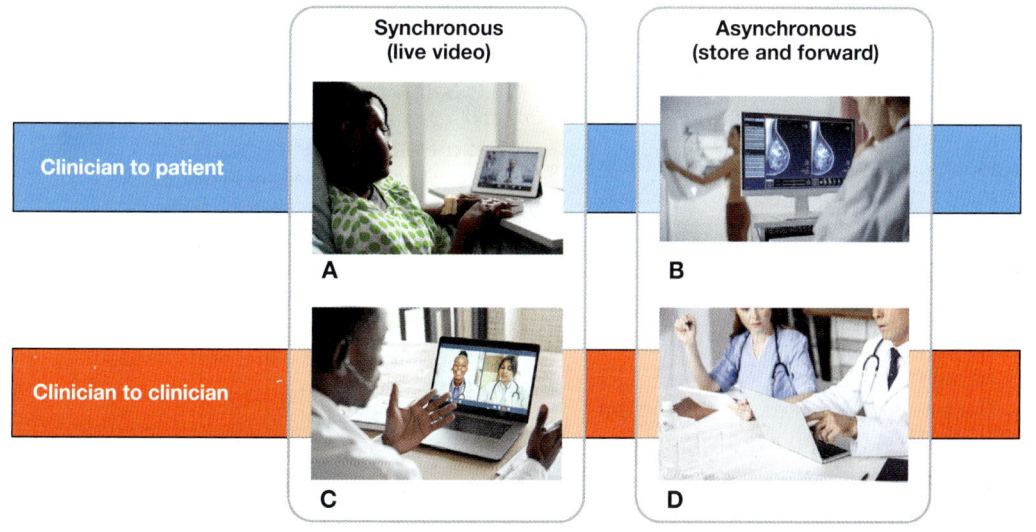

Figure 6-2. Synchronous and asynchronous telehealth technology. (**A.** Shutterstock/DC Studio; **B.** Shutterstock/Gorodenkoff; **C.** Shutterstock/Ground Picture; **D.** Shutterstock/Lightfield Studios.)

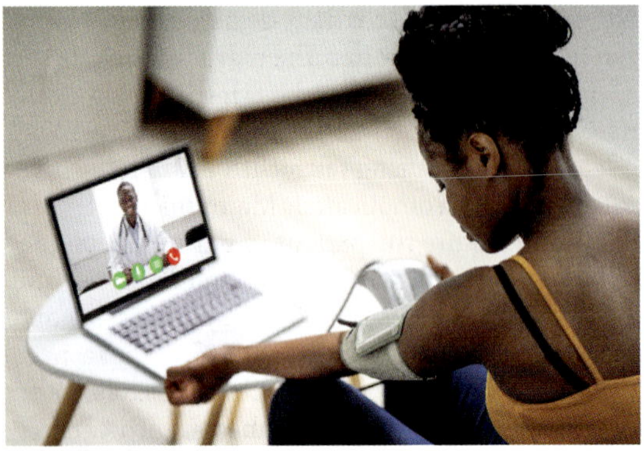

Figure 6-3. Person using home telehealth monitoring equipment. (Shutterstock/Andrey_Popov.)

which is the use of technology to provide the appearance of a person's presence, though they are located at a remote site. Holoportation was mentioned earlier in the chapter and is another type of telepresence.

Although video conferencing is possible with a modem and telephone service, a higher quality of service is usually preferred. Some services require at least a secure T1 fiberoptic line or a line on an integrated digital network, which must not only connect the sites but also extend to the rooms where both the patient and the distant consultant are located. Telehealth also may use large satellite systems that have a global audience.

Telenursing

Telenursing is the use of telehealth to provide home nursing care. The American Academy of Ambulatory Care Nursing (AAACN) notes that telehealth nursing is a complex and multifaceted nursing specialty that involves both independent and collaborative practice in patient encounters, using health information technologies in a virtual environment (AAACN, 2018). What began as the handling of basic healthcare questions over the phone in the 1970s has morphed into nursing specialists caring for patients across geographical distances. Nurses may also work as telepresenters, located with the patient and participating in a consultation with a provider at a distant location. Telenursing offers nurses a chance to create more collaborative and autonomous roles and at the same time reduces the overall cost of healthcare.

They can work in a variety of places including hospitals, local community clinics, and Federally Qualified Health Centers (FQHCs) (Rutledge & Gustin, 2021). As with other areas of nursing, it is important to set standards for providing care and to ensure nurses are educated about the appropriate delivery of telehealth.

Standards for Telenursing and Telehealth

To establish set standards in the subspecialty of telephone nursing in ambulatory care, the AAACN established the telehealth nursing practice special interest group in 1995. In 1997, the AAACN developed the *Scope and Standards of Practice for Professional Telehealth Nursing* that addresses six clinical practice standards for telenursing, including assessment, nursing diagnosis, identification of expected outcomes and goals, planning, implementation, and evaluation (AAACN, 2018).

The American Telehealth Association (ATA) focuses on advancing telehealth and has information about telehealth practice guidelines. The goals of this organization include the delivery of safe, equitable, affordable, and appropriate virtual healthcare (ATA, n.d.). ATA policy principles are outlined in Box 6-1.

BOX 6-1 ATA Policy Principals

- Ensure patient choice, access, and satisfaction.
- Enhance provider autonomy.
- Expand reimbursement to incentivize 21st-century virtual care.
- Enable healthcare delivery across state lines.
- Ensure access to nonphysician providers.
- Expand access for underserved and at-risk populations.
- Support older adults and expand "aging in place."
- Protect patient privacy and mitigate cybersecurity risks.
- Ensure program integrity.

(Adapted from The American Telemedicine Association (ATA). (2020, July 22). ATA policy principles. https://www.americantelemed.org/policies/ata-policy-principles/)

The U.S. Department of Health and Human Services (USDHHS) has best practice guides for practitioners getting started with telehealth. These cover strategies, preparation for staff, preparation for patients, and billing. These guides cover a variety of specialties, including behavioral health, cancer care, maternal health, and school-based services. Even physical therapy, which is traditionally considered as requiring in-person care, can benefit from telehealth services and has a best practice guide (USDHHS, n.d.).

The USDHHS created Medicare policy changes after the COVID-19 pandemic to support the use of telehealth. Rural emergency hospitals are now eligible originating sites, allowing patients to receive telehealth at these sites. For behavioral and mental health services, FQHCs and rural health clinics can serve as providers and Medicare patients can receive telehealth in the home. There are no geographic restrictions for behavioral and mental telehealth sites, and these services can be delivered using audio-only communication (USDHHS, 2023b).

In a classic international study completed between 2004 and 2005 that has not yet been replicated, most of the telenurses surveyed indicated they learned telenursing skills on the job (Grady & Schlachta-Fairchild, 2007). Most of the nurses had no prior experience with telehealth before their telenursing positions, but 89% of those surveyed indicated that telehealth should be included in basic nursing curriculum. Telehealth is still not a standard component for entry-level registered nurse education in the United States, though the American Association of Colleges of Nursing (AACN) Essentials now contains telehealth competencies in both the entry-level and advanced categories (2021).

Telehealth and Education

Patient education is one of the most important nursing duties. Most telehealth involves an educational component either delivered during synchronous visits or asynchronously through links to websites or videos. Several successful education projects support the use of telehealth. Fitzner and Moss (2013) reviewed the literature related to telehealth and emerging technologic tools that supported best practice for self-management of diabetes. Findings of their research supported the use of telehealth for education and training when it provides benefit, when it does not negatively affect the provider's care, and when costs are reimbursed. The researchers identified 10 areas of best practice for telehealth delivery of education and training, which have been used by the Centers for Disease Control and Prevention (CDC) to develop a guide for using telehealth technologies in diabetes self-management (CDC, 2022b). These principles are applicable to any use of telehealth for patient education, not just diabetes.

In a more recent telenursing example, a combination of telephone calls, video clips, and automatic reminders in the span of 3 to 12 months significantly increased patient self-care for diabetes. Health promotion activities included physical activity, blood sugar monitoring, diet, and foot care (Marlina et al., 2023).

Telehealth is also useful for educating healthcare professionals, for example, for continuing education and preparing practitioners. Telehealth education is especially useful in rural or remote areas where it is difficult to recruit healthcare professionals and where costs, difficulty of travel, and time away from the workplace are barriers to receiving care from specialists located in more populous areas. As described in the case study, Project ECHO uses videoconferencing via the internet to provide mentoring and education to providers caring for patients with COVID-19 on tribal lands (Begay et al., 2021). Since its creation in 2003, Project ECHO has grown globally with medical professionals from 193 countries now participating. Participants in Project ECHO are part of a virtual community with peers who share clinical challenges and get feedback, providing support and guidance to each other. In this way, it fosters an "all learn, all teach" approach (UNM Health Sciences, 2023).

EXAMPLES OF TELEHEALTH

As healthcare shifts away from the hospital and into home and community settings, the therapeutic uses for telehealth increase. A much broader range of healthcare professionals such as nurse practitioners, nutritionists, social workers, and home healthcare aides have roles in the provision of telehealth. Examples of settings in which education is delivered via telehealth include homecare, mental health and psychiatric services, primary care, intensive and trauma care, and care for those experiencing chronic diseases and disasters.

Telehomecare

Telehomecare refers to the ability to monitor data in the patient's home rather than the provider's work setting. Many of the telehealth examples that follow can be considered telehomecare but for specialty services. The advantages of telehomecare are that it allows the patient the comforts of home, improves quality of life, and avoids time-consuming and costly visits to office appointments or hospital admissions. Successful telehomecare provides comprehensive and coordinated care and accessible services, is patient-centered, and demonstrates a commitment to quality and safety (HRSA, 2021). Ongoing monitoring allows identification of potential problems before they become significant problems. Because telehomecare can eliminate unnecessary emergency room visits and hospital visits, it is cost-effective. Some of the duties of a home health nurse can be done through telehomecare.

Portable Monitoring Devices

Emerging monitoring technology facilitates a proactive approach to early identification of symptoms before problems develop. It can be used for tracking existing conditions to avoid complications. This has the potential for maintaining the patient's quality of life, reducing acute exacerbations of disease processes, and avoiding unnecessary medical costs. This type of monitoring can be achieved with **portable monitoring devices**, which include an input device and various types of peripheral monitoring equipment or accessories. Many of the input devices use a touch screen with text and audio to ask assessment questions about the patient's health. Examples of monitoring accessories include blood pressure cuffs, electrocardiograms, blood glucose meters, weight scales, fluid status monitors, pulse oximeters, monitors for prothrombin time/international normalized ratio, peak flow meters, and spirometers.

To monitor blood pressure without a cuff, a wearable skin patch made with flexible piezoresistive sensors and epidermal electrocardiogram sensors is available. These patches can detect changes in pulse and blood pressure with activity or at home. They use a very small amount of power (3 nanowatts) to maintain a steady pulse signal and measure those vital signs (Mukherjee et al., 2022). Other skin patch sensors can monitor the sweat of a person and determine the chemical makeup to virtually measure bodily fluids. For example, the polydimethylsiloxane (PDMS) dermal patch is a device that can read the body's interstitial fluid and detect molecules such as glucose without invasively extracting any fluid (Mukherjee et al., 2022).

In 2020, a wearable stethoscope was designed to capture patients' lung and cardiac sounds remotely via a specific garment implanted with piezoelectric film to capture and send thoracic sounds to the healthcare team (Yilmaz et al., 2020). By adding digital filters to mimic the filters on a physical stethoscope, differences between sounds on a digital versus physical stethoscope were minimized. The device is capable of picking up abnormal sounds (Yilmaz et al., 2020).

Smart clothing, also called e-textiles, contain biometric sensors that can measure sleep quality, activity and stress levels, temperature, and heart rhythms (Marr, 2021). Sensors are woven into fabric that can collect data and send it to an app that makes lifestyle recommendations based on the data. The data can also be shared with healthcare providers. Smart clothing can include underwear, socks, bras, leggings, and t-shirts. Advantages of smart clothing include comfort, washability, real-time data monitoring, and the ability to monitor a large amount of surface area. They may also be fashionable (Ahsan et al., 2022).

CASE STUDY

The case study described how smart thermometers have been used to predict future COVID-19 hotspots with accuracy. What other portable monitoring devices or wearables could be used to contribute to improved response times by healthcare providers? What role can wearables play in preventative health?

Self-Monitoring With Mobile Devices

Teaching patients to monitor their own health promotes wellness and prevents hospitalization and disease progression. Self-monitoring is growing in popularity with the release of low-cost or free health and wellness apps available without prescriptions. There are thousands of health and wellness apps for smartphones and tablets available. In addition to apps, wearable devices connect to mobile devices and can be used for self-monitoring. However, the data are not sent to a clinician. In one study, 74% of patients say using wearables and other mHealth tools helps them cope with and manage conditions (Franklin, 2021). Many apps and wearable monitoring devices used for disease monitoring and management were originally designed for fitness use and therefore are not regulated by the U.S. Food and Drug Administration (FDA), inhibiting official medical approval (Mattison et al., 2022). Without FDA approval and regulation, wearable technology cannot legally support clinical decision making.

Depending on the specific device, the wearable Fitbit assists the user in monitoring sleep quality, calories burned, and body activity (Fitbit, n.d.). Fitbit also has a WiFi-powered smart weight scale that allows the user to track their weight, body mass index, and percent body fat. The wearable Fitbit device and smart scales connect to the iPhone or Android smartphone app. Users can also use the social aspect of Fitbit to share and compare progress with others. Other smartwatches and wearables provide similar functions.

Cardiac rhythm devices are available for self-monitoring by consumers. For example, AliveCor KardiaMobile provides the ability to monitor one's heart rhythm using a touch pad that connects to an iPhone or Android smartphone app (Fig. 6-4), and it is available for purchase without a prescription (AliveCor, n.d.). The cardiac tracing, like Lead I, displays on the associated smartphone app noting the type of rhythm. Users can store their rhythm tracings in secure cloud storage as well as share the tracing with their healthcare providers. Additional features for purchase include blood pressure tracking using an associated blood pressure monitor, weight tracking, and medication tracking. The AliveCor monitoring device is FDA-approved for use and can detect the six most common arrhythmias.

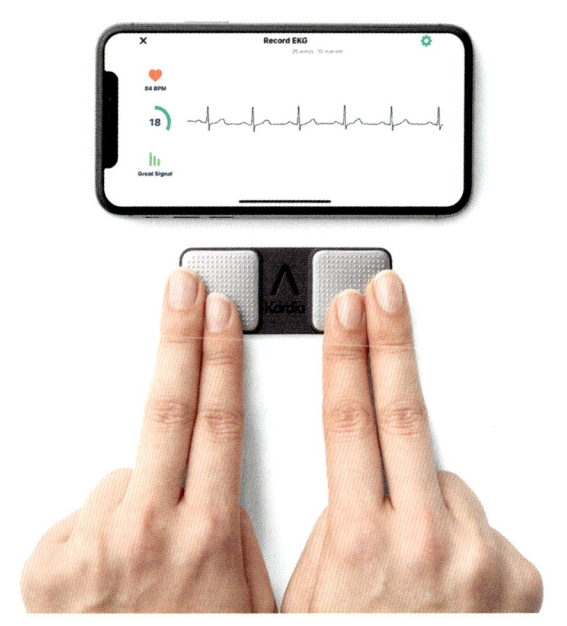

Figure 6-4. AliveCor heart smartphone case attachment. (Used with permission of AliveCor.)

Automatic Pill Dispensers and Reminders

Filling pill boxes and ensuring patients have taken their medications correctly is one of the duties of a home health nurse. Automatic pill dispensers and reminders are a way to do this using telehealth. Pill dispensers may include auditory reminders to prompt patients to take their medications, even if the medication is not a pill. Some automatic pill dispensers provide patient reminders to take the medication with food or to take an insulin injection. With some systems, if the patient does not dispense the medications within a specified time frame, the system notifies the caregiver by phone, email, or text message. If the caregiver does not answer the telephone, the device phones the support center. Other systems monitor compliance through a secure website. Several companies make automatic pill dispensers with and without reminders. Examples include Lifeline, ePill, MedaCube, and Hero.

Primary Care

The use of telehealth benefits people living in rural or remote areas where residents may have few options for healthcare and few, if any, specialists. The case study provides an example of how lack of access to healthcare providers led to the highest per capita death rate from COVID-19 for people in the Navajo Nation. In a Pew study, researchers reported that nearly a quarter of Americans living in rural areas say that access to good doctors and hospitals is a major problem in their communities (Lam et al., 2018). In Maine, there are many barrier islands inhabited by residents, many of whom make their livelihood from the lobster industry. Travel to the mainland for these residents can be inconvenient and result in a loss of income. To address the healthcare delivery problem, Sunbeam Health Services provides virtual doctors' visits by using a ship staffed by nurses and equipped with closed-circuit television (Maine Seacoast Mission, n.d.). Telehealth services are also provided from a renovated clinic on Swan's Island, one of the barrier islands.

Figure 6-5 shows the density of physicians, nurses, and midwives on a global scale, further demonstrating that the use of telehealth can potentially overcome problems associated with lack of access to healthcare providers.

Telemental Health

Telemental health is the use of telehealth to deliver mental health services, which may also be called telepsychiatry or telepsychology. Healthcare providers use telehealth to deliver care for various mental health concerns. Its use has increased substantially since the COVID-19 pandemic, especially in the veteran population (NIMH, n.d.). During the COVID-19 pandemic, many mental health services shifted to virtual appointments. Some veterans' clinics saw an increase in appointment volume and a decrease in no-show rates when the appointments moved to telehealth (Goetter et al., 2022). Other veterans' clinics saw a decline in new patient volumes but ongoing mental health appointments and prescribing remained stable (Zhang et al., 2022). Telemental health offers greater convenience and broader reach.

While there are many advantages of telemental health, barriers exist as well. Barriers related to access to technology, quality, cost, privacy, and insurance reimbursement and coverage of these services via telehealth persist (NIMH, n.d.). In a review of telehealth use by Indigenous populations, mental health was the most frequent focus of telehealth interventions (Moecke et al., 2023). The use of telemental health had the benefit of being anonymous and private, preventing feelings of shame due to stigma around mental health services. However, the lack of in-person human connection created difficulty with enhancing trusting relationships with medical professionals (Moecke et al., 2023). Despite barriers and limitations, telehealth is a promising way to facilitate broader mental healthcare.

e-Intensive Care Units

An aging population, advances in complex surgical procedures, and the recent exposure to a pandemic have increased the need for intensive care unit (ICU) beds across the United States, and that need is expected to continue growing (Straits Research, 2023). **E-intensive care** units are a form of telemedicine that are able to meet these needs and are designed to enhance the delivery of intensive patient care. The current use of telepresence of intensivists in ICUs is redefining the meaning of critical care remote monitoring. E-intensive care can be achieved with tele-intensive care units or robotics.

Tele-Intensive Care Units

The global tele-intensive care market is forecasted to be worth $12.4 billion in 2027 compared to $3.18 billion in 2022 (Straits Research, 2023). Additionally, reports on tele-intensive care units provide promising results for the use of telehealth in critical care. For example, a tele-intensive care unit introduced in Potomac Valley Hospital, a rural hospital in the mountains of West Virginia, decreased the need for critical patients to be transferred to a tertiary care center nearly 2 hours away by ambulance (Dudas et al., 2023). A cost-effective, collaborative effort increased the capacity of care the rural hospital could provide critically ill patients while allowing the team of providers to

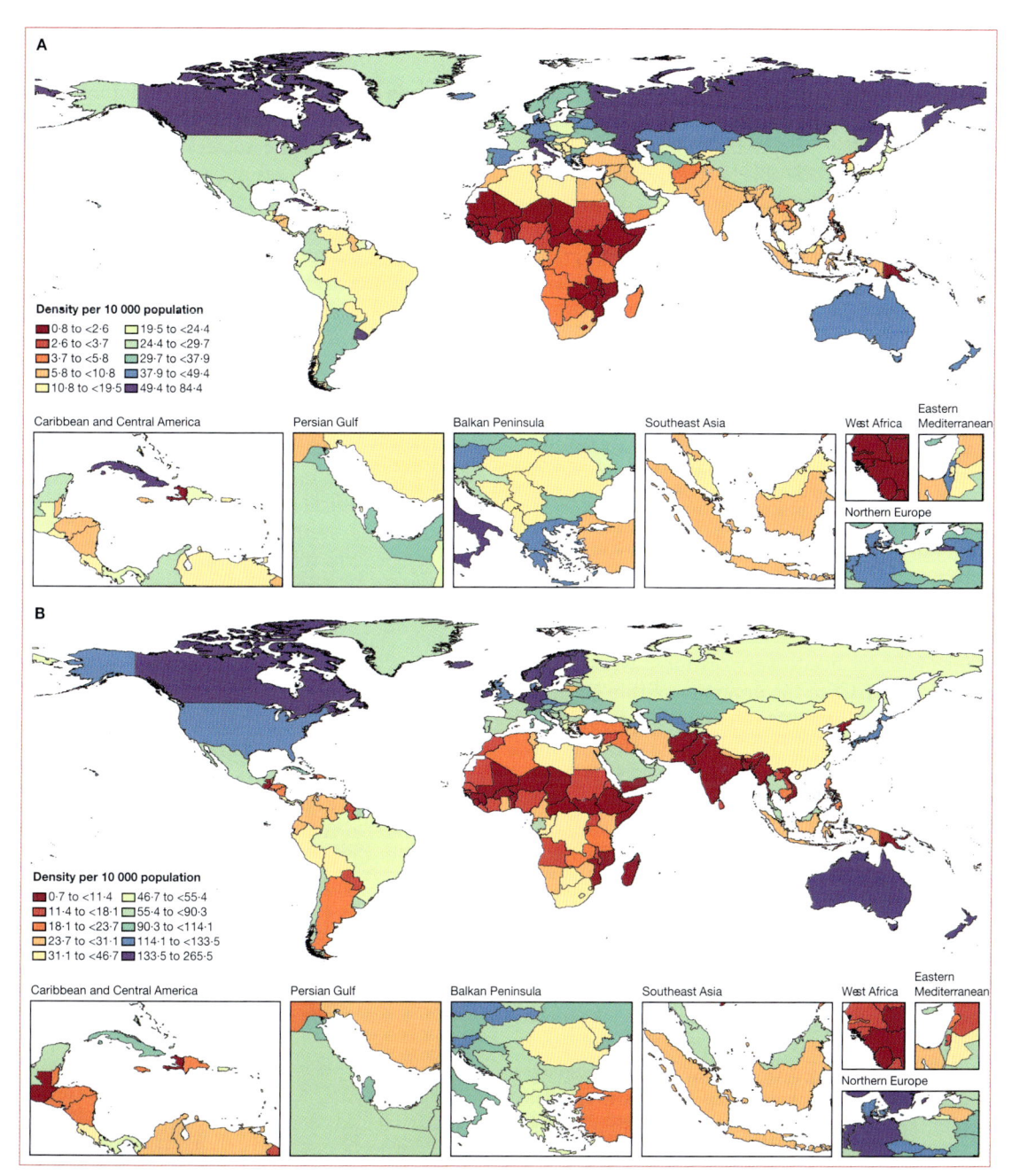

Figure 6-5. Density of access to healthcare workers by global location. **A.** Physicians. **B.** Nurses and midwives. (From GBD 2019 Human Resources for Health Collaborators. (2022). Measuring the availability of human resources for health and its relationship to universal health coverage for 204 countries and territories from 1990 to 2019: a systematic analysis for the Global Burden of Disease Study 2019. *The Lancet*, *399*(10341), P2129–P2154. https://doi.org/10.1016/S0140-6736(22)00532-3)

continue serving the community without turning patients away. A virtual ICU was developed to include daily rounding of an intensivist at the tertiary care center via video call with a hospitalist at Potomac Valley Hospital. The intensivist from the larger hospital was able to collaborate with the Potomac Valley physicians and create new plans of care and treatment options for ICU patients. After successful implementation of the program, Potomac Valley Hospital saw a decrease in transfer of patients to other hospitals, an increase in number of patients within the ICU, and more physician comfort with providing critical care (Dudas et al., 2023).

Telehealth has been shown to be effective in the intensive care setting when discharging a patient, as well. A nurse-led telehealth model in Florida was used to connect patients and families being discharged from the neonatal intensive care unit (NICU) with a NICU team. The program, called Baby Steps, included virtual visits of 15 to 60 minutes at 24 and 48 hours after discharge (Sarik et al., 2022). The families also had access to on-demand telehealth services for 2 weeks after discharge as part of the program. Within the first 18 months, 378 infants were enrolled in the program, and the rate of hospital readmissions within the first 30 days of discharge decreased 46% (Sarik et al., 2022). The rate of emergency care use within 4 weeks after discharge was 13.8% in families participating in Baby Steps compared to 30.9% in families who were not participating.

Nurses agree that improved patient outcomes are important, but implementing tele-intensive care has implications for the entire ICU environment. The use of these tele-intensive care unit tools requires extensive planning and communications as well as workflow redesign. The most important factor is buy-in by all affected departments, including not only the ICU staff but also attending physicians, hospital leadership, information services, and respiratory therapy.

A survey done on hospitals in the New England region found that while hospitals and emergency departments are willing to participate in teleconsultation programs and have the capacity to do so, these programs can be hard to execute. The lack of standardization between hospital systems could ruin many time-sensitive consults or procedures due to a delay in communication (Boyle et al., 2023).

A study by Wilkes et al. (2016) reinforced the importance of organizational and teamwork factors that influence the success of tele-intensive care units. The study results indicated the importance of addressing cultural and teamwork factors to reduce negative feelings and misunderstanding between care providers at collaborating sites. It also demonstrated the importance for intensive care nurses and physicians to have a mutual respect in order to best coordinate care.

Robotics

Robotic telepresence can allow providers and nurses not only to communicate with the patient (Fig. 6-6) but also to remotely assess their physical state using medical equipment like an ultrasound machine or a stethoscope (Teng et al., 2022). Telepresence via robotics reduces response time to a patient in distress and time-sensitive tasks for patients with critical care needs. Robotics can also help make up for staffing shortages in ICUs at night or in rural and remote areas by allowing physicians and nurses in other locations to provide care for patients. Hospitals using robotics are also able to save money with a higher patient turnover rate and lower external transfers to areas that can provide higher levels of care (Teng et al., 2022).

The CareDo robot and system were developed during the COVID-19 pandemic to deliver supplies, foster communication between the patient and care team or families, and recognize facial

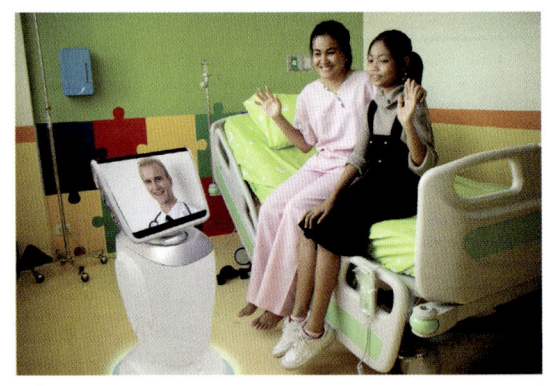

Figure 6-6. Telemedicine robots. (Shutterstock/MONOPOLY919.)

expressions in patients on isolation protocols to report back to the healthcare team (Yu et al., 2023). The robot was programmed to enter into isolation rooms alone and then use real-time communication solutions to initiate video calls, a convolutional neural network to recognize facial expressions, and incremental motion mapping to deliver supplies and operate remotely. During the trial period conducted by Zhejiang University, the CareDo robot was able to accurately read a happy facial expression on the patient 95% of the time, a neutral expression 92.8% of the time, and a sad expression 80% of the time. The robot's ability to deliver supplies and requested items to the patient in isolation decreased the chances of transmitting infection to the staff while providing the patient with what they needed (Yu et al., 2023).

Teletrauma Care

Teletrauma is used to obtain second opinions and advice from trauma care experts. A 2023 literature review found that not only did trauma patients save money when being treated with telehealth services but they were also more likely to stay and wait to be seen and treated by a physician (Alter et al., 2023). The length of time spent in the emergency department by trauma patients was either comparable or reduced when telehealth services were implemented before admission (Alter et al., 2023). Teletrauma care has also been used to deliver care in parts of the world affected by violence and war.

Remote hospitals and clinics have been able to use teletrauma and obtain reimbursement for these services (CMS, 2022a). Rural and remote physicians and staff want to provide the best possible care to the patients while keeping the inconvenience of care, travel and expense of care as low as possible. Without specialists available, however, patients are often transferred to larger metropolitan hospitals where specialized care is available. Telehealth equipment can bring specialty care to rural and remote hospitals virtually. A study of transfer rates of acutely ill children in rural emergency departments in Northern California found that telemedicine consultations resulted in significantly fewer transfers as compared to telephone consultations (Marcin et al., 2023). Near the Canadian border, Jackman, Maine has just one clinic, and the nearest emergency room is more than an hour away. To provide care around the clock, paramedics staff the clinic after hours to provide urgent care by using telehealth to connect with emergency room physicians at a hospital 100 miles away. By collaborating with trauma care experts, the paramedics have been able to treat wounds and heart attacks (Fitzgerald, 2022).

A survey of patients receiving trauma care and living in rural Mississippi revealed that for the 87% of patients surveyed with internet access at home, 60% would be interested in using telehealth to complete follow-up appointments and connect with their providers using technology versus commuting back to the hospital that treated them (Emily et al., 2022). This use of telehealth would help these patients connect with their providers about their traumatic injury and recovery and save them time and money commuting back and forth to their doctors' offices.

A 2022 survey of data found that the Midwest region uses telehealth in their emergency centers more than any other region in the United States, and that Maine, Alaska, and Missouri are the three individual states that use the most emergency room telehealth technology in the country (Castner et al., 2022). Since 2017, the use of telehealth in emergency rooms has grown and is predicted to continue growing as more nurses are gaining experience and comfort with the devices and their use (Castner et al., 2022).

Telehealth for Chronic Illness Management

Approximately 60% of Americans have one chronic illness, and 40% have two or more (CDC, 2022a). For patients with chronic diseases, telehealth can be a powerful self-management tool. Traditionally, chronic disease has been managed through an episodic office-based model rather than a care management model, which uses frequent patient contact and regular physiologic measurement. Especially since the COVID-19 pandemic, telehealth communication systems have facilitated better patient adherence to treatment programs and smoother communication with providers. Patients with chronic illnesses can have their statuses monitored remotely, with technology sending live updates to the healthcare team, requiring little to no self-reporting by the patient (Yu et al., 2023). Home health monitoring devices (Box 6-2) such as cardiac monitors and insulin pods can collect and transmit vital signs and other data to healthcare providers (Fig. 6-7).

A 2023 article notes patients with heart failure and their providers were satisfied with the use of teleheath for managing their conditions, and most felt that using telehealth instead of in-person services did not impair the quality of their healthcare (Leonard et al., 2023). Infrastructure support provided to the patients was vital in their use and approval of technology when managing their heart failure.

Research studies support the use of remote patient monitoring to reduce emergency department visits, reduce hospital readmission rates, improve care, and reduce costs. Lemelin et al. (2020) conducted a trial in which people with diabetes were recruited and randomized between a control and study group to determine the efficacy of telehomecare on disease management. They found that participants in the telehomecare group had better hemoglobin A1c results on future tests than did the control group.

While telehealth systems are effective in many ways at managing chronic illness, they require technologic access. Many patients lack the necessary digital access at home, and the inequities they experience in healthcare are only exacerbated when patients are expected or required to use this technology (Williams & Shang, 2023). These patients will continue to fall behind unless accommodations are made to increase their digital utilization as telehealth advances.

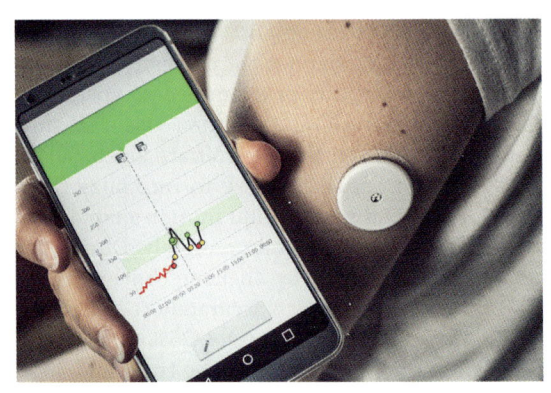

Figure 6-7. Person wearing remote blood glucose monitor. (Shutterstock/Lukasz Powel Szczepanski.)

Disaster Healthcare

Telehealth has been successfully used in providing healthcare during disasters. The North American Treaty Organization (NATO) developed a telemedicine system for use in combat zones and emergencies (NATO, 2017). The Centers for Medicare & Medicaid Services (CMS) has a toolkit detailing how to respond to public health emergencies, such as natural disasters and pandemics, including ways to make telehealth more flexible during these times (CMS, 2022b).

Telehealth played a large role in caring for the mental health of people working in healthcare during the COVID-19 pandemic. The U.S. government passed legislation to expand the use of telehealth to ease the stress of healthcare personnel caring for their patients, like reducing limitations on prescribing medications over telehealth visits or expanding the geographic locations where telehealth technology could be used (Gaiser et al., 2023). An online hotline for physicians to connect with licensed psychiatrists called the Physician Support Line was developed in response to the pandemic crisis to help the doctors deal with their own feelings of personal crisis and burnout.

Natural disasters have the potential to knock out power and eliminate the use of telehealth technology (Lokmic-Tomkins et al., 2023). However, when the digital technology is preserved, telehealth can function as a triage

---

BOX 6-2 Home Healthcare Devices
- Weight scales
- Pulse oximeters
- Blood glucose meters
- Blood pressure monitors
- Apnea monitors
- Heart monitors
- Monitors for dementia and Parkinson disease
- Breathing apparatuses
- Fetal monitors
- Medication dispensers

service after a disaster hits. After Hurricane Florence hit the coast of North Carolina in 2018, patients were able to use telehealth to connect with a provider virtually who could assess if they needed to be seen in an urgent care setting or emergency room for their conditions or injuries. This system was able to reduce the strain on emergency rooms after the disaster by deferring the transport of 35% of patients potentially requiring emergency room care to an urgent care or primary care office instead (Lokmic-Tomkins et al., 2023).

ISSUES WITH TELEHEALTH

Telehealth can provide many benefits such as enhanced patient care, reduced travel time, increased productivity, access to specialists, and expanded educational opportunities. However, many issues surround this mode of healthcare delivery. The four main issues are high-speed internet access, reimbursement, regulation, and fraud.

High-Speed Internet Access

With the introduction of new technologies, it is vital that there is the infrastructure to support these technologies. One of the key advancements needed to support telehealth is the expansion of internet connectivity. In Chapter 4, internet access was discussed as a social determinant of health, meaning access to the internet plays a role in health outcomes. It is estimated that approximately 21 million Americans are living in a "digital desert," meaning they do not have access to broadband internet (Cooke, 2020). This includes the Navajo Nation, which is the largest Native American reservation in the United States, spanning Arizona, New Mexico, and Southern Utah. Figure 6-8 shows the location of digital deserts in the United States and the location of the Navajo Nation.

The lack of internet access can exacerbate health disparities and other prominent socioeconomic factors that influence health outcomes (Bauerly et al., 2019). The Affordable Connectivity Program legislation was enacted in 2021 to help provide

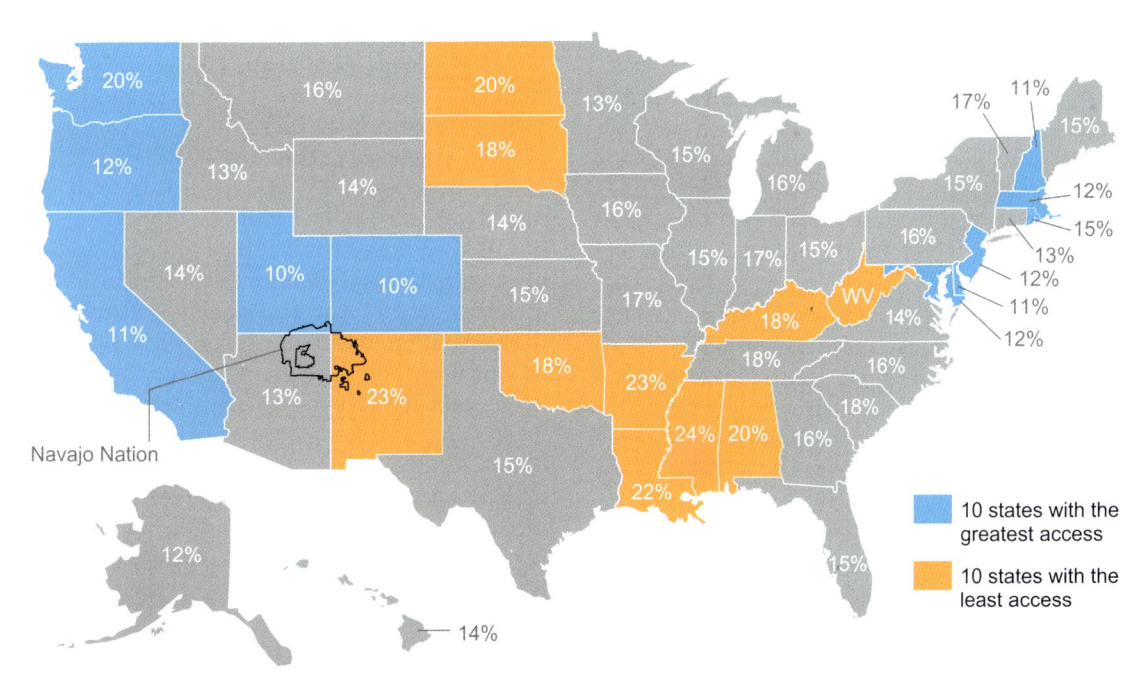

Figure 6-8. Digital deserts and the Navajo Nation. Percentages of households that do not have internet. (Data from Cooke K. (2020, April 27). The top internet deserts in the US. https://www.satelliteinternet.com/resources/top-internet-deserts/)

internet access to people in the United States living below the poverty threshold and/or in rural areas (Early & Hernandez, 2021). Improvements in access should be inclusive of cultural, literacy, and linguistic needs, follow federally regulated privacy standards, and track access and usage data across socioeconomic and demographic characteristics to monitor for increasing digital divides (Rodriguez et al., 2020).

Reimbursement

How healthcare providers are reimbursed for telehealth services can be a barrier to the widespread adoption of telehealth. The U.S. healthcare system is shaped by insurance providers (third-party payers), both government and private. Currently, there is no uniformity for the reimbursement of telehealth and telemedicine services. Conflict exists between federal- and state-regulated reimbursement systems (CCHP, n.d.a). While Medicaid is jointly funded by federal and state governments and largely developed by state policy, federal standards must be met in efficiency, economy, and quality of care. Because each state has the freedom to administer its policies, telehealth is reimbursed differently in each state. With private payers, there are no federal laws governing coverage and reimbursement, but many states do have state laws that regulate the coverage and payment parities (CTeL, 2022).

At the federal level, telehealth reimbursement is dictated by Medicare regulations in four key areas (CCHP, n.d.a):

- Who is providing the services: Those covered include physicians, nurse practitioners, clinical nurse specialists, certified registered nurse anesthetists, nurse midwives, physician assistants, registered dietitians or nutrition professionals, clinical psychologists, and clinical social workers.
- The type of service being delivered: Over 100 types of services are covered.
- The patient location: Medicare limits the use of telehealth to rural health professional shortage areas or outside metropolitan statistical areas.
- How services are delivered: Telehealth must be delivered via live video conferencing.

At the state level, telehealth reimbursement is dictated by Medicaid and/or local commercial payer systems. The same key areas must be addressed at the state level with the following variations or issues (CCHP, n.d.a):

- Who is providing the services: States vary on who can provide services, but most include physicians, nurse practitioners, and psychiatrists.
- The type of service being delivered: Some states follow federally regulated requirements for Medicare, while other states allow any services as long as they are medically necessary.
- How services are delivered: All 50 states and Washington, D.C., reimburse for live video as of September 2020; S&F is reimbursed in 17 states; and remote patient monitoring is reimbursed in 22 states.

The United States enacted the Coronavirus Aid, Relief, and Economic Security (CARES) Act in 2020 in response to the COVID-19 pandemic. The CARES Act specifies the implementation of a variety of programs, and addresses issues related to the pandemic. This legislation supports small businesses through tax credits and payroll protections, provides financial relief to families with low and moderate incomes, and financially supports states in the deployment of broadband internet in rural areas to support distance learning, telework, and telehealth/telemedicine efforts (U.S. Department of the Treasury, n.d.). In conjunction with the CARES Act, an emergency declaration known as the Stafford Act or the National Emergencies Act has changed several rules for telehealth, making it easier for patients and providers to utilize. Under the declaration, telephone without live video can now be used, and the patient can now be in their home when receiving telehealth services (CMS, 2022a).

The CARES Act dramatically improved the rates of telehealth reimbursement, which in turn increased telehealth utilization at the highest rate ever recorded. However, the CARES Act may be a temporary measure. Until providers are fully reimbursed for providing care through telehealth, much of the population will remain underserved post pandemic. Nurses should advocate for utilization and reimbursement since telehealth has the potential for treating illnesses in the early stages, preventing costly procedures and readmissions. Changes to Medicare reimbursement will require congressional actions to lift any limitations placed on the CMS. For telemedicine to survive/thrive, reimbursement must be a joint effort between states, the federal government, and private payers.

Regulation

Under the 10th Amendment of the U.S. Constitution, individual states have assumed the power to regulate healthcare practitioners for the protection of their citizens (Congress.gov, n.d.). No state, however, has the authority over practice in another state. Certification and licensure requirements are also state-level decisions. Because of this, travel nursing and telehealth both create difficult questions. If a nurse practicing and licensed in one state provides nursing care to a patient in another state, where should care be regulated? Should it be at the location of the provider or the patient? Should the healthcare provider be licensed in both states? These questions have created barriers to the expansion of telehealth.

The Federation of State Medical Boards (FSMB) has worked to develop a framework for regulating interstate practice. The work began in 1996 and was officially adopted in April 2022. In 2016, the FSMB reported that 75% of medical state boards listed telemedicine as their number one medical regulatory topic (FSMB, 2016). Their framework clearly states that the physician must be licensed to practice in the state where the patient is receiving care (FSMB, 2022). This has led to interstate compacts that expedite licensure for providers in order to provide care in that state or allow them to practice under a single multistate license. The decision to adopt the license is still left to the individual state boards (USDHHS, 2023a).

The National Council of State Boards of Nursing (NCSBN) endorsed the Nurse Licensure Compact (NLC) as a framework for regulating the interstate practice of nursing for registered nurses and licensed practical/vocational nurses. It was later upgraded to the Enhanced Nurse Licensure Compact (eNLC). The eNLC removes regulatory barriers for travel and telehealth nursing and reduces costs for licensing fees and renewals. Nurses meeting uniform licensure requirements are eligible for multistate licenses that can be used in all eNLC states (NCSBN, n.d.). They can practice both in person and through telehealth to assess and provide care in other states according to the rules and regulations of those states. The NCSBN maintains up-to-date information for current licensure as well as pending legislation on the NLC website. The system shares licensure and disciplinary history for nurses with participating states. Figure 6-9 shows the states that have enacted the eNLC.

It is important to stay abreast of laws and policies through the Center for Connected Health Policy (CCHP). Liability and malpractice can be issues when licensing and credentialing laws do not clearly specify the use of telehealth (Becker et al., 2019; CCHP, n.d.b). HealthIT.gov (2023) has links to information regarding licensure for telehealth.

Fraud

Many states have introduced bills that allow healthcare providers to be paid the same amount of money for online or in-person services to create incentives for providers to continue offering telehealth services. These services have grown exponentially since the COVID-19 pandemic. For example, Medicare visits conducted with telehealth increased from 840,000 in 2019 to 52.7 million in 2020 (Belloni, 2022). The rise in the use of telehealth has been accompanied by concerns about fraud. Some states are responding with provisions like that found in Texas which requires that "all physicians utilizing telemedicine medical services in their practices shall adopt protocols to prevent fraud and abuse through the use of telemedicine medical services" (Belloni, 2022). In California, where Assembly Bill 32 ensures payment equality for phone, video, and asynchronous patient monitoring, providers are responsible for determining if the services they are providing are appropriate according to established standards of care (Belloni, 2022).

In a nationwide coordinated law enforcement action to combat fraud, the U.S. Department of Justice (USDOJ) filed criminal charges against 36 defendants in 13 federal districts for more than

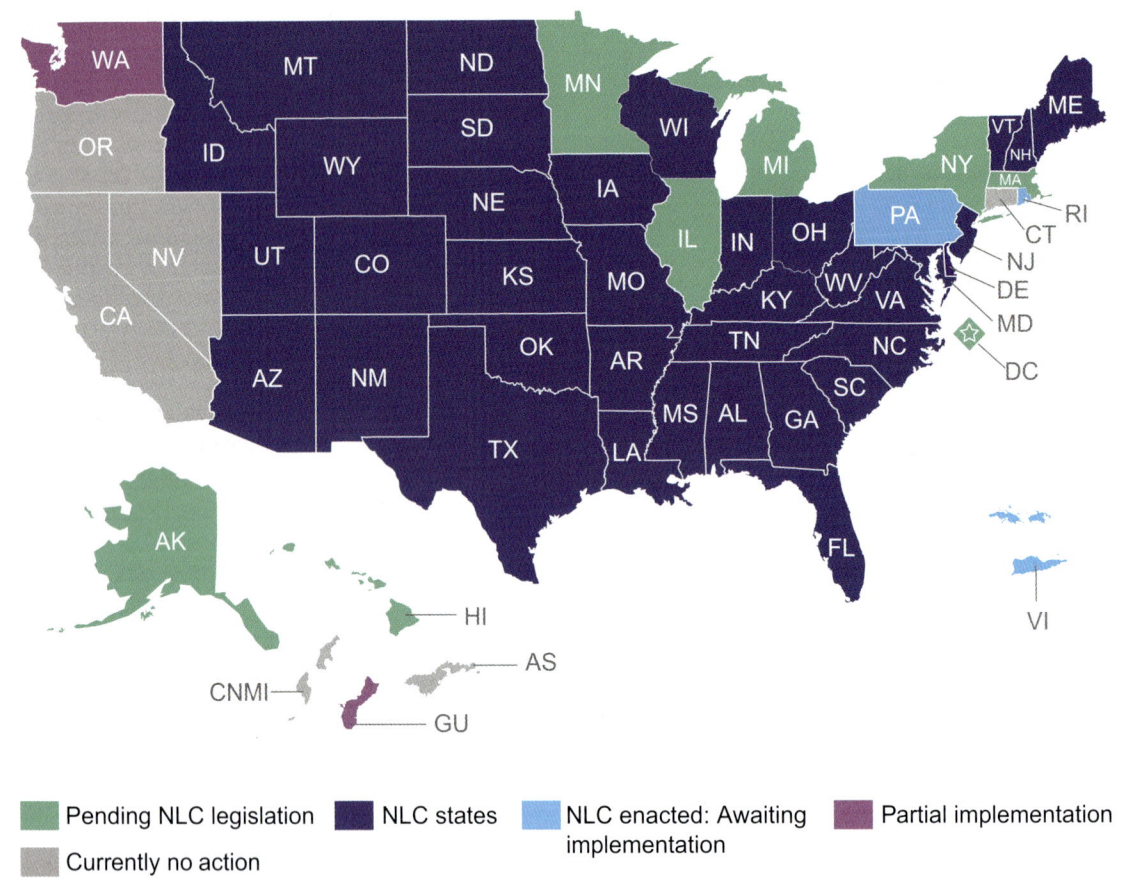

Pending NLC legislation ■ **NLC states** ■ **NLC enacted: Awaiting implementation** ■ **Partial implementation**
■ **Currently no action**

Figure 6-9. Nurse Licensure Compact states as of 2023. (Data from National Council of State Boards of Nursing (NCSBN). (2023). Nurse licensure compact. https://www.nursecompact.com/)

$1.2 billion in alleged fraudulent telemedicine, cardiovascular and cancer genetics testing, and durable medical equipment schemes (USDOJ, 2022). One case involved telemarketers who paid telemedicine companies and call centers to obtain doctor's orders for fraudulent cardiovascular genetic testing. The defendants used deceptive techniques to induce older adult and disabled patients to agree to cardiovascular genetic testing. The orders for testing were used to submit over $174 million in false Medicare claims (USDOJ, 2022). In 2023, the USDOJ charged 11 people with telehealth fraud schemes resulting in more than $2 billion in false claims. In this case, telehealth practitioners signed off on fraudulent orders for orthotic braces for older adult patients that were then submitted to Medicare as false claims (Vaidya, 2023).

Previous efforts to combat telemedicine fraud include Operation Brace Yourself, Operation Double Helix, and Operation Rubber Stamp. These efforts were all part of the 2021 National Health Care Fraud Enforcement Action. The Strike Force Operations division maintains 16 strike forces operating in 27 districts and has charged over 5,000 defendants attempting to defraud federal healthcare programs and private insurers of approximately $24.7 billion (USDOJ, 2022).

These schemes often target vulnerable populations. It is important to inform patients that if they are contacted as part of a fraudulent telemedicine scheme or suspect fraud to call 1-800-HHS-TIPS.

SUMMARY

- **Telehealth concepts.** Telemedicine is the delivery of remote clinical services through the electronic exchange of patient information between two sites. Telehealth includes and extends beyond the delivery of clinical services to include provider training and administrative meetings. Telehealth is used to treat patients when they cannot physically interact with healthcare providers for many reasons (location, mobility, or access). Telehealth can be synchronous or asynchronous (S&F) and can use remote patient monitoring to send patient data to healthcare providers. Telenursing is the use of telehealth to provide home nursing care. The *Scope and Standards of Practice for Professional Telehealth Nursing* addresses six clinical practice standards for telenursing. Telehealth can be used by nurses to provide patient education synchronously or asynchronously. Telehealth can also be used to educate healthcare providers.
- **Telehealth examples.** Telehomecare involves disease prevention in which patients can use automatic pill dispensers and reminders, smart wearables, and self-monitoring to promote health. Primary care delivered via telehealth benefits people living in rural and remote areas by increasing access to highly trained healthcare providers. Telemental health can be used to deliver psychiatric and psychological services like counseling or therapy. E-intensive care units enhance the delivery of intensive care and include the use of tele-intensive care units and robotics. Teletrauma care provides expert advice during emergencies. Telehealth can be a powerful tool for patients with chronic diseases. Portable monitoring devices can monitor glucose levels, weight, blood pressure, and even cardiac rhythms. These devices can save patients money, reduce hospitalization and readmission rates, and improve quality of life. Telehealth can also be used to care for those experiencing natural disasters.
- **Issues with telehealth.** People living in rural and remote areas are often not only those most in need of telehealth but also those who do not have access to high-speed internet. Both reimbursement and regulation for telehealth are complicated by state and federal regulations. Certification and licensure requirements are state-level decisions, but telehealth has no geographic boundaries. As the use of telehealth increases, the misuse of telehealth for fraudulent claims is also on the rise. The USDOJ is actively prosecuting criminal activity committed using telehealth, and individual states are using a variety of approaches to prevent fraud.

DISCUSSION QUESTIONS AND ACTIVITIES

1. Give examples of synchronous and asynchronous telehealth. Are either of these technologies used in your workplace? Discuss how the use of telehealth might improve patient care.
2. Search the internet for examples of current uses for telehealth. Identify at least one journal article. Summarize the findings using bullet points. Cite the source(s) you used.
3. Describe how you would educate a patient using telehealth about a chronic health problem other than diabetes using the information you have learned in this chapter.
4. Select a telehealth issue (telehealth reimbursement, federal and state regulation of telehealth, access to high-speed internet, or fraud), and discuss at least three potential solutions.
5. Analyze two research studies done with telehealth. Compare the findings for similarities and differences.
6. Explore telehealth regulations in your state and report your findings.
7. After sharing information about telehealth with a nursing colleague, the colleague asks you how the system affects the quality and safety of patient care. How should you respond?
8. You have an older adult family member who lives alone independently. The family member is medically complex and on several medications. You are researching automated medication dispensing solutions to assist with medication compliance.
    a. Identify the advantages of automated medication dispensing systems.
    b. Identify three possible solutions in order of your preferences.

c. What is the cost–benefit for each of the choices?

d. Do any of the possible solutions have alerts for non-pill medications?

e. Do the possible solutions you identified create alerts for caregivers?

PRACTICE QUESTIONS

1. Which term is defined as the delivery of remote clinical services through the electronic exchange of patient information between two sites for improving the patient's health status?

   a. Telehealth
   b. Telemedicine
   c. Store-and-forward technology
   d. Remote patient monitoring

2. What is the term for telehealth that involves the patient and the provider interacting at the same time by using interactive audio and sometimes video?

   a. Remote patient monitoring
   b. Asynchronous telehealth
   c. Synchronous telehealth
   d. Telehomecare

3. While telehealth is growing exponentially in its use, there are still barriers to overcome. What is one of the largest barriers to the widespread use of telehealth?

   a. Patient interest and engagement
   b. Provider interest and engagement
   c. Technologic advances
   d. Reimbursement

REFERENCES

Ahsan, M., Teay, S. H., Sayem, A. S. M., & Albarbar, A. (2022). Smart clothing framework for health monitoring applications. *Signals*, *3*(1), 113–145. https://doi.org/10.3390/signals3010009

AliveCor. (n.d.). AliveCor home. Retrieved from https://www.kardia.com/

Alter, N., Arif, H., Wright, D.-D., Martinez, B., & Elkbuli, A. (2023). Telehealth utilization in trauma care: The effects on emergency department length of stay and associated outcomes. *The American Surgeon*, *89*(11), 4826–4834. https://doi.org/10.1177/00031348231173944

American Academy of Ambulatory Care Nursing [AAACN]. (2018). *Scope and standards of practice for professional telehealth nursing* (6th ed.). American Academy of Ambulatory Care Nursing [AAACN].

American Association of Colleges of Nursing (AACN). (2021, April 6). Core competencies for professional nursing education. https://www.aacnnursing.org/Essentials

American Telehealth Association (ATA). (n.d.). About us. Retrieved September 16, 2023 https://www.americantelemed.org/about-us/

Bauerly, B. C., McCord, R. F., Hulkower, R., & Pepin, D. (2019). Broadband access as a public health issue: The role of law in expanding broadband access and connecting underserved communities for better health outcomes. *Journal of Law, Medicine and Ethics*, *47*(2 Suppl. l), 39–42. https://doi.org/10.1177/1073110519857314

Becker, C. D., Dandy, K., Gaujean, M., Fusaro, M., & Scurlock, C. (2019). Legal perspectives on telemedicine Part 1: Legal and regulatory issues. *The Permanante Journal*, *23*, 18–293. https://doi.org/10.7812/TPP/18-293

Begay, M., Kakol, M., Sood, A., & Upson, D. (2021). Strengthening digital health technology capacity in Navajo communities to help counter the COVID-19 pandemic. *Annals of the American Thoracic Society*, *18*(7), 1109–1114. https://doi.org/10.1513/AnnalsATS.202009-1136PS

Belloni, G. (2022, November 22). *Telehealth scores states' backing despite concerns on abuses*. Bloomberg Law. https://news.bloomberglaw.com/health-law-and-business/telehealth-scores-states-backing-despite-concerns-on-abuses

Boyle, T., Boggs, K., Gao, J., McMahon, M., Bedenbaugh, R., Schmidt, L., Zachrison, K. S., Goralnick, E., Biddinger, P., & Camargo Jr, C. A. (2023). Hospital-level implementation barriers, facilitators, and willingness to use a new regional disaster teleconsultation system: Cross-sectional survey study. *JMIR Public Health and Surveillance*, *9*, e44164. https://doi.org/10.2196/44164

Castner, J., Bell, S. A., Hetland, B., Der-Martirosian, C., Castner, M., & Joshi, A. U. (2022). National Estimates of workplace telehealth use among emergency nurses and all registered nurses in the United States. *Journal of Emergency Nursing*, *48*(1), 45–56. https://doi.org/10.1016/j.jen.2021.07.001

Center for Connected Health Policy (CCHP). (2022). *Medicaid and medicare: Store-and-forward*. Retrieved from https://www.cchpca.org/topic/store-and-forward/

Center for Connected Health Policy (CCHP). (n.d.a). Telehealth policy 101. Retrieved from https://www.cchpca.org/policy-101/

Center for Connected Health Policy (CCHP). (n.d.b). Cross-state licensing. Retrieved from https://www.cchpca.org/topic/cross-state-licensing-professional-requirements/

Center for Telehealth & e-Health Law [CTeL]. (2022). Policy. Retrieved from http://ctel.org/policy/#reimbursement/

Centers for Disease Control and Prevention (CDC). (2022a, July 21). About chronic diseases. https://www.cdc.gov/chronicdisease/about/index.htm#print

Centers for Disease Control and Prevention (CDC). (2022b, December 30). A guide for using telehealth technologies in diabetes self-management education and support and in the national diabetes prevention program lifestyle change program. https://www.cdc.gov/diabetes/programs/stateandlocal/resources/telehealth.html

Centers for Medicare & Medicaid Services (CMS). (2022a). New & expanded flexibilities for RHCs & FQHCs during the COVID-19 PHE. Retrieved from https://www.cms.gov/files/document/se20016-new-expanded-flexibilities-rhcs-fqhcs-during-covid-19-phe.pdf

Centers for Medicare & Medicaid Services (CMS). (2022b). Preparedness and response toolkit for state Medicaid and CHIP agencies in the event of a public health emergency or disaster. https://www.medicaid.gov/sites/default/files/2022-06/medicaid-chip-disastertoolkit.pdf

Congress.gov. (n.d.). Constitution of the United States: 10th amendment. https://constitution.congress.gov/constitution/amendment-10/

Cooke, K. (2020, April 27). The top internet deserts in the US. https://www.satelliteinternet.com/resources/top-internet-deserts/

Dudas, L. M., Bardes, J. M., Wagner, A. K., White, T., & Wilson, A. M. (2023). Cost effective virtual intensive care unit expanding capabilities in Critical Access Hospitals. *The American Surgeon, 89*(5), 1533–1538. https://doi.org/10.1177/00031348211062653

Early, J., & Hernandez, A. (2021). Digital disenfranchisement and COVID-19: Broadband internet access as a social determinant of health. *Health Promotion Practice, 22*(5), 605–610. https://doi.org/10.1177/15248399211014490

Emily, G. E., Anna, D., Jack, M., O'Brien, R., Kutcher, M., Morris, M., & Chinenye, I. (2022). Perceptions and barriers of telehealth services among trauma and acute care surgery patients. *Surgery in Practice and Science, 11*, 100138. https://doi.org/10.1016/j.sipas.2022.100138

Federation of State Medical Boards. (2016). FSMB survey identifies telemedicine as most important regulatory topic for state medical boards in 2016. Retrieved from https://www.fsmb.org/siteassets/advocacy/news-releases/2016/annual_state_board_survey_sesults.pdf

Federation of State Medical Boards. (2022). The appropriate use of telemedicine technologies in the practice of medicine. Retrieved from https://www.fsmb.org/siteassets/advocacy/policies/fsmb-workgroup-on-telemedicineapril-2022-final.pdf

Fitbit. (n.d.). What's new: Fitbit. Retrieved from https://www.fitbit.com/global/us/products/whats-new

Fitzgerald, B. (2022, November 15). FirstNet enables telehealth in the inland island of Jackman, Maine. https://firstnet.gov/newsroom/blog/firstnet-enables-telehealth-inland-island-jackman-maine

Fitzner, K., & Moss, G. (2013). Telehealth—an effective delivery method for diabetes self-management education? *Population Health Management, 16*(3), 169–177. https://doi.org/10.1089/pop.2012.0054

Franklin, R. (2021, October 25). 11 surprising mobile health statistics. https://mobius.md/2021/10/25/11-mobile-health-statistics/

Garcia, M. (2022, April 8). *Innovative 3D telemedicine to help keep astronauts healthy*. NASA. https://www.nasa.gov/feature/innovative-3d-telemedicine-to-help-keep-astronauts-healthy

Gaiser, M., Buche, J., Baum, N. M., & Grazier, K. L. (2023). Mental health needs due to disasters: Implications for behavioral health workforce planning during the COVID-19 pandemic. *Public Health Reports, 138*(1 suppl), 48S–55S. https://doi.org/10.1177/00333549231151888

Genes, N. (2018). *Alexander Graham Bell and the birth of telemedicine*. Telemedicine. Retrieved from http://www.telemedmag.com/article/alexander-graham-bell-and-the-birth-of-telemedicine/

Goetter, E. M., Iaccarino, M. A., Taney, K. S., Furbish, K. E., Xu, B., & Faust, K. A. (2022). Telemental health uptake in an outpatient clinic for veterans during the COVID-19 pandemic and assessment of patient and provider attitudes. *Professional Psychology: Research and Practice, 53*(2), 151–159. https://doi.org/10.1037/pro0000437

Grady, J. L., & Schlachta-Fairchild, L. (2007). Report of the 2004–2005 international telenursing survey. *Computers, Informatics, Nursing, 25*(5), 266–272.

Health Resources and Services Administration [HRSA]. (2021). Defining the PCMH. Retrieved from https://www.ahrq.gov/ncepcr/research/care-coordination/pcmh/define.html

Health Resources and Services Administration [HRSA]. (2023). *Uniform data system 2023 manual: Health center data reporting requirements*. https://bphc.hrsa.gov/sites/default/files/bphc/data-reporting/2023-uds-manual.pdf

HealthIT.gov. (2023). Frequently asked questions. Retrieved from https://www.healthit.gov/faqs

Lam, O., Broderick, B., & Toor, S. (2018, December 12). *How far Americans live from the closest hospital differs by community type*. Pew Research Center. https://www.pewresearch.org/fact-tank/2018/12/12/how-far-americans-live-from-the-closest-hospital-differs-by-community-type/

Lemelin, A., Paré, G., Bernard, S., & Godbout, A. (2020). Demonstrated cost-effectiveness of a telehomecare program for gestational diabetes mellitus management. *Diabetes Technology & Therapeutics, 22*(3), 195–202. https://doi.org/10.1089/dia.2019.0259

Leonard, C., Liu, W., Holstein, A., Alliance, S., Nunnery, M., Rohs, C., Sloan, M., & Winchester, D. E. (2023). Informing use of telehealth for managing chronic conditions: Mixed-methods evaluation of telehealth use to manage heart failure during COVID-19. *Journal of American Heart Association, 12*(4), e027362. https://doi.org/10.1161/jaha.122.027362

Lokmic-Tomkins, Z., Bhandari, D., Bain, C., Borda, A., Kariotis, T. C., & Reser, D. (2023). Lessons learned from natural disasters around digital health technologies and delivering Quality Healthcare. *International Journal of Environmental Research and Public Health, 20*(5), 4542. https://doi.org/10.3390/ijerph20054542

Maine Seacoast Mission. (n.d.). Sunbeam. https://seacoastmission.org/sunbeam/

Marcin, J. P., Sauers-Ford, H. S., Mouzoon, J. L., Haynes, S. C., Dayal, P., Sigal, I., Tancredi, D., Lieng, M. K., & Kuppermann, N. (2023). Impact of tele-emergency consultations on pediatric interfacility transfers: A cluster-randomized crossover trial. *JAMA Network Open, 6*(2), e2255770. https://doi.org/10.1001/jamanetworkopen.2022.55770

Marlina, T.T., Haryani, H., Widyawati, W., & Febriani, D.H. (2023). The effectiveness of telenursing for diabetes self-management education: A scoping review. *The Open Nursing Journal, 2023*, 17. https://doi.org/10.2174/18744346-v17-230815-2023-38

Marr, B. (2021, July 5). Smart underpants: A new "brief" in health monitoring. Forbes. https://www.forbes.com/sites/bernardmarr/2021/07/05/smart-underpants-a-new-brief-in-health-monitoring/?sh=62bd96f74570

Mattison, G., Canfell, O., Forrester, D., Dobbins, C., Smith, D., Töyräs, J., & Sullivan, C. (2022). The influence of wearables on health care outcomes in chronic disease: Systematic review. *Journal of Medical Internet Research, 24*(7), e36690. https://doi.org/10.2196/36690

Moecke, D. P., Holyk, T., Beckett, M., Chopra, S., Petlitsyna, P., Girt, M., Kirkham, A., Kamurasi, I., Turner, J., Sneddon, D., Friesen, M., McDonald, I., Denson-Camp, N., Crosbie, S., Camp, P. G. (2023). Scoping review of telehealth use by Indigenous populations from Australia, Canada, New Zealand, and the United States. *Journal of Telemedicine and Telecare, 0*(0), https://doi.org/10.1177/1357633X231158835

Mukherjee, S., Suleman, S., Pilloton, R., Narang, J., & Rani, K. (2022). State of the art in smart portable, wearable, ingestible and implantable devices for health status monitoring and disease management. *Sensors, 22*(11), 4228. https://doi.org/10.3390/s22114228

National Consortium of Telehealth Resource Centers (NCTRC). (2021) What is telehealth: Context for framing your perspective. Retrieved from https://telehealthresourcecenter.org/wp-content/uploads/2021/03/WhatIsTelehealth3.pdf

National Council of State Boards of Nursing (NCSBN). (n.d.). eNLC fast facts. https://www.ncsbn.org/public-files/NLC_Fast_Facts.pdf

National Institute of Mental Health [NIMH]. (n.d.) What is telemental health? Retrieved from https://www.nimh.nih.gov/health/publications/what-is-telemental-health

Nevada Intergenerational Healthy Aging Network (NIHAN). (2022). Telehealth. https://www.nihan.care/telehealth/

North American Treaty Organization [NATO]. (2017, February 24). NATO develops telemedicine system to save lives in emergencies. Retrieved from http://www.nato.int/cps/en/natohq/news_141822.htm

Reifegerste, D., Harst, L., & Otto, L. (2022). Sauerbruch, STARPAHC, and SARS: Historical perspectives on readiness and barriers in telemedicine. *Journal of Public Health, 30*(1), 11–20. https://doi.org/10.1007/s10389-021-01513-1

Rodriguez, J. A., Clark, C. R, Bates, D. W. (2020). Digital health equity as a necessity in the 21st century cures Act era. *JAMA, 323*(23), 2381–2382. https://doi.org/10.1001/jama.2020.7858

Rutledge, C. M., & Gustin, T. (2021). Preparing nurses for roles in telehealth: Now is the time! *The Online Journal of Issues in Nursing* (26). Retrieved from https://ojin.nursingworld.org/MainMenuCategories/ANAMarketplace/ANAPeriodicals/OJIN/TableofContents/Vol-26-2021/No1-Jan-2021/Preparing-Nurses-for-Roles-in-Telehealth-Now-is-the-Time.html

Sarik, D. A., Matsuda, Y., Terrell, E. A., Sotolongo, E., Hernandez, M., Tena, F., & Lee, J. (2022). A telehealth nursing intervention to improve the transition from the neonatal intensive care unit to home for infants & caregivers: Preliminary evaluation. *Journal of Pediatric Nursing, 67*, 139–147. https://doi.org/10.1016/j.pedn.2022.09.003

Simpson, A. T., Doarn, C. R., & Garber, S. J. (2020). A brief history of NASA's contribution to telemedicine. Retrieved from https://history.nasa.gov/NASAtelemedicine-briefhistory.pdf

Straits Research. (2023, August 7). *Tele-intensive care unit market size is projected to reach USD 12.40 billion by 2031, growing at a CAGR of 16.3%: Straits research*. GlobeNewswire News Room. https://www.globenewswire.com/en/news-release/2023/08/07/2720003/0/en/Tele-Intensive-Care-Unit-Market-Size-is-projected-to-reach-USD-12-40-billion-by-2031-growing-at-a-CAGR-of-16-3-Straits-Research.html

Teng, R., Ding, Y., & See, K. C. (2022). Use of robots in critical care: Systematic review. *Journal of Medical Internet Research, 24*(5), e33380. hhttps://doi.org/10.2196/33380

University of New Mexico (UNM). Health Sciences. (2023). Project ECHO 2022 annual report. https://projectecho-annualreport.unm.edu/wp-content/uploads/2023/04/Project-ECHO-2022-Annual-Report-FINAL.pdf

U.S. Department of Health and Human Services (USDHHS). (2023a, April 20). *Licensure compacts*. Telehealth.HHS.gov. Retrieved from https://telehealth.hhs.gov/licensure/licensure-compacts

U.S. Department of Health and Human Services (USDHHS). (2023b, August 31). *Telehealth policy: Changes after the COVID-19 public health emergency*. Telehealth.HHS.gov. https://telehealth.hhs.gov/providers/telehealth-policy/policy-changes-after-the-covid-19-public-health-emergency

U.S. Department of Health and Human Services (USDHHS). (n.d.). *Best practice guides*. https://telehealth.hhs.gov/providers/best-practice-guides

U.S. Department of the Treasury. (n.d.). Capital projects fund. Retrieved from https://home.treasury.gov/policy-issues/coronavirus/assistance-for-state-local-and-tribal-governments/capital-projects-fund

U.S. United States Department of Justice (USDOJ). (2022, July 20). Justice department charges dozens for $1.2 billion in health care fraud. https://www.justice.gov/opa/pr/justice-department-charges-dozens-12-billion-health-care-fraud

Vaidya, A. (2023, June 28). *DOJ charges 11 people in telehealth fraud schemes worth $2B*. Telehealth News. https://mhealthintelligence.com/news/doj-charges-11-people-in-telehealth-fraud-schemes-worth-2b#

Wilkes, M. S., Marcin, J. P., Ritter, L. A., & Pruitt, S. (2016). Organizational and teamwork factors of tele-intensive care units. *American Journal of Critical Care, 25*(5), 431–439. https://doi.org/10.4037/ajcc 2016357

Williams, C., & Shang, D. (2024). Telehealth for chronic disease management among vulnerable populations. *Journal of Racial and Ethnic Health Disparities, 11*(2), 1089–1096. https://doi.org/10.1007/s40615-023-01588-4

Yilmaz, G., Rapin, M., Pessoa, D., Rocha, B. M., de Sousa, A. M., Rusconi, R., Carvalho, P., Wacker, J., Paiva, R. P., & Chételat, O. (2020). A wearable stethoscope for long-term ambulatory respiratory health monitoring. *Sensors, 20*(18), 5124. https://doi.org/10.3390/s20185124

Yu, S., Wan, R., Bai, L., Zhao, B., Jiang, Q., Jiang, J., & Li, Y. (2023). Transformation of chronic disease management: Before and after the covid-19 outbreak. *Frontiers in Public Health, 11*, 1074364. https://doi.org/10.3389/fpubh.2023.1074364

Zhang, J., Boden, M., & Trafton, J. (2022). Mental health treatment and the role of tele-mental health at the veterans health administration during the COVID-19 pandemic. *Psychological Services, 19*(2), 375–385. https://doi.org/10.1037/ser0000530

UNIT III

Using Data to Improve Patient Outcomes

Chapter 7	Finding Information
Chapter 8	Collecting Data
Chapter 9	Analyzing Data
Chapter 10	Disseminating Data

You were first introduced to the data, information, knowledge, and wisdom (DIKW) model in Chapter 2. This unit discusses how the informatics nurse can convert data into information, contribute to nursing knowledge, and generate wisdom. You will learn how to use the Advancing Research and Clinical Practice Through Close Collaboration (ARCC) model to collect, critically appraise, analyze, and disseminate information, while keeping your focus on the most important goal—improving patient outcomes.

The AACN Essentials state that knowledge of the basic principles of research and evidence-based practice are essential to improve clinical practice, influence policy, and educate nurses (2021). Nurses must not only have the skills to engage in research but be able to find and evaluate research to determine how it applies to nursing practice. The application of EBP utilizes the best practice to inform clinical decision making. Understanding how data are collected, analyzed, and disseminated to improve patient outcomes is also an essential part of nursing practice.

Chapter 7, "Finding Information," begins with a case study on patient falls and provides step-by-step guidance for how to conduct an evidence-based practice (EBP) study using the ARCC model. The chapter compares EBP to research, covers how to rate articles using levels of evidence, and important sources of nursing knowledge. The chapter guides the learner through how to search library resources for high-level information to support research and EBP.

Chapter 8, "Collecting Data," begins with a case study that points out health disparities for people assigned female at birth and explores the importance of collecting demographic information in ways that are inclusive to all identities to improve patient outcomes on national and international levels. This chapter includes reasons, guidelines, and tools for data collection. Chapter 8 provides an explanation of how databases work. Ethical considerations for reducing health disparities with inclusive data collection and the importance of advocacy are also discussed.

Chapter 9, "Analyzing Data," gives learners an understanding of basic data analysis concepts. Types of data and how they are analyzed as well as major sources of standard data sets for benchmarking are discussed. Big data, artificial intelligence, and other current trends in data analytics are also covered. The case study explores an article in which the risk of uterine perforation from intrauterine device (IUD) insertion was calculated using multiple types of data.

Chapter 10, "Disseminating Data," starts with a case study demonstrating that the dissemination of data is important for improving patient outcomes. This chapter covers different methods of disseminating data, including presentations, posters, and publishing articles. Universal design is also discussed, showing the importance of accessibility, usability, and inclusivity in any material meant for an audience.

REFERENCE

American Association of Colleges of Nursing (AACN). (2021). *The essentials: Core competencies for professional nursing education*. https://www.aacnnursing.org/Portals/42/AcademicNursing/pdf/Essentials-2021.pdf

CHAPTER 7

Finding Information

Andrew Kearns, Meredith MacKenzie, and Kristi Miller

OBJECTIVES

After studying this chapter, you will be able to:

1. Explain the creation of nursing knowledge and distinguish between research and evidence-based practice.
2. Explain the importance of library resources and services to nurses and healthcare professionals.
3. Discuss how bibliographic databases are constructed and what databases are useful to discovering nursing knowledge.
4. Demonstrate effective electronic search strategies to support evidence-based practice.
5. Identify sources of nursing knowledge.

AACN Essentials for Entry-Level Professional Nursing Education

1.2a Apply or employ knowledge from nursing science as well as the natural, physical, and social sciences to build an understanding of the human experience and nursing practice.

1.2b Demonstrate intellectual curiosity.

1.3b Integrate nursing knowledge (theories, multiple ways of knowing, evidence) and knowledge from other disciplines and inquiry to inform clinical judgment.

4.1a Demonstrate an understanding of different approaches to scholarly practice.

4.1b Demonstrate application of different levels of evidence.

4.1e Participate in scholarly inquiry as a team member.

8.2c Use appropriate data when planning care.

8.3a Demonstrate appropriate use of information and communication technologies.

AACN Essentials for Advanced-Level Nursing Education

1.2f Synthesize knowledge from nursing and other disciplines to inform education, practice, and research.
1.3e Synthesize current and emerging evidence to influence practice.
4.1i Engage in scholarship to advance health.
4.2f Use diverse sources of evidence to inform practice.
4.2h Address opportunities for innovation and changes in practice.
8.2f Generate information and knowledge from health information technology databases.
8.3g Evaluate the use of information and communication technology to address needs, gaps, and inefficiencies in care.

HIMSS TIGER Competencies

Applied computer science

Information and knowledge management in patient care

Information management research

Teaching, training, education

KEY TERMS

Bibliographic database
Bibliographic record
Boolean connectors
Discovery search
Factual database
Full-text collection
Impact factor (IF)
Interface
Invisible web (deep web)
Limiter (filter)

Medical subject headings (MeSH)
Meta-analysis
Metadata
Natural language searches
Nursing knowledge
Nursing research
Open access
Plagiarism
Randomized control trial (RCT)

Reference manager
Scholarly nursing journals
Self-plagiarism
Seminal work
Stop words
Subject headings
Systematic review
Truncation
Visible web (surface web)
Wildcard

CASE STUDY

Two nurse researchers at a hospital in Florida noticed that despite the use of generalized standard fall prevention interventions like demonstrating call light use, ensuring the patient's personal possessions are within reach, and keeping the bed in the lowest position, the fall rate on their unit remained high. Using a patient-centered fall prevention toolkit called Fall Tailoring Interventions for Patient Safety (TIPS), the nurses explored its impact on patient knowledge of fall risk factors and interventions and how this influenced fall and injury rates. In the study, the authors explored fall risks and individualized interventions to engage patients and families in fall prevention at the bedside using a pre- and post-intervention design to compare patient's knowledge and the fall rate before and after implementing Fall TIPS. Thirty patients were interviewed before the study and at 1-, 3-, and 6-month time points (N = 120). The number and rates of falls per 1,000 patient days were calculated and audits were done to monitor use of Fall TIPS. After implementing Fall TIPS, patients were found to be more knowledgeable about falls and the fall rate dropped from 3.3% to 1.9% following study (Fowler & Reising, 2021).

Many healthcare organizations struggle with how to prevent patient falls. How did the authors of this paper decide to use the Fall TIPS approach? Why did they choose this intervention over others? The informatics nurse must be able to not only find information, but evaluate it. These competencies support research and EBP that can improve patient outcomes.

Providing the best care to patients demands continual engagement with research and evidence-based practice (EBP) that supports the most effective interventions. Gathering information to gain knowledge is related to the data, information, knowledge, and wisdom (DIKW) model discussed in Chapter 2. Given the vast amount of information available online, looking for information relevant to a specific situation can be frustrating and overwhelming. This is particularly true of research, much of which is only available behind passwords and paywalls on the internet, inaccessible to search engines like Google. Fortunately, library online resources provide a gateway to this knowledge. It is crucial, therefore, that nurses and healthcare providers proactively develop and practice information search competencies that allow them to find information using digital solutions. This chapter focuses on gathering information from libraries and other digital resources that can be used to support research and EBP projects to improve patient outcomes.

CREATING NURSING KNOWLEDGE

Nursing research is a systematic process of inquiry that involves collecting, documenting, analyzing, and reporting data to contribute to nursing knowledge. It is the scientific foundation for practice used to promote health, prevent diseases, manage illness symptoms, and assist with palliative and end-of-life care. Nursing research addresses individuals as well as populations (NINR, 2022).

Nurses are constantly involved in collecting data that build **nursing knowledge**, the information known to nursing practice that defines the profession. There are three ways to engage in data collection and analysis that contribute to nursing knowledge: research, EBP, and quality improvement (QI) studies. These terms are often used interchangeably, but they are different (Table 7-1). You can learn more about QI in Chapter 11.

The quest for new nursing knowledge involves recognizing an information need, discovering information to answer that need, understanding and analyzing that information, applying findings from literature to clinical practice, and assessing and disseminating the results so that others can utilize that knowledge.

The Cyclical Nature of EBP

The seven-step Advancing Research and Clinical practice through close Collaboration (ARCC) model is a way to guide EBP research (Melnyk & Fineout-Overholt, 2023). The seven steps are:

1. Step 0: Cultivate a spirit of inquiry.
2. Step 1: Ask a burning question in PICOT format.
3. Step 2: Search for the best evidence to answer the PICOT question.
4. Step 3: Conduct a critical appraisal of the studies found from the search.
5. Step 4: Implement best practice.
6. Step 5: Evaluate the outcome of the practice change.

TABLE 7-1 Differences Between Research, Evidence-Based Practice, and Quality Improvement

	Research	Evidence-Based Practice (EBP)	Quality Improvement (QI)
Definition	Scientific process to validate or generate new knowledge	Problem-solving to critically appraise best evidence to address a question	Data-driven approach to improve internal systems
Purpose	Reinforces existing knowledge and develops new knowledge	Foundation for integration of best evidence in patient care	Improves workflow quality and efficiency
Overlaps	Informs EBP and QI	Informs QI and opportunities for research and identifies research gaps	Informs EBP and opportunities for research
Generalizability	Yes, depending on design	Yes, results may be transferrable	No, not to other organizations

From Shirey, M. R., Hauck, S. L., Embree, J. L., Kinner, T. J., Schaar, G. L., Phillips, L. A., Ashby, S. R., Swenty, C. F., & McCool, I. A. (2011). Showcasing differences between quality improvement, evidence-based practice, and research. *The Journal of Continuing Education in Nursing, 42*(2), 57–68. https://doi.org/10.3928/00220124-20100701-01

7. Step 6: Disseminate the outcomes of the EBP change.

This chapter covers Steps 1 through 3. Step 0, cultivating a spirit of inquiry, will be developed within you as you read this entire book. You can learn more about Steps 4-6 in an EBP or research course.

Despite the ARCC model steps being presented in a list, research is not a linear process but rather cyclical and iterative (Fig. 7-1). In other words, the researcher may go back and forth through the several steps that define the process. Because the generation of new knowledge is continual, the process of research never stops, with new information modifying old answers and new questions constantly emerging. The more you engage with finding knowledge, the better you will understand the cyclical nature of the EBP process. The information you find in your library search may lead to modifications of your burning question and your PICOT (discussed in the following section). As you plan the implementation of your research, you may need to return to the library to find more information on how to roll out the implementation. Evaluation of the outcome may lead to changes in the burning question and the PICOT. Sharing the results with patients, staff, the public, academia, and others conducting similar research may lead to questions that need further research and inquiry.

The PICOT Question

A common mistake in nursing research is searching for evidence for a topic that is too broad. Formulating a well-thought-out research question and putting it in the form of a PICOT question will help to avoid this. The parts of a PICOT question include:

- *Population/patient/problem:* Who/what is the population, patient, or problem?
- *Intervention:* What is the intervention being considered?
- *Comparison:* What are the other interventions in place or being considered?

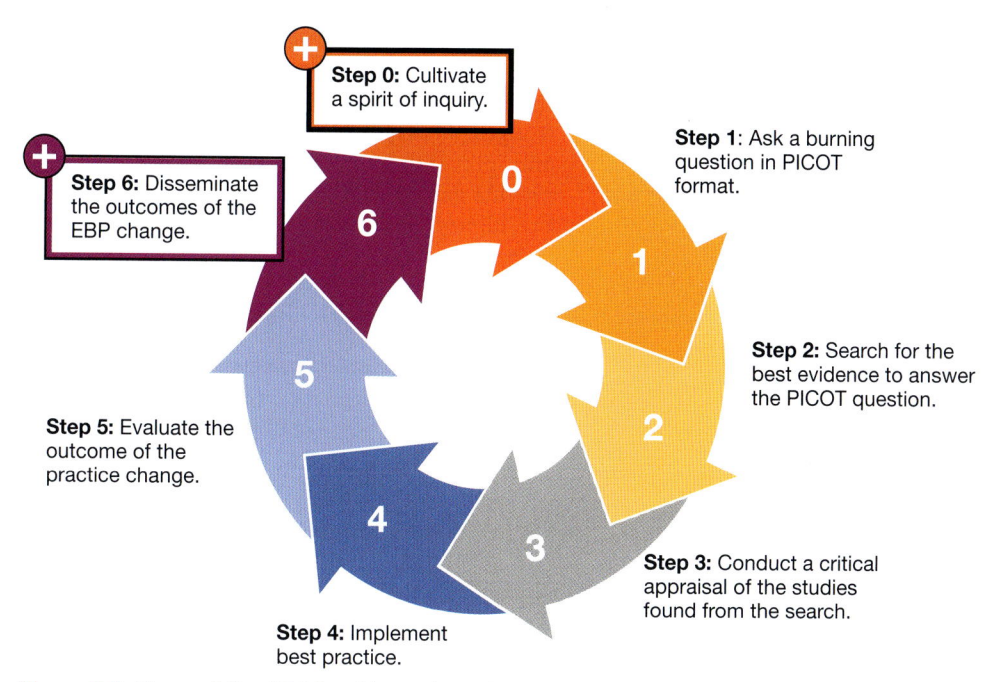

Figure 7-1. Steps of the ARCC evidence-based practice process leading to high-quality healthcare and best patient outcomes.

- Outcome: What is the desired outcome of the intervention?
- Time: How long will it take to reach the desired outcome?

To derive keywords from a PICOT question, the population, intervention, and outcome categories are usually the most important, followed by comparison and time. It is important to identify the most important words from the research question that might be used as search terms. Also, think of any synonyms, alternate terms, and different forms of words that may be useful in a search. For example, in a keyword search for "nurse," you will need to account for alternate forms: nurses and nursing.

CASE STUDY

Recall the Fowler and Reising article from the case study. Find the article using your university library. Read it and formulate the PICOT question they might have used to guide their study. Think of an issue in your work and formulate a PICOT question that would help solve the problem.

LIBRARY ADVANTAGES

Today, most of our information comes to us through the internet, specifically the public-facing portion of the web. The quantity of health information that search engines find on the web is vast, unorganized, and of varying quality, from useful government websites to advice from people with questionable medical authority. Finding research articles can be frustrating because while there is a growing number of open-access journals and government-funded research articles available online, it can be cumbersome finding them through Internet search engines. Furthermore, many conventionally published articles are not available for free. Finally, keyword searching on which internet search engines are built lacks precision and makes the comprehensive searches required for nursing research harder. For this kind of research, library resources are more effective and efficient.

Libraries have long had an online presence. They were among the first institutions to provide access to electronic databases and moved their catalogues online decades ago. Library catalogues have evolved over time to provide more direct access to digital materials, and today many university and school libraries have a discovery search feature. A **discovery search** (also known as a federated search) allows the user to simultaneously search select databases as well as physical and digital materials from the library's collection using one search box. Discovery searches can be a good first step to get an idea of what is available, but for comprehensive research, more specialized resources, such as databases that include medical and nursing literature, are necessary.

One of the most important things to do to facilitate research is to know what kind of library resources and services are available. Academic libraries at colleges and universities will have collections supporting the nursing curriculum, including subscriptions to core nursing databases. Institutions with large medical and nursing programs may even have a dedicated health sciences library. Larger healthcare institutions such as hospital systems often have libraries as well. If an institution or facility does not have a library, the facilities and resources of nearby academic sites may be available, and public libraries often have online resources available to the community. Bear in mind that most states now subscribe to a suite of databases, including scholarly and health sciences databases, that they make available to residents, often through programs run through the state library. Contact the nearest library to find out what is available.

As important as access to library resources is for nursing practice, almost equally important are the services libraries provide, including the service of professional librarians. Professional librarians have master's or doctoral degrees in library science, and many have second degrees in fields related to an area of specialization. All librarians have expertise in assisting users in accessing and utilizing library resources, including detailed advice on how to effectively search library databases. In addition, a librarian can provide information about services such as interlibrary loans, which enables researchers to get materials, including the full text of articles, not available through institutional resources.

Change in the library world is constant. Library collections and resources are dynamic rather than static, vendor interfaces undergo frequent improvements, and new technologies are often incorporated in library operations. Therefore, even the most experienced library patrons can benefit from the library guides, tutorials, and other guidance provided by librarians. These materials can provide guidelines on how to find information in the library, summarize important resources by subject, and give detailed instruction on search strategies or individual databases. A library's homepage will provide links to these materials as well as to library resources and services.

USING DATABASES FOR RESEARCH

In addition to their online catalogues, libraries provide access to other types of databases useful for nursing research, including factual databases, bibliographic databases, and full-text collections. Each database is specialized by the number and type of resources (e.g., journal or book names) indexed, the span of years indexed, and the words that the database uses to describe the resources for searching purposes. **Factual databases** contain point-of-need information and may include reference books such as dictionaries and encyclopedias, drug and laboratory manuals, and statistics and data sets. Examples include the Nursing Reference Center (an EBSCO product) and the multidisciplinary Credo Reference.

A **bibliographic database** is an index of published literature, often limited to a particular area such as health sciences, business, history, government, law, or ethics. A bibliographic database provides citations (a brief reference to an item of literature), abstracts (which summarize the information presented in an academic paper), and sometimes full text for articles from selected periodicals. Bibliographic databases are successors to the paper periodical indexes, which were systems used to file or catalogue references.

A third type of database is a **full-text collection** of publications by a single publisher. While these collections can be searched directly, users tend to learn about articles in them by searching a bibliographic database. The search screens of full-text collections often have fewer features to limit and refine the search than those of bibliographic databases.

Libraries purchase or subscribe to databases directly from library vendors or through library consortia. Often a subscription includes several of a vendor's databases bundled together, and the exact contents of a subscription may vary from one library to another. Each vendor provides a common interface (the search screen) for its databases, allowing the user to do a search across several databases simultaneously. (Look for a link near the search box to "choose" or "change" databases; this presents the option to select multiple databases from a list.) Three important library vendors that package health science databases are EBSCO, Ovid, and ProQuest. Discuss the databases available in the library with the librarian, who can also recommend specific health science databases for a particular research need.

Metadata and Records

Searching a library database is a different experience than using a web search engine. To effectively search a library database, it is important to understand how databases are put together. Most library databases rely on metadata to organize information. **Metadata** is information about other data, and it is used to create descriptions of items called **bibliographic records** ("records" for short). A typical record consists of fields such as author, title, journal name, date, subject, and so on. When searching in a database, the search terms are finding words in these records, not the actual text of articles or books (even when the full text is provided in the database). This allows for much more flexibility and precision in searching. The user can search different fields, such as title if they are looking for a specific article, or limit the search for keywords (tags used to identify topics) in the abstract field, for example. Databases often have **limiters (filters)**, which are ways to limit a search from the search interface or refine a search from the results screen. Limiters often include peer-reviewed journals, full-text availability, language, age of subjects of a research study, type of article, and years of publication.

Reference Managers

Reference managers allow for the collection and organization of citations from search findings. Other common features include storing digital copies of full-text articles, citing sources, capturing citations from multiple databases and the web, and automatically generating a formatted reference list while writing with word processing software. Many reference managers can interact with word processors and store files and other information on the cloud as well as the computer, which can allow the user to sync the research information on more than one device. When considering which reference manager to acquire, it is important to consider the kind of research needed, the kinds of resources used to find information, and what features will be most useful. Some vendors and publishers include versions of their reference managers as part of or an add-on to an institutional subscription. Others can be purchased or freely downloaded by individuals.

Two popular commercial reference managers available through institutional subscriptions are RefWorks by ProQuest, accessed online, and EndNote by Clarivate, which has both desktop and online components. The full version of EndNote is also available through individual purchase, while a more basic version, EndNote Online, is available through institutional subscription to the Web of Science database, also by Clarivate. Citavi by Swiss Academic Software is a similar product available in individual and institutional versions and widely used in the European Union.

Zotero is a popular open-source reference manager available as a free download with browser plug-ins for Firefox, Chrome, and Safari. It can capture citations from many databases and websites and allows for cloud storage and syncing among multiple devices. Mendeley is another popular free reference manager offering similar features. Elsevier owns it and offers a premium version for purchase.

Avoiding Plagiarism

The correct use of references and citations will prevent **plagiarism**, or using another's work as one's own. Three common types of plagiarism include:

1. Copying the exact text written by others without citing the source
2. Reordering the words of a source text without citing the source

3. **Self-plagiarism**, presenting one's own previously published work as new work

Unless the writer is presenting common, widely known information, they must cite the sources they used. The most common citation style used in the social and health sciences, including nursing, is American Psychological Association (APA) style.

To avoid plagiarism, never copy and paste to add content to a paper, even if the intention is to paraphrase it later; avoid changing a few scattered words from an original source; and never attribute information to a source that is cited in another source (Goodwin & McCarthy, 2020). In other words, always go to the original source of information, confirm what the original author said, and cite the original source.

Even if plagiarism occurs unintentionally, it is still a violation of scholarly ethics. There appears to be a potential shift in academic emphasis from punishment for plagiarism toward a more positively positioned culture of support for academic integrity in nursing education (Amsberry, 2022). To promote academic integrity in scholarship, use a plagiarism checker such as iThenticate or Turnitin to self-check a paper. Many instructors and editors use plagiarism checkers, so it is a good idea to self-check first.

Bibliographic Databases Pertinent to Nursing

There are numerous databases with information pertinent to nursing. Essential ones with a focus on nursing and health-related topics are Cumulative Index to Nursing and Allied Health Literature (CINAHL), MEDLINE/PubMed, Cochrane Library, JBI Evidence-Based Practice Database, and APA PsycINFO/PsycARTICLES. Although there may be some overlap in the journals and resources these databases index, there are important differences that may affect the search outcome. Furthermore, there are variations for each of the databases for each library system. EBSCO, for example, markets a basic version of CINAHL as well as versions designated Plus, Complete, and Ultimate, each reflecting an increase in the number of journals indexed and amount of full text included. Consult with a reference librarian to assist with refining the search question and selecting the best databases to search. See Table 7-2 for a list of databases according to nursing topic. The databases included in this table are commonly available through most medical and academic libraries.

CINAHL

When researching a nursing topic, the CINAHL database is an excellent place to start. CINAHL has roots as a paper periodical index that acquired its current name and focus in 1977. It first went online in 1984 and has been published exclusively by EBSCO since 2003 (CINAHL, 2021). CINAHL is an important database in any of its versions. The most comprehensive Ultimate version indexes more than 3,000 journals from around the world including more than 1,000 open-access journals (no fee for access) (EBSCO, n.d.). Full text is provided for many non–open-access journals. Depending on the version the library subscribes to, CINAHL may also include other materials such as evidence-based care sheets, book chapters, continuing education modules, newsletters, standards of practice, and nurse practice acts. To identify search terms, click the CINAHL "Subject Headings" link at the top of the page and enter the search word or phrase you are searching to get a list of the associated subject headings. Figure 7-2 shows the interface for CINAHL.

MEDLINE/PubMed

When researching a biomedical research topic that crosses healthcare disciplines, use MEDLINE in addition to CINAHL. MEDLINE is a journal citation database produced by the National Library of Medicine (NLM), the largest medical library in the world. MEDLINE provides citations to biomedical articles from over 5,200 journals from around the world, some dating back to 1946 (NLM, 2022b). Access to MEDLINE is available either through PubMed on the web or through versions by commercial vendors such as EBSCO and Ovid that facilitate searching MEDLINE content using the vendor's interface (and they may include links to the full text in the vendor's other databases). PubMed also includes citations to literature not yet included in MEDLINE, articles submitted by publishers to PubMed Central, and books available online through the National Center for Biotechnology Information (NCBI) Bookshelf (NLM, n.d.). PubMed Central

TABLE 7-2 Discovering Nursing Knowledge in Library Databases

Topic of Search Question	Examples of Databases to Search
Nursing	CINAHL Cochrane Library JBI Evidence-Based Practice Database ProQuest Nursing & Allied Health MEDLINE/PubMed
Biomedical research	MEDLINE/PubMed Embase CINAHL
Education	ERIC CINAHL
Evidence-based practice/systematic reviews	Cochrane Library JBI Evidence-Based Practice Database CINAHL MEDLINE/PubMed
Legal/ethical	LexisNexis Academic CINAHL MEDLINE/PubMed
Management	ABI/INFORM CINAHL
Oncology/cancer	MEDLINE/PubMed National Cancer Institute and Physician Data Query (PDQ) CINAHL
Psychological/mental health	CINAHL APA PsycINFO APA PsycARTICLES

is a full-text archive of the biomedical and life science journal literature comprising over 5 million full-text records (NLM, 2022a). Although PubMed Central can be searched directly, records in PubMed will link out to full text in PubMed Central and on publishers' websites. While many publishers provide open-access articles, they may charge for copies of an article; as an alternative to purchasing the article, the article can be requested from a library via interlibrary loan.

Nursing & Allied Health Premium (ProQuest)

Nursing & Allied Health Premium from ProQuest indexes more than 700 peer-reviewed journals, dissertations, and gray literature (research produced outside of normal publishing routes, such as working papers and government documents). It also includes over 350 clinical skills videos (ProQuest, 2021). While there is a large overlap with CINAHL in the journals indexed, Nursing & Allied Health Premium does contain several

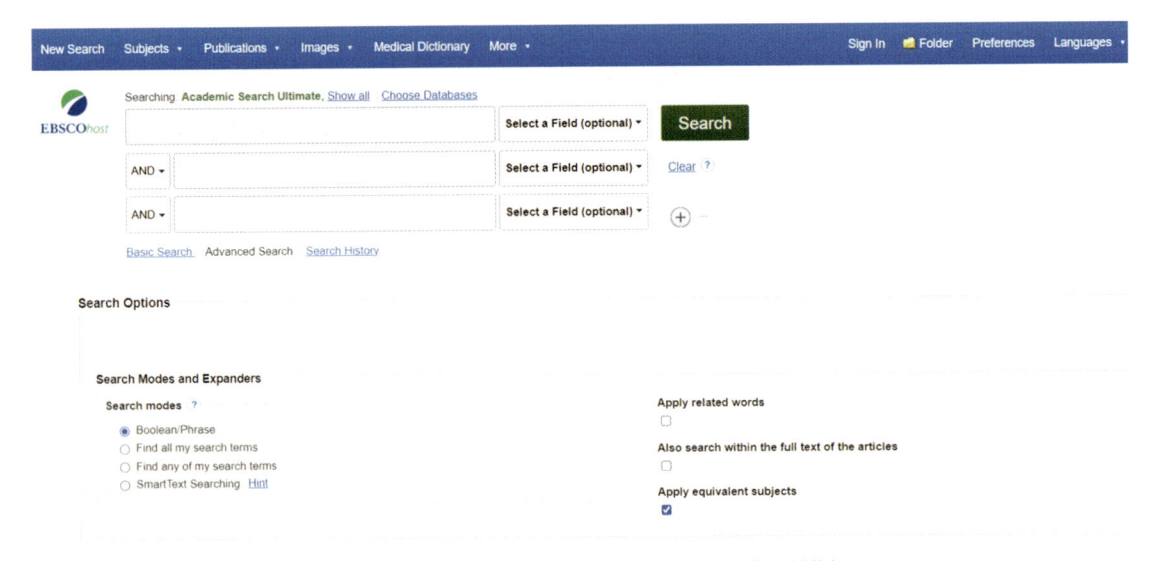

Figure 7-2. Cumulative Index to Nursing and Allied Health Literature (CINAHL).

journals not indexed in CINAHL and has a different selection of full-text articles, including full texts of dissertations. It is therefore worth searching if access is available.

Evidence-Based Practice Databases

While research studies of all kinds can be found in CINAHL and MEDLINE, there are some databases that specialize in **systematic reviews** (articles analyzing the results of multiple, similar research studies) and other materials specifically intended for EBP.

The Cochrane Library, published by John Wiley & Sons, is a product of Cochrane (formerly the Cochrane Collaboration). Founded in 1993, Cochrane is named after Dr. Archie Cochrane and was inspired by his advocacy for evidence-based medicine, particularly **randomized controlled trials** (RCTs; studies in which participants are assigned randomly to an intervention or comparison group) (Archie Cochrane, 2022). It has long been recognized as a gold standard for synthesis of medical research (Sackett et al., 1996).

Currently, Cochrane has review groups with thousands of volunteers around the world producing systematic reviews (Cochrane, 2022). The Cochrane Library consists of the Cochrane Database of Systematic Reviews, the Cochrane Central Registry of Controlled Trials, and Cochrane Clinical Answers, a database designed to inform point-of-care decision making by providing answers to clinical questions based on data and outcomes of systematic reviews (Cochrane Library, n.d.). The Cochrane Library is available through institutional or individual subscriptions. A growing number of its systematic reviews are available through open-access arrangements, and Cochrane has plans to move to an open-access model by 2025 (Cochrane, n.d.).

The JBI Evidence-Based Practice Database, available through Ovid, is also a good source of systematic reviews and related EBP materials. JBI was founded in 1996 as the Joanna Briggs Institute at the Royal Adelaide Hospital in association with the University of Adelaide in Australia. The institute was named for the first nurse at the hospital (JBI, n.d.-b). The organization currently has 75 collaborating centers in 40 countries producing materials for EBP (JBI, n.d.-a). In addition to systematic reviews, the JBI Evidence-Based Practice Database contains evidence summaries and recommended practices and best practice information sheets, all designed to summarize essential information from systematic reviews to aid in evidence-based decision making.

Other Useful Databases

For some topics, it may be meaningful to go beyond the core databases covered previously. Other non-healthcare disciplines have databases that may have content related to medical topics, and some of the more useful databases are listed here.

ABI/INFORM (ProQuest) is a comprehensive business and economics database. For nursing, it is a good source for topics pertaining to management and the business aspects of medicine.

The APA produces the PsycINFO and PsycARTICLES databases. PsycINFO is the primary citation and abstract database for the discipline, while PsycARTICLES is a full-text collection of journals published by the APA. These databases are useful when researching a question related to psychology, behavior, or mental health. Libraries often have several options for subscriptions through the APA PsycNet, EBSCO, Ovid, or ProQuest.

Embase (Elsevier) is a large biomedical database with citations from over 8,000 journals (many unique to this database), conference abstracts, and other materials. It incorporates all of the citations from MEDLINE.

Education Resources Information Center (ERIC) is a freely accessible government database sponsored by the U.S. Department of Education. In addition to indexing the scholarly education literature, it contains a series of ERIC reports. This is a useful database for topics related to nursing and patient education.

LexisNexis is an important commercial service for legal, news (including health and medical news), and business information. Nexis Academic is the version available to colleges and universities. For questions involving legal issues, including laws and legislation, this is an important source.

Physician Data Query (PDQ) is the comprehensive database of the National Cancer Institute (NCI). PDQ Cancer Information Summaries present evidence-based summaries on many cancer-related topics, while the NCI Drug Information Summaries provide information about cancer drugs and drug combinations. Access is through the publications page on the NCI website.

Searching the Invisible Web

Only a small portion (about 0.03%) of websites can be found on the **visible web (surface web)** using traditional search tools (Open Education Database, 2022). Despite this, there are plenty of scholarly documents on the visible web that you can use to support practice change. However, it is important for the informatics nurse to know about the existence of websites available on the **invisible web (deep web)** (sites not reachable by traditional search tools). There are several reasons for documents to be invisible, such as password protection or timed access. Not all pages are static or permanent. Some websites are dynamic, that is, created quickly in response to a question. An example is a schedule of flights required by a user or a list of resources in response to a question. These dynamic websites are often invisible to search engines.

Although thousands of online resources are invisible to standard searches, the searcher can discover them with a little ingenuity. As an example, advanced searches can retrieve specific file types, reading levels, and usage rights. Figure 7-3 shows an advanced search for health literacy resources with filters to annotate results with assessment content using the English language, in any file format, and usage rights that are free to use or share, even commercially. Specialized tools for searching the invisible web include the Internet Archive "Wayback Machine," USA.gov, and the WWW Virtual Library.

> **CASE STUDY**
>
> Try searching the invisible web for information about fall prevention strategies using the advanced search engine in Google. Did the results increase your understanding of the topic?

USING A SEARCH INTERFACE

Most database vendors offer a basic search **interface** consisting of a single search box and a few limiters, as well as an advanced search screen that allows users to enter multiple search terms and define fields to narrow the search. Database vendors have made these interfaces more intuitive over time. Although it is tempting to jump right in

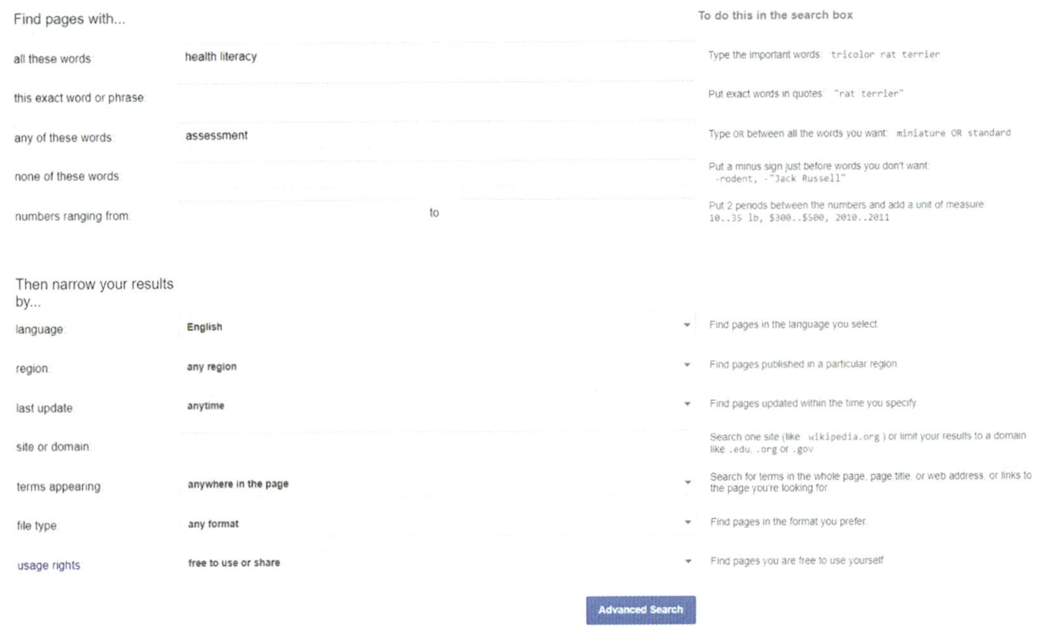

Figure 7-3. Example of using the Google advanced search feature.

and start searching, taking time to review a search interface guide and tutorials before embarking on a literature search may save time and prevent frustration and disappointing results. Each search interface links to a help menu (often identified by a "Help" or question mark link near the top of the interface) that will lead to online tutorials and guides to answer specific questions. It is important to understand that specific search features may differ by vendor and database.

Natural language searches, in which the user can search with the natural spoken phrasing rather than focusing on specific key terms, are becoming more common. However, key terms combined with Boolean searches, limiters, and the other strategies listed in the following sections are often more precise.

Boolean Connectors

When searching for nursing knowledge, be familiar with the way the vendor search engine handles Boolean connectors, named after the 19th-century mathematician George Boole. **Boolean connectors** are a form of algebra in which matches are either true or false. Three concepts make up Boolean logic: "AND," "OR," and "NOT." When used in database searching, these connectors function to find keywords in database records:

- "AND" finds records with all words (all records containing both terms).
- "OR" finds records with one or more words (all records with either or both terms).
- "NOT" finds records without the words (all records with one term but without another term).

Most databases are programmed to recognize these connecting words. Some search interfaces require Boolean connectors to be in capital letters. Other interfaces require setting the search mode to use Boolean connectors. Libraries usually have guides on how to construct a Boolean search.

Other Limiters

Stop words are words such as articles, pronouns, and prepositions that are not added to a search dictionary. The primary reason that stop words are not indexed is to allow for the most precise result list.

Truncation and wildcards can be used with many search engines. Truncation is often represented by an asterisk (*), while a common symbol for the wildcard is a question mark (?). However, these symbols vary among databases, so be sure to consult the help screens of the database you are using to find the correct symbols. Use **truncation** for searching variations in word endings. For example, a search for "nurs*" (adding an asterisk to the stem of the word) would result in citations with the words "nurse," "nurses," and "nursing." Use the **wildcard** to search for alternate spellings by replacing a single unknown character or letter anywhere in the word with the wildcard symbol. For example, a search for "colo?r" (if "?" is the wildcard symbol) will bring up results with the American spelling "color" and the British spelling "colour." A search for "wom?n" will bring results with both the singular "woman" and the plural "women."

As mentioned above, most search interfaces allow you to limit your search to attributes such as peer-reviewed journals, full-text articles, articles with references, articles with abstracts, or different types of articles from the beginning of your search. Generally, advanced search screens provide more options than basic search screens, and limiting options vary significantly from database to database, even among those offered by a single vendor. This is particularly true of subject databases that are among the primary indexes of literature in a discipline. For example, Figure 7-4 shows the options in the advanced search of CINAHL to limit and focus a search. These include such attributes as geographic subset (journals published in a given region), journal subset (journals from a particular discipline), publication type (types of articles, such as case studies or systematic reviews), and age groups (age of the subjects of study).

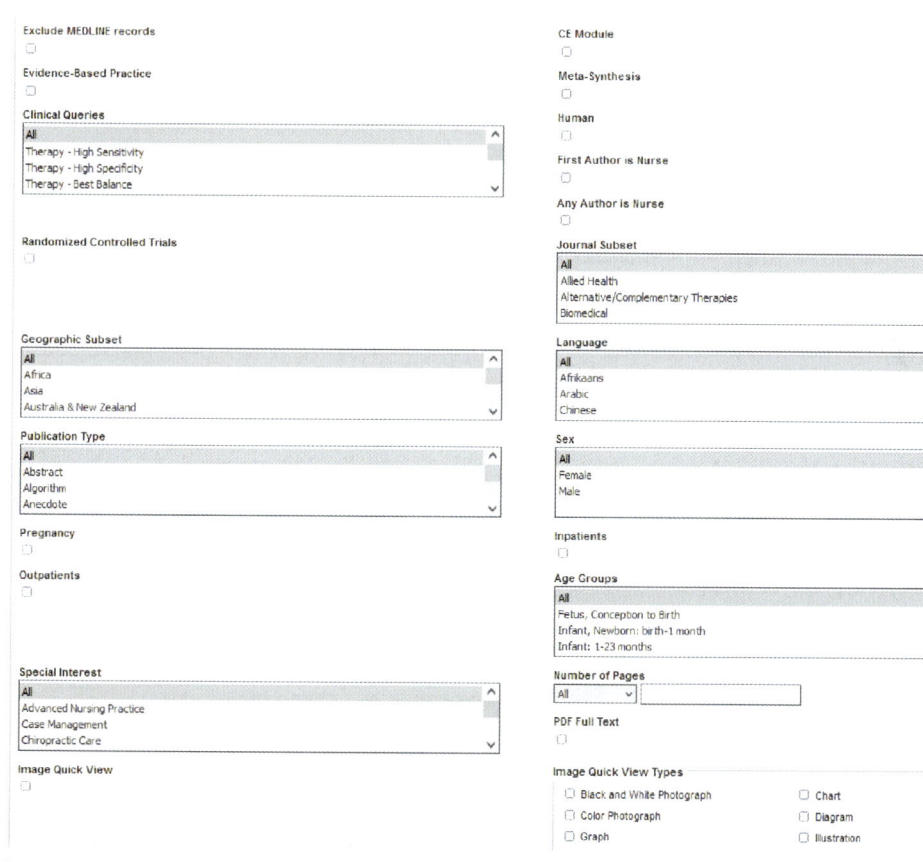

Figure 7-4. Advanced search options in CINAHL.

Many of these same limiters are available from the results list, usually as a column to the left or right of the search results, allowing the user to refine the search as they proceed. To find scholarly research articles, check what limiters are available in the database. Starting with the "peer review" or "scholarly journal" checkbox is a good start, but be aware that this limiter usually limits to a type of journal that may contain non–peer-reviewed content like book reviews. Limiting by type of article, when available, can be more precise.

Subject Headings

Searches on the web are limited to keyword searches with a few limiters available in advanced search screens. Most library databases allow for another powerful type of search, the subject search made possible by the metadata behind database records. One of the searchable fields of a database record is the subject field in which **subject headings** are entered. Subject headings form a "controlled vocabulary," that is, a standardized list of terms. During the cataloguing or indexing process, one or more terms are chosen from this list that best match the subject or subjects covered in the source. This means that all items in the database that relate to that subject can be found through searching one subject heading. It also makes combining subject and keyword searching possible.

Subject headings are sometimes called subject terms or descriptors in databases. They can usually be found in database records and the most common subject headings in a search often appear at the side of search results, among the options for refining searches. Subject headings are often hyperlinked in database records, allowing the user to quickly find other sources with the same heading. Many databases also allow the user to look up subject headings through an index, sometimes called a thesaurus, which suggests related concepts and synonyms. Once found, the user can begin a search with a subject heading by selecting the subject field in the search box (usually through a drop-down menu) and typing in the subject heading.

There are several lists of subject headings used by libraries and indexing services. Library of Congress (LC) subject headings are standard for academic library catalogues and form the basis of the subject heading lists in many library databases. Health sciences libraries and databases, on the other hand, may use the NLM medical subject headings (MeSH), sometimes in addition to LC subject headings.

Searching Using MeSH Terms

Medical subject headings (MeSH) refer to the controlled vocabulary of terms used to index materials in the PubMed and MEDLINE databases. CINAHL subject headings also follow the MeSH structure. Since CINAHL and MEDLINE are two primary databases of nursing literature, it is important to understand this search term structure. MeSH headings are organized in a "tree" structure with 16 top-level branches. Each branch has several levels of sub-branches, with each heading and subheading having a place in the hierarchy. Terms can appear in more than one branch. Searching on a broader term will automatically "explode" the search to include all narrower terms from the tree. For example, Figure 7-5 shows the hierarchy for "neoplasms," which falls under the main branch "diseases." A search for "neoplasms" will include all of the narrower terms and their subheadings from "cysts" down. A search for "neoplasms by site" will be more limited, including those terms grouped below it. A search for "abdominal neoplasms" will have an even narrower focus.

It is worth taking the time to understand how to use subject headings and MeSH terms before using a search interface. As MeSH headings are revised each year, it is also important to know how to use the NLM's MeSH database to look up subject headings. A link to the database can be found on the NLM homepage. The database is also linked to PubMed, and the PubMed Online Training page contains a MeSH tutorial.

Advantages of Search Interfaces

Most search interfaces have tools that allow emailing, exporting, printing, or saving citations and full-text files from the search results. Most also allow the user to select a common citation format, such as APA, the Modern Language Association

NIH National Library of Medicine

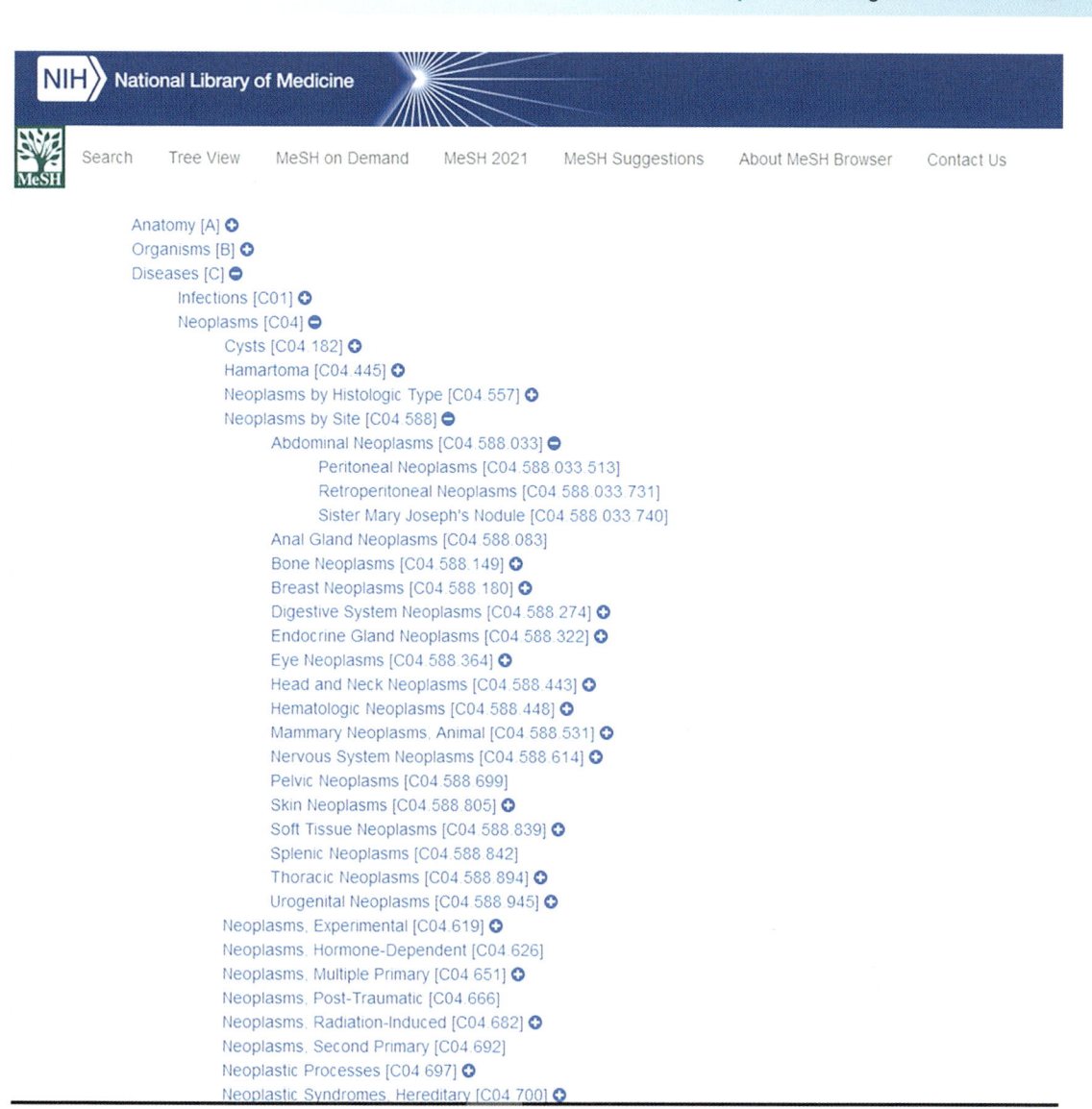

MeSH | Search | Tree View | MeSH on Demand | MeSH 2021 | MeSH Suggestions | About MeSH Browser | Contact Us

- Anatomy [A]
- Organisms [B]
- Diseases [C]
    - Infections [C01]
    - Neoplasms [C04]
        - Cysts [C04.182]
        - Hamartoma [C04.445]
        - Neoplasms by Histologic Type [C04.557]
        - Neoplasms by Site [C04.588]
            - Abdominal Neoplasms [C04.588.033]
                - Peritoneal Neoplasms [C04.588.033.513]
                - Retroperitoneal Neoplasms [C04.588.033.731]
                - Sister Mary Joseph's Nodule [C04.588.033.740]
            - Anal Gland Neoplasms [C04.588.083]
            - Bone Neoplasms [C04.588.149]
            - Breast Neoplasms [C04.588.180]
            - Digestive System Neoplasms [C04.588.274]
            - Endocrine Gland Neoplasms [C04.588.322]
            - Eye Neoplasms [C04.588.364]
            - Head and Neck Neoplasms [C04.588.443]
            - Hematologic Neoplasms [C04.588.448]
            - Mammary Neoplasms, Animal [C04.588.531]
            - Nervous System Neoplasms [C04.588.614]
            - Pelvic Neoplasms [C04.588.699]
            - Skin Neoplasms [C04.588.805]
            - Soft Tissue Neoplasms [C04.588.839]
            - Splenic Neoplasms [C04.588.842]
            - Thoracic Neoplasms [C04.588.894]
            - Urogenital Neoplasms [C04.588.945]
        - Neoplasms, Experimental [C04.619]
        - Neoplasms, Hormone-Dependent [C04.626]
        - Neoplasms, Multiple Primary [C04.651]
        - Neoplasms, Post-Traumatic [C04.666]
        - Neoplasms, Radiation-Induced [C04.682]
        - Neoplasms, Second Primary [C04.692]
        - Neoplastic Processes [C04.697]
        - Neoplastic Syndromes, Hereditary [C04.700]

Figure 7-5. MeSH heading tree for "neoplasms" in the MeSH database on the National Library of Medicine website.

(MLA), and the American Medical Association (AMA). Vendors such as EBSCO, ProQuest, and Ovid also offer free personal accounts as part of institutional subscriptions. (This means the user will retain access to the personal account only as long as they are affiliated with the institution.) These accounts require registration and are accessed through the vendor's interface. In addition to the tasks described previously, personal accounts allow users to save search histories for future reference, organize research into folders for multiple projects, and gather information from multiple databases provided by the vendor. However, if the user frequently moves between databases by different vendors or including web sources in addition to sources from databases, or if they want to consolidate their research in one place, a reference manager can be useful.

> **CASE STUDY**
>
> Look back to the case study. Do a library search for individualized fall prevention strategies published since 2020. Did the Fowler and Reising article come up in your search? Has there been additional research on the topic that supports the use of individualized fall prevention strategies?

SOURCES OF NURSING KNOWLEDGE

Reading articles (also called literature) about nursing research and EBP is one of the best ways to understand what is needed to conduct research and EBP. Searching for information to solve clinical problems, also known as a literature review or going to the literature, is covered in detail in Chapter 11. This section will provide a brief overview of the various places and ways that research and EBP are published to provide an idea for where to begin looking. Remember that nurses are often involved in research and EBP. Reading articles can be the inspiration to turn questions into research or EBP studies.

Scholarly Nursing Journals

Scholarly nursing journals contain articles about studies and research conducted by people with expertise in nursing. The peer-review process for scholarly journals is rigorous. Once received by the editorial office, the journal's editor screens each article. If the editor considers the subject matter appropriate for the journal readers, the editor sends a copy with the author's name removed (sometimes called a blind review) to two or more nurse experts for peer review to ensure the validity, quality, and reliability of information. If the article receives approval for publication, the authors are allowed to make final editing changes based on the comments of the reviewers and editors.

Be sure to differentiate a scholarly article from news or magazines. Scholarly articles usually have an abstract and include references. The name and credentials of the authors are listed in the article. When using a library database, the user can limit the search options to include resources that are peer reviewed.

Although academic libraries provide the most comprehensive nursing and medical knowledge, most journals and full-text scholarly journal articles are also available online. Many print journals are choosing to publish articles online before they are featured in a printed edition of the journal. Scholarly journal articles are often available online as a personal subscription benefit to print journal subscribers or with a small fee for nonsubscribers. The online presence of print journals also allows nonsubscribers who want to purchase and download individual articles to set up an account and purchase only what they need.

Impact Factors

The **impact factor (IF)** of a journal helps determine its scholarly merit. The IF is an index calculated by Clarivate, a British-American analytics company, that reflects the yearly mean number of citations of articles published in the last 2 years in a given journal. The IF is frequently used as a measure of the relative importance of a journal within its field; journals with higher IF values carry more prestige than those with lower values. The IF is frequently used by universities and funding bodies to decide on promotion and research proposals.

The top 10 journals ranked by IF, according to Journal Citation Reports for 2022 (University of Colorado Anschutz Medical Campus, 2023), are:

1. *International Journal of Nursing Studies*
2. *International Journal of Mental Health Nursing*
3. *Journal of Nursing Management*
4. *Intensive and Critical Care Nursing*
5. *Nursing Outlook*
6. *Worldviews on Evidence-Based Nursing*
7. *Journal of Clinical Nursing*
8. *Nursing Ethics*
9. *International Nursing Review*
10. *Nurse Education Today*

Online Journals

True online journals publish all their articles online with no print version. They feature peer-reviewed articles and maintain an archive. Bibliographic databases, such as CINAHL and MEDLINE, index some online journals but not all of them. The number of online nursing journals continues growing slowly.

In 1996, the *Online Journal of Issues in Nursing* (*OJIN*) became the first fully online nursing journal (OJIN, n.d.). The focus of *OJIN* is to provide different views on current topics relating to nursing practice, research, and education. *OJIN* is peer-reviewed and indexed in both CINAHL and MEDLINE. The American Nurses Association (ANA) now sponsors *OJIN*. The *Online Journal of Nursing Informatics* (*OJNI*) focuses on topics relating to nursing informatics. The Healthcare Information and Management Systems Society (HIMSS) sponsors *OJNI*.

There are many benefits to using online journals. When they are open access, there is broader readership. Articles published in online journals are instantly available, meaning dissemination of research happens more quickly. They are easily accessible and are often designed for mobile-friendly access. They can be more easily edited if errors are discovered or retractions are needed. They are also more environmentally friendly, requiring no material, printing, or shipping costs to publish (PubliMill, n.d.).

One difficulty with online journals is the perception that the quality of their content is lower than that of print journals. A few bibliographic indexes still refuse to index such journals for this reason. Part of this perception may result from the great variability in the quality of online journals, and part of it is a perception among researchers that online journals do not have as rigorous a peer-review process. However, as most print journals are turning to online options, scholars increasingly use online options to access journal articles. Acceptance of online-only journals is growing.

Another difficulty with online journals is the lack of awareness that the journals exist, especially the ones that are not indexed by services such as EBSCO, MEDLINE, or Embase. Although nurses in all specialties need to be information literate, some are not. A person who has not learned how to use the web is limited to print journals. In addition, search engine results do not necessarily make a distinction between a scholarly print journal with a web presence and a true online journal, magazine, or newspaper.

Unlike print journals, which are the product of a publishing company, many online journals start with little financial or organizational support. As a result, the life cycle of some online journals is short. Although it may seem easy to run an online journal, a large amount of work is involved in producing one of high quality. The journal staff must find writers, reviewers, and administrative staff to coordinate the progress of articles, someone to convert the articles into an online format, and staff to market the journal. All these tasks and responsibilities take time and money. Without strong financial backing, sustaining publication of the journal can become insurmountable.

Open-Access Journals

The term **open access** refers to free and open online access to academic information in the form of publications, images, and data. Open-access journals publish peer-reviewed articles with no user fees. Many open-access journals have limited copyright and licensing restrictions and allow anyone with an internet connection to download, copy, and distribute the articles. *BMC Nursing* is a peer-reviewed online open-access journal that publishes research on topics related to nursing research, training, practice, and education. Access to full-text articles from other medical journals is available from BioMed Central and from the Directory of Open Access Journals (DOAJ).

Some open-access journals charge processing fees to authors to cover publishing costs. In fact, some high-quality journals may charge several thousand dollars to publish an article. As a result, the publication setting shifts from high-priced access to journals to high-priced publication costs for the authors. There are benefits and drawbacks to open-access publication. Open-access publication undoubtedly increases the number of people who have access to research findings and articles. Open-access journals tend to be more widely read, shared, and cited (Cuschieri, 2018). However, the high costs for publication for the author may create an economic divide in which authors who cannot afford the costs of publication are not published. In addition, open-access publishing has spurred the growth of numerous questionable or predatory open-access journals. Many academic libraries maintain guidelines for identifying questionable open-access journals, often based on criteria from Beall (2012) and Prater (2017). Some questionable practices include a lack of a reputable editorial board, poor website quality, and article content that is not consistent with the stated scope of the publication.

Open-Access Journal Articles Resulting From Grant Funding

In 2005, the National Institutes of Health (NIH) issued a policy providing unrestricted open access to publications resulting from NIH-funded research within 12 months of publication (NIH, 2005). In 2022, the White House Office of Science and Technology (OSTP) updated policy guidelines to mandate taxpayer-supported research be made available to the public immediately and at no cost, eliminating the 12-month wait (The White House, 2022). As a result of mandates such as these, a large amount of high-quality peer-reviewed research is available to the public from the PubMed website. The trend for mandating open access to publications from grant funding continues to grow in the United States, Canada, the United Kingdom, and Europe.

Magazine, Newsletter, Newspaper, and Website Articles

Most online magazines, newsletters, and other online articles are available without charge because of advertising support. Newspapers with an online presence generally charge a subscription fee but may allow a certain number of free articles. Generally, these sources address current topics such as career information, jobs, and news items of interest to their audience. Only a few magazines maintain archives. Newspapers are more likely to have archives since they are often online versions of print products. On sites with no archives, information has a short life.

It is critically important for nurses to be able to differentiate a scholarly nursing article from an article in a magazine, newspaper, newsletter, or other website. In contrast to the expert writers of scholarly articles, reporters often write the articles in magazines, newsletters, and newspapers. Reporters are not required to be nurses or to have any expertise in nursing practice. Editors review and approve content for publication but they are not necessarily content experts and there is no peer-review process. Magazines and other news media may not cite specific references. The information online varies in quality, which is why nurses should carefully scrutinize websites using the currency, relevance, authority, accuracy, purpose (CRAAP) tool found in Chapter 9.

Government and Not-for-Profit Specialty Organization Information

Government-sponsored and not-for-profit health and disease specialty organizations include quality information that enhances nursing knowledge. The NIH's website has links to the associated 27 specialty institutes and centers providing information to the latest NIH research, clinical trials, and grants to promote health. The website of the Centers for Disease Control and Prevention (CDC) provides statistical data, information about diseases and disease control, and online disease control and prevention journals. The CDC WONDER website provides searchable online databases with public health data, morbidity tables, and the Healthy People 2030 initiative. The website for the Agency for Healthcare Research and Quality (AHRQ) provides information on EBP, grants, research, and quality and patient safety issues. Finally, the Centers for Medicare & Medicaid Services (CMS) provides access to manuals, a Medicare coverage database, CMS forms, communication of policy changes, and Medicare learning network resources.

Professional Nursing Organization Information

Each professional nursing organization has a website with general information for the public and password-protected information for its members. For example, the ANA website includes membership information and links to purchase the Nursing Code of Ethics and the Scope and Standards of Practice for nursing specialties. The ANA also includes links to information on continuing education modules, individual and Magnet certification, ANA-sponsored nursing journals and books, healthcare policy, and much more.

The website of the Sigma Theta Tau International (STTI) Honor Society of Nursing has membership information, links to STTI-sponsored journals and books, as well as continuing education modules. Examples of resources include grants, research, full-text journal articles and data sets, Doctor of Nursing Practice final projects, theses, and learning objects created by faculty.

Laws, Rules, and Regulations

Several sites relate to laws, rules, and regulations. The website of the National Council of State Boards of Nursing (NCSBN) includes links to all U.S. state boards of nursing and includes information about the National Council Licensure Examination (NCLEX). Each state board of nursing site includes clearly stated laws, policies, and rules and regulations. The state boards of nursing websites also provide services for license verification and license renewal online. Other regulatory websites include those of The Joint Commission, the CMS, and individual state departments of health and human services.

Online Evidence-Based Resources

The internet has an abundance of information about evidence-based care resources. As with other healthcare information found on the internet, the variation in quality is tremendous. The first step toward approaching a search for evidence-based care is to determine what one wants to learn. Some of the most comprehensive websites are in libraries and educational EBP centers. Clinical practice guidelines are available from government and educational websites in the United States, Canada, England, and Australia. Table 7-3 provides a starting point for nurses and healthcare professionals beginning to learn about EBP.

TABLE 7-3 Evidence-Based Practice Information on the Internet

Evidence-Based Practice Topic	Resources
Definition and history	*Crossing the Quality Chasm: A New Health System for the 21st Century* (Institute of Medicine Committee on Quality of Health Care in American Nurses Association, 2015), Chapter 6
Core competencies	Nursing Competency: Definition, Structure and Development (Fukada, 2018)
Education resources	• Introduction to Evidence-Based Practice • Evidence-Based Medicine Toolbox
Evidence-based nursing	Sigma Theta Tau International
Clinical practice guidelines	• AHRQ Clinical Practice Guidelines Online • Nursing Best Practice Guidelines (Registered Nurses of Ontario) • Joanna Briggs Institute: Best Practice Information Sheets
How to read, evaluate, and use research	• Critical appraisal tools by the Centre for Evidence-Based Medicine • Critical Appraisal Skills Programme (CASP) • Evidence-Based Practice for Nursing: Evaluating the Evidence

> **BOX 7-1** Rating System for the Hierarchy of Evidence
>
> Level I: Evidence from a systematic review or meta-analysis of all RCTs or evidence-based clinical practice guideline based on systematic review of RCTs
> Level II: Evidence obtained from at least one well-designed RCT
> Level III: Evidence obtained from well-designed controlled trials without randomization
> Level IV: Evidence from well-designed case–control and cohort studies
> Level V: Evidence from systematic reviews of descriptive and qualitative studies
> Level VI: Evidence from single descriptive or qualitative studies
> Level VII: Evidence from the opinion of authorities and/or reports of expert committees
>
> From Melnyk, B. M., & Fineout-Overholt, E. (2023). *Evidence-based practice in nursing & healthcare: A guide to best practice* (5th ed.). Philadelphia, PA: Wolters Kluwer Health/Lippincott Williams & Wilkins.

Levels of Evidence

When evaluating published articles about research, EBP, or QI, Melnyk and Fineout-Overholt's (2023) rating system for hierarchy of evidence can be useful (Box 7-1). The lower the number, the more credible the information is for making decisions about clinical care.

The most credible evidence is from systematic reviews, **meta-analyses** (research on previous research, similar to systematic reviews), and RCTs. EBP is based on the most credible, rigorously researched evidence.

EXAMPLE OF CONDUCTING A LITERATURE SEARCH

Imagine working on a unit where the fall rate is high despite best efforts. The burning question might be, "What is the most effective nursing intervention for preventing patient falls on my unit?" Perhaps an initial idea is to use something the unit has not tried before, like video monitors to oversee patient movements. However, a researcher needs to go into the literature search with an open mind.

Search for the Best Evidence

Once the research question has been formulated, put it into PICOT format to guide the literature search. For example, the PICOT question may be formatted like this:

- Population/patient/problem: Adult patients receiving care on a medical-surgical unit who are falling
- Intervention: Develop a novel fall prevention strategy, such as video monitoring, suitable for nurses on the unit
- Comparison: The fall prevention interventions already in place on the unit
- Outcome: Reduction in the fall rate on the unit
- Time: Within 3 months

Next, decide what kind of information is needed to answer the question and where the best place to find that information might be. When focusing on a question of nursing practice, a good place to begin is with systematic reviews found in CINAHL. Using the PICOT format, the key concepts are "P," "hospital patients" and "falls," and "I," "prevention strategy." Try out the following steps on CINAHL. Be aware that the following figures were generated from searches performed in the fall of 2023. The appropriate date range for the past 5 years and the number of results are likely to have changed.

1. *Find the* "Advanced Search" *screen.* If you see three search boxes that allow you to select fields to search on the right and Boolean connectors on the left, you are on the "Advanced Search" screen. If you see only one search box, click on "Advanced Search" under it.
2. *Arrange key terms in the search boxes.* In the top box, type "hospital patients," in the next box, type "falls," and in the third box, type "prevention." The initial search yields 837 results. Under "Search Options," check the boxes for "Full Text," "Academic Journals," and under "Subject: Major Heading," check the box for

"inpatients." Limit the published date range to the past 5 years. The "Apply Equivalent Subjects" box is already checked. This works as an expander, adding additional words mapped to the keywords, so it is usually a good idea to keep it. Make sure the Boolean "AND" connector is selected.

3. *Review the* "Search Results" *screen.* This search yielded 55 results (Fig. 7-6). Notice that the current search phrases and limiters appear to the left of the search results with additional ways to limit and refine the search in the column below. (Clicking on "Show More" under the date range will bring up the comprehensive search options menu.)

4. *Review the individual records.* Clicking on a title will lead to the database record, which usually includes an abstract. When available, full text can be accessed from links in the search results or database record. Although the option of limiting to available full text is available, this is not recommended for a comprehensive literature search. First, you will want to know about all the literature available, and second, you will often find the full text of articles in other databases or will be able to order them through interlibrary loan.

5. *Review the subject options.* While entering search terms, other words are suggested. These are the subject headings used in the MeSH database. As indexing terms, these words can often prove invaluable to refine a search. For example, as you type in the word "fall," you may see a MeSH term like "fall prevention in hospitals." Redoing the search with this new term yields 23 results.

After thorough searching in CINAHL, you may decide to expand your search by searching PubMed, the freely available government database.

1. *Enter the key concepts into the search.* PubMed's search interface automatically maps search

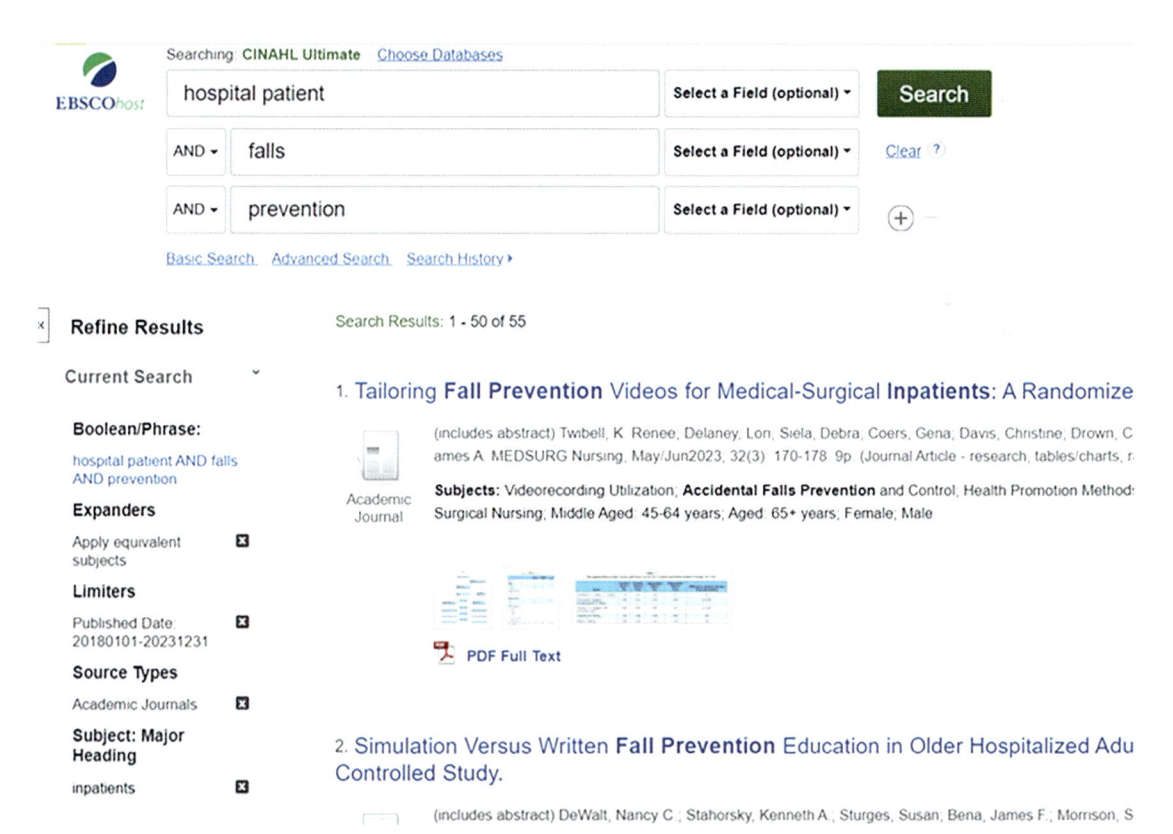

Figure 7-6. CINAHL search results showing "Advanced Search" at the top and limiting options on left.

terms to MeSH headings when they're entered in the search box. Therefore, it is recommended not to use punctuation, Boolean connectors, or truncation symbols when using the main search box. (Using them turns off the automatic mapping.) Because the scope of PubMed is much broader than nursing, you might want to include "nursing" as a keyword. Thus, you enter "inpatient falls prevention nursing" into the search box.

2. *Review the search results screen.* The results screen shows 534 results. As with CINAHL, you can limit to a date range and article type on the left side of the search results. Limiting to the past 5 years and "Systematic Reviews" yields 198 results (Fig. 7-7).

3. *Use the advanced search builder.* If you want to search by MeSH terms or other fields, or combine subject and keyword searching, use the Advanced Search Builder, which also allows for Boolean connectors (typed in all capital letters) and truncation.

It is important to remember that a comprehensive search must never be limited to the web, online library full-text resources, or even one database. Although a wide range of information resources is available online, libraries, librarians, and bookstores are vital to help borrow or purchase the knowledge-based resources needed for nursing education and practice. Always check with the librarian to see what your options are.

While searching for and finding relevant citations, it is advisable to save or download the citation information for use in the analysis and summary of the literature search. A reference manager or personal account with the library database would be useful for this purpose. PubMed also has options to save, email, or export citations. A personal NCBI account has the ability export citations to "My Bibliography" by selecting the

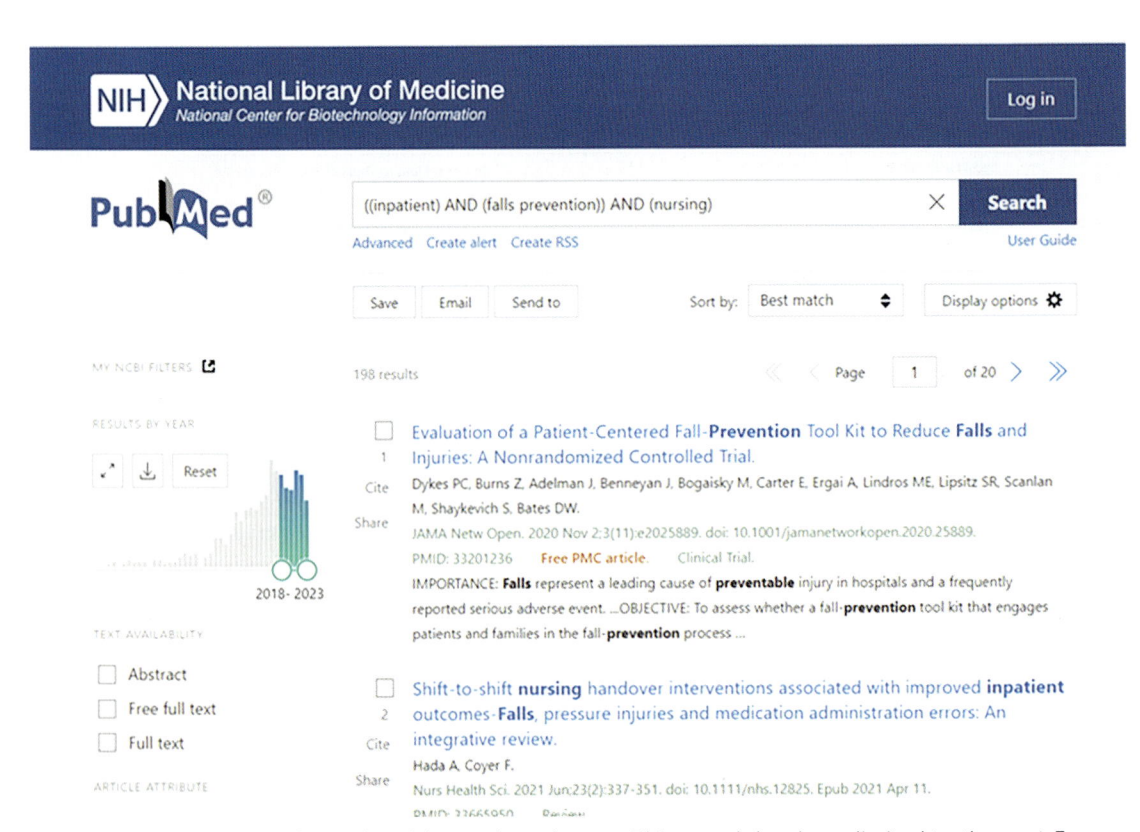

Figure 7-7. PubMed search results with search at the top. This search has been limited to the past 5 years with article type "Systematic Review."

"Send to" button above the search results. The same button allows the user to select "Citation Manager" to create a file for export to any reference manager.

Conduct a Critical Appraisal of the Studies

Although clinical judgment (a combination of critical thinking and clinical reasoning) is required for each step in the search process, it is especially important when analyzing the information from the search results. A critical appraisal should be done to make sure that it provides the appropriate evidence to answer the information need. Reading abstracts and browsing the conclusions of articles can be a good way to determine which ones can answer your research question in whole or part. After reviewing the abstracts, decide on the articles that could be potentially useful and download or request the full text of each article to read.

Select the most recent articles possible. A rule of thumb is to use the sources published within the past 3 to 5 years. Literature reviews and references within articles are a good way to learn about additional sources, especially important older articles that may represent seminal work. **Seminal work** refers to work frequently cited by others or influences the opinions of others. The Sackett et al. (1996) article about evidence-based medicine, cited in the section on the Cochrane Library in this chapter, is an example of seminal work.

The next step is to read each article in full to analyze the findings critically. Highlight key points pertinent to the search question. Identify any gaps in knowledge. For example, were any age groups of patients omitted? Was there an omission of any practice settings? Look for agreements and differences in research findings using the literature review, discussion, and conclusion sections of the research articles. Assess whether the literature findings are current and relevant to answer your search topic question.

Finally, assess the quality of the evidence. Analyze the literature using the seven-level rating system from Box 7-1. The most credible form of evidence is derived from meta-analyses of RCTs and evidence-based clinical guidelines based on systematic reviews of RCTs. When searching and reviewing the literature, look for the search terms "systematic review" and "meta-analysis." Be aware that the least credible forms of evidence are from the opinion of authorities and/or reports from expert committees.

Although the original idea was to use video monitors to address the problem of falls, after reading all the articles, developing a comprehensive education toolkit seems like the best option. Many of the important interventions discovered in the literature, such as toileting, complimentary health interventions, and high-risk medication, can be included in the educational intervention. The literature also shows how important it is to push this education out to all staff, not just nurses. Many of the articles measure falls on a month-to-month basis, so the same can be done when measuring new outcomes. The PICOT now looks like this:

- Population/patient/problem: Adult patients receiving care on a medical-surgical unit who are falling
- Intervention: Develop a *fall prevention education toolkit* suitable for *all hospital staff*
- Comparison: The fall prevention interventions already in place on the unit
- Outcome: Reduction in the *monthly* fall rate on the unit
- Time: Within 3 months

SUMMARY

- **Creating nursing knowledge.** Nursing research is a process done to collect data that build nursing knowledge, the information known to the nursing practice which defines the profession. Nursing knowledge is collected and analyzed through research, EBP, and QI. The seven-step ARCC model guides EBP research, which is cyclical in nature in that researchers may move back and forth through different steps to refine ideas. To narrow down research, a well-thought-out research question should be put into PICOT format.
- **Library advantages.** Libraries provide access to resources and services essential for finding current research to support research and EBP. Digital library basics involve understanding how to find useful information in the vast amount of knowledge on the internet. Discovery searches are a good place to begin and are usually available

on university library websites. Librarians are highly qualified to help find resources.

- **Using databases for research.** Databases contain metadata, information about other data in the form of bibliographic records. Reference managers are software programs that allow users to keep track of their research. They can capture citations from databases. Avoiding plagiarism involves the correct use of references and citations and using a plagiarism checker like iThenticate or Turnitin. Bibliographic databases pertinent to nursing include CINAHL, MEDLINE/PubMed, Cochrane Library, JBI Evidence-Based Practice Database, and APA PsycINFO/PsycARTICLES.
- **Using a search interface.** Using a search interface to look for references is more useful and accurate with good search strategies. Review guides and tutorials can help with this. Boolean terminology is used to search databases with "AND," "OR," and "NOT" conventions. Truncation and wildcards also facilitate effective searching. When searching, use MeSH to access the controlled vocabulary of terms associated with subject headings. Search interfaces facilitate saving search results for future access.
- **Sources of nursing knowledge.** Sources of nursing knowledge need to be carefully examined by student researchers to ensure they are accurate and credible. Sources include scholarly nursing journals with a high IF; online journals with peer-reviewed articles; open-access journals; magazine, newsletter, newspaper, or website articles; government and not-for-profit health and disease specialty organizations; professional nursing organizations; laws, rules, and regulations; and online evidence-based resources. When evaluating published articles, use the rating system for the hierarchy of evidence. The higher the level, the more credible the information is for making decisions about clinical care.
- **Conducting the literature search.** The literature search is a critical component of the research process. After developing a PICOT question, search for the best evidence and then conduct a critical appraisal of the evidence. When searching for evidence, use key concepts and narrow the topic. It helps to begin with systematic reviews to get an idea of the current state of the research. Use resources that are as recent as possible, but it is acceptable to also cite seminal works. Looking at abstracts can help narrow results. Then read each article looking for gaps in knowledge and evaluate the evidence with the hierarchy of evidence. Finally, update the PICOT question with new information discovered in the search.

DISCUSSION QUESTIONS AND ACTIVITIES

1. Look at the steps of the ARCC model in Figure 7-1. Which step seems to be the most challenging? Which seems to be the easiest? Explain your answers.
2. Think about a clinical issue you have observed other than fall prevention, and decide if research, EBP, or QI are most appropriate for solving this problem.
3. Choose a nursing topic and conduct several searches for information in CINAHL or another nursing database. Try searching by keyword, then by subject. Try combining subject headings with keywords in a single search. Experiment with the search options by choosing limiters, a date range, and using some of the search techniques (e.g., Boolean connectors, truncation, wildcard) mentioned in this chapter. Which searches were most effective? How did different modes of searching and using different search techniques affect the search?
4. Search for personal reference management software. Summarize the findings using information from:
   a. Recent articles and reviews discussing personal reference management software, both online and journal articles retrieved with the search
   b. Pertinent online tutorials and support for users of the personal reference management software

   Based on your research, identify a personal reference management software that best meets your needs.
5. How does knowing about bibliographic records, subject headings, limiters, and other search

options affect your search strategy for finding information in library databases? How does this differ from the strategy you might use in a web search? Choose a topic and briefly compare and contrast the way you would go about searching for information in a library database and a search engine such as Google.

PRACTICE QUESTIONS

1. The PICOT acronym is used to help guide the formulation of research questions. The "C" in PICOT stands for:
   a. clinician.
   b. clinical setting.
   c. comparison.
   d. cost.

2. Databases that index the periodical literature of a particular discipline, providing citations, abstracts, and sometimes full text, are:
   a. factual databases.
   b. bibliographic databases.
   c. full-text journal collections.
   d. library catalogues.

3. A description of an item in a database organized in searchable fields is known as a(n):
   a. bibliographic record.
   b. citation.
   c. subject heading.
   d. abstract.

4. An example of a "controlled vocabulary" or standardized list of words used in indexing is a:
   a. keyword.
   b. limiter.
   c. subject heading.
   d. stop word.

5. A service available in most libraries that allows the user to borrow materials from other libraries, including the full text of articles, is:
   a. interlibrary loan.
   b. library guides.
   c. discovery search.
   d. metadata.

REFERENCES

American Nurses Association. (2015). *Code of ethics for nurses*. American Nurses Publishing. https://www.nursingworld.org/practice-policy/nursing-excellence/ethics/code-of-ethics-for-nurses/

Amsberry, S. (2022). Promoting academic integrity in nursing education: An integrative review. *Journal of Nursing Education, 61*(6), 303–307. https://doi.org/10.3928/01484834-20220404-14

Archie Cochrane. (2022). In *Wikipedia*. Retrieved July 8, 2022. https://en.wikipedia.org/wiki/Archie_Cochrane

Beall, J. (2012, December 1). *Criteria for determining predatory open-access publishers*. Retrieved from https://scholarlyoa.files.wordpress.com/2012/11/criteria-2012-2.pdf

CINAHL. (2021). In *Wikipedia*. Retrieved July 8, 2022. https://en.wikipedia.org/wiki/CINAHL

Cochrane Library. (n.d.). *About the Cochrane Library*. Retrieved July 8, 2022. https://www.cochranelibrary.com/about/about-cochrane-library/

Cochrane. (n.d.). *Our open access strategy*. Retrieved July 8, 2022. https://www.cochrane.org/about-us/our-open-access-strategy

Cochrane (organisation). (2022). In *Wikipedia*. Retrieved July 8, 2022. https://en.wikipedia.org/wiki/Cochrane_(organisation)

Cuschieri, S. (2018). WASP: Is open access publishing the way forward? A review of the different ways in which research papers can be published. *Early Human Developmental, 121*, 54–57. https://doi.org/10.1016/j.earlhumdev.2018.02.017

EBSCO. (n.d.). *CINAHL ultimate*. Retrieved July 8, 2022. https://www.ebsco.com/products/research-databases/cinahl-ultimate

Fowler, S. B., & Reising, E. S. (2021). A replication study of fall TIPS (tailoring interventions for patient safety): A patient-centered fall prevention toolkit. *MedSurg Nursing, 30*(1), 28–34.

Goodwin, J., & McCarthy, J. (2020). Explaining plagiarism for nursing students: An educational tool. *Teaching and Learning in Nursing, 15*(3), 198–203. https://doi.org/10.1016/j.teln.2020.03.004

JBI. (n.d.-a). *JBI collaboration*. University of Adelaide. Retrieved July 8, 2022 https://jbi.global/global-reach/collaboration

JBI. (n.d.-b). *Our history*. https://jbi.global/our-history

Melnyk, B. M., & Fineout-Overholt, E. (2023). *Evidence-based practice in nursing & healthcare: A guide to best practice* (5th ed.). Wolters Kluwer Health/Lippincott Williams & Wilkins.

National Institute of Nursing Research (NINR). (2022). *The National institute of nursing research 2022-2026 strategic plan*. https://www.ninr.nih.gov/aboutninr/ninr-mission-and-strategic-plan

National Institutes of Health (NIH). (2005). *Policy on enhancing public access to archived publications resulting from NIH-funded research*. https://grants.nih.gov/grants/guide/notice-files/NOT-OD-05-022.html

National Library of Medicine (NLM). (2022a). *About PMC*. Retrieved July 8, 2022. https://www.ncbi.nlm.nih.gov/pmc/about/intro/

National Library of Medicine (NLM). (2022b). *Medline: Overview*. Retrieved July 8, 2022. https://www.nlm.nih.gov/medline/medline_overview

National Library of Medicine (NLM). (n.d.). *PubMed overview*. Retrieved July 8, 2022. https://pubmed.ncbi.nlm.nih.gov/about

Open Education Database. (2022). *The ultimate guide to the invisible web*. http://oedb.org/ilibrarian/invisible-web/

Prater, C. (2017). *8 ways to identify a questionable open access journal*. American Journal Experts. Retrieved from http://www.aje.com/en/arc/8-ways-identify-questionable-open-access-journal/

ProQuest. (2021). *Introducing nursing & allied health premium*. Retrieved July 8, 2022. https://go.proquest.com/nursing-and-allied-health-premium/

PubliMill. (n.d.). *Benefits of online journal publishing*. https://publimill.vtex.lt/benefits-of-online-journal-publishing/

Sackett, D. L., Rosenberg, W. M., Gray, J. A., Haynes, R. B., & Richardson, W. S. (1996). Evidence based medicine: What it is and what it isn't. *British Medical Journal, 312*(7023), 71–72. https://doi:10.1136/bmj.312.7023.71

The Online Journal of Issues in Nursing (OJIN). (n.d.). *Author submission guidelines*. https://ojin.nursingworld.org/about-ojin/author-guidelines

The White House. (2022). *OSTP issues guidance to make federally funded research freely available without delay*. https://www.whitehouse.gov/ostp/news-updates/2022/08/25/ostp-issues-guidance-to-make-federally-funded-research-freely-available-without-delay/

University of Colorado Anschutz Medical Campus. (2023.) *JCR top 20 nursing journals*. Strauss Health Sciences Library. https://library-cuanschutz.libguides.com/c.php?g=259536&p=6935490

CHAPTER 8

Collecting Data

Kristi Miller

OBJECTIVES

After studying this chapter, you will be able to:
1. Follow data collection guidelines when collecting data.
2. Discuss the importance of collecting data that represent the diversity of healthcare consumers.
3. Compare data collection tools.
4. Explain the role of databases for improving patient care outcomes in nursing.

AACN Essentials for Entry-Level Professional Nursing Education

- 8.1a Identify the variety of information and communication technologies used in care settings.
- 8.2b Explain how data entered on one patient impacts public and population health data.
- 8.2c Use appropriate data when planning care.
- 8.3a Demonstrate appropriate use of information and communication technologies.
- 8.3e Identify impact of information and communication technology on quality and safety of care.
- 9.1a Apply principles of professional nursing ethics and human rights in patient care and professional situations.

AACN Essentials for Advanced-Level Nursing Education

- 8.1g Identify best evidence and practices for the application of information and communication technologies to support care.
- 8.2f Generate information and knowledge from health information technology databases.
- 8.2i Clarify how the collection of standardized data advances the practice, understanding, and value of nursing and supports care.
- 8.3g Evaluate the use of information and communication technology to address needs, gaps, and inefficiencies in care.
- 8.5h Assess potential ethical and legal issues associated with the use of information and communication technology.

HIMSS TIGER Competencies

Applied computer science

Communication

Data analytics

Data protection and security

Documentation

Ethics in health internet technology

Information and communications technology systems applications

Project management

Quality and safety management

KEY TERMS

- Data
- Database
- Data mining
- Data scraping
- Data warehouse
- Database management system (DBMS)
- Database model
- Demographics
- Field
- Flat database
- Focus group
- Hierarchical database
- Hypothesis
- Interview
- Network model
- Object-oriented model
- Observation
- Parameter query
- Poll
- Primary data
- Qualitative
- Quantitative
- Record
- Relational database
- Secondary data
- Structured query language (SQL)
- Survey

CASE STUDY

In a survey conducted in 2019, more than 50% of female participants compared to 33% of male participants stated they believed that gender discrimination in patient care is a serious problem (Paulsen, 2020). People who identify as female and need cardiac care or pain management may get different treatment than those who identify as male, resulting in poorer outcomes. Much of medical science is based on the belief that male and female physiology differ only in terms of sex and reproductive organs. This has led to research being largely limited to male animals and humans. Additionally, females have been historically excluded from clinical trials, especially those of childbearing age to protect them and any potential fetuses from possible adverse events. Researchers have also avoided trying to control for variability in female sex hormones.

Because females have been less studied, there is less known about how to treat them effectively. Now, people assigned female at birth constitute about 50% of clinical research supported by the National Institutes of Health (NIH), and we now know that sex has an impact on cell physiology, metabolism, and other biologic functions including how diseases manifest and what symptoms arise (Paulsen, 2020).

Collecting demographic information in ways that are inclusive to all identities is a positive step toward greater accuracy and equity and is necessary to improve patient outcomes. In 2019, the World Health Organization (WHO) global health statistics were disaggregated by sex for the first time (WHO, n.d.). When data on individuals are broken down in this way, it better facilitates addressing inequalities. These data can also show how sex interacts with other factors like age, ethnicity, sexual orientation, gender identity, economic resources, and geographic location. For example, the WHO 2022 report found that female participants were much more likely to believe that wearing a face mask is moderately effective for preventing the spread of COVID-19 (females: 84.7% vs. males: 78%). This information is useful for planning health education directed at changing perceptions (WHO, 2022).

In healthcare, **data** (individual facts) are collected from various sources to improve people's health and well-being. Data collection occurs at many levels. In Step 5 of the Advancing Research and Clinical practice through close Collaboration (ARCC) Model (see Chapter 7), a nurse researcher might design a fall prevention study and collect data from patients on a unit over a 6-month time period. As you can see from the case study, millions of pieces of data can be collected at the population or even a global level. No matter what the scale of your data collection is, the type of data collected is just as important as how the data are collected. Omitting a data collection point when making healthcare decisions can result in an entire group of people being ignored.

An example of how large amounts of data can be gathered and used for many different purposes is the census. The U.S. Census Bureau has been gathering large amounts of data on the U.S. population every 10 years since 1790. Among other decisions, these data are used to plan where and when to build new hospitals and to allocate funding for programs that benefit families with limited resources and older adults. Census data have been used by researchers to associate lower family income with morbidity (illness) and mortality (death) among children and adolescents. But not even the census is perfect. The U.S. Census Bureau is working to enhance health data by identifying gaps in federal statistics (U.S. Census Bureau, 2022).

Data collection can be used to improve health outcomes. Global data collected during the COVID-19 pandemic helped address a wide variety of issues, including the availability of ventilators; who, when, and how often to test for COVID-19; and how to prevent infection. In a 2022 paper about lessons learned from the COVID-19 pandemic, Lee et al. state that addressing the pandemic was dependent on a "coherent and accessible data infrastructure." During the pandemic, researchers needed to identify the data elements that contributed to optimal outcomes for each individual patient. However, critical healthcare data sources are not as functional as they need to be (Lee et al., 2022). For example, data were often shared in the early stages of the pandemic on social media due to a lack of data-sharing options. This is an example of why it is important for nurses to understand the best methods for data collection and sharing.

This chapter will cover ways to collect and manage data spanning from a simple poll and ending with database creation and utilization. You will explore and use tools that will allow you to collect data that represent the diversity of the human experience and to advocate for data collection and management that will improve outcomes for all patients.

DATA COLLECTION GUIDELINES

A nurse manager who has just made changes in the way holiday requests are handled might want to create a survey asking staff how satisfied they are with the new process. An undergraduate nursing student is doing a research project on the frequency and type of self-care used by nursing students. An oncology physician wants to create a clinical trial to test an experimental chemotherapy agent. All of these are examples of setting goals and using data to reach those goals. It is important to consider many factors when designing a data collection strategy to ensure you meet your goals. Data collection guidelines include setting goals, identifying opportunities for collecting data, planning an approach and method, and collecting data while capturing diversity of those being served.

Setting Goals

It is important to know the reason behind collecting data and what the desired outcome of the data collection is. Imagine a nurse working to reduce the rate of falls in their unit. To discover if there is anything that could be done to reduce the fall rate, the nurse could look at the characteristics of patients on the unit who fell to identify commonalities. If the nurse found that many of the people who fell had vision impairments, they could work with the information technology (IT) department to add a question about eyewear to the assessment tool. The nurse could then observe the fall rate over the course of several months to see if the fall rate decreased when eyewear needs were better addressed. After determining a reason to collect data (in this example, to reduce falls), the nurse can determine the best way to collect, utilize, and analyze data.

The goal of data collection may depend on a **hypothesis** or guess about something using limited evidence: Gathering data can test that hypothesis. For example, a hospital may receive feedback from patients who identify as lesbian, gay, bisexual, transgender, questioning/queer, intersex, and asexual/agender (LGBTQIA) about unwelcome treatment from staff. The hypothesis may be that the hospital staff lack awareness of how to communicate respectfully with patients who are part of this community. The goal is to gather data to test this hypothesis. Questions to ask that might achieve this goal include:

- Is there evidence of discrimination on the basis of sexual orientation or gender identity at this hospital?
- Are there any training opportunities about treating patients from diverse populations offered to staff at this hospital?
- What percentage of patients identify as part of the LGBTQIA community?
- What are the perceptions of the service received by self-identified LGBTQIA patients?

Knowing the goal of the data will help guide the data collection.

Identifying Opportunities for Collecting Data

It may seem obvious at first what data need to be collected to reach a certain goal, but ask the following questions to identify all possible opportunities (OHRC, n.d.):

- About which opportunity will the data be collected?
- With whom will the group of interest be compared?
- What categories will be used to identify the group of interest and comparison group?
- How should data be collected?
- What sources should be used to collect data?
- From what locations or geographical areas will the data be gathered?
- How long will the data be collected?
- What data are others collecting on the topic?

As demonstrated in the case study, it can be easy to overlook important information. To avoid missing useful data, conduct a review of all policies, practices, and procedures, as well as the environmental or cultural aspects that may apply to the data. For example, imagine wanting to investigate the complaint procedures for discrimination, harassment, or systemic barriers at a healthcare organization. You might begin by reviewing the written policies and procedures regarding complaints. But you should also explore organizational culture from a human rights, diversity, and equity lens. Is the organization diverse? Does it represent the community it serves? Were the policies created by a representative sample of the people at the organization to ensure everyone's needs were being met? Asking questions like this can reveal potential opportunities for data collection.

Consider a student investigator designing a research project that explores nursing student self-care activities. The investigator might want to consider not only collecting data from the students but also collecting data on how much the nursing program is promoting self-care. Exploring the culture of the nursing program will help the student investigator design a more thorough data collection strategy. The more opportunities identified to collect data, the more robust and useful the data will become.

It is also important to consider types of data. **Qualitative** data are about experiences and relies on descriptions from interviews, observations, and focus groups. A qualitative question could be, "What is your experience with hospital staff?" **Quantitative** data involve numbers and are collected using polls, surveys, and measurements. A hospital researcher could collect the number of patients who identify as LGBTQIA. Qualitative data excel at telling the story of the participants but are subjective and often difficult to analyze. Quantitative data are objective and excel at summarizing information and showing trends but do not easily show complex situations or realities. Thus, these data types rely on each other to produce meaningful results.

Qualitative and quantitative data can provide a good basis for creating an action plan or deciding on next steps. Data collection can be viewed as part of a cyclical process. The results of data collection can lead to additional questions or the need to collect data again after an intervention to determine success. For example, if a hospital finds evidence of discrimination against those who identify as LGBTQIA, it may decide to begin a training program, which will be followed by a second round of data collection to determine if the intervention has been effective.

CASE STUDY

In the case study, you learned that the WHO has begun processing data for both males and females for the first time. If you discovered an inequity in data you collected, what steps might you take to alert your organization about the inequity and advocate for using data to enact changes?

Capturing Diversity

It can be helpful to collect demographic data from the population of interest. **Demographics** are the social characteristics and statistics of a human population including information like gender, age, and socioeconomic status. Collecting in-depth demographic data will facilitate generalizing the results to a wider variety of people and validating the data as representative of the population being served.

Data collection is an important tool for understanding and addressing challenges faced by those in underserved or underrepresented communities. For example, although strides have been made in recent years, a persistent lack of routine data collection on sexual orientation, gender identity, and variations in sex characteristics (SOGISC) is still a barrier for policymakers, researchers, healthcare providers, and advocates seeking to improve the health and well-being of LGBTQIA people. More comprehensive demographic data on SOGISC are crucial. Involving LGBTQIA people in question development, testing, and evaluation is important for collecting the most valuable data (Medina & Mahowald, 2022).

Race is another potential factor for consideration in data collection. It is important to remember that race is a sociopolitical system of categorization without a biologic basis. Despite this, race has continued to play a role in clinical decision making within healthcare. It can play a role in providers' attitudes and implicit biases, disease stereotyping, and clinical treatment guidelines. While some diseases have higher prevalence among individuals with certain genetic ancestry, genetic ancestry is poorly correlated with commonly used social racial categories. The use of race to inform clinical diagnoses and decision making may reinforce disproven notions of race as a biologic construct and contribute to ongoing racial disparities in health and healthcare (Tong & Artiga, 2021).

Read the Ethical Considerations box to learn about how knowledge of data collection supports the American Nurses Association (ANA) Code of Ethics.

Overcoming Obstacles

Data collection can involve logistical challenges. Anticipating and preparing for these challenges

ETHICAL CONSIDERATIONS FOR DATA COLLECTION

Provision 8 of the ANA Code of Ethics states that "the nurse collaborates with other health professionals and the public to protect human rights, promote health diplomacy, and reduce health disparities" (ANA, 2015). One way the nurse can reduce health disparities is to advocate for inclusive data collection. Interpretive Statement 8.1 asserts that health is a universal human right. It goes on to tell us that nurses have an obligation to promote the right to health and well-being for all people regardless of their sex, gender, race, religion, ethnicity, color, socioeconomic status, or sexual preference. Nurses must use their voices to collaborate with the healthcare team to ensure that data collection reflects optimal health goals for everyone. Explore the diversity of data collected in your workplace or clinical environment. Ask your IT and informatics colleagues about efforts to make data collection more inclusive.

make data collection an easier process. Sometimes senior leadership and key stakeholders must approve a project. It may help to get a more senior member of the team or a committee to help make decisions and present ideas to leadership. Strategies are necessary to protect the privacy of respondents. Collecting data, especially if it is sensitive information, can raise concerns of distrust and confidentiality in respondents. Plan to clearly communicate the rationale, data collection method, the people who have access to the data, and how it will be securely stored. It is also necessary to minimize the impact and inconvenience for the people from whom data are being collected, including picking the best time and method for collecting the data. A pilot or test project on a small scale can be helpful for identifying unforeseen issues (OHRC, n.d.).

DATA COLLECTION TOOLS

Informatics nurses collect data in many ways, from simple to complex. The choice of data collection tool is dependent on what information is being sought. When collecting data in the moment, polls can be given while presenting, in a workshop, or in a team meeting. When collecting data from a wider audience, surveys are useful and are used extensively in nursing research to collect data on a wide variety of topics. Focus groups and interviews are other common ways to collect research data.

Other data collection tools include inspection of documents, inquiry (asking questions of other people), formal interviews, observations, data collection instruments, and computer-generated reports. In addition, look to see what data others have collected on a given topic.

Polls

A **poll** is a simple way to record an opinion or collect votes quickly. Polls are typically limited to one question so there is no demographic information or other details collected. A poll may be used during a presentation to gauge audience interest or engagement; nurse educators often use polls in the classroom to engage students. You could poll nursing staff to discover interest in changing the process of requesting time off, or you could put a poll on a nursing student Facebook page asking about engagement with self-care activities. Figure 8-1 shows the results of a CBS News poll asking

CASE STUDY

In the case study, you read about how health outcomes for people assigned female at birth have been impacted by the type of data historically collected. What are some examples of data that have been collected from the LGBTQIA community that have impacted their care? Think about gender and sexuality questions on surveys. For example, how would an LGBTQIA person who has been with the same partner for 50 years have responded to a survey question about marital status before same-sex marriage became legalized? Would their response about their marital status have been reflective of their actual status?

Americans if they are for or against a government health insurance plan for all.

When using polls, keep things simple. Anyone should understand the question and how to respond. Save complex questions for surveys. Limit the multiple choice options to facilitate a quick response.

There are numerous ways to create polls. Social media applications like Facebook, Instagram, and X have polling functions as does Forms in Microsoft or Google. There are many free polling apps, such as SurveySparrow, SurveyMonkey, and EasyPolls. There are also web-based poll creators, such as Poll Maker and Doodle. Use the internet to research and choose the poll creator that works the best for your data needs.

Surveys

A **survey** is a data collection method that uses a questionnaire to gather data from a set of respondents. Surveys and questionnaires are not the same thing. A survey requires a questionnaire, but a questionnaire is not a survey; a questionnaire is a tool used in a survey. Surveys have a lot of advantages. Using online platforms, they are easy to create and distribute and can be accessed anywhere with an internet connection. Surveys can collect a wide range of data types, including opinions, values, and preferences. Also, survey data can often be downloaded into a spreadsheet for easy data analysis. A disadvantage to surveys is that without physically seeing respondents, there is the potential for them to falsify their identities or information they provide.

The most common type of survey used in healthcare is the patient satisfaction survey. These surveys are used to measure the patient experience with the goal of improving the patient experience. The Hospital Consumer Assessment of Healthcare Providers and Systems (HCAHPS, pronounced "H-caps") survey is a national, standardized, publicly reported survey of patients' perceptions of their hospital experience (CMS.gov, n.d.). Other surveys that are commonly used in healthcare include health risk assessment (often used before a visit to identify teaching points for providers); gaps in care (identifies which preventative services patients are not using); medication adherence; and remote health monitoring (monitors high-risk patients and those with chronic conditions) (Brogan, 2019).

In the past, physical copies of surveys were sent out to participants, but now surveys are almost exclusively electronic, making them an inexpensive option for gathering data if a free tool is used. The difficulty can be in getting an electronic survey into the hands of the target audience. A patient who is being discharged from the hospital. They may be given a hand-held device that contains the HCAHPS survey, and they are asked to complete it before they leave. If you wish to target a specific group of people, you may need to partner with a market research firm to get your survey to your target demographic. Organizations may also offer their email lists for a fee. For example, to survey nursing students about self-care activities you might approach the National Student Nurses' Association who will send out surveys to their members for a fee.

When creating a survey, many types of questions can be used, facilitating the collection of exactly the type of data needed to achieve one's goals. Some types of survey questions include (Mahmutovic, 2021):

1. Multiple choice questions (several answer options to choose from)
2. Rating scale questions (may use stars, 1-to-5 grading, thumbs up or down)

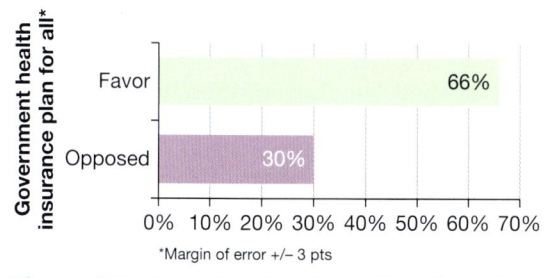

Figure 8-1. Example of poll results. (Data from Backus, F., De Pinto, J. [2019, October 15]. *CBS news poll: most Americans favor a national health plan.* https://www.cbsnews.com/news/2020-polls-national-health-care-plan-favored-by-most-americans-cbs-news-poll-finds/).

Government health insurance plan for all*
- Favor: 66%
- Opposed: 30%

*Margin of error +/− 3 pts

3. Likert scale questions (questions with a range of answers, such as "strongly agree," "agree," "neutral," "disagree," and "strongly disagree")
4. Matrix questions (column of questions to the left and a row of answers across the top)
5. Drop-down questions (drop-down menu allows selection of an answer; birth year is a common demographic drop-down)
6. Ranking questions (rank items in order of preference)
7. Slider questions (allow participants to slide a bar across a scale, such as 1-to-10 range)
8. Fill in questions (open area to type to capture information not covered elsewhere, often used for "Other comments" questions)

When writing survey questions, be aware of the potential for bias. A survey question is biased if it is phrased or formatted in a way that skews respondents toward a certain answer. Survey question bias also may occur if a question is hard to understand or overly broad. See Box 8-1 for examples of biased survey questions and suggestions for improving them.

> **BOX 8-1** Biased Survey Questions
>
> **Leading questions:** Sways the participant to answer one way or another, lacks objectivity.
> Example: What problems do you have with the staff at our hospital?
> Fixed: How likely are you to recommend our hospital to someone else?
> **Loaded questions:** Contains assumptions about a customer's habits or perceptions.
> Example: When do you plan to quit smoking?
> Fixed: Do you smoke? Do you plan to quit smoking? (The fix often involves breaking the question down into smaller questions so that no assumptions are made.)
> **Double-barreled questions:** Asking two questions in one.
> Example: Were your discharge instructions easy to understand and did you follow them?
> Fixed: Were your discharge instructions easy to understand? Did you follow your discharge instructions? (The fix involves making two simpler questions.)
> **Jargon:** A word or phrase that is difficult to understand or not widely used by the general population, including slang, catchphrases, clichés, colloquialisms, or any other words that could be misconstrued or offensive.
> Example: How was face time with your CSR?
> Fix: How would you rate your experience with the customer service representative?
> **Double negatives:** Using two negatives in the same sentence.
> Example: Is the patient portal not easy to use unless you use the search bar?
> Fix: Is the patient portal easy to use? Did you need to use the search bar to find information on the patient portal?
> **Confusing answer scale options:** Survey questions or answer options that are confusing.
> Example: How often do you engage with the patient portal? 0-1, 1-2, 2-3, More than 3
> Fix: How many times each week do you use the patient portal? 0, 1-2, 3-4, More than 4
> **Unbalanced answer scale options:** Survey answer options that are unbalanced and will provide skewed data.
> Example: How was our service today? Okay, Good, Fantastic, Unforgettable, Mind-blowing (Note that these options are all positive answers.)
> Fix: How satisfied were you with our service today? Very dissatisfied, Dissatisfied, Neutral, Satisfied, Very satisfied
> **Overly broad answer scale:** Providing too many answer options that could dilute the data.
> Example: How likely are you to recommend this clinic to other people? 1, 2, 3, 4, 5, 6, 7, 8, 9, 10
> Fix: How likely are you to recommend this clinic to other people? Unlikely to recommend, Would maybe recommend, Likely to recommend

Examples of online survey platforms include SurveyMonkey, Jotform, and Formstack. You can create a questionnaire in Google or Microsoft Forms that will provide you with a sharable link to post online or email to participants..

Observation

Observations involve directly visualizing how people are behaving. Instead of relying on proactive self-reporting from surveys or polls, the information comes directly from participants. It is also difficult for subjects to falsify information about their identities. Examples of the use of observation in healthcare include monitoring for hand hygiene and medication errors. Both issues are underreported due to unawareness, shame, and fear of repercussions and thus are good opportunities for gathering data through direct observation.

Observations provide the ability and freedom to be as detail-oriented as possible when it comes to describing or analyzing behaviors and actions. It typically involves watching and taking notes, so it is a data collection method that requires no technology and little training. Observers should remain in the background and not insert themselves into the situation. In some cases, the goal is for those being observed to be unaware of the observation. It is important to be aware of the ethical implications of observing someone who is not aware they are being observed. If an investigator intends to publish the results of an observation, they will need to get permission from the participants, if not before the observation, then afterward.

There are three primary methods of observations (McLeod, 2023):

- Structured (controlled): The researcher sets specific conditions (location, time, circumstances, participants) and uses a standardized procedure. This allows for greater control of the data, which are often collected with a coded scale system, but participants who know they are being watched may act differently.
- Naturalistic: The researcher studies the spontaneous behavior of participants in natural settings and records what they see. This leads to more realistic behaviors from participants and may generate new ideas for the researcher. However, it may require training to recognize behaviors that should be recorded, and the observations are less reliable because they cannot be repeated in the exact same way.
- Participant: This method is similar to naturalistic, but the researcher becomes part of the group they are studying, either overtly (the participants are aware) or covertly (the participants are unaware). This gives researchers deeper insight into the lives and behaviors of the participants, but the researcher may lose objectivity and become biased.

Interviews

An **interview** is defined as a formal meeting between two individuals in which the interviewer asks the interviewee questions to gather information. The interviewer can ask subjects anything about their opinions, motivations, and feelings regarding their experience. They can also ask follow-up questions to better understand the subject.

Interviews are often used by those doing qualitative research who are looking for the lived experience of a patient. An example would be a study done that explores the experience of nurses who have made medication errors. An interview of a small number of nurses can provide rich data on what it is like to deal with having made a medication error. Interviewing can be a good tool to gather preliminary data about a subject. Interviews can assist in explaining, understanding, and exploring the perspectives, behavior, and experiences of participants.

As with surveys, a disadvantage with interviews is that there is the potential for bias, so questions should be worded in ways that do not lead participants in a particular direction. Another difficulty is that the interviewer may need training on how to conduct interviews to obtain data that meet the project goals. Plus, interviewing can be time-consuming and expensive. There are companies that will conduct interviews on the researcher's behalf for a fee. However, often only a small number of individuals are interviewed compared to survey data collection, which can involve thousands or even millions of subjects.

Focus Groups

A **focus group** has all the characteristics of an interview but involves a larger group. Focus groups tend to function best with six to 12 subjects who have similar qualities or shared interests. A moderator creates an atmosphere that encourages people to discuss their thoughts and opinions. The moderator leads the group through a series of planned topics but must be careful to avoid bias. The moderator is also critical in getting answers from all participants and not letting one or several participants dominate or sidetrack the group.

Like interviews, focus groups are a type of qualitative data collection in which the information is descriptive and cannot be quantified statistically. Focus groups are sometimes used in healthcare to determine the acceptability of a new product or process. Conducting focus groups with a small number of staff from different areas of the hospital could yield data to assist the organization with making a decision about how to proceed.

Experimentation

Experimentation involves collecting data in a systematic and planned way and with oversight from an institutional review board (IRB), a group of people who vet research projects to ensure they are being conducted ethically. Clinical trials are an example of experiments often done in healthcare. After researchers have obtained IRB approval for a project, they carefully screen applicants before obtaining their consent and then randomizing them to a control (no treatment) or experimental (treatment) group. Statistical analysis is performed on the data that are gathered. The results of clinical trials are considered extremely reliable and trustworthy due to the large number of participants required to make a final conclusion about the data.

Data from Data

So far, we have discussed primary data. **Primary data** are generated by the researcher from surveys, interviews, and experiments that were designed for answering specific research questions. **Secondary data** come from existing data generated by large government institutions, healthcare facilities, and other organizations. That information is then extracted and used for other purposes. Using secondary data involves data collection and analysis, which is covered in Chapter 9.

Records and Documents

Investigators may also choose to analyze an organization's existing records or documents to track or predict changes over a specific time. Data collected from a healthcare organization could include:
- Email logs
- Call logs
- Staff reports
- Databases such as electronic health records (EHRs)
- Information logs
- Minutes of meetings

An advantage of using organizational records and documents is that the data are already available. Using records and documents also allows rechecking the history of a specific event. For example, if you wanted to know how often medication errors are being made, one piece of data you could collect is the number of times diphenhydramine was given as a stat or emergency medication. This medication is commonly given for allergic reactions, and its usage can indicate that a patient has been given the wrong drug or a drug that has caused an allergic reaction. A disadvantage of this type of data collection is that it is limited to what data have already been collected, which may limit the scope of the project.

Other Methods

Online tracking, social media monitoring, and online marketing analytics are other ways to obtain data that can inform healthcare decisions. For example, tools are available that can tell an organization about public perception of the company or about financial considerations when planning marketing strategies. **Data mining** is the process of finding anomalies, patterns, and correlations within large data sets to predict outcomes. Using a broad range of techniques, this information can be used to increase revenues, cut costs, improve customer relationships, reduce risks, and more.

Data scraping is a technique in which a computer program extracts data from output generated from another program. Data scraping is commonly manifest as web scraping, the process of using an application to extract valuable information from a website. Some advantages of web scraping include speed, profitability, flexibility, and the automatic delivery of structured data (Pawar et al., 2023). However, data scraping can be malicious, so be mindful of ethical issues. It can be used to obtain contact details for bulk mailing lists, robo calls, or malicious social engineering attempts by scraping websites that contain email addresses and phone numbers in plaintext. This is one of the primary methods both spammers and scammers use to find new targets. Chapter 4 has more information about cyber criminals and how to protect information from attacks.

DATABASES

A **database** is a tool for collecting and organizing information. Databases can store information about people, products, orders, or anything else. Examples of databases nurses use include web search engines, library databases, and EHRs. An EHR (Chapter 13) database facilitates comparisons among patients or searching patient data for useful information. With electronic records, data retrieval can provide tools for improving patient outcomes. A database can be as simple as a tool for organizing patient records at a primary care clinic or as complex as the U.S. Census. Understanding how a database works and how to manipulate data facilitates influencing patient care outcomes.

Nurses use a variety of digital databases to access data for nursing education and in healthcare settings. In nursing education, students often use databases to track their clinical requirements, such as immunizations or cardiopulmonary resuscitation certifications. Nursing students may also use databases to schedule clinical laboratory experiences or create e-portfolios with examples of learning and technical competencies. The learning management system used for course work is another example of a database. In the healthcare setting, nurse educators may use databases to track licensure and clinical competencies. Databases may also be used for scheduling nursing unit staffing. In nursing administration, databases may be used to track patient adverse events, such as falls, code blue events, and pressure injury rates. In risk management, databases are used to track incident reports for medication errors and other risk incidents.

Many databases begin as a list in a word processing program or spreadsheet (such as Microsoft Excel). As the list grows, redundancies and inconsistencies can make it harder to understand the data in list form and there are limited ways to search or retrieve data for review. Once these problems appear, it is a good idea to transfer the data to a database.

A database table looks similar to a word processing table or spreadsheet formatted as a list with only column headings, but there are distinct differences. Whereas a spreadsheet is helpful for manipulating numbers, a database is best for analyzing information that may include nonnumerical data. Data in a spreadsheet are displayed in different cells, whereas data in a database relate to **records** (rows) and **fields** (columns). Spreadsheet workbooks can contain a variety of unrelated worksheets, but the objects in a database are all related (Oracle, n.d.). Common database terminology is outlined in Table 8-1.

Anecdata is a collection of databases developed to gather data from citizen observations. This free online community provides a platform to collect, manage, and share data (Anecdata, n.d.). In 2023, a search of the Anecdata website revealed 13,906 users and 288 projects collecting data on a wide variety of topics. A litter journal encourages citizens to track and remove plastics and other debris from both land and water. This data set could be used by a public health nurse to design localized interventions to reduce water contaminants that impact health. All About Arsenic (arsenic is a naturally occurring groundwater contaminant) engages students and communities to sample well water while building data literacy skills. The informatics nurse could use these data for education or prevention interventions to reduce the impact of arsenic on health. Orchards, Gardens, and Fields asks citizens to collect soil and well water samples for heavy metal analysis in Washington and Maine. The data from this project could be used to identify areas of contamination and lead to nursing interventions that improve the

TABLE 8-1 Common Database Terminology

Database Term	Definition
Data	Facts without meaning, for example, the number 37
Field	Smallest structure in a database (a column in a spreadsheet)
Field name	The label applied to a field
Form	Used to add, edit, and view data from a database table or query
Parameter query	Queries that require the user to enter a constraint to define data output; only records that match the parameter are returned
Primary key	The unique identifier of a record in a table of a database
Query	The search function for a relational database; one of the characteristics that make databases powerful
Record	All the information about a single "member" of a table (a row in a spreadsheet)
Report	Used for printing information from data in a table(s) or query, it provides data organized to fulfill user need
Table	A collection of related information consisting of records, each record is made up of fields
Validation or lookup table	A database table that provides a list of allowable entries for a field that is linked to that field

health of the community. You can learn more about how to create and use the Microsoft Access database in Appendix A.

Database Management System

A **database management system (DBMS)** is system software for creating, manipulating, and managing databases. A DBMS makes it possible for users to create, protect, read, update, and delete data. The DBMS serves as an interface between databases and users or application programs, ensuring that data are organized and accessible. A healthcare **data warehouse** is a type of DBMS that serves as a centralized repository for all the healthcare information retrieved from multiple sources like EHRs, electronic medical records (EMRs), enterprise resource planning systems, radiology and lab databases, and wearables (Mullins, 2022).

Database Models

A **database model** is the way data are organized. Several models exist, each with advantages and disadvantages. A database model should be chosen based on the tasks that the database must perform.

A **flat database** has all the data located in one table. A spreadsheet worksheet is the simplest flat database model. Flat databases are simple to construct and use, but they have limitations when it comes to tracking items when there are more than one of the same item in a single record. For example, if you wanted to track the infections that occurred in a unit using a flat database, you would need to enter multiple records for each patient who had more than one pathogen causing the infection. Multiple records can create errors if the data are not input identically to the related record.

A **hierarchical database** has tables that are organized in the shape of an inverted tree, like an organizational chart. In this organizational plan, often called a tree structure, records are linked to a base, or root, but through successive layers in a hierarchical structure. The difficulty with this structure is that it is hard to link data from one branch of the tree with another (e.g., nursing diagnoses to demographics). Because of its structure, this model is complex and inflexible.

The **network model** is like the hierarchical model, but the trees can share branches. Although this is somewhat more useful than the hierarchical database, because of the structure, this network model is also complex and inflexible.

A **relational database** is more flexible than the hierarchical and network models. In a relational database model, there can be two or more tables that are connected by identical information in fields in each table. These are called key fields. This allows the data in a record from one table to be matched to any piece or pieces of data in records in another table. Desktop software, such as Microsoft Access, Apple FileMaker Pro, and Apache OpenOffice Base, are examples of relational databases. Today, most business and personal computer databases use the relational database model (Oracle, n.d.).

Queries can be used as a basis for a report with the relational model. A query produces information based on the current data in the tables, not the data that were there when they were originally created. **Structured query language (SQL)** is a programming language for storing and processing information in a relational database. You can use SQL statements to store, update, remove, search, and retrieve information from the database. For queries for which you will want information at routine intervals, such as monthly, you would design a **parameter query,** which constrains the data to a certain span of dates. In this way, you can use the same report each month to show only the information for the identified time.

The true **object-oriented model** combines database functions with object programming languages, making a more powerful tool. Because it provides better management of complex data relationships, it is more suited to applications such as hospital patient record systems, which have complex relationships among data. To create such a database requires knowledge of programming languages and is not suited to the application software in an office suite. Data from object-oriented database models, however, can be exported and analyzed in a relational database.

Database Design

Learning the correct database design method is essential to maximize productivity and success. There are three important steps in the database design process:

1. Identify the purpose of the database. Consider what data will be included as well as data that will be excluded.
2. Identify the questions or queries that aggregated data can answer.
3. Make a list of all data requirements necessary to draw conclusions from the questions asked of the data.

It is helpful to write out the purpose, questions, and data requirements before constructing the database. A common error that novices make when designing a clinical database is to replicate a paper form. The database should contain only the data that will be aggregated for analysis. Efficient database design requires the use of consistent terminology (naming conventions). This applies to column headings and names of tables, forms, queries, and reports. It is important to understand how to best design the database for efficient analysis, how to use the built-in powerful query functions, and how to display analyzed data with reports and charts.

Designing databases for large organizations is outside the scope of this chapter, but it is important to know the components of a database. End users like nurses, physicians, and other healthcare providers need to be involved in the design of databases to ensure functionality. Knowing the way a database works and the terminology involved can help you provide much needed input into the design process.

Database Software

Database software is designed specifically for creating databases. Generally, there are two types, those used in the healthcare industry, such as EMRs, and those used for home and small businesses. Industry databases can manage huge volumes of data and thousands of users. Examples of industry software include Oracle, Microsoft SQL Server, and Sybase. Database software for homes and small businesses can handle smaller volumes of data and number of users. Examples of home and small business database software include commercial desktop software, such as Microsoft Access and Apple FileMaker Pro, as well as free software, such as Zoho Creator and Apache OpenOffice Base (Oracle, n.d.).

SUMMARY

- **Data collection guidelines.** Data collection is important, complex, and multifaceted and can result in improved health outcomes. Nurses have an obligation to ensure that data collection captures information that can reduce poor health outcomes. Data collection guidelines include setting goals, identifying opportunities for collecting data (quantitative and qualitative data), capturing diversity, and overcoming obstacles. Asking questions about data collection in your organization is a good way to begin. Guidelines for asking questions about demographics can help with inclusivity.
- **Data collection tools.** Tools to collect primary data include polls, surveys, observations, interviews, focus groups, and experimentation. You can also extract secondary data from primary data sources such as records and documents, social media, and online methods like data mining and data scraping. There are advantages and disadvantages of every method, and it is important to be mindful of bias in written or verbal questions.
- **Databases.** A database is a tool for collecting and organizing information. Examples of uses in nursing include EHRs, web search engines, and learning management systems. A database management system is software for creating and managing databases. There is a wide variety of database software for use in healthcare organizations, homes, and businesses. Database models organize data in five ways: flat, hierarchical, network, relational, and object-oriented. Database design involves identifying the purpose of the database, any questions that need to be answered, and a list of all data requirements needed to draw conclusions.

DISCUSSION QUESTIONS AND ACTIVITIES

1. What is the most important step in designing a data collection strategy? Defend your answer.
2. Identify two potential problems with data collection and how you would address them.
3. Compare two ways nurses collect data and discuss how you would use those methods to improve patient outcomes.
4. Create a simple poll and share it with the class or your colleagues. What software did you choose and why?
5. Create a survey and gather at least 10 responses. How could you use the information you gathered to improve patient outcomes?

PRACTICE QUESTIONS

1. The nurse wants to collect data on patient falls. Which step in the data collection strategy involves reviewing the unit definition of a patient fall?
    a. Identifying opportunities for collecting data
    b. Setting goals
    c. Planning an approach and methods
    d. Acting on results

2. Which data collection method would be best for collecting qualitative data about the experience of caring for patients during the COVID-19 pandemic?
   a. Poll
   b. Survey
   c. Interview
   d. Observation

3. A Microsoft Excel table is an example of what kind of database?
   a. Flat
   b. Hierarchical
   c. Network model
   d. Relational database

REFERENCES

American Nurses Association. (2015). *Code of ethics for nurses*. American Nurses Publishing. https://www.nursingworld.org/practice-policy/nursing-excellence/ethics/code-of-ethics-for-nurses/

Anecdata. (n.d.). *About Anecdata*. Retrieved February 10, 2023 from https://anecdata.org/pages/about

Brogan, N. (2019, April 4). Industry Voices—6 types of healthcare surveys that can improve patient experiences. https://www.fiercehealthcare.com/practices/industry-voices-6-types-healthcare-surveys-can-improve-patient-experiences

Centers for Medicare and Medicaid Services (CMS.gov). (n.d.). *HCAHPS: Patients' perspectives of care survey*. Retrieved November 19, 2022 from https://www.cms.gov/Medicare/Quality-Initiatives-Patient-Assessment-Instruments/HospitalQualityInits/HospitalHCAHPS

Lee, P., Abernethy, A., Shaywitz, D., Gundlapalli, A. V., Weinstein, J., Doraiswamy, P. M., Schulman, K., & Madhavan, S. (2022). *Digital health COVID-19 impact assessment: Lessons learned and compelling needs*. NAM Perspectives. Discussion Paper, National Academy of Medicine. https://doi.org/10.31478/202201c

Mahmutovic, J. (2021, February 26). *3 different types of data collection: Survey vs questionnaire vs poll*. https://www.surveylegend.com/customer-insight/survey-questionnaire-poll/

McLeod, S. (2023, July 31). *Observation method in psychology: Naturalistic, participant and controlled*. Simply Psychology. https://www.simplypsychology.org/observation.html

Medina, C., & Mahowald, L. (2022, May 24). *Collecting data about LGBTQI+ and other sexual and gender-diverse communities*. The Center for American Progress. https://www.americanprogress.org/article/collecting-data-about-lgbtqi-and-other-sexual-and-gender-diverse-communities/

Mullins, C. S. (2022, July). *Database management systems*. TechTarget. https://www.techtarget.com/searchdatamanagement/definition/database-management-system

Ontario Human Rights Commission (OHRC). (n.d.). *What is involved in collecting data – six steps to success*. Retrieved on November 18, 2022 from https://www.ohrc.on.ca/en/count-me-collecting-human-rights-based-data/6-what-involved-collecting-data-%E2%80%93-six-steps-success

Oracle. (n.d.). *What is a database?* Retrieved November 20, 2022 from https://www.oracle.com/database/what-is-database/

Paulsen, E. (2020, January 14). *How can you improve care for female patients?* https://physicians.dukehealth.org/articles/recognizing-addressing-unintended-gender-bias-patient-care

Pawar, S., Chandran, P., & Salvi, P. (2023) Issues and challenges of web scraping: Healthcare industry case study approach. *The Online Journal of Distance Education and E-Learning*, 11(1), 770–775.

Tong, M., & Artiga, S. (2021, December 9). *Use of race in clinical diagnosis and decision making: Overview and implications*. Kaiser Family Foundation. https://www.kff.org/racial-equity-and-health-policy/issue-brief/use-of-race-in-clinical-diagnosis-and-decision-making-overview-and-implications/

U.S. Census Bureau. (2022, November 2). *Health*. https://www.census.gov/topics/health.html

World Health Organization (WHO). (2022). *World health statistics 2022*. https://cdn.who.int/media/docs/default-source/gho-documents/world-health-statistic-reports/world-healthstatistics_2022.pdf

World Health Organization (WHO). (n.d.). *Closing data gaps in gender*. Retrieved November 20, 2022 from https://www.who.int/activities/closing-data-gaps-in-gender

CHAPTER 9

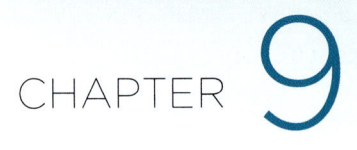

Analyzing Data

Meredith Mackenzie, Jean Mellum, and Kristi Miller

OBJECTIVES

After studying this chapter, you will be able to:
1. Discuss the importance of data analysis in nursing.
2. Explain the role of data analysis in evidence-based practice and research.
3. Identify different types of data.
4. Discuss big data and how it can be used to improve patient outcomes.
5. Explore sources of data that can be used for comparison and benchmarking.
6. Identify tools such as artificial intelligence for the analysis of structured data, unstructured data, and big data.
7. Discuss current trends in data analytics.

AACN Essentials for Entry-Level Professional Nursing Education

3.1b Assess population health data.
5.1d Interpret benchmark and unit outcome data to inform individual and microsystem practice.
8.1a Identify the variety of information and communication technologies used in care settings.
8.2a Enter accurate data when chronicling care.
8.2b Explain how data entered on one patient impacts public and population health data.
8.2c Use appropriate data when planning care.
8.3a Demonstrate appropriate use of information and communication technologies.
8.3b Evaluate how decision support tools impact clinical judgment and safe patient care.
8.3e Identify impact of information and communication technology on quality and safety of care.
8.3d Examine how emerging technologies influence healthcare delivery and clinical decision making.

AACN Essentials for Advanced-Level Nursing Education

2.7d Analyze data to identify gaps and inequities in care and monitor trends in outcomes.

2.7e Monitor epidemiological and system-level aggregate data to determine healthcare outcomes and trends.

2.7f Synthesize outcome data to inform evidence-based practice, guidelines, and policies.

3.1k Analyze primary and secondary population health data for multiple populations against relevant benchmarks.

5.1i Establish and incorporate data-driven benchmarks to monitor system performance.

7.3f Design system improvement strategies based on performance data and metrics.

8.2f Generate information and knowledge from health information technology databases.

8.2j Interpret primary and secondary data and other information to support care.

HIMSS TIGER Competencies

Communication

Data analytics

Information and communications technology systems applications

Information management research

KEY TERMS

- Aggregate data
- Artificial intelligence (AI)
- Bar chart
- Benchmarking
- Big data
- Clinical decision support system (CDSS)
- Column chart
- Continuous data
- Dashboard
- Descriptive data analysis
- Discrete data
- Electronic health record (EHR)
- Healthcare data analytics
- Health information technology (HIT)
- Health portal
- Information governance
- Likert scale
- Line chart
- Natural language processing (NLP)
- Nominal data
- Nonrelational databases (NoSQL)
- Ordinal data
- Pie chart
- Stacked bar chart
- Statistical analysis
- Structured data
- Unstructured data

CASE STUDY

Intrauterine devices (IUDs) are effective, safe, long-acting reversible contraceptives, but the risk of uterine perforation occurs with an estimated incidence of one to two per 1,000 insertions (Anthony et al., 2021). A retrospective study was designed to evaluate the risk of IUD-related uterine perforation and device expulsion among people who were breastfeeding or within 12 months after delivery at insertion. Structured (quantitative) and unstructured (qualitative) data were obtained from three healthcare systems with electronic health records (EHRs) plus an organization with access to a health information exchange with access to EHRs. Study sites were included based on their ability to access population-based EHR data, data quality, and variation in demographics. Algorithms were developed to identify potential risk factors and outcomes using operational definitions, natural language processing, and medical record review. The study population included 326,658 people. Combining retrospective data from multiple sites allowed for a large and diverse study population. Pooling data across multiple sites provided demographic variation and confirmed results across sites. Collaboration with clinicians at different organizations ensured the results reflected current clinical practice (Anthony et al., 2021).

As you read this chapter, think about whether there are additional benefits to collecting and comparing data from several settings when conducting research. What software might be needed to analyze the data? How might patient privacy be a concern?

Every day, a vast number of data points that can inform healthcare decision making are generated. Census data, morbidity and mortality data, data from insurance companies, the results of research studies, and data generated within clinical environments are just some examples of sources of data. Data collected from **electronic health records** (**EHRs**, digital records of a patient's health history) such as vital signs, laboratory values, medication orders, the number of nurses who are clocked in for a shift, and the number of times a nurse has overridden a medication dispenser alert are all example pieces of a puzzle that, when put together, can shed light on how to improve patient outcomes. Data are increasingly stored electronically, making it easier to access and analyze. In this data-rich healthcare environment, the need to turn data into useable information to inform decisions on quality and safety of care is imperative.

Because data are readily available in healthcare settings today, nurses have an obligation to use them responsibly. Nurses must collect, aggregate, analyze, and interpret data correctly. Data are just facts and figures. Informatics nurses are needed to analyze and interpret data to tell a story—a story that can improve patient outcomes. Statistical analysis of data has become easier over the years with software options that can perform high-level statistical functions on large quantities of data. Nurses have access to publicly available data sets for benchmarking with quality improvement initiatives.

For large data sets, advanced data analytic solutions, including software, can be used to monitor trends including care delivery and outcomes across a variety of settings. With increasing amounts of data being collected, innovative technologic tools have been introduced to analyze the vast amount of data available.

This textbook contains a wide variety of information on how to collect, store, and present data. The purpose of this chapter is to develop basic competencies in data analysis to support research and evidence-based practice (EBP) with the goal of improving patient outcomes. From the Advancing Research and Clinical practice through close Collaboration (ARCC) Model discussed in Chapter 7, this chapter addresses Step 5, evaluate the outcome of the practice change

(Melnyk & Fineout-Overholt, 2023). You can also think about the Data, Information, Knowledge, and Wisdom (DIKW) model (see Chapter 2) and how analysis of data can transform information into knowledge, and knowledge into wisdom.

In this chapter, you will explore data analysis in nursing, including types and sources of data, tools for data analysis, how to interpret research findings to guide decision making in healthcare, and how data analysis is currently being used to improve patient care.

DATA ANALYSIS IN NURSING

Nurse informatics specialists are increasingly engaged in healthcare data analysis and need to consider how data are entered, stored, and accessed to support meaningful analysis. Moreover, nurses in all roles need skills and tools to summarize sets of data into understandable pieces of information and to interpret the meaning of evidence produced through research.

Although technologic innovations have changed the pace of data accumulation and the amount of data to analyze, data analysis is not a new concept in healthcare or nursing. In the 1830s, French doctor Pierre-Charles-Alexandre Louis collected and compared data from hospitalized patients who underwent bloodletting and those who did not. After examining the outcomes of 83 patients, 47 who received bloodletting and 36 who did not, he argued that the higher mortality rate among those who received bloodletting suggested that the practice was more dangerous than helpful (Matthews, 2016).

As discussed in Chapter 2, Florence Nightingale, widely regarded as the founder of modern nursing, was also a highly regarded statistician (Richardson et al., 2020). As part of her work analyzing mortality data during the Crimean War, she pioneered new methods of data visualization to communicate the results of her analysis more readily (Fig. 9-1). Following the Crimean War, she used these same skills to advocate for reformations in public health that resulted in legislature leading to improved access to clean water, safer building codes, and better-built sewer systems (Andrews, 2022). Nightingale's work was groundbreaking in large part because she focused on the systematic collection of data; for example, by collecting data

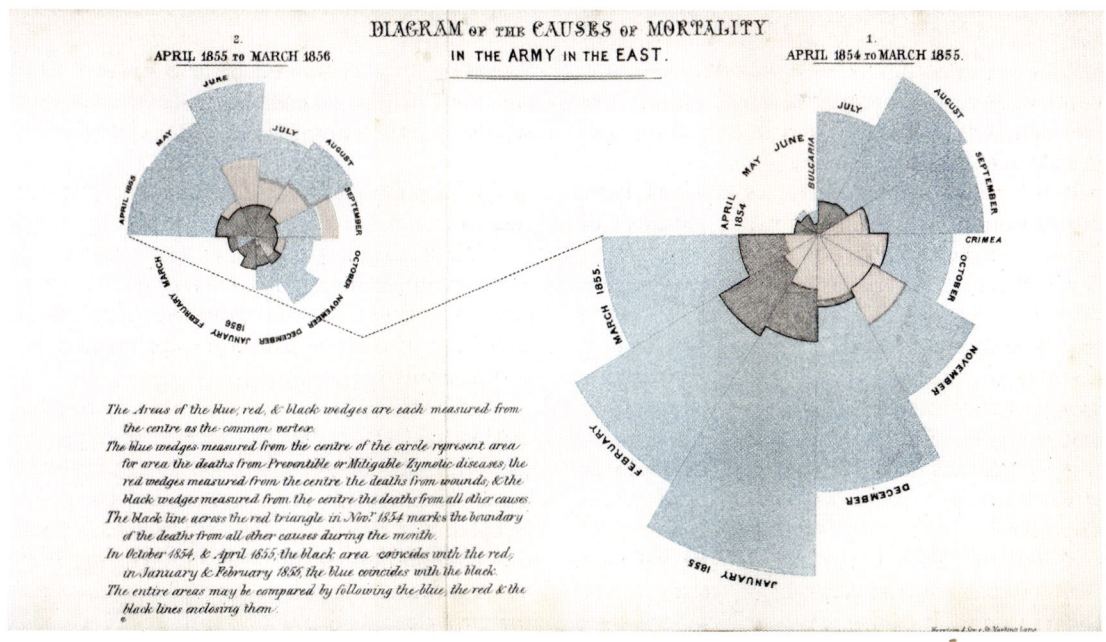

Figure 9-1. Polar area diagram of the causes of mortality in the Army in the East. (Florence Nightingale, 1858. Public Domain.)

on the age, location, and cause of death for each soldier, she was able to demonstrate that many more soldiers were dying of unhygienic conditions than of battlefield wounds (Andrews, 2022).

Despite Nightingale's work, the emergence of nursing as a clinical science did not develop until the 1980s. The National Institute of Nursing Research (NINR), established in the mid-1980s, provides federal funding to nursing studies aimed at prevention of illness, promotion of healthy lifestyles, and support of quality of life. The NINR has five research lenses that leverage the strengths of nursing research to enact change: health equity; social determinants of health; population and community health; prevention and health promotion; and systems and models of care (NINR, n.d.). Since the establishment of NINR, nurse scientists have been providing research evidence to change traditional ways of caring for patients to provide better patient outcomes. The NINR website includes resources for research and funding, training opportunities, and NINR publications that provide the latest scientific evidence on clinical topics.

DATA ANALYSIS IN EBP AND RESEARCH

Data analysis is frequently used to guide decision making for clinical units and healthcare systems. But it is also used as part of research studies that are published to inform broader practice. Emphasis on EBP is an important step in the development of nursing science and the improvement in patient care. EBP is a process that incorporates the best evidence from research, along with clinical expertise and patient preferences, into clinical practice to support clinical decision making (Dang et al., 2022). The use of EBP can bring about scientifically sound changes in nursing practice. Just as data analysis is used in the research studies that generate evidence, it is also used to measure the impact of EBP projects. For example, when implementing a new intervention intended to reduce patient falls, the investigator would want to analyze the fall rate before and after the intervention was initiated. Data analysis is a key component of the entire EBP process.

It is the responsibility of every nurse to keep current in practice by using research evidence. There are several ways to stay current, including reading research literature; subscribing to clinical practice journals, electronic apps, and professional blogs; attending professional meetings; networking; reviewing clinical practice guidelines; and participating in quality improvement or clinical practice committees.

TYPES OF DATA

Understanding what kind of data you are looking at will help you decide how to analyze it. Data exist in many different forms and sizes (Fig. 9-2).

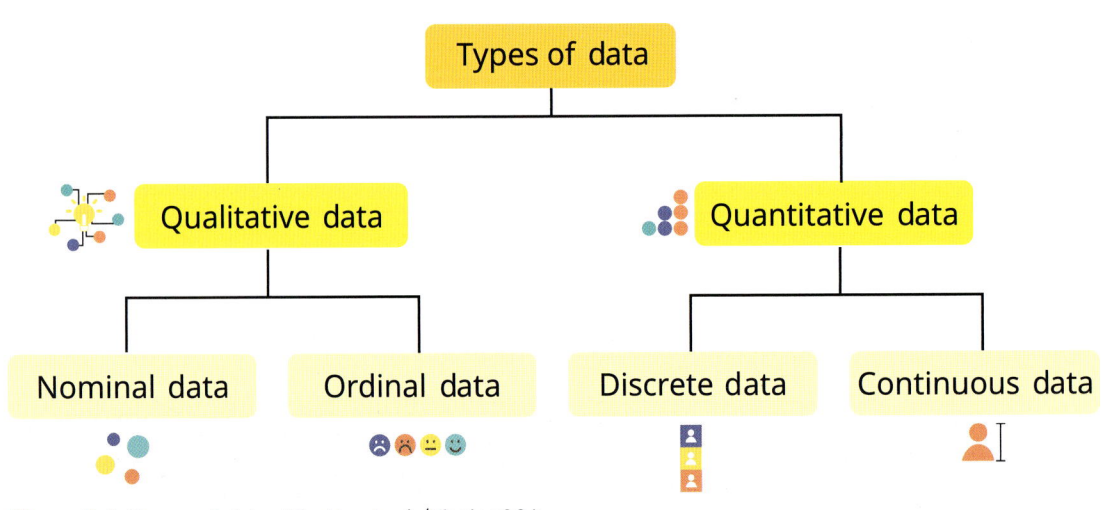

Figure 9-2. Types of data. (Shutterstock/Piscine26.)

In the case study, the researchers looked at both structured and unstructured data. Structured (quantitative) data can be further broken down into discrete and continuous data. Unstructured (qualitative) data can be broken down into nominal and ordinal data (Valcheva, n.d.).

Structured Data

Structured data are quantitative in nature, meaning they answer questions like, "how many," "how much," and "how often." Quantitative data are considered objective, meaning they are not influenced by opinion and can be measured as a number and analyzed with statistical software. Recall from Chapter 8 that the programming language used to store structured data is called structured query language (SQL). Structured data can be stored in tables like Microsoft Excel spreadsheets or Google spreadsheets or in databases (Chapter 8). Examples of structured data can be found in the research from the case study on IUDs, including the average age and weight of the participants and the number of IUD insertions in the previous year (Anthony et al., 2021).

There are two types of structured data: discrete and continuous. Knowing what type of data is available helps determine what type of statistical analysis to perform and what conclusions can be made about the data. **Discrete data** involve only integers, meaning they cannot be subdivided into parts. The number of people in the IUD study was 326,658. This number is made up of discrete values, only countable as whole individuals—it is not possible to count 1.5 people. **Continuous data** are measured on a scale or continuum, meaning they can be divided into smaller parts and have any numeric value. The body mass index (BMI) of the participants in the study is an example of continuous data.

Unstructured Data

Unstructured data are qualitative in nature, meaning they can answer questions like, "How did this happen?" or "How do you feel about what happened?" Unstructured data are descriptive and conceptual and cannot be expressed as a number. They are subjective in nature (influenced by personal feelings or opinions) and consist of words, pictures, and symbols. As mentioned in Chapter 8, qualitative data can come from interviews, focus groups, surveys, emails, and observation notes. Qualitative data can be categorized depending on their characteristics and traits (they are sometimes called "categorical data" for this reason). This type of data makes up the majority of all data.

Unstructured data can be divided into two types: nominal and ordinal. **Nominal data** are used for labeling variables that have no specific order. Race and gender are common examples of nominal data. **Ordinal data** are also used to label variables, but the data can be placed in order. From the case study, the calendar year of IUD insertion would be an example of ordinal data. Other examples include satisfaction ratings or economic status. A **Likert scale** is a way to collect ordinal data using a five- to seven-point linear scale, for example, a continuum from strongly agree to strongly disagree. Keep in mind that it is not possible to do arithmetic or statistical analysis of nominal or ordinal data. Tools for analyzing data will be discussed in a later section.

> **CASE STUDY**
>
> Review the article by Anthony et al. (2021) from the case study (see the reference list at the end of the chapter). Make a list of the data collected and determine if the data are structured (discrete or continuous) or unstructured (nominal or ordinal). What type of data featured most prevalently in this particular study? Think about how other types of data could have been used to influence the conclusions of this study.

Big Data

Big data consist of massive collections of both structured and unstructured data that can be used to reveal relationships and dependencies or to perform predictions of outcomes and behaviors. Big data in healthcare involve collecting and analyzing millions of data points generated every second in the medical field, whether in patient care delivery

them. The European Union's General Data Privacy Regulation (GDPR) was introduced in 2018 and governs how personal data can be processed and transferred. More government agencies and regulatory organizations are following suit. In the United States, the California Consumer Privacy Act (CCPA) became effective in 2020 and is the equivalent of the GDPR. This act gives residents of California more control over how businesses collect and use their personal information (Pop, 2022).

Management of data privacy involves four critical data management activities:

1. Data collection
2. Retention and archiving
3. Data use, including testing of new applications
4. Creating and updating disclosure policies and practices

Healthcare systems must assess data-related risks and benefits to take decisive action based on trusted data. Examples of companies that offer big data information privacy protection include Palo Alto, Check Point, ColorTokens, Commvault, and IBM. These companies can prevent data breaches by identifying sensitive data assets, detecting risks and preventing data exposure, providing policy enforcement for sensitive data, and protecting across multiple data repositories (BasuMallick, 2021). You can learn more about data security breaches in Chapter 4 and how to protect data in Chapter 15.

> ### CASE STUDY
> Review the study of intrauterine perforation from IUDs discussed at the beginning of the chapter. Was there a need to protect the privacy of the patients whose data were used for the study? Why or why not?

Big Data in Action

Leaders in healthcare can use big data by integrating publicly available data sets with communication technologies to improve patient care management in primary or specialty practices. For example, one of the data sets commonly used is the U.S. Chronic Disease Indicator (CDI), which allows for the collection of chronic disease data relevant to public health. The CDI contains information such as asthma-related deaths and hospitalizations for each state (CDC, 2023).

For example, this big data can be put into action in the care of patients with asthma or chronic obstructive pulmonary disease (COPD). In these patients, environmental conditions can trigger exacerbations resulting in an office or emergency room visit (Rutland, 2021). A common trigger for people with asthma and COPD is poor air quality, which is a particular problem in large cities in the summer months. With knowledge of air quality problems and a free mobile warning system from the U.S. Environmental Protection Agency, a nurse could encourage patients with asthma and COPD to download the AirNow app (a mobile app that provides air quality information for planning daily activities) to receive air quality warnings, sign up for free email messages with notifications about air quality, or sign up for text messages on days with poor air quality. Nurses can emphasize the need for patients to use their individualized asthma action plan on days with poor air quality warnings.

SOURCES OF STANDARD DATA

When analyzing data, it is useful to have something to compare it to. **Benchmarking** is a process for comparing or evaluating something with a standard. National and international data are often needed to provide a comparison to an individual unit, clinic, or health system. For example, in the case study about uterine perforation, structured data were analyzed using the International Classification of Diseases, Clinical Modification (ICD-9 or ICD-10-CM) diagnosis and procedure codes, Current Procedural Terminology (CPT) codes, and Healthcare Common Procedural Coding System Codes. Benchmarking is part of many quality improvement initiatives.

There are many online resources available to provide data for comparative purposes. The U.S. Government (through data.gov), the U.S. Census Bureau, the Agency for Healthcare Research and Quality (AHRQ), and Centers for Medicare & Medicaid Services are among the most prominent

In the case study, the researchers looked at both structured and unstructured data. Structured (quantitative) data can be further broken down into discrete and continuous data. Unstructured (qualitative) data can be broken down into nominal and ordinal data (Valcheva, n.d.).

Structured Data

Structured data are quantitative in nature, meaning they answer questions like, "how many," "how much," and "how often." Quantitative data are considered objective, meaning they are not influenced by opinion and can be measured as a number and analyzed with statistical software. Recall from Chapter 8 that the programming language used to store structured data is called structured query language (SQL). Structured data can be stored in tables like Microsoft Excel spreadsheets or Google spreadsheets or in databases (Chapter 8). Examples of structured data can be found in the research from the case study on IUDs, including the average age and weight of the participants and the number of IUD insertions in the previous year (Anthony et al., 2021).

There are two types of structured data: discrete and continuous. Knowing what type of data is available helps determine what type of statistical analysis to perform and what conclusions can be made about the data. **Discrete data** involve only integers, meaning they cannot be subdivided into parts. The number of people in the IUD study was 326,658. This number is made up of discrete values, only countable as whole individuals—it is not possible to count 1.5 people. **Continuous data** are measured on a scale or continuum, meaning they can be divided into smaller parts and have any numeric value. The body mass index (BMI) of the participants in the study is an example of continuous data.

Unstructured Data

Unstructured data are qualitative in nature, meaning they can answer questions like, "How did this happen?" or "How do you feel about what happened?" Unstructured data are descriptive and conceptual and cannot be expressed as a number. They are subjective in nature (influenced by personal feelings or opinions) and consist of words, pictures, and symbols. As mentioned in Chapter 8, qualitative data can come from interviews, focus groups, surveys, emails, and observation notes. Qualitative data can be categorized depending on their characteristics and traits (they are sometimes called "categorical data" for this reason). This type of data makes up the majority of all data.

Unstructured data can be divided into two types: nominal and ordinal. **Nominal data** are used for labeling variables that have no specific order. Race and gender are common examples of nominal data. **Ordinal data** are also used to label variables, but the data can be placed in order. From the case study, the calendar year of IUD insertion would be an example of ordinal data. Other examples include satisfaction ratings or economic status. A **Likert scale** is a way to collect ordinal data using a five- to seven-point linear scale, for example, a continuum from strongly agree to strongly disagree. Keep in mind that it is not possible to do arithmetic or statistical analysis of nominal or ordinal data. Tools for analyzing data will be discussed in a later section.

> **CASE STUDY**
>
> Review the article by Anthony et al. (2021) from the case study (see the reference list at the end of the chapter). Make a list of the data collected and determine if the data are structured (discrete or continuous) or unstructured (nominal or ordinal). What type of data featured most prevalently in this particular study? Think about how other types of data could have been used to influence the conclusions of this study.

Big Data

Big data consist of massive collections of both structured and unstructured data that can be used to reveal relationships and dependencies or to perform predictions of outcomes and behaviors. Big data in healthcare involve collecting and analyzing millions of data points generated every second in the medical field, whether in patient care delivery systems, in nurse administrator daily reporting plans, or in management processes such as utilization review, case management, and infection control. The amount of data needed to be termed "big data" is evolving over time. In 1999, 1 gigabyte (GB) was considered big data. Today they are defined in petabytes (1,024,000 GB) or exabytes (1,024 petabytes) of information that include billions or even trillions of data points (IT Chronicles, n.d.).

Healthcare data analytics (also known as business intelligence, or the integration of financial, patient, and quality data) benefits from the use of big data. You can use big data to analyze clinical models to improve medical research, improve patient outcomes, gain operational insights, and improve staffing. When studies like the intrauterine perforation research in the case study use **aggregate data** (combined data from more than one source) collected from multiple sites, the results can be used to better identify the warning signs of uterine perforation and prevent it before it happens. Box 9-1 summarizes some of the benefits of big data to healthcare.

Big data are associated with a list of characteristics: volume, variety, velocity, veracity, value, variability, and visualization (Batko & Ślęzak, 2022). Volume refers to the quantity of data that are generated and stored. The size of the data determines whether they can be considered big data or not. The size of big data is usually larger than terabytes and petabytes. Variety refers to the type and nature of data. Relational databases (discussed in detail in Chapter 8) are capable of handling structured data; however, analysis of semistructured or unstructured data challenges existing tools and technologies. Velocity refers to speed and frequency of data generation and the frequency of handling, recording, and publishing data points. Compared to small data, big data are produced continuously and are often available in real time. Veracity is the quality of data, or its truthfulness and reliability. Value is the worth of the information, and the goal is to discover hidden knowledge in huge sets of data. Variability addresses inconsistency, both in the data and in the context in which data are interpreted. Finally, visualization covers the interpretation of data and the resulting insights.

Big Data Management

The biggest impediments to utilizing big data are at the organizational level: organizational alignment, change management, and resistance or lack of understanding. A major challenge when dealing with big data is ensuring that there is infrastructure to manage it. It can be difficult to separate relevant from irrelevant data. To use big data efficiently, focus on measurements that are key drivers of effective, quality care. There needs to be alignment of decisions about quality measurements throughout the healthcare organization to provide information about the outcomes of patient care, patient satisfaction, costs, and revenue.

Developing a plan for healthcare data analytics is a strategic process that benefits from the engagement of stakeholders like nurses, providers, administrators, and leadership. Other key positions in a healthcare organization include information management specialists, informatics nurse specialists, and statisticians who have the knowledge required to develop or select data warehousing software, data integration software, querying software, and dashboard software to present performance indicators. All must work together to have a robust healthcare analytics process that

---

BOX 9-1 Examples of How Big Data Improve Patient Outcomes in Healthcare

- Enhance patient experiences
- Reduce costs
- Increase efficiency allowing more time for patient care
- Provide real-time alerts and data
- Improve treatment plans and follow-up care
- Improve patient tracking
- Minimize medical errors
- Improve diagnostics and predictions
- Identify trends and patterns
- Improve strategic planning
- Reduce time in developing treatments
- Improve research
- Streamline administrative processes
- Reduce fraud

can be used to collect, store, and analyze data to answer relevant clinical and management questions and to track outcomes (Wang & Alexander, 2020).

The delivery of data analytics must be user-friendly for viewers. Often, these are in the form of dashboards. **Dashboards** are a user-friendly way to deliver real-time visually dynamic information on key performance indicators to drive decision making in healthcare (Randell et al., 2020). With healthcare focused on providing high-quality care at reasonable rates, administrators of complex healthcare organizations rely on these dashboards to be populated with streamlined data. Dashboards can focus on finances, patient care, or services depending on the needs of the user. The use of dashboards in healthcare is playing an important role at senior administrative levels, but dashboards are not just for executives. Anyone who has decision-making responsibility should have access to information in the timeliest manner possible. The use of dashboards has been linked to improvements in quality, particularly when they are customized to a unit or personal level and clinicians believe that they are able to act on the data being presented (Randell et al., 2020). Figure 9-3 shows an example of a patient dashboard.

Information Privacy

It is crucial to properly manage big data to minimize risk and protect sensitive information. Healthcare information is data that often drive organizational decision making, and as healthcare information is valued and placed as a critical organizational asset, it becomes an asset that requires high-level oversight to ensure that the information is handled securely and used appropriately. Because big data are made up of both large and complex data sets, many traditional privacy processes cannot handle the scale and velocity required. **Information governance** refers to the management of information at an organization. According to the America Health Information Management Association (AHIMA), information governance is one way to manage this exponentially expanding volume of healthcare information so that it is secure, reliable, and useable for consumers and stakeholders alike (AHIMA, 2022). Chapter 15 discusses how to protect the privacy and confidentiality of patient data in detail.

As organizations store more types of sensitive data in larger amounts over longer periods of time, they will be under increasing pressure to be transparent about what data they collect, how they analyze and use them, and why they need to retain

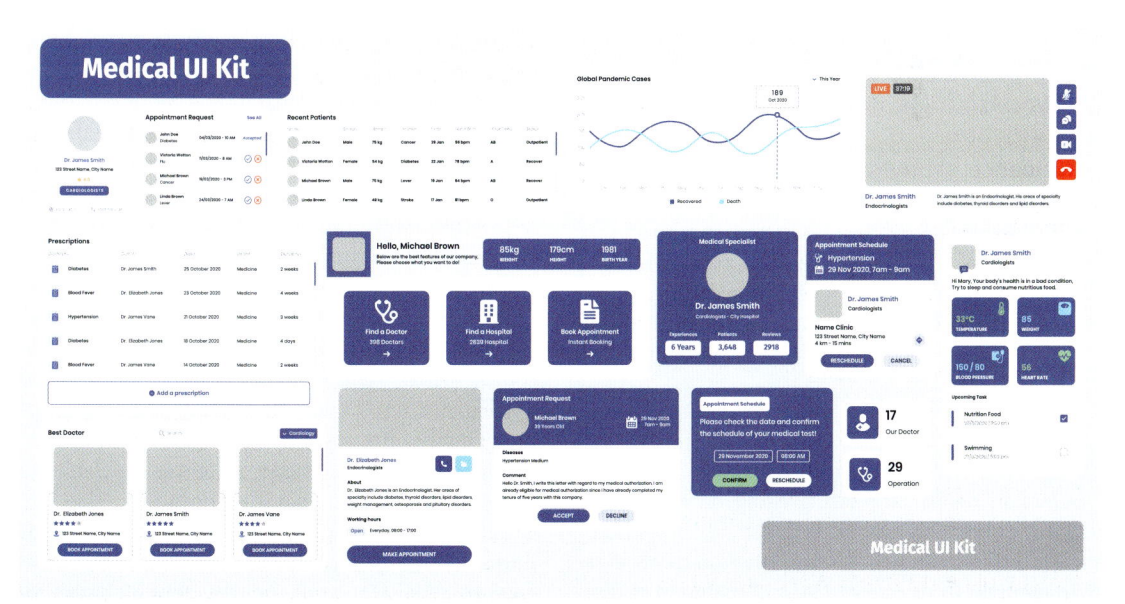

Figure 9-3. Patient dashboard. (Shutterstock/hasanstudio.)

them. The European Union's General Data Privacy Regulation (GDPR) was introduced in 2018 and governs how personal data can be processed and transferred. More government agencies and regulatory organizations are following suit. In the United States, the California Consumer Privacy Act (CCPA) became effective in 2020 and is the equivalent of the GDPR. This act gives residents of California more control over how businesses collect and use their personal information (Pop, 2022).

Management of data privacy involves four critical data management activities:

1. Data collection
2. Retention and archiving
3. Data use, including testing of new applications
4. Creating and updating disclosure policies and practices

Healthcare systems must assess data-related risks and benefits to take decisive action based on trusted data. Examples of companies that offer big data information privacy protection include Palo Alto, Check Point, ColorTokens, Commvault, and IBM. These companies can prevent data breaches by identifying sensitive data assets, detecting risks and preventing data exposure, providing policy enforcement for sensitive data, and protecting across multiple data repositories (BasuMallick, 2021). You can learn more about data security breaches in Chapter 4 and how to protect data in Chapter 15.

> **CASE STUDY**
>
> Review the study of intrauterine perforation from IUDs discussed at the beginning of the chapter. Was there a need to protect the privacy of the patients whose data were used for the study? Why or why not?

Big Data in Action

Leaders in healthcare can use big data by integrating publicly available data sets with communication technologies to improve patient care management in primary or specialty practices. For example, one of the data sets commonly used is the U.S. Chronic Disease Indicator (CDI), which allows for the collection of chronic disease data relevant to public health. The CDI contains information such as asthma-related deaths and hospitalizations for each state (CDC, 2023).

For example, this big data can be put into action in the care of patients with asthma or chronic obstructive pulmonary disease (COPD). In these patients, environmental conditions can trigger exacerbations resulting in an office or emergency room visit (Rutland, 2021). A common trigger for people with asthma and COPD is poor air quality, which is a particular problem in large cities in the summer months. With knowledge of air quality problems and a free mobile warning system from the U.S. Environmental Protection Agency, a nurse could encourage patients with asthma and COPD to download the AirNow app (a mobile app that provides air quality information for planning daily activities) to receive air quality warnings, sign up for free email messages with notifications about air quality, or sign up for text messages on days with poor air quality. Nurses can emphasize the need for patients to use their individualized asthma action plan on days with poor air quality warnings.

SOURCES OF STANDARD DATA

When analyzing data, it is useful to have something to compare it to. **Benchmarking** is a process for comparing or evaluating something with a standard. National and international data are often needed to provide a comparison to an individual unit, clinic, or health system. For example, in the case study about uterine perforation, structured data were analyzed using the International Classification of Diseases, Clinical Modification (ICD-9 or ICD-10-CM) diagnosis and procedure codes, Current Procedural Terminology (CPT) codes, and Healthcare Common Procedural Coding System Codes. Benchmarking is part of many quality improvement initiatives.

There are many online resources available to provide data for comparative purposes. The U.S. Government (through data.gov), the U.S. Census Bureau, the Agency for Healthcare Research and Quality (AHRQ), and Centers for Medicare & Medicaid Services are among the most prominent

> **BOX 9-2** Organizations with Resources for Standard Healthcare Data
>
> - U.S. Government
> - Agency for Healthcare Research and Quality (AHRQ)
> - U.S. Bureau of Labor Statistics (BLS)
> - Centers for Medicare & Medicaid Services (CMS)
> - Federal Interagency Council on Statistical Policy (FedStats)
> - Health Resources and Services Administration (HRSA)
> - Office of Disease Prevention and Health Promotion (ODPHP)
> - National Cancer Institute (NCI)
> - National Center for Health Statistics (NCHS)
> - World Bank
> - World Health Organization (WHO)
> - The Centers for Disease Control and Prevention (CDC)
> - The Cochrane Library
> - National Institutes of Health (NIH)
> - United Nations (UN)
> - U.S. Census Bureau

organizations with available healthcare data. A list of these and other resources can be found in Box 9-2.

U.S. Government

Data.gov is the home of the U.S. government's open data and includes data, tools, and resources to conduct research, develop web and mobile applications, and design data visualizations (Data.gov, n.d.). Over 258,000 data sets are available on Data.gov from multiple agencies at the state and national levels. For example, crime data are available from the city of Los Angeles, fruit and vegetable prices are available from the U.S. Department of Agriculture, and a walkability index is published by the U.S. Environmental Protection Agency. The site can be searched by location, topic, format, organization, and publisher.

U.S. Census Bureau

The U.S. Census Bureau provides data related to several social determinants of health, including age, sex, racial and ethnic identity, housing, and commute. Their website also has several user-friendly tools for data visualization, including easily buildable tables, maps, and profiles that can be tailored to specific geographic regions. In addition, their Census Academy is an online learning hub that walks users through how to use the data available in multiple ways. An example of how to use these data would be to help identify the racial and ethnic makeup of a healthcare system's patient population, which could inform decisions around what languages to use for health brochures or identifying higher risk for a particular disease. By comparing research data with Census data, a researcher can determine if their sample (the participants in their study) is representative of the general population. In addition, these data sets can provide excellent practice for nurses who are learning statistics and data analysis.

Agency for Healthcare Research and Quality

Another useful site for standard data is the AHRQ. The AHRQ provides software downloads, evaluation toolkits, and databases for conducting research. Tools such as the Medical Expenditure Panel Survey (MEPS) and the Healthcare Cost and Utilization Project (HCUP) facilitate mining for data from several national initiatives.

In addition, nurses can find research on quality, access, cost, and information technology at the AHRQ website. Research findings are synthesized or provided in fact sheets for easy reading. Figure 9-4 shows a sample of emergency room visits data sets available from HCUP along with prices for purchasing them.

Centers for Medicare & Medicaid Services

The Centers for Medicare & Medicaid Services (CMS) has a website titled Research, Statistics, Data & Systems, which provides information on patient satisfaction, outcomes of care, and costs. Findings from the required Hospital Consumer Assessment of Health Providers and Systems (HCAHPS) survey, a national, standardized, publicly reported survey of patients on hospital care, are available for review and comparison. A wide variety of data related to healthcare system and clinician quality from the CMS website are also available for download into a spreadsheet or statistical analysis program.

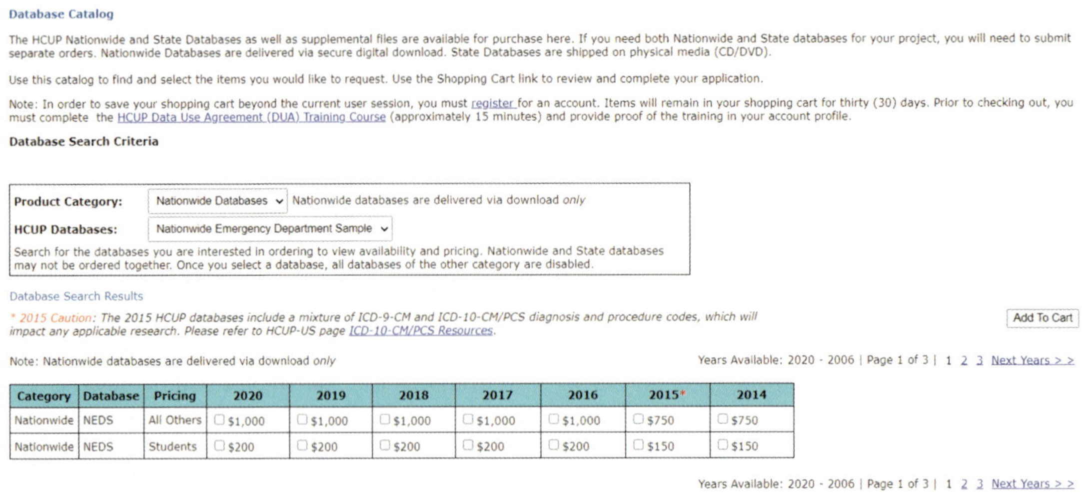

Database Catalog

The HCUP Nationwide and State Databases as well as supplemental files are available for purchase here. If you need both Nationwide and State databases for your project, you will need to submit separate orders. Nationwide Databases are delivered via secure digital download. State Databases are shipped on physical media (CD/DVD).

Use this catalog to find and select the items you would like to request. Use the Shopping Cart link to review and complete your application.

Note: In order to save your shopping cart beyond the current user session, you must register for an account. Items will remain in your shopping cart for thirty (30) days. Prior to checking out, you must complete the HCUP Data Use Agreement (DUA) Training Course (approximately 15 minutes) and provide proof of the training in your account profile.

Database Search Criteria

Product Category: Nationwide Databases — Nationwide databases are delivered via download *only*

HCUP Databases: Nationwide Emergency Department Sample

Search for the databases you are interested in ordering to view availability and pricing. Nationwide and State databases may not be ordered together. Once you select a database, all databases of the other category are disabled.

Database Search Results

* 2015 Caution: *The 2015 HCUP databases include a mixture of ICD-9-CM and ICD-10-CM/PCS diagnosis and procedure codes, which will impact any applicable research. Please refer to HCUP-US page ICD-10-CM/PCS Resources.*

Add To Cart

Note: Nationwide databases are delivered via download *only*

Years Available: 2020 - 2006 | Page 1 of 3 | 1 2 3 Next Years > >

Category	Database	Pricing	2020	2019	2018	2017	2016	2015*	2014
Nationwide	NEDS	All Others	$1,000	$1,000	$1,000	$1,000	$1,000	$750	$750
Nationwide	NEDS	Students	$200	$200	$200	$200	$200	$150	$150

Years Available: 2020 - 2006 | Page 1 of 3 | 1 2 3 Next Years > >

Figure 9-4. Example of searching emergency room visits data sets with pricing from the AHRQ website.

TOOLS FOR DATA ANALYSIS

Data analysis can be simple or complex depending on the type and amount of data. Analysis could involve making a chart of the types of self-care activities students engage in to show which are the most common. A hospital working on discrimination could compare results of a patient satisfaction survey before and after training. The results could be stratified by sexual orientation and gender identity to support identification of specific discrimination issues. As the amount of data increases, the way the data are managed changes. Simple analysis can be done with a calculator or an Excel spreadsheet, but analysis of vast amounts of data like that collected during the COVID-19 pandemic requires the use of databases. Data are only numbers and words until analyzed.

Analyzing Structured Data

Statistical analysis is a mathematical approach to analyzing and interpreting structured data and helps to guide decision makers in understanding how they can apply knowledge gained from a representative sample to a larger population. Nurses who wish to analyze structured (quantitative) data should refresh their knowledge of statistics either through an academic course or by using reliable sources. Several websites are excellent sources of information about the basics of statistics and correct application of statistical procedures to data. Consider reviewing one of the following online sources to understand statistical concepts before undertaking an analysis:

- *Online Statistics: An Interactive Multimedia Course of Study*, developed by Rice University, University of Houston Clear Lake, and Tufts University
- *Research Methods Knowledge Base*, a web-based free textbook by Dr. William M.K. Trochim
- *Statistics Online: Review of Basic Statistical Concepts*, an interactive self-assessment and tutorial by Penn State Eberly College of Science Statistics

Software for Statistical Analysis

As the need for data analysis to support decision making grows, healthcare is faced with the challenge of selecting software that will meet analytical needs, is cost-efficient, and is user-friendly. Ultimately, the goal is to analyze data and translate that information into improved patient care outcomes. Software options for statistical analysis include purchasing commercial statistical analysis programs, using free web-based programs, or using spreadsheet programs. Cost, user preference, and ease of use are likely to be the deciding factors.

Even though spreadsheets can be used to calculate many descriptive statistics, data analysis will be more efficient when using a program designed for that purpose. Examples of popular commercial analysis programs include Statistical Package for Social Sciences (SPSS provided by IBM), Statistical Analysis Software (SAS provided by SAS Institute Inc.), and Minitab (provided by Minitab Inc.).

If a healthcare facility does not own a copy of a commercially available data analysis program, free online software is available for statistical analysis. For example, R (provided by the R Foundation for Statistical Computing) is a language and software that provides statistical computing and graphics. SEER*Stat Software is a statistical analysis program available at no cost from the National Cancer Institute after filling out a request form. Most free statistical software offer users manuals or video tutorials on how to use the application.

Spreadsheet Software

Spreadsheets are widely used to complete simple **descriptive data analysis** (a meaningful description of data points). Spreadsheet programs such as Microsoft Excel often come with the purchase of software for an office or home computer. Numbers is spreadsheet software available with the free version of Apple iCloud. There are many other free spreadsheet software apps available. Web-based options, such as Google Sheets, also allow for a limited amount of descriptive data analysis. Appendix B contains detailed information for how to use Microsoft Excel to organize and analyze data.

Spreadsheet Functions That Facilitate Analysis

A spreadsheet formula is a mathematical equation that calculates data, cutting down on manual calculations. For instance, a formula can be developed to convert temperatures from Fahrenheit to Celsius. That formula can then be copied and used anywhere in the spreadsheet. Conditional formatting changes the appearance of a cell based on certain criteria, making it easy to highlight certain values or make cells easy to identify. For example, you could use conditional formatting to highlight high temperature values in red. You can use the text-to-columns function to separate multiple words within a cell into separate columns. The text-to-columns feature is useful when using data from other information systems that may have complex data in single cells: you can organize it into separate columns to meet your needs. When there are more rows or columns than can fit on a computer screen, spreadsheets provide a way to freeze or hide rows, columns, or both. Freezing keeps one part of the spreadsheet visible while scrolling to another area on the spreadsheet, which can be especially helpful for keeping column headers visible while scrolling down a long list of data. Hiding makes areas temporarily invisible to fit more useful data on a computer screen. Sometimes, spreadsheet design requires sequential data such as numbering 1 to 10. Excel allows users to make a few entries and then have the computer complete the series.

In healthcare, it is especially important to provide data protection and/or security when storing patient data. Data protection is achieved by locking cells to prevent the user from changing the cell value. This feature is helpful for preventing accidental changes to cell text, numbers, or formulas. Security means that the user must provide a password to view and/or edit the spreadsheet. Security is especially important when using a laptop to work with spreadsheets that contain patient-associated data. The Health Insurance Portability and Accountability Act (HIPAA) must be considered, as well as the protection, confidentiality, and privacy issues associated with patient data.

Charts

Spreadsheets allow for creating many different types of charts. Charts are visual representations of data and often work to get information across more easily than lists of data. When using chart variations, be certain that they reflect the point to communicate, as different charts have different strengths and purposes. Although it is important for nurses to demonstrate competencies in preparing charts for data visualization, it is also important to know how to read charts. Nurses must also understand how to use data visualization as a tool for understanding quality issues and other opportunities associated with improving nursing practice.

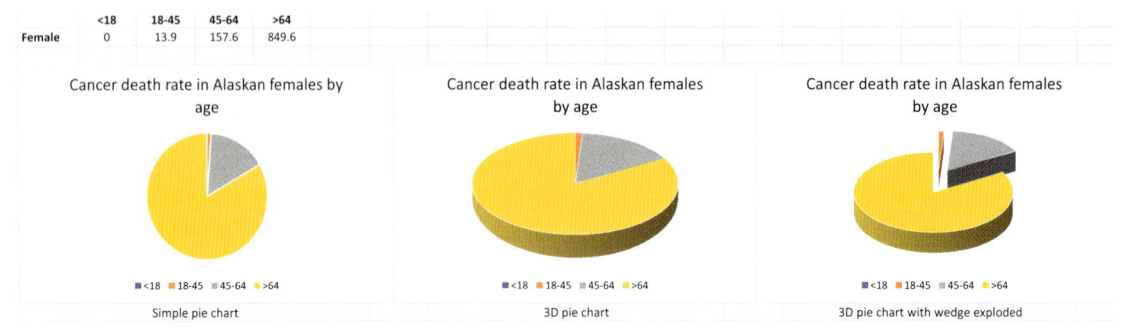

Figure 9-5. Pie chart variations.

When displaying charts in color, use bright and dark colors to emphasize key data. When possible, avoid the use of too many fill patterns, as they can distract from the data. Lines should be bold and clear, and labels should have only necessary information to keep them short.

Pie Charts

A **pie chart** communicates the proportion of various items in relation to the whole: a part-to-whole chart. They are designed to show percentages, not amounts, and thus the sectors should add up to 100%. A pie chart can also show a proportional relationship between a slice and a whole. Pie charts are good tools for visualizing proportions and differences among groups.

Figure 9-5 illustrates different types of pie charts, all representing the same data. Notice how the exploded and three-dimensional views are tilted, altering the perspective and making the segments look like different sizes than in the simple version. Without the percent values, it is difficult to approximate the value of each slice. If a pie chart will best depict the data, be mindful of the chart design, limit the number of slices, and include percentages as labels.

Column and Bar Charts

Column charts are commonly used to compare data over time, or to show comparisons among two or more sets of data. Data are usually presented vertically, and to prevent a distortion of value, it is best if the y-axis starts with a zero. If it does not start with a zero, include an explanation in the chart. **Bar charts** are generally associated with comparisons of amounts and are displayed horizontally. Figure 9-6 depicts column and bar charts that compare the death rate from cancer in Alaska by age and sex.

A **stacked bar chart**, like a pie chart, is a part-to-whole chart. Each data set uses the previous data set as its baseline. For a 100% stacked chart, each data set is a percentage of the whole. Stacked bar charts compare differences in groups of clustered data. However, a stacked chart is harder to understand than a simple bar chart, so be mindful

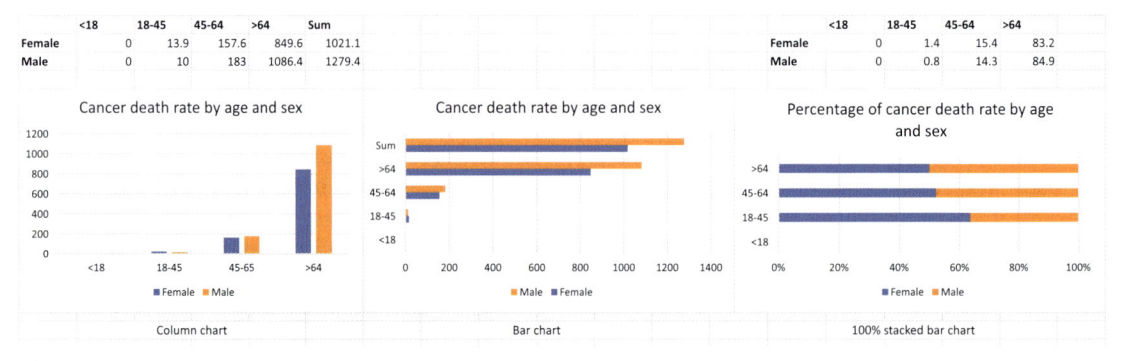

Figure 9-6. Column and bar charts.

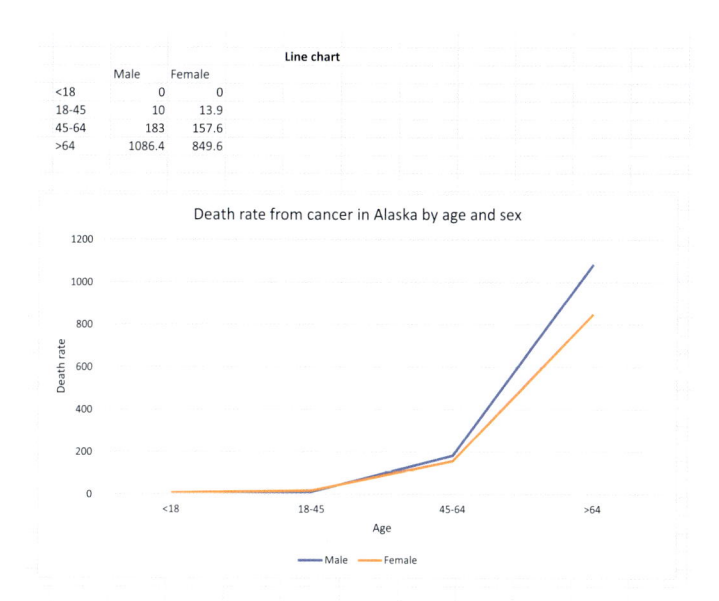

Figure 9-7. Line chart.

	Male	Female
<18	0	0
18-45	10	13.9
45-64	183	157.6
>64	1086.4	849.6

Death rate from cancer in Alaska by age and sex

when using them. The 100% stacked bar chart in Figure 9-6 compares the percentage by sex of age groups who died from cancer.

Line Charts

A **line chart** communicates changes in data over time. When creating a line chart, place the category data on the horizontal axis and the data values on the vertical axis. Use lines to connect individual data points to communicate changes in data over time. Multiple lines can be placed on the same chart to show a comparison between two sets of data. Figure 9-7 shows a line chart depicting trends by sex in death rates from cancer related to age.

Sparklines

Sparklines are small line graphs that fit within a single cell. Sparklines show comparisons of data from individual data criteria. Figure 9-8 illustrates how to view data trends using a single spreadsheet cell to the right of the data. Sparklines with data in the EHR can display variances visually in laboratory or vital signs. Like other standard chart features, markers can be added to depict specific periods.

Analyzing Unstructured Data

Up to 90% of healthcare data may be unstructured, but much of this goes unanalyzed because of the difficulties with this type of data (Kambies et al., 2017). Traditional methods and tools cannot be used to analyze and process unstructured data. It is stored in raw form in **nonrelational databases** (NoSQL), but specialized data analysis software is required for analysis. In healthcare, unstructured information can be extracted

New HIV infections in Ethiopia by decade

	Data on new HIV infections in young adults	Data on new HIV infections in male adults	Data on new HIV infections in female adults	Data on new HIV infections in children	Data on new HIV infections in all ages	Data on new HIV infections in adults	Sparkline
1900	81000	36000	51000	16000	100000	88000	
2000	37000	16000	24000	24000	64000	40000	
2010	17000	7000	11000	8900	27000	18000	
2020	8500	2900	6100	2800	12000	8900	

Figure 9-8. Sparklines.

from the free-text clinical notes entered into EHRs, free-text radiology reports, medical images from scans, comments on social media related to healthcare organizations, audio recordings from therapy sessions, and data found in paper records (TrueNorth, n.d.). Researchers engaged in qualitative research commonly analyze unstructured data gathered from interviews, focus groups, and observational studies.

Numerous software programs are available to analyze unstructured data. At one time, these tools were used only by statistical specialists, but as data have become easily available, even nonexperts can find programs with functionality they can use. Because unstructured data are nonnumerical, many software tools require manually coding data before analysis, but some programs provide more automation in data coding (Wolf, 2021).

Artificial Intelligence

Artificial intelligence (AI) refers to a machine's ability to imitate human behaviors, like reasoning and problem solving (Douthit et al., 2022). AI is increasingly being used in healthcare to interpret data from patient records, claims, or images. AI-powered text analysis tools can sift through billions of pieces data and inform clinical or operational decision making.

AI is an umbrella term that encompasses machine learning, natural language processing (NPL), and speech recognition. Machine learning is one of the most common forms of AI. It is a statistical technique that allows machines to "learn" by fitting models to data. In healthcare, machine learning is used for precision medicine to predict what treatments are most likely to work for a patient based on an analysis of their attributes and needs. Neural networks are a type of machine learning that have been used to predict whether a patient will acquire a particular disease. Deep learning is the most complex form of machine learning and can be used to scan x-rays for potentially cancerous lesions. Deep learning is also increasingly used for speech recognition (NPL) (Davenport & Kalakota, 2019).

Natural language processing (NLP) refers to the branch of AI concerned with giving computers the ability to understand text and spoken words in much the same way human beings can. NLP combines computational linguistics—rule-based modeling of human language—with statistical, machine learning, and deep learning models. Together, these technologies enable computers to process human language in the form of text or voice data and to "understand" its full meaning, complete with the speaker's or writer's intent and sentiment (IBM Cloud Education, n.d.). In healthcare, NLP is used to analyze clinical documentation such as unstructured clinical notes. It can also transcribe and analyze patient interactions and even conduct conversations with those who need information translated into another language.

Technologies used in healthcare may encompass several AI branches. For example, ambient clinical intelligence uses machine learning, speech recognition, and NLP. Ambient intelligence is commonly understood in devices like Google Assistant and Amazon Alexa, which automatically respond to a person's voice (Nelson, 2021). Ambient clinical intelligence can listen to the conversation between a provider and patient, use machine learning to interpret the collected data, and use NLP and speech recognition to automatically create clinical documentation.

Big Data Technology

Tools for analyzing big data enable organizations to perform deeper analysis of data, discover uses for which the data were not originally intended, and combine them with new data sources. The term "big data" comes not just from the sheer volume of data, but from the complexity, diversity, and exponential velocity at which data sets are growing. As more and more data are continuously generated, it raises concerns about the accuracy of aging data and the ability to track down entities for consent to use their information in new ways. Other big data analysis challenges include data capturing, storage, search, sharing, transfer, visualization, querying, updating, information privacy, and source. These challenges are driving the invention of new ways to analyze data, as well as technology to handle the fast pace with which the data changes over time (Wang & Alexander, 2020).

Big data requires novel methods of analysis compared to what has been used traditionally (Shilo et al., 2020). Big data technology encompasses the software tools for analyzing, processing, and extracting data from extremely complex and large data sets. Having access to big data technologies creates opportunities for researchers to find patterns and make predictions based on real data. Big data may require parallel software running on tens, hundreds, or even thousands of servers while many zettabytes of data are analyzed.

There are many types of software and applications that are useful for analyzing big data. Some types of applications that have been developed to handle big data include (Tyagi, 2020):

- AI: Accomplishes tasks that have in the past required human intelligence, such as analyzing unstructured data (covered in more detail later in the chapter)
- Data mining: The process of finding anomalies, patterns, and correlations within large data sets to predict outcomes
- Predictive analytics: Attempts to predict future behavior using machine learning technologies, data mining, and statistical models
- NoSQL databases: Used to accumulate, retrieve, and analyze unstructured data
- Cloud computing: Delivers computing services over the internet to offer speed and flexibility (covered in more detail in Chapter 3)
- Data lakes: Repositories of all formats of data, the term is typically applied to storage of unstructured data, but data lakes can store any type of data
- R programming: Open-source programming language used for statistical computing and visualization

CURRENT TRENDS IN DATA ANALYTICS

Successful healthcare systems and health communities know that data are the key to success. What is most amazing about the exploding trend in data capture and analysis is that as a society, we are at the crossroads of providing healthcare to help diagnose, treat, or even avoid a treatment, thanks to the advancements in technology, the internet, and vast amounts of data that before were inaccessible. Any healthcare consumer or provider can comb vast amounts of data that can change healthcare faster and in more directions than ever before. Current trends in data analytics include the use of health information technology (HIT), AI, information governance, and clinical decision support systems (CDSS).

Health Information Technology

Health information technology (HIT) is information technology used specifically for healthcare. It involves the processing, storage, and exchange of health information in an electronic environment. HIT has made data analysis faster and more accessible, often directly in the hands of patients. Mobile technology devices (discussed in more detail in Chapter 5) can continuously analyze health data such as blood sugar levels, heart rhythms, heart rates, and cardiac artery pressures in a patient's home. The COVID-19 pandemic triggered significant increases in the use of telehealth and the development of newer technologies to allow for remote analysis and monitoring, including remote blood sample collection to monitor COVID antibodies (Koulman et al., 2022). Monitoring patients' health with HIT data analysis at home can reduce costs and unnecessary visits to the healthcare setting, especially for those in underserved areas where accessing healthcare is more difficult.

Artificial Intelligence to Improve Healthcare

As AI becomes more robust and more readily available for public use, the benefits will expand. AI is already used to improve healthcare, and new technologies are expected to make even greater improvements as time goes on.

For example, the AI-based tool artificial immune recognition system uses AI to predict tuberculosis. Another AI tool has been used to diagnose malaria by automating the complex process of analyzing diagnostic laboratory samples (Malik et al., 2021). AI has been used for the prediction of epileptic seizures by analyzing patient data from wearable sensors (Nicoletti, 2023) and to analyze images gathered during diagnostic imaging scans to detect precancerous colorectal polyps during colonoscopy. This study showed that using AI reduced missed polyps by 50% when compared to a standard colonoscopy (Wallace et al., 2022). AI can also be used to improve the accuracy of mobile health technology by identifying false alerts for atrial fibrillation (AF) with insertable cardiac monitors. Using an algorithm, the use of AI has increased the identification of false AF alerts by 74.1% and preserved 99.3% of true AF alerts (Radtke et al., 2021).

ChatGPT is an example of emerging AI that can assist with healthcare data analysis. ChatGPT is a chatbot developed by OpenAI and launched in 2022 that uses an NLP model (Marr, 2023). It is capable of analyzing written or spoken word and outputting human-like responses. It can analyze global health data from a variety of sources to look for the emergence of new disease patterns, and then create automated health alerts. ChatGPT can analyze patient health data to help select ideal candidates for clinical health trials. It can also assist with remote patient monitoring by analyzing patient data from wearable devices and sending alerts to healthcare providers if a patient's condition is deteriorating (Marr, 2023).

Clinical Decision Support Systems

A **clinical decision support system (CDSS)** is a computer application that analyzes patient health information and makes recommendations for care that will result in the best possible outcomes (USF Health, 2021). According to the AHRQ, CDSSs provide information to clinicians, patients, and others to inform decisions about healthcare. CDSSs can positively affect patient outcomes, improve quality of care, and prevent the third leading cause of death in America—medical errors (AHRQ, 2019).

Examples of CDSSs include:

- Computerized EHR alerts and reminders for both the provider and patient such as allergies, drug–drug interactions, or drug–food interactions
- Chatbots embedded in medication management software that can support clinical decisions with information
- Evidenced-based clinical practice guidelines
- Condition-specific order sets
- Documentation templates, including additional data or restrictions for ordering high-risk medications, such as nephrotoxic medications or anticoagulants
- Diagnostic support

Like any other system put into place in healthcare, a CDSS is best used in conjunction with clinical judgment. If a CDSS is used in a silo without the employment of the human brain for clinical judgment, then failure can occur. The clinical reasoning skills of practitioners rely on knowledge and judgment. CDSSs support evidence-based clinical practice by assisting with information management to support clinicians' treatment plans.

Research about the effect of CDSSs on nursing processes and outcomes is more difficult to find. A systematic review examining the impact of CDSSs on nursing pressure injury management found that most studies did not report statistically significant improvements in decreasing pressure injury formation (Araujo et al., 2020). In contrast, a systematic review examining the impact of CDSSs on nurse and allied health performance and patient outcomes identified that CDSS use positively improved care processes in 47% of the measures adopted, including improvements in nurse hand hygiene, documentation, and timeliness of blood sampling (Mebrahtu et al., 2021). In addition, CDSS use was found to decrease the number of patient falls. More information about clinical decision support can be found in Chapter 11.

SUMMARY

- **Data analysis in nursing.** Data analysis requires an understanding of how data are entered, stored, and accessed to support improved patient outcomes. Florence Nightingale was the first nurse to advocate for data collection and analysis. Her work resulted in many lives being saved by increasing understanding of the role of germs in the disease process. The NINR provides funding to nurses interested in conducting research. Data analysis is often used in EBP studies to guide decision making and in research to support the growth of nursing knowledge.

- **Types of data.** Data can be structured (quantitative) and unstructured (qualitative). Structured data can be described as discrete or continuous. Unstructured data are either nominal or ordinal. Knowing what type of data are available is necessary for choosing how to analyze it. Big data consist of massive collections of complex data that can be structured and/or unstructured. They can be used to improve patient outcomes. Collecting and analyzing aggregate data can better identify issues and trends in healthcare. Special consideration must be given for the security and privacy of big data given the complexity and size of the data. Information governance is one way to manage the expanding volume of healthcare information so that it is secure, reliable, and useable.

- **Sources of standard data.** When analyzing data, it is helpful to have other sources of data to compare data to. Benchmarking is comparing healthcare data with national and international standards. Organizations with databases that provide useful data sets for comparison include the U.S. Government, U.S. Census Bureau, AHRQ, and CMS.
- **Tools for data analysis.** Analyzing structured data involves statistical analysis, which can be done with free or commercial software. Spreadsheet software can analyze structured data with functions that facilitate analysis and with the creation of charts. Unstructured data require specialized software to analyze. AI, including machine learning, NPL, and speech recognition, is becoming a popular way to analyze unstructured data. Some applications that help with big data analytics include AI, data mining, predictive analytics, NoSQL databases, cloud computing, data lakes, and R programming.
- **Current trends in data analytics.** HIT has put the ability to analyze data into the hands of patients, allowing them to manage complex diseases like diabetes and heart failure in the home. AI can be used to improve healthcare with early detection of disease and improvement of existing healthcare technology. A CDSS is a computer application that provides information to clinicians, patients, and others to inform decisions about healthcare.

DISCUSSION QUESTIONS AND ACTIVITIES

1. A public health nurse is concerned about the percentage of adults who use tobacco locally and wonders if the rate of tobacco use in the county is higher than national or international rates. What online resources could the nurse use to find comparison rates?
2. Consider your clinical or healthcare agency work setting. How are healthcare data analytics used to inform decisions?
3. Identify a clinical problem in your clinical or healthcare agency work setting. What data would you need to collect to define the problem?
4. If you were to select a statistical software program to analyze data for an EBP project, what would you consider when making your selection?
5. Look for a recent article about AI and how it can improve patient outcomes and discuss your findings.

PRACTICE QUESTIONS

1. The nurse is looking for U.S. data related to patient falls along with tools to assist with an EBP project focused on improving the patient fall rate. What resource would be best for the nurse to access?
   a. The U.S. Census Bureau
   b. The Agency for Healthcare Research and Quality
   c. The World Health Organization
   d. The Canadian Research Data Centre Network
2. What is a common concern that the nurse needs to consider when it comes to big data and HIT?
   a. The risk for patient privacy to be compromised
   b. The lack of technology to support appropriate data analysis
   c. The general lack of accessibility
   d. Both are too new to fully understand the benefits and risks.
3. Which statement about charts and graphs is true?
   a. "The y-axis should begin with the lowest number."
   b. "The segments of a pie chart are designed to show amounts."
   c. "Sparklines are used to communicate changes in data over time."
   d. "Bar charts are generally associated with comparison of amounts."

REFERENCES

Agency for Healthcare Research and Quality [AHRQ]. (2019, September 7). *Clinical decision support systems*. https://psnet.ahrq.gov/primer/clinical-decision-support-systems

American Health Information Management Association [AHIMA]. (2022). *IG 101: What is information governance?* Retrieved from https://library.ahima.org/doc?oid=300881#.YuH4juzMLFo

Andrews, R. J. (2022) Florence Nightingale's data revolution. *Scientific American, 327*(2), 78–85. https://doi.org/10.1038/scientificamerican0822-78

Anthony, M. S., Reed, S. D., Armstrong, M. A., Getahun, D., Gatz, J. L., Saltus, C. W., Zhou, X., Schoendorf, J., Postlethwaite, D. A., Raine-Bennett, T., Fassett, M. J., Peipert, J. F., Ritchey, M. E., Ichikawa, L. E., Lynen, R., Alabaster, A. L., Merchant, M., Chiu, V. Y., Shi, J. M., ... Asiimwe, A. (2021). Design of the association of uterine perforation and expulsion of intrauterine device study: A multisite retrospective cohort study. *American Journal of Obstetrics and Gynecology, 224*(6), 599.e1–599.e18. https://doi.org/10.1016/j.ajog.2021.01.003

Araujo, S. M., Sousa, P., & Dutra, I. (2020). Clinical decision support systems for pressure ulcer management: Systematic review. *JMIR Medical Informatics*. 8(10), e21621. https://doi.org/10.2196/21621

BasuMallick, C. (2021, September 2). *Top 10 cloud data protection companies in 2021*. https://www.spiceworks.com/tech/cloud/articles/cloud-data-protection-companies/

Batko, K., & Ślęzak, A. (2022). The use of big data analytics in healthcare. *Journal of Big Data, 9*(1), 3. https://doi.org/10.1186/s40537-021-00553-4

Centers for Disease Control and Prevention (CDC). (2023). *U.S. Chronic disease indicators*. https://catalog.data.gov/dataset/u-s-chronic-disease-indicators-cdi

Dang, D., Dearholt, S., Bissett, K., Ascenzi, J., & Whalen, M. (2022). *Johns Hopkins evidence-based practice for nurses and healthcare professionals: Model and guidelines* (4th ed.). Sigma Theta Tau International.

Data.gov. (n.d.) *The home of the U.S. government's open data*. https://data.gov/

Davenport, T., & Kalakota, R. (2019). The potential for artificial intelligence in healthcare. *Future Healthcare Journal, 6*(2), 94–98. https://doi.org/10.7861/futurehosp.6-2-94

Douthit, B., Shaw, R., Lytle, K., Richesson, R., & Cary, M. (2022). *Artificial intelligence in nursing*. American Nurse Today. https://www.myamericannurse.com/ai-artificial-intelligence-in-nursing/

IBM Cloud Education. (n.d.). *Natural Language processing*. https://www.ibm.com/cloud/learn/natural-language-processing

IT Chronicles. (n.d.). *What is big data?* https://itchronicles.com/what-is-big-data/

Kambies, T., Mittal, N., & Sharma, S. K. (2017, February 7). *Dark analytics: Illuminating opportunities hidden within unstructured data*. https://www2.deloitte.com/us/en/insights/focus/tech-trends/2017/dark-data-analyzing-unstructured-data.html

Koulman, A., Rennie, K. L., Parkington, D., Tyrrell, C. S., Catt, M., Gkrania-Klotsas, E., & Wareham, N. J. (2024). The development, validation and application of remote blood sample collection in telehealth programmes. *Journal of Telemedicine and Telecare, 30*(4), 731–738. https://doi.org/10.1177/1357633X221093434

Malik, Y.S., Sircar, S., Bhat, S., Ansari, M.I., Pande, T., Kumar, P., Mathapati, B., Balasubramanian, G., Kaushik, R., Natesan, S., Ezzikouri, S., El Zowalaty, M. E., & Dhama, K. (2021). How artificial intelligence may help the Covid-19 pandemic: Pitfalls and lessons for the future. *Reviews in Medical Virology, 31*(5), 1–11, https://doi.org/10.1002/rmv.2205

Marr, B. (2023, March 2). *Revolutionizing healthcare: The top 14 uses of ChatGPT in medicine and wellness*. https://www.forbes.com/sites/bernardmarr/2023/03/02/revolutionizing-healthcare-the-top-14-uses-of-chatgpt-in-medicine-and-wellness/?sh=24bc25366e54

Matthews, J. R. (2016). History of biostatistics. *Medical Writing, 25*(3), 8–11.

Mebrahtu, T. F., Skyrme, S., Randell, R., Keenan, A. M., Bloor, K., Yang, H., Andre, D., Ledward, A., King, H., & Thompson, C. (2021). Effects of computerised clinical decision support systems (CDSS) on nursing and allied health professional performance and patient outcomes: A systematic review of experimental and observational studies. *BMJ Open, 11*(12), e053886. https://doi.org/10.1136/bmjopen-2021-053886

Melnyk, B. M., & Fineout-Overholt, E. (2023). *Evidence-based practice in nursing & healthcare: A guide to best practice* (5th ed.). Wolters Kluwer Health//Lippincott Williams & Wilkins.

National Institute of Nursing Research (NINR). (n.d.) *2022-2026 strategic plan (fact sheet)*. https://www.ninr.nih.gov/sites/files/docs/NINR_One-Pager12_508c.pdf

Nelson, H. (2021, October 20). *Ambient clinical intelligence: What it means for the EHR industry*. TechTarget. Retrieved July 12, 2022, from https://ehrintelligence.com/features/ambient-clinical-intelligence-what-it-means-for-the-ehr-industry

Nicoletti, A. (2023, October 11). *Predicting epileptic seizures with AI*. FIU Research Magazine. https://news.fiu.edu/2023/predicting-epileptic-seizures-with-ai

Pop, C. (2022, September 27). *EU vs US: What are the differences between their data privacy laws?* Endpoint Protector. https://www.endpointprotector.com/blog/eu-vs-us-what-are-the-differences-between-their-data-privacy-laws/

Radtke, A., Ousdigian, K., & Haddad, T. (2021). Artificial intelligence enables dramatic reduction of false atrial fibrillation alerts from insertable cardiac monitors. *Heart Rhythm, 18*(8), S47.

Randell, R., Alvarado, N., McVey, L., Ruddle, R. A., Doherty, P., Gale, C., Mamas, M., & Dowding, D. (2019). Requirements for a quality dashboard: Lessons from national clinical audits. *AMIA Annual Symposium Proceedings*. 2019, 735–744.

Richardson, A., Kasza, J., & Lamb, K. (2020, May 11). *The healing power of data: Florence Nightingale's true legacy*. The Conversation. Retrieved from https://theconversation.com/the-healing-power-of-data-florence-nightingales-true-legacy-134649

Rutland, C. (2021, March 16) *Expert perspective: Managing asthma on poor air quality days*. Retrieved from https://www.healthline.com/health/asthma/expert-perspective-managing-asthma-on-poor-air-quality-days

Shilo, S., Rossman, H., & Segal, E. (2020). Axes of a revolution: Challenges and promises of big data in healthcare. *Nature Medicine, 26*(1), 29–38. https://doi.org/10.1038/s41591-019-0727-5

TrueNorth. (n.d.). *Healthcare unstructured data*. https://www.truenorthitg.com/healthcare-unstructured-data/

Tyagi, N. (2020, March 11). *Top 10 big data technologies.* https://www.analyticssteps.com/blogs/top-10-big-data-technologies-2020

University of South Florida (USF) Health. (2021, November 16). *The relationship between analytics and clinical decision support.* https://www.usfhealthonline.com/resources/healthcare-analytics/the-relationship-between-analytics-and-clinical-decision-support/

Valcheva, S. (n.d.). *6 types of data in statistics & research: Key in data science.* Intellspot. Retrieved February 16, 2023 from https://www.intellspot.com/data-types/

Wallace, M., Sharma, P., Bhandari, P., East, J., Antonelli, G., Lorenzetti, R., Vieth, M., Spernaza, I., Spadaccini, M., Desai, M., Lukens, F. J., Babameto, G., Batista, D., Singh, D., Palmer, W., Ramirez, F., Palmer, R., Lunsford, T., Ruff, K., ... , Hassan, C. (2022). Impact of artificial intelligence on miss rate of colorectal neoplasia. *Gastroenterology, 163*(1), 295–304.e5.

Wang, L., & Alexander, C. A. (2020) Big data analytics in medical engineering and healthcare: Methods, advances and challenges. *Journal of Medical Engineering & Technology, 44*(6), 267–283. https://doi.org/10.1080/03091902.2020.1769758

Wolf, R. (2021, September 29). *8 great tools to perform qualitative data analysis in 2022.* https://monkeylearn.com/blog/qualitative-data-analysis-software/

CHAPTER 10
Disseminating Data

Kristi Miller, Joni Tornwall, Meredith Mackenzie, and Sarah Rusnak

OBJECTIVES

After studying this chapter, you will be able to:

1. Explain why disseminating data is important and appropriate ways to disseminate your data.
2. Discuss strategies for making presentations engaging and effective.
3. Apply best practice design principles when creating presentations and posters.
4. Explain why publishing is important and how to choose an appropriate journal.
5. Explain legal concerns for the educator including the use of Universal Design for Learning (UDL) principles.

AACN Essentials for Entry-Level Professional Nursing Education

1.2f Synthesize knowledge from nursing and other disciplines to inform education, practice, and research.
2.2c Use a variety of communication modes appropriate for the context.
4.1g Communicate scholarly findings.
6.1b Use various communication tools and techniques effectively.
8.1c Effectively use electronic communication tools.
8.1d Describe the appropriate use of multimedia applications in health care.
8.3a Demonstrate appropriate use of information and communication technologies.

AACN Essentials for Advanced-Level Nursing Education

1.1e Translate evidence from nursing science as well as other sciences into practice.

2.2g Demonstrate advanced communication skills and techniques using a variety of modalities with diverse audiences.

4.1i Engage in scholarship to advance health.

4.1k Collaborate to advance one's scholarship.

4.1l Disseminate one's scholarship to diverse audiences using a variety of approaches or modalities.

4.2h Address opportunities for innovation and changes in practice.

8.4e Assess best practices for the use of advanced information and communication technologies to support patient and team communications.

HIMSS Competencies

Assistive technology

Communication

Information and communications technology systems applications

Information and knowledge management in patient care

Information management research

Learning techniques

Legal issues in health IT

Process management

Resource planning and management

Teaching, training, education

KEY TERMS

Academic paper
Accessibility
Alt-text
Assessment
Author guidelines
Bloom's Taxonomy of Learning
Closed caption
Impact factor
Instructional design
Journal article
Journal manuscript
Universal design for learning (UDL)
Scholarly writing

CASE STUDY

When you consider the question of whether to disseminate or share data, consider the implications for patient outcomes. Many researchers have confirmed that it takes an average of 17 years for research evidence to reach clinical practice (Morris et al., 2011). Only 20% of evidence-based interventions make it to routine clinical practice (Rubin, 2023). In historically marginalized populations, this gap is often larger. However, when research focuses on patient problems and interventions, changes are more quickly implemented (Munro & Savel, 2016). An example is early mobility in intensive care units (ICUs). Research done on the importance of implementing early mobility protocols that began in 2006 was widely implemented by 2016. Other examples of rapid translation of research to practice include nursing research in oral care, infection control, communication, and team processes (Munro & Savel, 2016).

In Chapter 7, you read a case study about the use of a tailored intervention (FallTIPS) to reduce the fall and injury rate on a medical telemetry unit. To better understand the importance of disseminating data, imagine you are a nurse who just finished a similar project. You and your colleagues designed a project that included several different hospital systems. In addition, you have data that show differences in fall rates between males and females as well as by ethnicity and race. You are interested to find that the FallTIPS intervention is perceived differently by people with different identities. You and your colleagues believe that the results of your study are important, and you want to share it, but you are not sure how to begin the process of disseminating the information. As you read this chapter, think about the best ways to disseminate data, whether publishing or presenting data would be more effective, and how to tailor your information to maximize accessibility.

As you learned in Chapter 7, the Advancing Research and Clinical practice through close Collaboration (ARCC) Model has seven steps (Melnyk & Fineout-Overholt, 2023). The focus of this chapter is on the final ARCC step, disseminating and sharing information with others. The process of changing data from information into knowledge (a step in the data, information, knowledge, and wisdom, or DIKW, model) only results in value across practice settings when the knowledge is shared with others in the profession. The maturation of professional nursing practice is dependent on the development and dissemination of nursing knowledge. Knowledge sharing allows nurses to influence nursing practice, drive health policy, and guide interdisciplinary health practices.

When nurses disseminate information, it allows others to learn from what they have done, increasing nursing knowledge and improving patient outcomes. It is important to share the results of studies with stakeholders such as nursing staff, administration, patients and their families, and the community at large. Sharing the results of quality improvement projects can inspire other nurses to ask their own burning questions and begin the process of adding to nursing knowledge on their own units. In addition, disseminating data can help advance one's career. Nurses working in academic settings may be required to publish or present as part of their job expectations. In most states, publishing and presenting is a way to earn continuing education (CE) credits required to maintain licensure.

You can disseminate data to your peers through institutional newsletters or in-service events, to a wider audience through publishing in an academic journal, or by presenting a poster or oral presentation at local, regional, national, or international conferences. Your institution may have a public relations department to assist in sharing information with the public, or you may want to contact local news outlets.

DATA DISSEMINATION

After gathering and analyzing data from a study, there are many options for what to do with the results. You might choose to create a poster about your work and share it with coworkers at a lunch and learn. You could create a PowerPoint presentation to share at a monthly research club at your hospital, at a regional falls prevention consortium, in an online meeting of the local chapter of the American Nurses Association (ANA), or at a national conference on nursing research. You might decide to write about your work in a blog or newsletter that is shared at your healthcare organization, on social media, or through an organization like the ANA, which has a website that publishes research and nursing news updates. You might also consider submitting the results to a journal like the *American Journal of Nursing* or the *Journal of Clinical Nursing*.

An important role of data dissemination comes in the development of clinical practice guidelines. Clinical practice guidelines are developed from rigorous, systematic syntheses of evidence. They are digestible guides that provide practical steps for applying the evidence to the clinical setting. Resources to find clinical practice guidelines include the National Guideline Clearinghouse from the Agency for Healthcare Research and Quality (AHRQ) and the Canadian Best Practice Portal. Other resources include specialty nursing organizations, such as the Oncology Nursing Society.

In addition, disseminating data can help build your career. Being a published nurse writer or presenter can help you stand out in the workplace and increase your value to your organization. Remember to add any efforts at disseminating data to your resume, no matter how small they may be. Disseminating data is valued by leadership and can support applications to graduate school or for new positions.

When considering the question of when, where, and how to disseminate data, it is important to remember that nurses have valuable insight into patient care. If you remind yourself that you have experiences and knowledge that others want and need to know about, it can help you find the confidence to share your data with a wider audience.

Finding a mentor in research or evidence-based practice (EBP) may help you get started and will become important as you progress in your career. If you are enrolled in school, you have access to a wide variety of nurse researchers who may be excited to mentor a student interested in disseminating EBP findings. Many hospitals or larger healthcare organizations have nursing research councils with EBP experts who are ready and willing to help with data dissemination. Nursing organizations are another source of research and EBP mentors.

CASE STUDY

As you read in the case study, disseminating data is important for improving patient outcomes and reducing healthcare disparities. Think about times when you have been the recipient of dissemination of evidence—maybe it was an in-service on smart beds, a presentation on new wound healing technology by a colleague, a screen saver describing how documentation on a unit is changing, or continuing education on fall prevention in an online meeting. How did what you learned change the way you performed your job? Was there an impact on patient outcomes? How have you disseminated information? Did it have an impact on patient care?

PRESENTING DATA

A falls prevention training video with narration, an instructor presenting a lecture on heart failure, and a poster presentation at a research conference on climate change and health outcomes are examples that illustrate the variety of options for presenting data. Sharing knowledge with others is essential in nursing education and practice, and presentations are a common way to do this in educational, research, and clinical settings. You might be asked to create a poster or slideshow to present information to your organization, or you may be encouraged to apply to present research findings at a local, national, or international conference.

Choosing a Venue

Nurses who are new to EBP and research may choose to share in smaller venues with people they know and trust. After getting positive feedback in those venues, they might then consider taking data to a wider audience.

Joining a nursing organization is a good first step in getting ideas for how to widely share data. For example, nurses who are members of the American Association of Critical-Care Nurses (AACN) have access to online discussion boards, virtual CE events, newsletters, and opportunities to present at conferences, collaborate with other professionals, and publish in reputable journals. Most nursing organizations provide these perks with membership. For example, you can search for local and national events on the AACN website (AACN, n.d.). Besides the ability to present your work, other benefits of attending a nursing conference include the chance to network with other nurses, the ability to earn CE credits for attending workshops, and the exposure to other nurses' EBP findings and research studies. Attendees often come home with new ideas for how to improve patient outcomes in their facilities.

The choice of where to share depends not only on one's willingness, but on funding sources. Nursing conferences can be expensive. Registration can cost anywhere from $100 to $1,000 to attend a conference that may last between a few days to a week. Expenses also include the cost of travel to and from the conference, meals, and hotels. Explore whether your healthcare organization has funds available to send employees to conferences. If you are in school, explore the possibility of a travel scholarship to attend conferences and research for discounts and attendance options. For example, the 2023 annual conference for the North Carolina Nurses Association (NCNA) offered discounts for NCNA members, first-time attendees, students, and early registrants and provided the option of attending the full conference or only single days (NCNA, 2023).

The rigor of a research study is another factor to consider in deciding where, when, and how to share data. A study done on one unit over a short period of time with only a few patients is a good way to get experience with research. Data from small studies are useful to individual organizations and other nurses who work on similar units. Studies done with larger numbers of participants at multiple sites and for longer periods of time are more valuable sources of nursing knowledge and will be of greater interest to a wider audience.

If you choose to present at a local, regional, national, or international conference, you will need to research submission guidelines. Nursing organizations send out emails and social media posts to advertise when they are accepting applications, termed a "call for abstracts." Applications are likely to require an abstract (a short summary of the study). For example, a local event listed on the AACN website is the Horizons 2024 call for poster abstracts. The eighth edition of the Nursing World Conference (NWC) was scheduled for 2024. Prior to the event, the website listed poster, speaker, and virtual presentation guidelines detailing how and when to submit materials, how long presentations should be, and how large posters could be (NWC, 2024, 2023).

Presentations

Presentations are an effective way to communicate data and knowledge to a group of people. The group may be small if the presentation is given in one unit or organization, or it can be large if delivered at a nursing conference. An effective presentation provides the audience with an overview of the upcoming information, the information itself, and then a summary of the important points. More than that, an effective presentation will be based on sound instructional design, have clear learning objectives, and be well designed. An effective presenter always keeps the audience in mind. Engage the audience to enhance their understanding and reduce cognitive overload by chunking complex topics into smaller components. This section will provide an overview of how to give an effective presentation.

Software for Creating Presentations

There are many different presentation software platforms, such as Microsoft PowerPoint, CustomShow, ClearSlide, Haiku Deck, Prezi, Google Slides, Adobe Spark, Apple Keynote, and Apache OpenOffice Impress. Each platform has different features, advantages, and disadvantages

(Turner et al., 2022). Presentation software usually includes many of the same features as word processing menus, like font style, size options, and the ability to create tables and insert graphics and multimedia. The implementation of specific features will vary by software type and version. Most slideshow software is compatible with other slideshow software. For example, you can import slides developed with PowerPoint into Keynote for Mac and into Google Slides. Although the slides import, the added special effects, like sound, transitions, and animations, may not import. For more information about how to create a slide presentation using Microsoft PowerPoint, see Appendix C.

Instructional Design

When creating a presentation, consider an **instructional design** model to guide the development of the activity. One example is the ADDIE model, a method widely used to create highly effective online courses (Chappell, 2018). Each of the five components of the ADDIE model—analyze, design, develop, implement, and evaluate—reflect an important stage of instructional design:

1. Analyze: Identify the educational or instructional problem, the goals, the current state of the learning environment, and the learner's existing knowledge and skills.
2. Design: Design a proposal that is systematic and specific with learning objectives, assessment instruments, activities, content, and media selection.
3. Develop: Create or find content with consideration of how technology is integrated; pilot testing can aid development.
4. Implement: Deliver the educational intervention, taking training and facilitator preparation into consideration as well as learning outcomes, method of delivery, and assessment procedure.
5. Evaluate: Determine if the learners have achieved the objectives.

Instructional design is a cyclical, flexible process. As one part of the presentation is completed, other parts may need to be modified (Fig. 10-1).

Learning Objectives

An effective presentation begins with learning objectives that clearly state what participants can expect to learn from the activity. Learning objectives are best when they are specific, measurable, actionable or achievable, reasonable or relevant, and time-bound (SMART) (Fig. 10-2).

Bloom's Taxonomy of Learning (Anderson et al., 2001; Bloom, 1956), a model showing how learning progresses from simple to complex, can

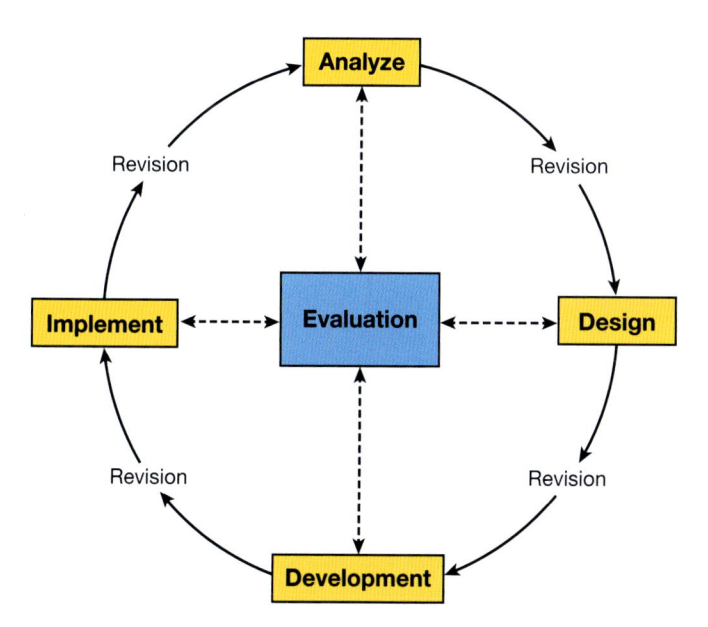

Figure 10-1. ADDIE instructional design model.

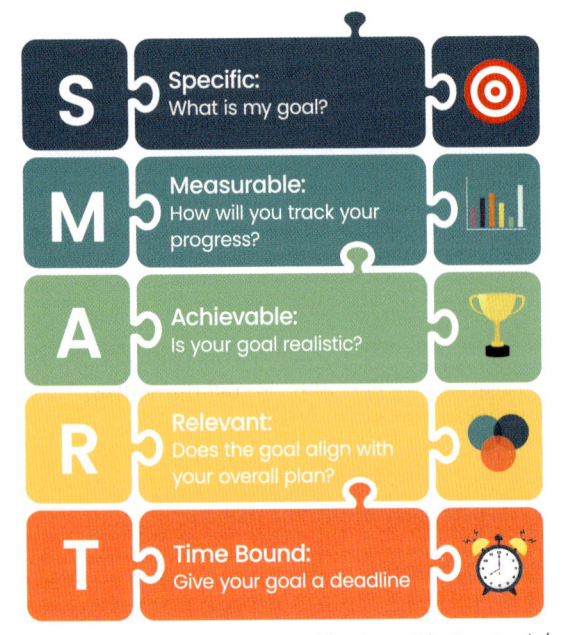

Figure 10-2. SMART learning objectives. (Shutterstock/Julee Ashmead.)

be used to help create learning objectives that are appropriate for the content. Learning something new starts at the most basic level of the taxonomy, remembering, and progresses through understanding, applying, analyzing, evaluating, and creating (Fig. 10-3). With each level, the learner has a deeper understanding of the information:

- Remembering: The learner can recite discrete facts.
- Understanding: The learner can explain the concept.
- Applying: The learner can understand the concepts well enough to apply them to a new situation.
- Analyzing: The learner can break apart the concept and compare the parts or identify relationships between the parts.
- Evaluating: The learner can make judgments about the quality or validity of something based on standards or predetermined criteria.
- Creating: The learner can put elements together to form new ideas and models that function.

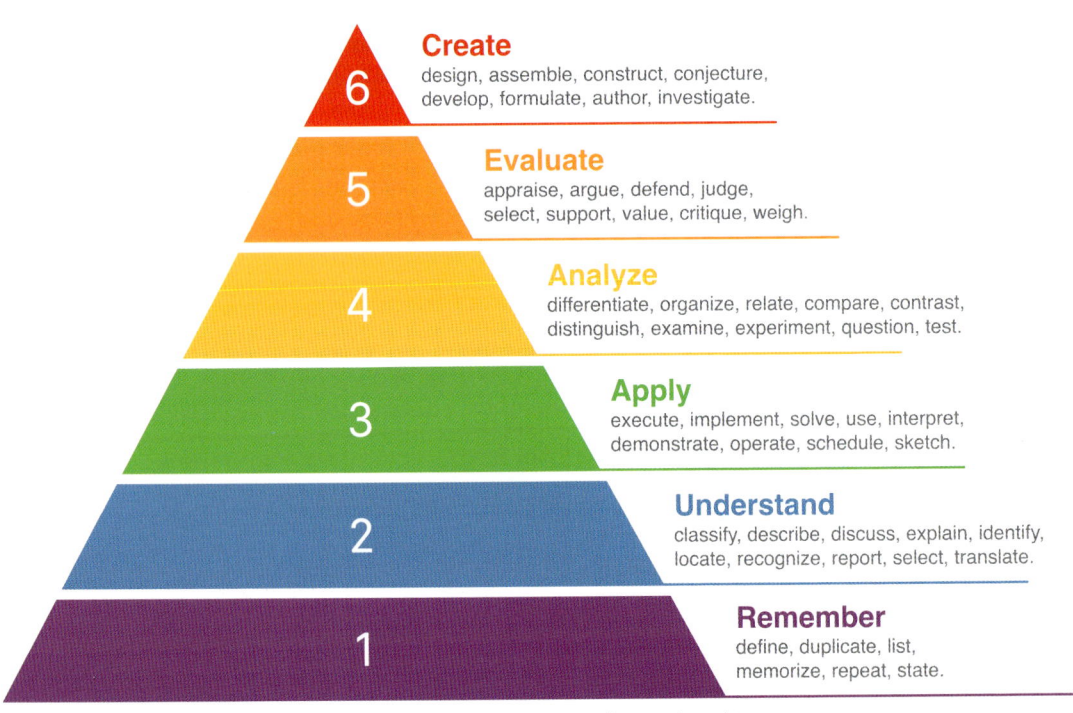

Figure 10-3. Bloom's Taxonomy of Learning. (Shutterstock/Martial Red.)

Nurses are expected not only to remember or understand facts and concepts but also to make sound clinical judgments about patient care by analyzing and evaluating information and creating solutions.

Making a Presentation Engaging

At a minimum, a slideshow and presentation achieve a one-way transfer of information: The presenter speaks, and the learners listen. Lecturing in this style remains an effective way to convey a lot of information, but it does not help the learner retain the information. Active learning techniques can enhance learning and reduce cognitive load. Any lecture can incorporate active learning by asking the audience to participate (Babik & Luther, 2020). The audience will find it easier to pay attention knowing they will be engaged.

The key feature in active learning is a required response from the learner. Consider a learning experience in a virtual discussion in which the learner can express their viewpoint through text, voice, or images. Whether this discussion takes place on an asynchronous discussion forum or in a synchronous class meeting via video conference, the learner is engaged because of the required interaction. In contrast, video lectures are, by themselves, passive learning. However, they can be made more active through reflection questions, embedded quiz questions, or other strategies that require a response from the learner.

Oral Presentation

There are some important considerations for presenting a slideshow to a live audience. You may feel nervous about doing a live presentation despite practicing and rehearsing. One way to calm down at the start is to give the audience 5 seconds to read the title slide while you breathe. After reading the title, introduce yourself and give the audience an icebreaker or an anecdote. It can help to make eye contact with various people in the audience and to nod and smile. The audience will relax as you relax. If someone asks a question that you are not ready to answer, make a note of it and tell the audience you will get to the question later or inform them that you are covering the information in a future slide. You can always communicate after the presentation about a difficult question. Some tips for improving presentation skills can be found in Box 10-1.

Asking Questions

Budgeting time for audience questions throughout the presentation or saving 5 to 10 minutes at the end of the talk for questions ensures learners can ask for clarification. Checking in with the audience is important, and how you open the presentation up for questions matters. Instead of asking "Does anyone have questions?" or "Does that make sense?" try a prompt like "What questions do you still have about (the topic)?" This encourages learners to speak up, rather than making them feel foolish for not "getting it" the first time (Rosenshine, 2012).

BOX 10-1 Tips for Improving Presentation Skills

- Practice, practice, practice.
- Attend other presentations to get ideas for what works and what does not.
- Arrive early and adjust your environment to meet your needs.
- Begin with a strong, interesting, entertaining introduction.
- Transform any nervous energy into passion and enthusiasm.
- Use positive visualization; imagine the presentation going well.
- Remember that most audiences are sympathetic.
- Take deep breaths to get oxygen to your brain.
- Pause to take a sip of water to gather your thoughts; audiences need pauses too.
- Limit the amount of material you are covering; leave them wanting more.
- Admit when you do not have all the answers.

Data from Kim, L. (2022, December 12). *20 ways to improve your presentation skills*. Wordstream. https://www.wordstream.com/blog/ws/2014/11/19/how-to-improve-presentation-skills

You can also embed questions in the presentation using anonymous polling, which lowers the stakes for learners who do not understand a concept. When polling is anonymous, participants can express honest beliefs and views different from others. Polling the audience will both engage them and provide feedback to the presenter. Synchronous audience members can respond to questions embedded into slide presentations using smartphones or a web browser. Asynchronous learners can respond to questions embedded into online lectures.

Sharing Access

Printing copies of the materials for audience members can result in wasted paper. With cloud hosting of files, you have the option to provide handouts, guided notes, or the presentation itself via a hyperlink or quick response (QR) code. Given the proliferation of cloud-based presentation software and cloud hosting of files, many presenters provide a copy of their presentation as a file or via hyperlink. To keep the audience's attention focused on the message rather than reading handouts, tell attendees at the beginning of the presentation that you will make materials available after the presentation.

If you are creating a presentation as lecture replacement or to share with audience members following a presentation, you can record narration as you move through the slides so you can explain the information to the learner. Storing video on the cloud is a way to avoid having to deal with large file sizes. You can create a free YouTube account and upload the video, making it possible to access it anywhere there is internet access.

Designing a Presentation

When creating a presentation, you may want to start right away with designing slides, but planning before the first slide is created will save time and result in a more interesting presentation. A traditional presentation style uses slides with the standard slide title and bullet design, but this is not always the most engaging design. Design principles that apply to all slide presentations will help the audience engage and retain more information.

Images

Presentation software provides an easy way to include images on your slides. As you design your slides, consider whether a picture, graph, or table will communicate the message better than words. Images are often more effective in a slideshow, allowing you to fill in the narrative through your oral presentation. A table or chart may make data easier to interpret. A simple table with rows and columns labeled or simple chart with different aspects labeled is accessible to all learners. Labels should be clear and concise and visible enough to be easily seen from a distance. Be wary of complex tables as they may not resize well on mobile devices and are difficult for those using screen readers to access. Slides that are unreadable create learner frustration. Also be careful of overusing charts and tables. Over reliance on these graphics can make a presentation too busy.

When searching for images, keep in mind that pictures and photographs can elicit both strong emotional responses and more subtle biases. Do your images represent the diversity of providers and patients that nurses will encounter? Stock photo sites that provide free images that represent and respect diverse communities including Nappy, the Disabled and Here Collection, and the Gender Spectrum Collection.

Though an endless number of images are available on the internet, be sure to give credit to the original creator of the image. It is essential to check the copyright permission and license terms of any images, video, or sound that you use and did not create yourself. By default, all content creators own copyright on their works. Some creators are happy to share their work and will designate how their creations can be reused. A Creative Commons license clarifies what uses the creator will allow, and whether they require credit in the presentation (Creative Commons, n.d.). If you plan to include an image, it is best to create your own or find images that are labeled for reuse.

Special Effects

You can enhance slideshow presentations using special effects such as sound, video, animations, and transitions. However, use moderation when adding special effects to a presentation. You want the viewers to pay attention to the message, not the special effect. If a presentation uses special effects, such as sound and video, test the presentation in the setting where viewers will see it. Remember that special effects are sometimes incompatible between different software, so if slides need to be imported to another software, check the presentation carefully to be sure it works as intended.

Fonts and Colors

The most important thing to remember when selecting fonts (the typeset of the letters) is to be consistent and intentional. Sans serif fonts are more widely used for presentations because they are easier to read on a digital screen, but titles or headings may be acceptable in a serif font since they are larger in size. One font can be used for the whole presentation, or one font for the headings and another for the body text as long as they are consistent throughout. For a slideshow accompanying an oral presentation, there will be less text on screen and a greater distance between the screen and audience, so use a larger font size for headings and body text (for example, 24 points for headings and 18 points for body text) to effectively fill the space. For a presentation intended to be read, a smaller font can be used for headings and body text (for example, 18 points for headings and 14 points for body text) because learners will often be reviewing these individually on personal screens.

Although you can use a few colors to draw attention to a feature, always include additional means of expression so that viewers with limited color vision or low or no vision are also able to comprehend the content. This may mean adding a pattern to bars in charts, adding data labels, or adding text descriptions. Note that providing multiple means of comprehension helps all learners. As with fonts, it is important to be consistent in using color. When viewers grasp the implications of a given color, the result is improved comprehension of the meaning of the visuals.

Posters

Poster presentations are common in academic and professional organization conference settings to share and discuss the results of research. A poster is a visual presentation of an abstract (Hess et al., 2009). The visual appeal helps draw in the audience (Siedlecki, 2017). The content of a well-designed poster is quickly understood by the viewer and relies on photos and charts with minimal words. The New York University Library has examples of well-designed and poorly designed posters (NYU Library, 2023). Guidelines for how to create a research poster can be found on many university websites. For specific events, professional organization conferences will have poster presentation guidelines online.

A poster presentation can be done electronically or it can be printed. Electronic posters are displayed from a laptop or large monitor. If displayed from a laptop, the poster sections are presented as a slideshow. If displayed on a large screen (50 in or greater) the design of the poster is a single slide. Electronic presentations have the advantage of multimedia and the internet. Electronic posters are economical to produce, though at present, their use is limited by costs and access to computers or large monitors.

Print posters are popular but can be expensive to create. They can also be cumbersome when traveling to conferences. When using print posters, pay attention to the presentation guidelines to know if the posters are displayed on a tabletop or a bulletin board posting format. If the latter, be sure to bring extra push pins. Guidelines should also be followed for sizing. Standard print poster sizes are 3 by 4 ft and 5 by 7 ft (SUNY Brockport, n.d.). You can create a printed poster presentation from a single electronic slide by using Google Slides, OpenOffice Presentation, and the commercial versions of PowerPoint and Keynote by changing the document size from a slide size to the desired poster size. Since multimedia features cannot be included with printed posters, the inclusion of a QR code on a printed poster allows viewers to easily access these resources on their own device (Faridi, et al., 2021).

For both electronic and print posters, you will be assigned times to stand with your poster to

> ### CASE STUDY
>
> After reading about what makes a presentation effective, describe experiences you have had with effective and ineffective presentations. What components of a good presentation do you find most valuable for your learning? What do you find most distracting? Imagine you are one of the researchers who worked on the FallsTIPS research mentioned in the case study and discussed in Chapter 7 (Fowler & Reising, 2021). Use what you have learned to create a title slide and a slide with three learning objectives about the research in the article.

answer questions. For times when you are not present, it is helpful to provide a QR code or email contact on your poster so that those who view it can reach out if they have questions.

As with slideshow presentations, be judicious with the use of color on posters. White or light backgrounds with black text are easiest to read. Adding two to three accent colors enhances visual appeal. You do not need to be a graphic design professional to add color; free color wheel tools such as Adobe Color and Canva color wheel simplify the process of selecting complementary colors. The visual appeal and relevance of the topic are crucial for successful knowledge transfer of the presentation (Siedlecki, 2017).

General Guidelines for Poster Design

Several guidelines apply to the creation of a printed poster or electronic poster presented on a large monitor (Berg & Hicks, 2017; Faridi et al., 2021; Siedlecki, 2017). See Box 10-2 for some of these guidelines.

Poster Handouts

Print poster handouts can be taken home by participants. Handouts will reiterate the poster message and will include a way of contacting the presenter with questions or comments on the presentation. The 8.5-by-11-in handout should have a small version of the poster on one side and any additional information on the other side. If the mini version is difficult to read, it is probably difficult to read on the poster. In that case, modify the poster.

Consider creating a website or download link with more information. You can link to this resource with a QR code that viewers can scan from the poster or handout. Once you have created

---

BOX 10-2 General Poster Guidelines

Design
- Start with your institution's poster template and/or the conference poster guidelines.
- Use no more than three different fonts throughout, and all fonts should be easy to read.
- Use a white or light background with black text, adding two to three accent colors to enhance visual appeal.
- Allow for up to 40% of empty space (also known as negative space) so that the poster elements are not crowded.
- Use empty space to separate sections, not borders.
- Design the presentation in three columns.
- Do not allow fonts, colors, or other design elements to interfere with the message.
- Your title and headings should stand out so people can quickly see what the poster is about and how it is structured. The font sizes you should use depend on the size of and amount of content on your poster. Suggested font sizes for a print poster of 48 in by 36 in are:
  - Title: 88 to 120 points
  - Names and affiliations: 70 to 90 points
- Major headings: 54 to 80 points
- Sub headings: 48 to 72 points
- Text: 36 to 52 points

Content
- Content should be organized into sections: the title, purpose, methods or summary of what is known, results, conclusion, and references.
- Place a succinct title at the top of the poster that communicates research results.
- Use minimal text (fewer than 600 to 800 words).
- Write text information succinctly and in lay terms when possible.
- Begin bullets with an action verb.
- Use consistent punctuation for bullets.
- Include descriptive captions beneath charts and graphs.
- Include your contact information (or a QR code with the information) so that viewers can request a copy of the poster or additional information and/or videos related to the poster.

a website, the amount of additional information you can provide is endless. However, consider limiting the website to your contact information, a digital copy of the poster, and a few supplemental resources or videos that may be of interest.

Assessment and Evaluation

After providing patient education, nurses are taught to assess whether the patient has learned the information. You may want to include an assessment or evaluation of your poster or presentation. An **assessment** is a systematic strategy for gathering data and measuring learning outcomes achieved by learners from the instruction. Evaluations are designed to document the level of achievement attained with a competency or skill. In addition, assessing and evaluating participants can provide you with direction for improving future performance.

To assess learner understanding, you could create an online quiz using learning objectives, ask informal questions, or have learners fill out an evaluation of their understanding (Fig. 10-4). When using evaluations, include a section for an open-ended response to allow participants to share suggestions or questions about the presentation.

PUBLISHING DATA

Writing is an essential communication tool for nurses. It is a learned skill and, like other nursing skills, takes practice. Nurses are expected to produce scholarly writing at all levels of practice (AACN, 2021). In nursing, **scholarly writing** is related to the generation, synthesis, translation, application, and dissemination of nursing knowledge to improve health and transform healthcare (AACN, 2021). Nurses regularly conduct EBP, quality improvement projects, and research, depending on their professional roles, but they don't always write about their findings (Stucky, 2020). Scholarship, especially scholarly writing in the nursing discipline, is key to sharing knowledge with nurse colleagues and advancing nursing science.

Try not to be intimidated by the concept of publishing ideas. Every nurse who has been published began their career in nursing school. To develop the skills necessary to produce practice scholarship, development of foundational skills in nursing-specific scholarly writing should begin at the undergraduate level and continue throughout a nurse's career. When students engage in nursing-specific writing beginning at the undergraduate level, they develop critical thinking skills they can apply to practice (Jefferies et al., 2018). For more information about scholarly writing using Microsoft Word, see Appendix D.

How Do Scholarly and Academic Writing Differ?

It is important to understand how academic and scholarly writing are similar and different as you move between your educational and professional experiences. An **academic paper** is generally written by students, and the audience is the instructor or professor. For example, students may be asked to write in a scholarly style for online discussion

Please share your opinion about the presentation:

	Strongly agree	Agree	Neither agree nor disagree	Disagree	Strongly disagree
I understand how to implement falls prevention interventions	○	○	○	○	○

Figure 10-4. Sample evaluation question for presentation learners.

postings, assignment submissions, master's theses, and doctoral dissertations. Criteria for preparation of an academic paper depends on the course, program, and instructor preferences. In academic writing, follow instructor and program guidelines for preparation of the document.

In contrast, scholarly writing by nurses is focused on publication of **journal manuscripts**. A manuscript is a research writing submitted to journal publications. Manuscripts are reviewed by peer reviewers assigned by journal editors to maintain the quality of the publication. A **journal article** is a manuscript that has been published. It will be read by an audience of nursing students, nurse leaders, and researchers.

Although both types of papers tend to follow a strictly defined style, submitting an academic paper to a journal for publication may result in rejection, even if the content is sound (Morton, 2020). When preparing a manuscript, it must follow the style of the journal or publication to which it was submitted and conform to the preferences of the publisher or editor. Follow the **author guidelines**, also known as instructions to authors or submission guidelines, for all papers intended for publication in any venue. These guidelines outline how to prepare the manuscript, and they must be followed exactly or the submission will be rejected or returned for further editing. For example, the author guidelines for the *American Nurse Journal* have specific instructions for article length, number and style of references, figures, and tables, plus guidelines on what to do before and after submission (ANA, 2023). Author guidelines are typically available on a journal's website.

Choosing a Journal for Publication

Choosing the most appropriate journal for a manuscript can be difficult. There are several strategies for finding the right journal. For each reference on the topic of interest, take note of the journal that publishes it. Search for suitable journals by searching topic keywords in a library database. Which journals are represented repeatedly and have a good reputation among professionals in your discipline? The Nurse Author & Editor Directory of Nursing Journals (2022) is an online resource that may be helpful in identifying a suitable target journal for given article.

Keep in mind that even reliable journal identification tools can unintentionally present options related to predatory journals. Predatory journals publish articles that are unvetted, do not meet rigorous standards of disciplinary science and scholarship, and give readers content that has not passed ethical or quality standards. They make money by charging article authors a significant fee to publish. Jeffrey Beall's list of predatory journals and publishers is available online along with strategies for recognizing predatory journals (Beall, 2012, 2021).

All reputable nursing journals have an online presence where they describe their scope, editorial board, author guidelines, and publishing practices on publicly available websites. It is possible that some or all the published articles are available only by subscription (either individual or institutional). If you identify the best fit between the paper you want to write and the journal in which you want to publish it before you begin writing, your writing task will be easier. By following the author guidelines for format, sections and headings, citations and references, article length, and other journal-specific requirements from the outset, you will have a paper that is ready for submission sooner.

Journal editors look for uniqueness in manuscripts. They tend to look more favorably at papers that add new ideas to the literature. In research, this means editors are looking for new knowledge that adds to the science and practice of nursing. In a broader context beyond research scholarship, editors are looking for innovative or EBPs implemented in new contexts or with new populations. They will usually not accept a paper that closely resembles a paper published recently in the same journal. Be sure to search the recent (in the previous year or two) publications in the target journal for articles that are similar to yours. Editors strictly avoid republishing articles in whole or in part, and your paper will be run through plagiarism-checking software before it is officially accepted by the journal.

You may also want to consider the impact factor of the journal. Impact factors are calculated by several companies including Clarivate, Google, and Scimago. The **impact factor**, or journal impact factor, is an objective method for comparing the relative influence and prestige of competing journals.

Traditionally, journals with higher impact factor values carry more prestige in their respective fields than those with lower values; however, the quality of a journal should be assessed holistically and not based on metrics alone. The impact factor is frequently used by universities and funding bodies to decide on promotion and research proposals (ImmunoFrontiers, 2022). See Chapter 7 for more information on journal impact factors.

> **CASE STUDY**
>
> In the case study, you were asked to imagine that you conducted FallsTIPS research and that you obtained data about the impact of sex and ethnicity on how FallsTIPS is received by patients. Would it be appropriate to submit an article on your research to the *MEDSURG Nursing* journal? Why or why not? Find two other journals to which you might submit and discuss your reasoning. Describe how the publication guidelines for each journal are the same or different.

UNIVERSAL DESIGN

Universal design for learning (UDL) principles guide the design of content and active-learning methods with accessibility, usability, and inclusivity in mind (Davis et al., 2022). UDL used in combination with active learning gives all learners more equal opportunities to succeed by supporting learning self-regulation, providing options for engaging with content, and giving the learner choices in the assessment process. A key feature of UDL is purposeful engagement with representation of the learner through action and expression (Davis et al., 2022).

Accessibility

The Centers for Disease Control and Prevention (2020) reports that approximately one quarter of adults in the United States have some type of disability. The American Disabilities Act (ADA), Section 508 (U.S. Access Board, 2017), ensures equal access to educational opportunities for people with disabilities, including educational opportunities supported by technology. As part of their work and in compliance with federal law, nurse educators routinely integrate strategies to design the most inclusive, accessible education possible.

Accessibility involves removing barriers that prevent interaction with digital tools and technologies (like presentations) by people with disabilities (Georgetown Law, n.d.). Learners with low or no vision use screen readers, an assistive technology that allows learners to navigate digital content by listening. With videos, the software you use to create videos likely includes the use of **closed captions** (textual representation of video narration) so that those who are deaf or hard of hearing can learn from the presentation.

By providing accommodations for nursing students and nurses with disabilities, you make it possible to help diversify the nursing workforce, reduce barriers for everyone, and meet the critical demand for nurses in healthcare. This applies to learning and technology in ways that address visual, auditory, motor, and cognitive disabilities. Accessibility in online instruction means that people with disabilities can perceive and engage with digital instruction in equally effective and integrated ways as people who do not have disabilities and with equivalent ease of use (W3C, 2023). Common instructional design features that support accessibility are captioned videos, documents that can be read by a screen reader, and learning technologies that have clear accessibility statements online demonstrating their transparency about and commitment to an accessible and inclusive learning experience.

Imagine the experience of a learner who wishes to review the slides provided, but cannot access the information in images or cannot navigate a slide presentation because titles and slide numbers are missing. Modern operating systems include screen readers, but it is the presenter's responsibility to effectively communicate the information to all learners. Before you begin creating your slides, familiarize yourself with the accessibility features included in presentation software.

Accessibility is measured in degrees rather than "yes, it's accessible" or "no, it's not accessible." There is no definitive line to cross that makes a presentation or course fully accessible. There is always a chance that a learner with a disability will not be able to use some component of a presentation. The goal is to design it so it is accessible, useable, and inclusive for the largest possible number of potential learners. Answering the questions in Box 10-3 will support accessibility design.

Everyone benefits from slides that are designed to be accessible, including the presenter. Adding accessibility features can help you think through what you will emphasize to learners. When you use default layouts in presentation software, you can quickly make changes to the overall appearance of your slides by editing the theme, and all slides in the presentation within the layouts will change simultaneously. When you design your visuals with strong color contrast, slides will be easy to view in any setting, regardless of the quality of the projector or screen or the lighting in the room. Accessibility is covered in more depth in Chapters 5, 9, and 21).

Checking Accessibility

Checking for accessibility has become easier over time. Microsoft 365 includes accessibility checkers throughout the suite of applications, including PowerPoint (Microsoft, 2022a; 2022b). The accessibility checker will automatically review headings, fonts, hyperlinks, color contrast, and readability by a screen reader and provide a report listing any potential problems. For example, tables may trigger warnings, but keeping tables as simple as possible can facilitate accessibility. The checker also checks for meaningful use of color and sufficient contrast in the document to assist readers with low vision or color blindness. It looks for built-in headings and styles that are in a logical, hierarchical order because screen readers use them to navigate through a document.

Alt Text

Images should include alternative text, commonly abbreviated as alt text. **Alt text** describes an image or table and the information it conveys. For example, an illustration of the heart that shows the flow of blood through the chambers must include alt text that describes the same level of detail that learners without visual impairment obtain from the image itself. Simply stating *drawing of a heart*

BOX 10-3 Questions to Ask About Accessibility

- Are there any components in your presentation that are not useable by someone with a visual or hearing impairment? If the component cannot be made accessible immediately, it is imperative to include a statement near the component that tells the learner how to go about obtaining accommodations to engage in the content in an equally effective and user-friendly way.
- Do all images have alt text? Text will appear when a cursor hovers over an image that has alt text. Always type a simple description of the image in this box that pops us when you upload an image.
- Have you used text and graphics that add function to the course and are not distracting? An example of a distracting element is blinking text or a rapidly cycling GIF image.
- How will a person who is colorblind perceive your presentation? Is there sufficient contrast for individuals with low vision?
- Can screen reader software read the text? If you compose your text using common editors like the one in Microsoft Word, or if you save your documents in PDF, you should be able to use the tools in the document processing software to ensure accessibility. Search the internet for instructions to do this within the software you use. Always use heading styles in web-based editors or word processors.
- Do learners have opportunities to engage in different learning strategies and a variety of ways to demonstrate their learning through different kinds of assessments? Not every objective needs to have multiple strategies and assessments; rather, the presentation should include a reasonable variety of approaches to learning and demonstrating proficiency.

does not allow learners with low or no vision to fully engage with the content. Alt text should be provided on all shapes, images, graphics, icons, smart art, flow charts, and any other visual media. If an object is purely decorative, it can be marked as such. However, if an image does not convey any meaning to the learner, it may be worth asking if the image should be on the slide at all.

Color

Keep in mind that a significant number of people have some degree of color perception problem or color blindness (American Optometric Association, n.d.). These conditions may make it difficult to distinguish the difference between colors, to perceive the brightness of colors, or to distinguish different shades of colors (National Eye Institute, n.d.). Color is often used to convey meaning, and because people perceive color differently, it should not be the only means by which information is provided. For example, a chart with different shades of red indicating the prevalence of various conditions in a population may be inaccessible to some viewers. Adding text descriptions via data labels ensures that all learners without visual impairment can understand the information presented and including alt text ensures that users with low or no vision are also able to fully engage.

Using strong contrast between colors assists viewers to read the text. To check the level of contrast between the background and any text or icons in the foreground, search for browser-based color contrast checkers such as those provided by Web Accessibility in Mind (WebAIM). The accessibility checker in Microsoft 365 will flag any text that has poor color contrast with the background.

Usability

Usability is a concept closely related to accessibility and UDL and includes user experience design and applies to everyone regardless of ability (W3C, 2023). Intentional strategies in digital content design that increase ease of use support the usability of instructional content for all users. Examples of strategies that support usability are use of heading styles, meaningfully hyperlinked text, and user-friendly navigation. Formal or informal usability testing of presentations is always a good practice. Resources for understanding how to conduct usability testing for all types of content are readily available on the internet.

Inclusivity

Inclusive instruction fully supports active involvement of everyone in the educational experience. Features of inclusive instruction include diverse materials that contain visual and textual representations of people from different backgrounds, appearances, ages, and cultures. Inclusive design also allows learners to experience a variety of approaches to learning within one unit of instruction (i.e., a combination of teaching strategies and methods of assessment that fit a variety of learning preferences). Nonthreatening opportunities for self-assessment and reflection on learning give learners a chance to identify gaps and seek support when needed. These strategies move the center of power in education—and the responsibility for learning—toward a more learner-centered model that is supportive and open to differences in the overall learning experience (The Derek Bok Center for Teaching and Learning, 2022).

Table 10-1 is an example of an inclusive language style guide for universal terms that apply to content on multiple devices and for learners with diverse abilities. This inclusive language should be used when writing instructions to access online content.

There is considerable overlap among accessibility, usability, and inclusive design and the instructional design strategies used to optimize each one. It is well worth the time and effort to design a presentation from the outset to include common features for accessibility, usability, and inclusion (Box 10-4) because when you address one of them, you

TABLE 10-1 Inclusive Language Examples for Simple Instructions

Less Inclusive Language	More Inclusive Language
Click the link.	Select the link. Choose the link.
Look at the table.	Reference the table.
Watch the video.	Play the video.

> **BOX 10-4** Common Design Features Supporting Accessibility, Usability, and Inclusion
>
> **Accessibility**
> - Textual content is readable with a screen reader.
> - Audio content is closed captioned with accurate captions.
> - Alt text is applied to images.
> - Extra time is allowed on quizzes.
>
> **Usability**
> - Content is organized with appropriate headings and heading structure.
> - Where color is used, contrast is strong and meaning is conveyed in alternate ways to accommodate colorblindness.
> - Distinguish hyperlinks from text with a different color and underline; link text is meaningful on its own.
> - Form controls have labels, instructions, and error messages.
>
> **Inclusion**
> - Alternative formats are available for viewing multimedia content using low-bandwidth connections.
> - There is support for gaps in computer literacy and skills.
> - Images and content contain representations of people from multiple backgrounds, age groups, and cultures.
> - Content is available in multiple languages or resources are provided for translation.
>
> WebAIM (webaim.org) and W3C (w3.org) are important resources with more information about accessibility, usability, and inclusion for instructional designers.

are likely addressing more than one. WebAIM, a website on disability services, and the World Wide Web Consortium (W3C) offer resources to support educators, including web accessibility checklists, tutorials, training, technical assistance, and other freely available resources.

SUMMARY

- **Data dissemination.** Data can be disseminated through poster or slideshow presentations, scholarly journals, or other written publications and can be done on local, state, national, or international levels. Disseminating data improves patient outcomes and reduces healthcare disparities. A research or EBP mentor can help determine how and where to disseminate data.
- **Presenting data.** Data can be presented to an organization or at a nursing conference. For presentations, the ADDIE model of instructional design includes analyze, design, develop, implement, and evaluate and can be used to define the activities needed to guide development of educational activities. Learning objectives should be specific, measurable, actionable, reasonable, and time-bound (SMART) and should utilize Bloom's Taxonomy. Presentations are more engaging when they use active learning, or engaging the audience respond and interact. Slideshow design should have impact and be thoughtful without overwhelming the audience with too many images, special effects, fonts, and colors. Poster presentations are common in academic settings and should follow best practice and specific conference guidelines for size and design to maximize impact. An assessment of audience members following a presentation can gauge learner knowledge and provide feedback for future presentations.
- **Publishing data.** Academic writing is done for school assignments with an instructor as the audience. Scholarly writing is related to the generation, synthesis, translation, application, and dissemination of knowledge to a large audience to improve health and transform healthcare. Manuscript submitted to a journal for publication must follow the journal's author guidelines. Strategies for choosing a journal for publication

include noting what journals similar articles appear in, searching for suitable journals using the Nurse Author & Editor Directory of Nursing Journals, or researching journals with high impact factors. Avoid predatory journals.

- **Universal design.** UDL principles guide teaching and learning activities to ensure accessibility, usability, and inclusion. Accessibility should be a goal for every presentation. Design your presentation so that those with vision or hearing impairments can understand the material. You can check accessibility using presentation software. Add alt text for images and judiciously use color to ensure everyone can access the material. Use intentional heading styles, meaningfully hyperlinked text, and user-friendly navigation to enhance usability. Inclusivity involves representations of people from different backgrounds, appearances, ages, and cultures in instructional material.

DISCUSSION QUESTIONS AND ACTIVITIES

1. Choose a nursing organization that would be useful to your nursing career and list ways the organization could help with disseminating research or EBP data.
2. Review a slideshow or poster you have created for an assignment. Review:
   a. Whether the text is readable.
      - Background color shows text to best advantage.
      - Font used is easily readable.
   b. Whether the visuals are appropriate.
      - Images do not upstage the presentation.
      - Slides do not present a message different from the content.
      - Slides make the presentation easy or difficult to follow.
      - Images add to the message.
3. Reflect on a specific academic paper you have written for a course in the past. What would you need to do to develop that paper into an article for a journal? How might you go about finding a suitable journal and the author guidelines that will help you answer this question?
4. For a topic of interest to you, find a journal in which you might want to publish. What is the impact factor? Locate the author guidelines. Are there any guidelines that surprise you?
5. Describe ways that scholarly writing differs from academic writing. Compare scholarly and academic writing to creative writing. Why is it important to follow scholarly writing guidelines?
6. Find a nursing presentation online and evaluate it for UDL principles. What recommendations would you make to the authors to increase usability and accessibility?
7. Take another look at Figure 10-2 and try to write alt text for the figure. Think about the key components needed to understand this figure and try to briefly explain them in words to someone with low or no sight.

PRACTICE QUESTIONS

1. Which is a basic rule for designing a slide presentation that will be presented at a conference?
   a. Use a serif font for headings and text.
   b. Use large tables of data.
   c. Use no more than a few colors per presentation.
   d. Use special effects for every slide.
2. Which statement is true about publishing?
   a. A journal manuscript is an article that has been published.
   b. The impact factor is a subjective method for comparing competing journals.
   c. Library databases will automatically prevent you from viewing predatory journal articles.
   d. Author guidelines tell you the exact font style, size, spacing, and format for your article.
3. As the unit informatics nurse, you have helped create a learning module on septic shock. A learner with hearing loss reports that an embedded YouTube video in a training module has captions that do not seem to reflect what is being said in the video. What is your best course of action?

a. Consult your organization's disability services office to find out if they can assist with correcting the captions or producing an accurate transcript.
b. Explain that the video is not an important component of the instructional unit, they will not be tested on the video content, and they can skip viewing it for now.
c. Explain to the learner that the captions were autogenerated in YouTube, and so the organization's obligation is met because the video is captioned.
d. Create an in-house video to replace the YouTube video.

REFERENCES

American Optometric Association. (n.d.). *Color vision deficiency*. Eye and Vision Conditions. Retrieved August 4, 2022, from https://www.aoa.org/healthy-eyes/eye-and-vision-conditions/color-vision-deficiency?sso=y

American Association of Colleges of Nursing. (2021). *The essentials: Core competencies for professional nursing education* [PDF]. AACN. https://www.aacnnursing.org/Portals/42/AcademicNursing/pdf/Essentials-2021.pdf

American Association of Critical-Care Nurses (AACN). (n.d.) *Events calendar*. https://www.aacn.org/conferences-and-events/events-calendar

American Nurses Association (ANA). (2023). *American Nurse Journal author guidelines*. https://www.myamericannurse.com/wp-content/uploads/2023/06/Author-Guidelines-2023.pdf

Anderson, L. W., Krathwohl, D. R., & Bloom, B. S. (2001). *A taxonomy for learning, teaching, and assessing: A revision of Bloom's taxonomy of educational objectives* (complete edition). Longman.

Babik, J. M., & Luther, V. P. (2020). Creating and presenting an effective lecture. *Journal of Continuing Education in the Health Professions, 40*(1), 36–41. https://doi.org/10.1097/CEH.0000000000000281

Beall, J. (2012, December 1). *Criteria for determining predatory open-access publishers*. Retrieved from https://scholarlyoa.files.wordpress.com/2012/11/criteria-2012-2.pdf

Beall, J. (2021). *Beall's list of potential predatory journals and publishers* [webpage]. Beall's List. https://beallslist.net/

Berg, J., & Hicks, R. (2017). Successful design and delivery of a professional poster. *Journal of American Association of Nurse Practitioners, 29*(8), 461–469. https://doi.org/10.1002/2327-6924.12478

Bloom, B. S. (1956). *Taxonomy of educational objectives, handbook 1: Cognitive domain*. Addison-Wesley.

Centers for Disease Control and Prevention. (2020). *Disability and health promotion* [webpage]. https://www.cdc.gov/ncbddd/disabilityandhealth/infographic-disability-impacts-all.html

Chappell, M. (2018, September 26). *Instructional design using the ADDIE Model*. eLearning Industry. https://elearningindustry.com/addie-model-instructional-design-using

Creative Commons. (n.d.). *About the licenses*. Retrieved August 4, 2022, from https://creativecommons.org/licenses/

Davis, D., McLaughlin, M. K., & Anderson, K. M. (2022). Universal design for learning: A framework for blended learning in nursing education. *Nurse Educator, 47*(3), 133–138. https://doi.org/10.1097/NNE.0000000000001116

Faridi, E., Ghaderian, A., Honarasa, F., & Shafie, A. (2021). Next generation of chemistry and biochemistry conference posters: Animation, augmented reality, visitor statistics, and visitors' attention. *Biochemistry and Molecular Biology Education, 49*(4), 619–624. https://doi.org/10.1002/bmb.21520

Fowler, S. B., & Reising, E. S. (2021). A replication study of fall TIPS (tailoring interventions for patient Safety): A patient-centered fall prevention toolkit. *MedSurg Nursing, 30*(1), 28–34.

Georgetown Law. (n.d.). *Digital accessibility*. Retrieved August 4, 2022, from https://www.law.georgetown.edu/your-life-career/campus-services/information-systems-technology/digital-accessibility/

Hess, G. R., Tosney, K. W., & Liegel, L. H. (2009). Creating effective poster presentations: AMEE guide no. 40. *Med Teach, 31*(4), 319–321. https://doi.org/10.1080/01421590902825131

ImmunoFrontiers. (2022, July 17). *Top 20 nursing journals of 2022*. Research Hub. https://research.immunofrontiers.com/top-20-nursing-journals-of-2022/

Jefferies, D., McNally, S., Roberts, K., Wallace, A., Stunden, A., D'Souza, S., & Glew, P. (2018). The importance of academic literacy for undergraduate nursing students and its relationship to future professional clinical practice: A systematic review. *Nurse Education Today, 60*, 84–91. https://doi.org/10.1016/j.nedt.2017.09.020

Melnyk, B. M., & Fineout-Overholt, E. (2023). *Evidence-based practice in nursing & healthcare: A guide to best practice* (5th ed.). Wolters Kluwer Health//Lippincott Williams & Wilkins.

Microsoft. (2022a). *Create accessible PowerPoint presentations*. Microsoft Office Support. https://support.microsoft.com/en-us/office/video-create-slides-with-an-accessible-reading-order-794fc5da-f686-464d-8c29-1c6ab8515465

Microsoft. (2022b). *Make your PowerPoint presentations accessible to people with disabilities*. Office Accessibility. https://support.microsoft.com/en-us/office/make-your-powerpoint-presentations-accessible-to-people-with-disabilities-6f7772b2-2f33-4bd2-8ca7-dae3b2b3ef25

Morris, Z. S., Wooding, S., & Grant, J. (2011). The answer is 17 years, what is the question: Understanding time lags in translational research. *Journal of the Royal Society of Medicine, 104*(12), 510–520. https://doi.org/10.1258/jrsm.2011.110180

Morton, P. G. (2020). Why was my manuscript rejected? *Journal of Professional Nursing, 36*(2), 1–4. https://doi.org/10.1016/j.profnurs.2020.02.006

Munro, C. L., & Savel, R. H. (2016). Narrowing the 17-year research to practice gap. *American Journal of Critical Care, 25*(3), 194–196. https://doi.org/10.4037/ajcc2016449

National Eye Institute. (n.d.). *Color blindness*. Eye Conditions and Diseases. Retrieved August 4, 2022, from https://www.nei.nih.gov/learn-about-eye-health/eye-conditions-and-diseases/color-blindness

New York University (NYU) Libraries. (2023). *How to create a research poster*. https://guides.nyu.edu/posters

North Carolina Nurses Association (NCNA). (2023). *2023 annual convention*. https://ncnurses.org/events/annual-convention/registration/

Nurse Author & Editor. (2022). *Nursing journals directory [webpage]*. Wiley Online Library. https://onlinelibrary.wiley.com/page/journal/17504910/homepage/journals-directory

Nursing World Conference 2024 (NWC 2024). (2023). *Guidelines*. https://nursingworldconference.com/information/guidelines

Rosenshine, B. (2012). Principles of instruction: Research-based strategies that all teachers should know. *American Educator, 36*(1), 12.

Rubin, R.. (2023). It takes an average of 17 Years for evidence to change practice—the burgeoning field of implementation science seeks to speed things up. *JAMA: The Journal of the American Medical Association, 329*(16), 1333–1336. https://doi.org/10.1001/jama.2023.4387

Siedlecki, S. L. (2017). Original research: How to create a poster that attracts an audience. *Am J Nurs, 117*(3), 48–54. https://doi.org/10.1097/01.NAJ.0000513287.29624.7e

Stucky, C. H. (2020). Advancing nursing leadership through writing: Strategies for publishing success. *Journal of Continuing Education in Nursing, 51*(10), 447–449. https://doi.org/10.3928/00220124-20200914-04

SUNY Brockport. (n.d.). *How to design & print a poster with PowerPoint*. Retrieved February 8, 2023 from https://www2.brockport.edu/academics/scholars-day/power-point/

The Derek Bok Center for Teaching and Learning (Harvard University). (2022). *Inclusive course design [webpage]*. https://bokcenter.harvard.edu/inclusive-course-design

Turner, B., DeMuro, J. P., & Fearn, N. (2022, November 2). *Best presentation software of 2023*. TechRadar. https://www.techradar.com/best/best-presentation-software

U.S. Access Board. (2017). *Information and communication technology: Revised 508 standards and 255 guidelines [web document]*. https://www.access-board.gov/ict/

World Wide Web Consortium (W3C). (2023, August 8). *Accessibility fundamentals overview*. https://www.w3.org/WAI/fundamentals/

UNIT IV

The Role of The Informatics Nurse

Chapter 11	Roles and Responsibilities of the Informatics Nurse
Chapter 12	Interoperability at the National and the International Levels
Chapter 13	Electronic Health Records and Standardized Nursing Terminology

Unit IV covers information for the nurse who is interested in specializing in informatics. It covers the wide variety of roles and responsibilities of informatics nurses, including their involvement in interoperability and electronic health records (EHRs). In 2004, President George W. Bush set a goal for every American to have an EHR by 2014. And though most U.S. hospitals and primary care providers now have EHRs, barriers remain around their use by practitioners and the public (Diaz, 2023). Informatics nurses can facilitate the use of EHRs in all aspects of healthcare. To ensure patients get the best possible care, nurses must advocate for interoperability and the use of standardized terminology.

This unit provides instruction on how to design and manage quality improvement projects, how to educate nurses using informatics skills, and the importance of applying nursing informatics to patient safety. "The field of nursing informatics has helped drive healthcare's application of technologies such as [electronic medical records] and computerized provider order entry. Nursing informatics professionals work with a diverse group of stakeholders across the care continuum, ultimately helping to bridge the gap between clinical and technical perspectives. Their number one priority is maintaining focus on patient safety" (HIMSS, 2019). The National Academy of Sciences, Engineering, and Medicine emphasizes the importance of aligning the approaches and intentions of healthcare organizations with patient safety and equity (2021).

Chapter 11 (The Roles and Responsibilities of the Informatics Nurse) gives nurses a deeper understanding of the job duties of the informatics nurse, pulling data from the HIMSS Nursing Informatics Workforce Survey that was done in 2022. Career titles and job responsibilities are discussed, including quality improvement projects and the importance of leadership skills. The case study provides an example of a quality improvement study that sought to detect sepsis in a better way by adapting the EHR. The importance of leadership and interprofessional communication are new topics. The ethics of combating misinformation in the pandemic infodemic is also discussed.

Chapter 12 (Interoperability at the National and the International Levels) begins with a case study on the impact of the lack of interoperability of COVID-19 test results and strategies for future success. This chapter covers how the informatics nurse can support interoperability at the National and International level, how U.S. and informatics organizations are supporting the interoperability of healthcare information technology and explores ethical considerations for protecting human rights, permitting health diplomacy, and promoting health equity.

Chapter 13 (Electronic Health Records and Standardized Terminology) discusses the history, trends, and types of EHRs including the importance of using standardized terminology. The role of the informatics nurse in the design, selection and implementation of EHRs is discussed, as well as certified EHR standards, adoption strategies, and design considerations. The case study highlights how the tennis star Serena Williams experienced a pulmonary embolism after giving birth and includes evidence for the potential for EHRs to reduce racial disparities in maternal morbidity and mortality. The chapter covers the ethical mandate for nurses to evoke the shared meaning of nursing by communicating nursing values to the public.

REFERENCES

Diaz, N. (2023, March 7). *96% of US hospitals have EHRs, but barriers remain to interoperability, ONC says*. https://www.beckershospitalreview.com/ehrs/96-of-us-hospitals-have-ehrs-but-barriers-remain-to-interoperability-onc-says.html

Healthcare Information and Management Systems Society (HIMSS). (2019, May 14). *What is Nursing Informatics?* https://www.himss.org/resources/what-nursing-informatics

National Academies of Sciences, Engineering, and Medicine. (2021). *The Future of Nursing 2020-2030*. Charting a Path to Achieve Health Equity.

CHAPTER 11

Roles and Responsibilities of the Informatics Nurse

Kristi Miller, Neal Reeves, Marilyn Faye Hughes, and Heather Shirk

OBJECTIVES

After studying this chapter, you will be able to:

1. Compare nursing informatics job roles.
2. Explain the role of the informatics nurse in systems implementation and how the Iowa Implementation Framework can be used to support the adoption of new technology.
3. Explain the role of the IN in system optimization and utilization and give examples.
4. Explain the role of the IN in systems development and give examples.
5. Discuss quality improvement aims, priorities, and strategies to achieve quality care.
6. Describe the steps of project management and how the IN can use these to manage new healthcare information technology projects.
7. Discuss the importance of the role of the IN in leadership and ways the IN can achieve leadership competencies.

KEY TERMS

Benchmarking
Best-of-breed approach
Big bang conversion
Business continuity plan
Change control
Clinical decision support system (CDSS)
Computerized provider order entry (CPOE)
Cost-benefit analysis
Enterprise system integration
Intangible assets
Integrated interface approach
Interoperability
Iowa Implementation Framework (IIF)
Model for Improvement
National Database of Nursing Quality Indicators (NDNQI)
Needs assessment

(Continued)

Parallel conversion
Phased conversion
Picture archiving and communication system (PACS)
Pilot conversion
Plan-do-study-act (PDSA) cycle
Process improvement
Project management
Project scope
Quality improvement (QI)
Quality measures
Regression testing
Request for information (RFI)
Request for proposal (RFP)
Return on investment (ROI)
Scope creep
Skills assessment
Strategic planning
Systems life cycle
Tangible assets
The Joint Commission (TJC)
User interface (UI)
Workflow

CASE STUDY

Kangas et al. (2021) used the quality improvement (QI) process to modify screening tools in an electronic health record (EHR) for the recognition and early detection of sepsis and septic shock. Sepsis occurs when harmful microorganisms in the blood release chemicals that can cause organ system failure and death. Rapid recognition of sepsis symptoms can result in improved patient outcomes and survival rates.

The authors created a screening tool for sepsis based on three tools published in the literature: the systemic inflammatory response syndrome (SIRS) criteria, the modified early warning score (MEWS), and the national early warning score (NEWS) criteria. They tested their work in an inactive version of the EHR where they were able to modify and optimize warnings. With software enhancements, they were able to track the documented reasons that nurses did not implement the hospital sepsis protocol. They also identified an opportunity for improvement to lock out the warning for 48 hours after a patient left the operating room and decrease nurse alarm fatigue. Their modified tool decreased the number of alerts the nurses received and improved the accuracy of EHR sepsis alerts.

Kangas et al. (2021) used the plan-do-study-act cycle for this QI project. They used data to modify alerts, making the sepsis alert more specific. They balanced the sensitivity of the screening tool with its specificity by testing their changes in an inactive version of the EHR using real patient data. As you read this chapter, think about the processes you encounter or perform routinely. How could they be done more efficiently or more effectively? These are some of the questions that an informatics nurse will ask when supporting a QI project—just one of many roles of the IN.

AACN Essentials for Entry-Level Professional Nursing Education

3.5c Define stakeholders, including members of the community and/or clinical populations, and their level of influence.

5.1e Compare quality improvement methods in the delivery of patient care.

5.1f Identify strategies to improve outcomes of patient care in practice.

5.1g Participate in the implementation of a practice change.

5.1h Develop a plan for monitoring quality improvement change.

6.2a Apply principles of team dynamics, including team roles, to facilitate effective team functioning.

6.2c Engage in the work of the team as appropriate to one's scope of practice and competency.

7.1d Recognize internal and external system processes that impact care coordination and transition of care.

7.2c Describe the impact of healthcare cost and payment models on the delivery, access, and quality of care.

7.2d Explain the relationship of policy, regulatory requirements, and economics on care outcomes.

7.2e Incorporate considerations of efficiency, value, and cost in providing care.

7.3a Demonstrate a systematic approach for decision making.

7.3b Use reported performance metrics to compare/monitor outcomes.

8.1f Explain the importance of nursing engagement in the planning and selection of healthcare technologies.

8.3b Evaluate how decision support tools impact clinical judgment and safe patient care.

8.3d Examine how emerging technologies influence healthcare delivery and clinical decision making.

8.3f Identify the importance of reporting system processes and functional issues (error messages, mis-directions, device malfunctions, etc.) according to organizational policies and procedures.

8.4a Explain the role of communication technology in enhancing clinical information flows.

8.4d Explain the impact of health information exchange, interoperability, and integration on health care.

9.1a: Apply principles of professional nursing ethics and human rights in patient care and professional situations.

9.5a Describe nursing's professional identity and contributions to the healthcare team.

10.2c Commit to personal and professional development.

10.3c Demonstrate leadership behaviors in professional situations.

AACN Essentials for Advanced-Level Nursing Education

2.9j Participate in system-level change to improve care coordination across settings.

3.6h Collaborate with interdisciplinary teams to lead preparedness and mitigation efforts to protect population health with attention to the most vulnerable populations.

3.6j Contribute to system-level planning, decision making, and evaluation for disasters and public health emergencies.

4.1j Discern appropriate applications of quality improvement, research, and evaluation methodologies.

4.2h Address opportunities for innovation and changes in practice.

5.1k Integrate outcome metrics to inform change and policy recommendations.

5.1l Collaborate in analyzing organizational process improvement initiatives.

5.1m Lead the development of a business plan for quality improvement initiatives.

6.1g Evaluate effectiveness of interprofessional communication tools and techniques to support and improve the efficacy of team-based interactions.

6.1h Facilitate improvements in interprofessional communications of individual information (e.g., EHR).

6.1k Provide expert consultation for other members of the healthcare team in one's area of practice.

6.2g Integrate evidence-based strategies and processes to improve team effectiveness and outcomes.

7.1e Participate in organizational strategic planning.

7.1f Participate in system-wide initiatives that improve care delivery and/or outcomes.

7.1g Analyze system-wide processes to optimize outcomes.

7.2g Analyze relevant internal and external factors that drive healthcare costs and reimbursement.

7.2h Design practices that enhance value, access, quality, and cost-effectiveness.

7.2i Advocate for healthcare economic policies and regulations to enhance value, quality, and cost-effectiveness.

7.2j Formulate, document, and disseminate the return on investment for improvement initiatives collaboratively with an interdisciplinary team.

7.2k Recommend system-wide strategies that improve cost-effectiveness considering structure, leadership, and workforce needs.

8.1i Propose a plan to influence the selection and implementation of new information and communication technologies.

8.1j Explore the fiscal effect of information and communication technologies on health care.

8.3h Formulate a plan to influence decision-making processes for selecting, implementing, and evaluating support tools.

9.1i Model ethical behaviors in practice and leadership roles.

9.4e Assess the interaction between regulatory agency requirements and quality, fiscal, and value-based indicators.

9.4f Evaluate the effect of legal and regulatory policies on nursing practice and healthcare outcomes.

9.5f Articulate nursing's unique professional identity to other interprofessional team members and the public.

10.3j Provide leadership to advance the nursing profession.

HIMSS TIGER Competencies

Care processes and IT integration.

Change/stakeholder management.

Ethics in health IT.

Financial management.

Information and knowledge management in patient care.

Leadership.

Process management.

Project management.

Quality and safety management.

Resource planning and management.

Strategic management.

System lifecycle management.

Teaching, training, education.

According to the U.S. Bureau of Labor Statistics (2022), healthcare information technology (HIT) positions are expected to grow by 15% from 2021 to 2031, much faster than the average for all occupations. The American Medical Informatics Association (AMIA) estimated an increased need for 70,000 nursing informatics positions due to the ongoing technologic advancements and requirements in healthcare (Gaines, 2022). Since the implementation of the Patient Protection and Accountable Care Act (PPACA) in 2008 and the Health Information Technology for Economic and Clinical Health (HITECH) Act in 2009, there has been an increased need for nurses to be adept in the current technology. This need creates more opportunities for nurses interested in informatics.

In Chapter 1, you learned that an informatics nurse (IN) is a registered nurse (RN) who works at the intersection of technology and nursing. This nursing specialty combines the knowledge of nursing, communications, computer science, and information science. This role is usually taken on early in the career and does not involve educational specialization (Stobierski, 2021). Often, an RN interested in informatics takes on the role of a "super user" on their unit and is involved in supporting staff with integrating new HIT. Most INs work for a hospital or large health system, but INs also work in academic settings, ambulatory care centers, consulting firms, information technology (IT) companies, the government and military, and research facilities (Gaines, 2022).

The Healthcare Information Management and Systems Society (HIMSS) conducts a Nursing Informatics Workforce Survey every several years, most recently in 2022. The survey data provide insight into the functions, responsibilities, and compensation in nursing informatics (HIMSS, 2023). The results of this survey have

Chapter 11　Roles and Responsibilities of the Informatics Nurse　**223**

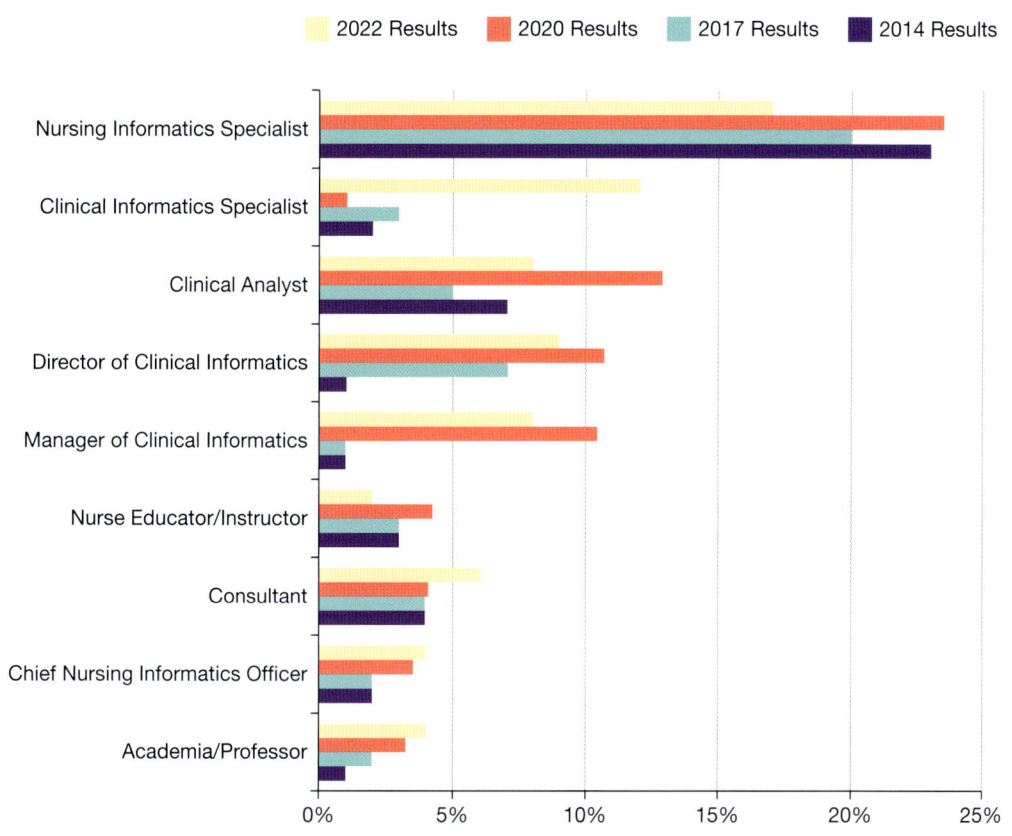

Figure 11-1. Top nursing informatics job titles from the HIMSS Nursing Informatics Workforce Survey. (Data from Healthcare Information and Management Systems Society (HIMSS). (2023). *2022 nursing informatics workforce survey.* https://www.himss.org/sites/hde/files/media/file/2023/04/05/2022-nursing-informatics-workforce-survey.pdf)

helped guide this chapter, which presents many of the most common job titles (Fig. 11-1) and job responsibilities (Fig. 11-2) of INs. The leadership and collaboration roles of the IN are also discussed.

IN JOB TITLES

There are many opportunities for the IN as they develop and progress in their role. While nursing informatics specialist remains the most common job title, clinical informatics specialist, clinical analyst, director or manager of clinical informatics, and chief nursing informatics officer are titles increasingly being used (HIMSS, 2023). INs may also find careers as nurse educators, professors, and consultants. Refer to Figure 11-1 for the most common IN job titles.

IN Specialist and Clinical Informatics Specialist

Recall from Chapter 2 that an IN specialist (also known as a nursing informatics specialist) is an RN with a graduate-level degree or certification in informatics. This job title is often defined by the organization for which the IN works. Box 11-1 shows a list of daily tasks that might be undertaken by an informatics nurse specialist.

A clinical informatics specialist is a type of IN specialist as they require a graduate degree in informatics. Clinical nurse specialists work with healthcare data entry, storage, and analysis. They often train staff on how to use data entry systems, build interfaces, and troubleshoot software applications. Clinical informatics specialists often have backgrounds in both healthcare and clinical informatics. Job duties vary widely and can include project management, consulting, or support (WGU, 2023).

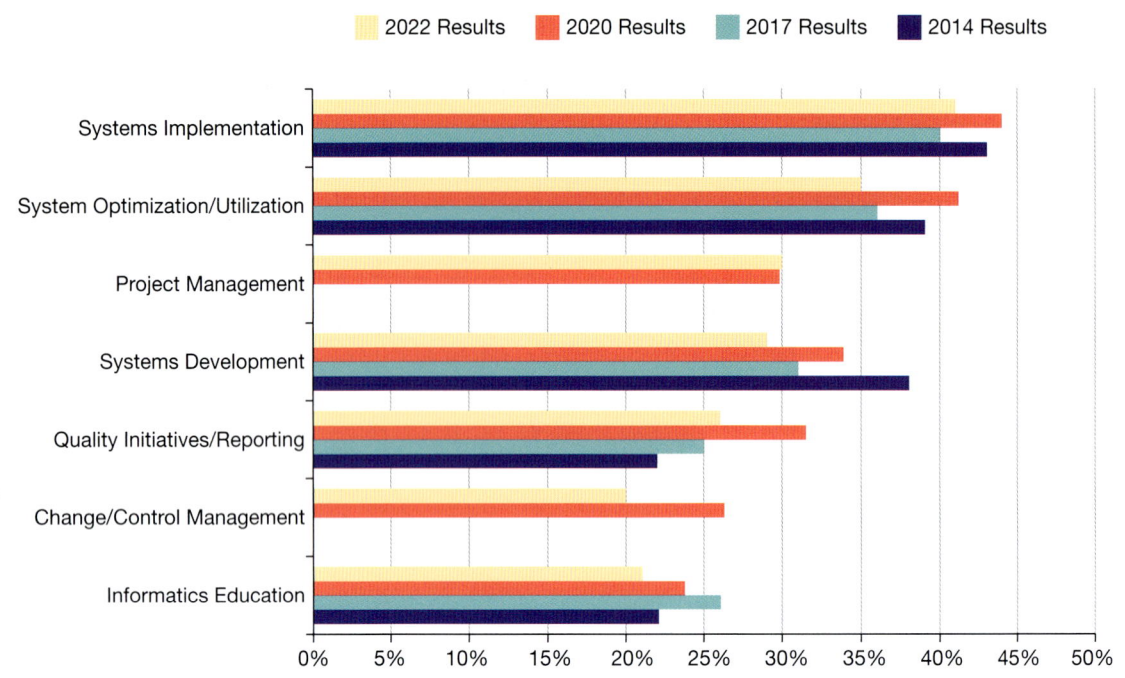

Figure 11-2. Top nursing informatics job responsibilities from the HIMSS Nursing Informatics Workforce Survey. (Data from Healthcare Information and Management Systems Society (HIMSS). (2023). *2022 nursing informatics workforce survey*. https://www.himss.org/sites/hde/files/media/file/2023/04/05/2022-nursing-informatics-workforce-survey.pdf)

Clinical Analyst

The need for clinical analysts has risen due to the large amount of data that has become available with the widespread adoption of EHRs. A clinical analyst collects and analyzes data to improve patient outcomes by adjusting practices, processes, and workflows. For example, if a hospital sees a rise in hospital-acquired infections, a clinical analyst can identify methods for reducing them.

Director or Manager of Clinical Informatics

Directors and managers oversee the design of HIT systems to facilitate health information collection, management, and analysis. Data analysis may include patient medical records, such as symptoms, diagnosis, and records of procedures and outcomes. These roles are often the "next step" for an IN as they gain experience.

Nurse Educator or Instructor

Nurse educators have advanced nursing degrees and are responsible for teaching and instructing nurses at colleges, universities, and in clinical settings such as hospitals or primary care offices. An IN who is a nurse educator often works in a hospital setting to support staff with developing and maintaining HIT competencies, such as how to use a new feature of an EHR or the correct use of a glucometer at the bedside.

Chief Nursing Informatics Officer

The chief nursing informatics officer is an executive position. This IN is responsible for overseeing initiatives related to health informatics and patient records. They can be involved in launching new software, new process development, and drafting and implementing strategic plans related to long-term IT infrastructure.

BOX 11-1 Sample of Daily Tasks of an Informatics Nurse Specialist

- Meet with educator and training team on upcoming implementation of a new smart bed.
- Review requests for assistance in meeting new regulatory guidelines.
- Review reports after the TJC regulatory survey to fix areas of opportunity.
- Develop plans for ways to improve the EHR system to meet new requirements.
- Review high-alert medications in interdisciplinary patient safety meeting. Determine who needs the alerts and who can bypass them. Who will educate the staff about the change?
- Make rounds on clinical units to answer questions and find opportunities for improvement. Ask staff, "What is working and what can be improved?"
- Meet with the chief of medicine about building a monthly report on patient volumes, postoperative length of stay, and infection rates. Set up meetings with other teams such as QI, case management, and admissions and registration to find out what might already exist and what needs to be built.
- Meet with chief nursing officer and nursing leadership to discuss input from nursing staff during clinical rounding and discover nurse-led initiatives with which informatics could assist.

EHR Implementation Manager

An EHR implementation manager designs, implements, and optimizes EHR software. Duties may include developing custom templates, making recommendations for software enhancements, and training others to use new EHR software. An EHR manager might attend IT governance meetings in which new project requests come for approval and resource allocation. They also address tickets or issues reported to the help desk, review enhancement requests, plan for system upgrades, and meet with interdisciplinary teams such as IT, billing and finance, medical records, and clinical teams. Chapter 13 covers EHRs in more detail.

SYSTEM RESPONSIBILITIES OF THE IN

Many of the responsibilities of INs revolve around HIT systems (see Fig. 11-2). Organizations adopt a **systems life cycle** methodology governing the process of developing, acquiring, implementing, and maintaining computerized information systems and related technology (Fig. 11-3). The systems life cycle is analogous to the nursing process because it begins with assessment, has multiple places for iteration, and ends with evaluation. Similar to the nursing process, it never really ends because changes are made in response to evaluation findings; thus, a new cycle begins. Some organizations have dedicated information technology employees, but in healthcare organizations, the IN provides a valuable bridge between IT and healthcare, making them an integral part of the systems life cycle.

System Implementation

According to 41% of the responses to the HIMSS Workforce Survey (2023), systems implementation is the most common job responsibility of INs (see Fig. 11-2). System implementation involves selecting and adopting new HIT and then training and supporting nursing staff on how to use it. The **Iowa Implementation Framework (IIF)**, which includes 81 implementation strategies within four implementation phases, can be used to guide technologic system changes (Cullen et al., 2022). Figure 11-4 shows the four phases of the IIF.

Selecting a System

Selecting HIT is a complex task with the potential to improve or disrupt complex care delivery processes. HIT implementation can come with a significant financial investment in the multiple millions of dollars (Drees, 2020). Project planners can mitigate the risks of making a mistake by using a structured process, performing effective risk and needs analyses, and carefully investigating products. HIT selection committee members must educate themselves to be able to make informed decisions.

Selection committee members should also interview current users through site visits or phone or electronic communication to elicit both

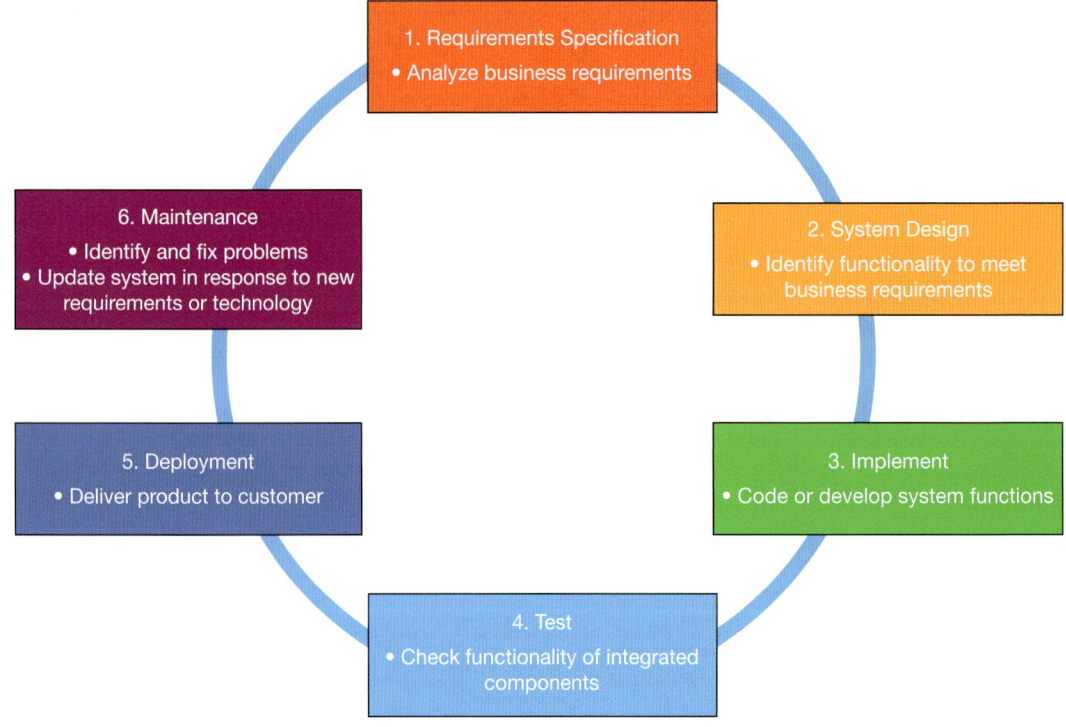

Figure 11-3. Systems life cycle.

```
1. Requirements Specification
• Analyze business requirements

2. System Design
• Identify functionality to meet business requirements

3. Implement
• Code or develop system functions

4. Test
• Check functionality of integrated components

5. Deployment
• Deliver product to customer

6. Maintenance
• Identify and fix problems
• Update system in response to new requirements or technology
```

good and bad feedback. No HIT system is perfect, and the success of HIT may have as much to do with the organization as the vendor. The selection team must be open-minded and listen carefully to what is said but also be attuned to what is not said.

Ideally, implementation of new HIT is planned with consideration for its impact on societal, medical, commercial, ethical, and socioeconomic concerns (van Gemert-Pijnen, 2022). The authors of a study on the effect of patient portals reported that after the implementation of patient portals, 86% of patients who accessed their information digitally felt more informed, 80% reported better ability to manage their health, and 43% reported accessing their information digitally had allowed them to avoid in-person visits to the healthcare agency. These findings equate to improved patient satisfaction, reduction in utilization of office visits, and improved self-care management (Bhyat et al., 2021).

Two approaches are used when selecting a system: best-of-breed or integrated interface. The **best-of-breed approach** refers to the selection of systems that best meet the needs of services or departments from different vendors to obtain the best offering for each application area. For example, organizations may purchase a human-resource package from one vendor and an accounting package from another. Using best-of-breed ensures the best of each system is purchased but requires building an integrated interface at the institutional level. The **integrated interface approach** refers to the selection of a collection of systems

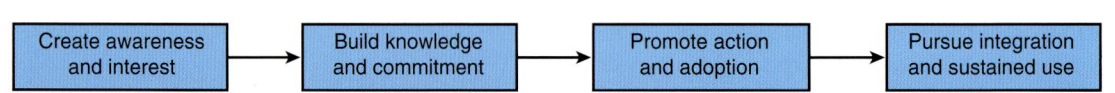

Create awareness and interest → Build knowledge and commitment → Promote action and adoption → Pursue integration and sustained use

Figure 11-4. Implementation strategies for evidence-based practice. (Data from Cullen, L., Hanrahan, K., Edmonds, S. W., Reisinger, H. S., & Wagner, M. (2022). Iowa implementation for sustainability framework. *Implementation Science, 17*(1), 1. https://doi.org/10.1186/s13012-021-01157-5.)

that are already interfaced; however, the systems may not all be the best choice for each application.

To support user adoption of the new HIT, it is important to engage stakeholders. Anyone with an interest or concern about the new HIT, such as people on the board of directors, support staff, administration, community members, and healthcare providers, should be able to give their opinions and input to garner a variety of perspectives. It is crucial to have the support of the leadership at the healthcare institution to ensure there is a plan with a vision, the creation of policies, accountability for unforeseen issues, and oversight for making any new HIT meet interoperability standards. It is important to try to predict the effect new HIT will have on a healthcare organization, including maintenance and the need for upgrades. Knowing how the implementation of the new HIT has affected other facilities and how they have dealt with issues can be helpful. Information about real-time use of technology, user feedback, and assessment of risks are important data to collect (van Gemert-Pijnen, 2022).

Recall that the American Nurses Association (ANA) Code of Ethics Provision 9 states that nurses have a duty to advocate for patient-centered technology (ANA, 2015). The rate of adoption of technology solutions continues to grow but is still far behind the rate of innovation, causing patients to be deprived of potential clinical benefits and leading to health inequities by limiting state-of-the-art care to patients with greater resources (Scarbrough & Kyratsis, 2022).

Approaches to Implementation

Four main approaches are used to convert from one HIT to another: parallel conversion, pilot conversion, phased conversion, and big bang conversion (Fig. 11-5). **Parallel conversion** requires the operation and support of new and old HIT simultaneously for a set time. It involves decreased risk but increased workload for users. The implementation plan typically addresses specific operational needs and defines the timing of the implementation. Project planners may target certain departments or care units with specific dates for a switch over to the new HIT. Training can be done with just those who will be using the new HIT.

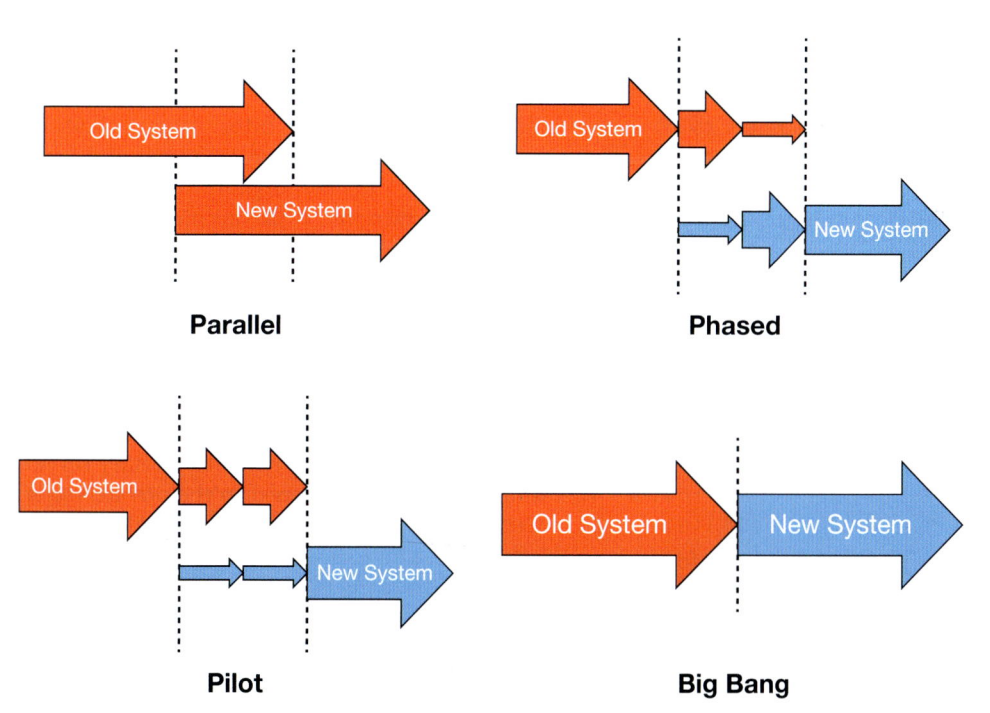

Figure 11-5. HIT conversion methods.

A **pilot conversion** is done to test the HIT to see what issues might occur when transitioning to new HIT. This approach enables testing on a smaller scale. For instance, in the case study, modifications to the sepsis tool were tested on an inactive portion of the sepsis warning system within the EHR, which gave the researchers the chance to measure the tool in real time as compared to the tool already in use (Kangas et al., 2021). A pilot test should be completed within a defined period. Pilot conversion could be useful when transitioning from a paper chart to an electronic charting system or when switching charting system vendors. Usually, a pilot helps determine operational or training needs for future system implementations and involves the least risk.

The **phased conversion** refers to HIT roll-out that takes place incrementally. A phased conversion offers a degree of control since it is done in stages and usually refers to HIT at the systems level such as a new EHR. The organization may implement a system of one module at a time, or the entire system can go live one unit at a time. The choice of the initial phased rollout area is usually made with the staff members who are most likely to champion the system. Personnel implementing the system learn from training sessions and go-lives and apply those learnings to future phases.

The **big bang conversion** refers to all users transitioning to or using new HIT at the same time. This method is most frequently used when there is no initial HIT, the HIT in use is failing or is highly integrated, or there is a requirement for implementation on a specific date, such as at the beginning of a new fiscal year. This conversion can involve the most amount of risk. However, risk and required support for this significant transition depend on the organization's size, the availability of support resources, and users' tolerance for considerable disruption.

Interoperability and System Integration

Interoperability is the ability of information systems, devices, and applications to access, exchange, integrate, and cooperatively use data in a coordinated manner, within and across organizational and geographic boundaries for optimal patient outcomes. Interoperability will be covered in more detail in Chapter 12, but it is introduced here because it is a significant issue with system implementation. Purchasing HIT from a single vendor does not ensure that the system is seamlessly interoperable since many vendors purchase smaller applications and design interfaces. These interfaces help but do not fully communicate, which creates a failure point in the system. The resulting lack of complete communication requires nurses to document the same data in more than one area or application. These duplications may seem minor, but the differences become apparent when attempting to see a complete picture of a patient from interfaces of disparate systems.

An example of a system that an IN may need to implement is a clinical information system (CIS). A CIS is a mix of integrated and interoperable information systems and technologies that provide information about patient care. Historically, the U.S. Department of Veterans Affairs (VA) used a CIS named VISTA in all their facilities. However, each facility was allowed to make changes to VISTA as needed, causing variations that made communication among facilities difficult. In 2018, the VA decided to use Cerner, a system that allows for **enterprise system integration**, the process of connecting existing systems to share and communicate information (U.S. Department of Veterans Affairs, 2018). Integrating applications enables data to flow among systems and facilities with ease. It allows organizations to track all patient interactions, while keeping it linked to basic patient details, such as demographics and insurance information, medical record numbers, care providers, and next of kin.

Once the VA implemented Cerner, they were able to communicate healthcare data with the U.S. Department of Defense, the U.S. Coast Guard, and community partners, giving a more complete picture of care during a patient's military service and after they transitioned to the private sector. Cerner implementation included the transition of nearly 24 million veteran records, making this the largest integrated health system in the country (U.S. Department of Veterans Affairs, 2020). Imagine the strategies needed to promote action and adoption; after trying the practice change, there was a need for education, skills competency, incentives for use, multidisciplinary discussion, and troubleshooting.

The third phase of implementation (promoting action and adoption) requires organizational system support from IT for the integration of multiple system components. Other components to consider in CIS implementation include:

- **Computerized provider order entry (CPOE)**, the process of providers entering and sending treatment instructions via a computer application rather than paper, fax, or telephone (HealthIT.gov, n.d.)
- Electronic medication administration record (eMAR)
- Positive patient identifier (PPID) systems, such as the use of barcode medication administration system (BCMA) discussed in Chapters 5 and 16
- Ancillary services and supplies not provided by the healthcare organization (e.g., long-term care facilities, home health, pharmacy, laboratory, and radiology systems)
- **Picture archiving and communication system (PACS)**, medical imaging technology that provides storage and easy access to images from multiple different machine types; the images are transmitted digitally via PACS, eliminating the need to manually file, retrieve, or transport radiologic images such as the film jackets used to store and protect x-ray films

The fourth phase of the framework involves pursuing integration and sustained use. This applies to upgrades or changes made to a CIS by vendors who, like other software companies, continuously work to improve the quality of their products. Major upgrades to CISs are usually associated with fees and may require equipment upgrades. Major software upgrades could also introduce new software defects, so it is important to test any changes or upgrades before introducing them into the patient environment.

System Optimization and Utilization

System optimization and utilization was the second most commonly cited job responsibility by INs (HIMSS, 2023) (see Fig. 11-2). System optimization and utilization is an example of the fourth phase of the IIF: to pursue integration and sustained use. To optimize a plan, system, or machine means to arrange or design it so that it operates as smoothly and efficiently as possible. Providing the best possible patient care requires making changes to systems when needed and ensuring access to data from all systems to monitor for known problem areas and anticipate others.

Electronic Health Record

An EHR is an electronic record of a patient's health history, maintained and accessed by providers and patients. Ongoing performance improvements to the EHR should be made through optimization. Siwicki (2020) maintains that optimization should be a thoughtful process in which functionality, workflow, and end users are considered. Some of the best ideas for optimization come from people who use an EHR daily. Listening to pain points and collaborating with stakeholders help drive changes to the system in a direction that benefits people who use it the most.

EHR Super Users

As the EHR system is optimized and software updates are installed, EHR super users provide ongoing support to end users by explaining and training new functionality and system changes. Super users are staff members who receive training on using the system and the workflows specific to where they work. During implementation, the primary duty of the super user is to provide immediate coaching and support to other users. Super users provide support during implementation, reducing end user anxiety and building end user confidence. For some roles and remote workers, super users can be accessible to end users through setting up team chats or giving a direct means to contact super users for assistance. Super user feedback during and after implementation is crucial to determine the successes and challenges of the implementation.

Super users can also help identify pain points or areas where the system may not be working as expected. Super users may also participate in several activities during the project and after its completion. Although most often nurses, super users might also be selected from within other healthcare professions to work with that profession (e.g., a physician super user provides support for other physicians). Super users might also assist in HIT system building and testing.

The super user role should not end with implementation; ongoing super user engagement and training are critical for upgrade and optimization support. Maintaining super user engagement can be challenging as priorities start to shift following implementation. Super users should be given many opportunities to engage. Offering super users virtual and in-person training for updates, providing training documents they can take back to their unit or office, granting early access to tip sheets and guides, and opening chat forums on platforms such as Teams or Yammer pages helps provide additional support and connection opportunities.

Electronic Medical Records Adoption Model

HIMSS developed the Electronic Medical Records Adoption Model (EMRAM), which scores the digital maturity of healthcare organizations and then provides a roadmap to guide adoption and optimization of electronic medical record technology. The model can serve as a guide for organizations that are transitioning from paper to electronic records or who are in the early stages of this process and need to utilize the available technology better. There are eight stages of digital maturity (Stages 0 to 7), and the goal of EMRAM is to level up organizations into the final stage (Table 11-1). By implementing and optimizing electronic medical records using EMRAM, healthcare organizations can improve care delivery and clinical outcomes (HIMSS, 2021).

EHR Task Force

The AMIA EHR-2020 Task Force made recommendations for improving HIT. These included improving interoperability and the exchange of data; speeding up, simplifying, and reducing the need for data entry; focusing on patient safety and patient outcomes; improving usability; promoting software application innovation; and improving integration and interfaces for health information systems (Payne et al., 2015). Following this successful initiative, the new AMIA 25 × 5 Task Force is working to reduce medical professional documentation burden by 25% in 5 years (2022 to 2026). Their goals come with the added priorities of not shifting work to others, not eroding care standards, leveraging existing technology and data inputs, and maximizing clarity (AMIA, 2023). A nurse choosing a career in informatics must be prepared to provide leadership in all these areas.

EHR Certification

As discussed in Chapter 13, use of certified EHR technology (CEHRT) is a quality measure to ensure interoperability and healthcare data communication. Certification programs were developed specifically to meet the requirements set forth by the HITECH Act. The original purpose of certification was to standardize EHR systems to allow extraction of data for meaningful use. Certification programs develop standard testing tools, test cases, procedures, and test data for interoperability required to meet meaningful use objectives. Use of CEHRT is still voluntary, but most vendors participate in some way to stay competitive and viable (HealthIT.gov, 2021). Theoretically, certification resolves issues associated with the EHR. However, the IN may need to support optimization and utilization with commercial vendor EMR products, which must communicate with the EHR.

> **CASE STUDY**
>
> In the case study, the authors identified a need to improve the sepsis screening tool embedded in the EHR. What changes would make the EHR where you work more effective? What process would you use to begin system optimization of the proposed changes? Identify whom you would contact, what support you would need, and what tools and strategies are available at your place of work for optimizing your EHR.

System Development

You can see in Figure 11-2 that systems development was identified as a job responsibility by 29% of INs in 2022 (HIMSS, 2023). Systems development is the process of defining, designing, and testing new HIT. There are only a few nurses who are also trained in writing code for software programs. Most INs are involved in

TABLE 11-1 Electronic Medical Record Adoption Model (EMRAM)

Stage	Cumulative Capabilities
7	Data from multiple external sources is integrated into the system, digital infrastructure enables dynamic patient engagement, and priorities are improving patient safety, increasing patient satisfaction, supporting clinicians, and securing data
6	HIE allows external data to be integrated into the CDR, digital tools are accessible to patients (patient satisfaction, personal clinical data, self-reported outcomes and progress), outcomes data are actively assessed, medical devices are integrated into system, and patient safety and quality of care priorities are identified
5	More than 75% of documentation is created via online tools available through CDR, electronic system continuously monitors at least one patient condition, HIE allows external documents to be integrated into the CDR, telehealth and virtual care are available, and clinical outcome and patient satisfaction targets inform changes and improvements
4	More than 50% of documentation created via online tools is available through CDR, more than 50% of medical orders are placed with the CPOE that is supported by CDS, clinicians have access to regional or national patient databases, patient information is accessible even during downtimes, and clinical outcome and patient satisfaction targets are identified and monitored
3	More than 25% of documentation created via online tools is available through the CDR with access based on staff role, eMAR is implemented, access to external data sources is available, infrastructure for bedside scanning is planned or installed, scheduled outages are communicated, and downtime/recovery plans are defined
2	Clinicians have access to the CDR to view results and reports, workflow and objectives are defined, policies and procedures are in place, and change management includes a review of proposed changes and a rollback plan
1	All major ancillary systems are installed and business resilience plans for each are in place
0	All key ancillary department systems have not been installed (e.g., laboratory, pharmacy, cardiology, radiology)

CDR: clinical data repository; CDS: clinical decision support; CPOE: computerized provider order entry, eMAR: electronic medication administration record, HIE: health information exchange.

Adapted from Healthcare Information and Management Systems Society (HIMSS). (2021). *Electronic Medical Record Adoption Model (EMRAM)*. https://www.himss.org/what-we-do-solutions/digital-health-transformation/maturity-models/electronic-medical-record-adoption-model-emram

identifying useful systems, testing them, and suggesting new developments. The IN works with computer programmers to develop optimal systems for their healthcare organization. This could include the internal development of customized systems, the creation of database systems, or the acquisition of third-party–developed software. Examples that benefit from IN involvement include user interface and communication system development.

User Interface

A **user interface (UI)** in healthcare systems is the space where interactions between humans and HIT occur to allow effective operation and control of HIT from the human end while HIT simultaneously feeds back information that aids the user's decision-making process. The UI needs to be designed mindful of issues that can arise when humans and technology interact. Examples of design issues in HIT include lack of uniform pain scales, terminology, pressure injury prevention programs, and falls prevention programs. These design issues can make documentation of care challenging for nurses who float to other units or who work for temporary assistance agencies. They can also affect the ability to analyze the data for evidence-based practice decisions.

Historically, nurses and other healthcare providers were not part of the teams that developed UIs. Even more recently when they are involved, healthcare providers may have no background knowledge of or skills with database design. Most computer programmers do not understand the context in which the UI will be used. Therefore, it is often the responsibility of the IN to bridge this gap in knowledge to help develop effective HIT.

Communication Systems

Hospitals and healthcare providers are increasingly using smartphones for communication, but personal smartphones cannot be used in healthcare settings due to privacy and confidentiality concerns and because they cannot be integrated into existing systems. INs can play a role in the development of communication devices while ensuring patient privacy and confidentiality are protected (Ahad et al., 2020). The IN should be involved in developing, acquiring, implementing, and maintaining these devices to ensure integration with current systems, that they best serve the nurses who use them, and that patients understand what they are. INs have the healthcare background to consider features of communication technology that would make it more appropriate for healthcare settings, such as the ability to disinfect the device, data encryption and antitheft prevention, and the ability to integrate with electronic medical records and EHRs.

Change/Control Management

Change/control management is a more recent addition to IN responsibilities, only appearing in the HIMSS workforce survey that began in 2020 (see Fig. 11-2). **Change control** is a systematic approach to managing all changes made to a product or system. The IN can assist with identifying, documenting, and authorizing changes to HIT with the goal of minimizing disruptions to patient care or errors. Change management is the practice and process of supporting people through change, with the goal of ensuring that the change is successful in the long-term. The role of the IN in change control is to determine who has the authority to authorize changes to the system, which members of the interdisciplinary team need to be involved in the changes, who will program the changes, and how to coordinate any changes with ancillary systems. An important role of the IN is to use change control processes to ensure minimal disruptions from issues that arise.

Unintended Consequences

One way changes that need to be made to systems are discovered is through unintended consequences. With the rapid adoption of EHRs and other systems, nurses and other healthcare professionals have faced many challenges and unintended consequences. An unintended consequence refers to an outcome, positive or negative, that was not planned or deliberate. INs may be tasked with managing unexpected consequences of systems implementation. Learning how others handled these problems can help manage unintended consequences and recognize compromises that must be made to ensure patient safety.

When CPOE was initially being implemented, the driving focus for decision making was patient safety by way of improved decision support and reduction in alert response and medical errors. However, because of this push, little attention was being paid to the potential negative consequences of CPOE implementation. A seminal research study by Ash et al. (2009) revealed nine types of unintended consequences with the implementation and use of CPOE (Box 11-2).

CPOE can be linked to a **clinical decision support system (CDSS)**, which enhances medical decision making using specific clinical knowledge and patient information with software designed to consider the characteristics of an individual patient (Chapter 9). Patient data are matched to an online clinical knowledge base and patient-specific assessments or recommendations are presented to the clinician (Sutton et al., 2020). Prescription CDSSs link electronic drug prescriptions from CPOEs with drug databases and provide alerts to the prescriber to reduce potential prescription errors. Despite the benefits of CDSSs, unintended negative consequences have been revealed.

Straichman et al. (2017) looked at misleading alerts that occurred for medication prescription errors in CDSSs. Of 390,841 prescriptions evaluated by the authors, 37% triggered an alert, while only 5% of alerts were accepted. The high rejection rate was largely justified by an expert panel, suggesting that many alerts were inaccurate or misleading. There were also problems with "alert fatigue," the phenomenon of too many alerts causing providers to pay less attention to them.

CDSSs could be a solution to many of these issues, but refinements should be made using these unintended consequences as data points to guide improvement. An IN must be vigilant with data following systems implementation, initiating changes to improve systems.

Business Continuity Plan

While preparing to implement a new system, a plan must be developed to address when the system is not available during planned or unplanned downtimes. Planned downtimes occur during software upgrades and system maintenance. Unplanned downtimes may include hardware failure, malicious software, natural disaster, or power failure (Roush et al., 2021). The importance of a **business continuity plan,** the term used by IT for disaster recovery plans, is crucial for patient safety and the continued delivery of patient care.

BOX 11-2 Unintended Consequences of CPOE Implementation

- *More and new work*: The providers were responsible for entering orders instead of the nurses or secretaries rendering tasks take longer as the users adjusted.
- *Workflow*: Mismatches between the CPOE and normal workflow
- *System demands*: Unintended system design, support, and maintenance that involved personnel, software, and hardware requirements
- *Paper persistence*: Amount of paper was not necessarily reduced
- *Communication*: Once information was put into the computer, face-to-face communication would be skipped when physical communication was necessary.
- *Emotions*: Personnel who were comfortable with automated systems acclimated to CPOE, but those who were uncomfortable experienced strong negative emotions.
- *Power shifts*: The provider or pharmacist was perceived as losing power, while information technology specialists and nurses were perceived as gaining power.
- *Dependence on technology*: Productivity loss was associated with computer failures.
- *New kinds of errors*: Computers had the potential to result in new errors, such as inadvertent selection of the wrong patient, medication dosing errors, and orders that overlapped.

Data from Ash, J. S., Sittig, D. F., & Dykstra, R. (2009). The unintended consequences of computerized provider order entry: findings from a mixed methods exploration. *International Journal of Medical Informatics, 78*(Suppl 1), S69–S76. doi:10.1016/j.ijmedinf.2008.07.015.

Healthcare providers need to be prepared to continue patient care, whether the downtime lasts a few minutes or several weeks. Training and awareness of the business continuity plan is crucial for patient safety. Preparation for downtime should include developing a downtime policy, downtime checklists to ensure downtime items are readily available, downtime forms, review of downtime reports, and downtime process maps. All EHR users must be familiar and comfortable with downtime procedures (Roush et al., 2021).

Business continuity planning should be an ongoing process of evaluating how electronic processes should be completed during downtimes. All departments that use the EHR and other systems should know how to apply the plan and what documents and equipment they need to complete their tasks during a downtime. When developing a business continuity plan, consider what operations are performed electronically and how documentation will be completed during downtime; also consider how staff and departments communicate and what information is communicated to other users and departments (Roush et al., 2021).

Even with the best plan, flexibility is needed as end users are suddenly pulled from their typical workflow. Business continuity planning must be an organizational priority so that the staff have the resources to continue operations through unexpected events. See Box 11-3 for questions that can be used to prompt business continuity planning.

OTHER RESPONSIBILITIES OF THE IN

The job duties of the IN are dependent on the needs of the healthcare organization. Larger healthcare organizations may have INs who focus solely on EHR development, implementation, utilization, and optimization. In other organizations, the IN may be involved in leading QI initiatives such as the one you read about in the case study. No matter what the job duties entail, the IN needs project management and leadership skills to ensure the healthcare information technology needs of the organization are met.

> **BOX 11-3** Questions to Prompt Business Continuity Planning
> - How are patients admitted during a downtime? How is the medical record number obtained? How are downtime labels obtained?
> - How are patients discharged during downtime? How are discharge documents prepared? Do patients have prescriptions they will need? How will housekeeping know to clean the room?
> - How will the pharmacy know orders are written? How will nurses know orders are written? Do nurses know how to transcribe orders to a paper medication administration record?
> - How will lab results be received and reviewed by clinical staff?
> - Do staff have enough downtime forms? Do they know where to get downtime forms?
> - For extended downtime, how will documentation be filed? Are there enough charts available?
> - For extended downtime, how will information in the paper record be reconciled when the system is back online?

Quality Improvement

Quality improvement (QI), also known as quality initiative planning, is a job task of 26% of informatics nurses surveyed by the HIMSS (2023). QI is a set of focused activities designed to monitor, analyze, and improve the quality of processes to improve the healthcare outcomes in an organization. QI is the systematic improvement of patient care using a framework of standardized processes and technology to reduce variations in care, achieve predictable results, and improve outcomes (CMS, 2023). By gathering and analyzing data in key areas, a hospital can effectively implement change. Analyzing patient data and using data-driven approaches to reduce postoperative infections, shorten the average length of hospital stays, reduce medication errors, or improve EMR documentation are examples of QI initiatives.

> **CASE STUDY**
>
> In the case study, the researchers did a QI project to determine whether the modification of a sepsis and septic shock screening tool improved the early detection of sepsis and patient deterioration (Kangas et al, 2021). What QI projects are happening in your place of work? Interview nurse leaders, read posters, attend conferences, or research club meetings at your place of work to identify what QI is happening and how you can get involved. QI projects involve collecting and analyzing data to create information for dissemination to improve patient outcomes. What QI project is most needed on your unit or at your place of work?

Models for Quality Improvement

When beginning a QI project, it is important to use a model for guidance and to provide feedback on your progress. The **plan-do-study-act (PDSA) cycle** is based on the scientific method and is widely used for small-scale QI projects. The Kangas et al. (2021) research from the case study used the PDSA cycle, as noted in the PDSA cycle steps:

1. *Step 1: Plan the test or observation.* Make predictions, plan for collecting data, and determine the objectives of the test. In the case study, the authors predicted that modification of a sepsis and septic shock screening tool using Institute for Healthcare Improvement (IHI) guidelines would improve the recognition of sepsis and early detection of patient deterioration.
2. *Step 2: Do the test.* Try out the test on a small scale and document problems and unexpected observations. In the case study, the authors gathered vital signs and laboratory values from patients older than 18 years admitted to medical-surgical and telemetry/progressive care units during a 2-week period.
3. *Step 3: Study the results.* Analyze the data and compare it to your predictions. In the case study, after the first round of data collection, they found the sensitivity of the tool was not high enough (there were too many false positives).
4. *Step 4: Act on the results.* Refine implementations or interventions based on what was learned from the test to determine what modifications should be made, then prepare a plan for any future tests. In the case study, after the sensitivity was found to be low, modifications were made including raising the thresholds for respiratory rate, heart rate, and temperature. With this, the authors found that though the tool was still not sensitive enough to identify sepsis, it did identify sick patients who needed further interventions. They will need to continue to look for the right combination of criteria that will have a positive predictive value for diagnosing sepsis but will not give false positives too often.

The **Model for Improvement** is based on the PDSA and was developed by the Associates for Process Improvement in conjunction with the IHI to accelerate improvement (Langley et al., 2009). The Model for Improvement adds the following three questions (Fig. 11-6):

1. What are you trying to accomplish?
2. How will you know that a change is an improvement?
3. What change can you make that will result in an improvement?

After answering the three questions, follow up with the PDSA cycle.

Benchmarking

Benchmarking is used in QI as a means of comparing the performance of an organization or provider with another to identify areas for improvement (ASQ, n.d.a). **Quality measures** are tools that help an organization measure or quantify healthcare processes, outcomes, patient perceptions, and organizational structure and/or systems that are associated with the ability to provide high-quality healthcare that relates to one or more quality goals. The data for these measures are collected from claims, chart abstractions, registries, and assessment instruments. An important role of INs is to ensure their organization meets benchmarking standards. Comparing data by benchmarking is an opportunity to investigate

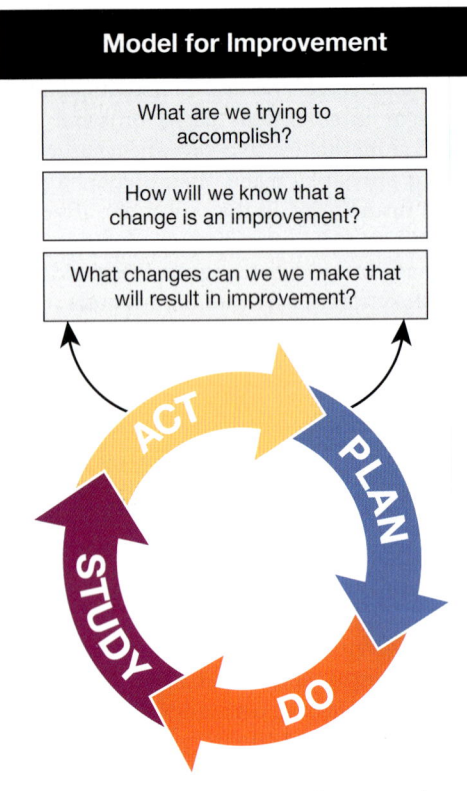

Figure 11-6. The plan-do-study-act cycle can be enhanced with the model for improvement questions. (Data from Langley, G. L., Moen, R., Nolan, K. M., Nolan, T. W., Norman, C. L., & Provost, L.P. (2009). *The improvement guide: A practical approach to enhancing organizational performance* (2nd ed.). San Francisco: Jossey-Bass Publishers.)

how other organizations or providers approach similar challenges and improve processes.

Benchmarks are set by organizations or providers based on their unique strengths or weaknesses. QI projects often focus on areas of weakness discovered through the benchmarking process. Clinical nurses and nurse leaders should be familiar with nationally recognized quality measures used for benchmarking. Healthcare benchmarking data sets include hospital data such as expenses, tangible and intangible assets; physician data such as postoperative infection or readmission rates; nursing data such as length of stay or labor costs; and clinical analytics that include any measure affecting patient care such as preventable medical errors. Benchmarks can be financial, operational, clinical, internal, external, competitive, or performance-related.

National Quality Forum

The National Quality Forum (NQF) is a nonprofit membership organization working to improve healthcare outcomes, safety, equity, and affordability (NQF, 2023a). Their mission is to be a trusted resource that drives measurable health improvements. When a healthcare organization joins the NQF, they have access to all data and quality measures available through the organization. An example of how the NQF supports hospitals includes an implementation guide to prevent hospital-onset bloodstream infections (NQFb, 2023). They bring together suppliers, purchasers, and insurance and healthcare providers to collaborate and promote best practices. Membership dues and application materials are available on their website.

Centers for Medicare & Medicaid Services

QI in a hospital setting that utilizes Medicare and Medicaid has additional meaning. The Centers for Medicare & Medicaid Services (CMS) develop quality measures for public reporting, QI measurement, and pay-for-reporting programs (CMS, 2023) known as the Measures Management System (MMS). The MMS is a set of business processes and decision criteria that CMS-funded organizations follow in the development, implementation, and maintenance of quality measures.

The Quality Payment Program was the result of the Medicare Access and CHIP Reauthorization Act of 2015 (CMS, 2021). The Quality Payment Program was designed to provide clinicians with tools and resources focusing on quality patient care. The Merit-Based Incentive Payment System (MIPS) is one of the two tracks of the Quality Payment Program (CMS, 2018). The purpose of MIPS is to provide financial incentives to eligible providers reporting data on quality measures. MIPS uses incentive payments for quality reporting and payment adjustments for unsatisfactory reporting. Detailed information about MIPS is available on the CMS website.

The other track of the Quality Payment Program is advanced alternative payment models (APMs). Providers who bill through Medicare Part

B can earn incentive payments for participating. Historically, healthcare systems in the United States paid for the number of patients served and the number of resources consumed. There were no financial incentives to improve care—just moral and ethical ones—meaning quantity (over quality) was being rewarded. Through the Quality Payment Program, advanced APMs provide payment incentives to clinicians who provide and report quality and efficient patient care. Information for clinicians to assist in maximizing reimbursement for services through participation in the APMs track of the Quality Payment Program can be found at the CMS website (CMS, 2021).

Beginning in 2008, the CMS in collaboration with the Hospital Quality Alliance (HQA), required hospitals to survey patients and families to gather information about their experiences with healthcare (CMS, 2021). The Agency for Healthcare Research and Quality (AHRQ) developed the Hospital Consumer Assessment of Healthcare Providers and Systems (HCAHPS), a standardized survey tool designed for administration to a sample of discharged patients. Hospitals are required to submit data from the survey to the CMS website so that patients' experiences can be trended over time in one hospital and benchmarked to other hospitals. These data are available to the public to provide accountability in healthcare. These data can be found by searching "HCAHPS Care Compare" in a search engine.

HCAHPS asks about patients' experiences, including communication with nurses and doctors, the responsiveness of staff, cleanliness, and quietness of the environment, and whether they would recommend the hospital (CMS, 2021). Hospitals can add other questions to customize the survey to meet their own needs for data measurement of the patient experience. The 2010 PPACA requires HCAHPS measurements to be used as a factor when calculating value-based payments to hospitals (CMS, 2021).

The quality of nursing care influences a hospital's performance in some of the areas measured by HCAHPS. A more direct measurement of the quality of nursing care is possible when nurse administrators choose to participate in the **National Database of Nursing Quality Indicators (NDNQI)**. The NDNQI data include nursing hours per patient day, staff mix, nursing turnover, and rates of falls, pressure injuries, infections, restraint use, intravenous infiltration, and nosocomial infection, to name a few (Lockhart, 2018).

The Joint Commission

The Joint Commission (TJC) is a U.S. nonprofit organization that accredits more than 22,000 healthcare organizations and programs. The main goals of TJC are to ensure quality healthcare for patients, prevent harm, and improve patient advocacy. TJC has specific quality measures holding healthcare organizations accountable for patient outcomes (Wadhwa & Huynh, 2022). Hospitals and healthcare facilities are reviewed every 2 to 3 years and gain in reputation by being awarded TJC accreditation. Failure to meet standards results in a plan of action and delay in accreditation. Onsite surveys can cause stress in organizations. An important role of the IN is to ensure organizations are always ready for a TJC site visit. TJC may review standards, policies, procedures, and processes during unannounced visits.

An example of quality measures set by TJC is the annual National Patient Safety Goals (NPSG) (TJC, 2023). Each year, TJC gathers data about emerging patient safety issues and creates a list of goals for various programs for the following year. The 2024 goals are for:

- Ambulatory healthcare
- Assisted living communities
- Behavioral health care and human services
- Critical access hospitals
- Home care
- Hospitals
- Laboratories
- Nursing care centers
- Office-based surgery

As an example, the goals for nursing care centers include identifying patients and residents correctly, using medicines safely, preventing infection, preventing patients and residents from falling, and preventing pressure injuries (TJC, 2023). The IN can help with designing projects to meet the NPSGs.

> **CASE STUDY**
>
> The case study describes a QI project on sepsis prevention. Review the TJC NPSGs for 2024 to see what specific goals would be addressed by the sepsis study.

Tools for Quality Improvement

There are many tools available to launch a successful QI project, including spreadsheets (Chapter 9) and several types of diagrams. Additional resources are available from QI organizations such as the AHRQ, the IHI, and the National Association for Healthcare Quality (NAHQ). The IHI has a QI Essentials Toolkit that contains directions, templates, and tools (IHI, n.d.). Creating spreadsheets, inserting formulas to perform calculations, and displaying data in charts are useful skills for QI projects for monthly budgets, schedule management, organizing or reviewing data, and creating reports.

Quality Improvement Organizations

Quality improvement organizations (QIOs) are nonprofit organizations that support QI in healthcare. Joining a QIO has many benefits, including the ability to connect with other professionals engaged in QI through message boards, meetings, and conferences; access to webinars, resources, articles, updates, and policy alerts; and some opportunities for certification. National QIOs include the AHRQ, the American Health Quality Association (AHQA), the American Society for Quality (ASQ), the IHI, and the NAHQ. Type "find your QIO" into your internet search bar to find local and regional organizations and ways to get involved.

Certification

Certification can distinguish you from other professionals and improve your opportunities to advance in your current role at your organization. The ASQ offers a Certified Quality Improvement Associate (CQIA) certification through examination. Someone with a CQIA certification has a basic knowledge of quality tools and is involved in QI projects but does not necessarily come from a traditional QI area (ASQ, n.d.b). Candidates must have worked full-time for 2 years and have an associate degree. Although this is not specific to healthcare, it still provides a solid foundation of QI.

The NAHQ offers the Certified Professional in Healthcare Quality (CPHQ) certification. The CPHQ certification is the only accredited certification in healthcare quality and is, therefore, valued by employers (NAHQ, n.d.). The CPHQ is based on a job task analysis to ensure relevancy. There are no formal eligibility requirements for the examination, though it is recommended that candidates have at least 2 years of experience in healthcare (NAHQ, n.d.).

Quality Improvement and Staffing

QI can be used for nurse staffing. Research shows that optimized professional nurse staffing is important for patient outcomes, better patient and family experiences, and nurse well-being. Adding assistive personnel without professional nurse qualifications may contribute to preventable deaths, compromise the quality of care, and contribute to nursing shortages.

Nurse staffing has become an even greater problem since the COVID-19 pandemic. The total supply of RNs decreased by more than 100,000 from 2020 to 2021, the largest drop over the past four decades (Auerbach et al., 2022). Factors include a shortage of nursing faculty, nurses near retirement age, increased acuity of an aging population, and nurse burnout. Increasing numbers of nurses are leaving the profession due to stress and job dissatisfaction (Rosseter, 2022). A national nurse staffing think tank was launched in 2022 to develop solutions to address this crisis (American Association of Critical Care Nurses, 2022). The team identified the following six priority areas that need urgent action:

1. Healthy work environment
2. Diversity, equity, and inclusion
3. Work schedule flexibility
4. Stress injury continuum
5. Innovative care delivery models
6. Total compensation

The think tank recommended building a staff scheduling approach that encompasses flexible scheduling, shifts, and roles. To do this requires several staffing systems, all of which would benefit from IN expertise and input.

Human Resource Management Systems

A human resource management system (HRMS) is essential for appropriately planning and staffing nursing services. HRMSs generally contain four categories: personnel profiles; daily work schedules and time-off requests; payroll data; and education, skill qualifications, and licensure information. An HRMS can serve as a scheduling system, which accounts for scheduling rules, shift rotations, and repeating shift patterns to create a draft schedule that can be modified for special circumstances. Scheduling systems can often prevent errors such as unintentional double shifts or overtime, overlapping shifts, or shifts during requested time off. Often, scheduling systems can generate reports to show the number of productive hours, education, vacation, and family medical leave hours in a period. Some scheduling systems allow managers to share the schedule with nurses via intranets, internet, email, or printing. With an intranet or internet interface, nurses can interact with scheduling systems to make requests, view schedules, or fill open shifts.

Not only can an HRMS serve as a scheduling system and repository of personnel data, but purchasing a productivity module can allow the system to pull nursing data (hours of care and skill mix) together with patient data (e.g., patient days, average length of stay, patient acuity). This productivity information is critical for nurse managers and nurse administrators to track, trend, and analyze for meaning within their organizations and to benchmark against similar organizations across the United States.

Because regulators and accreditation agencies require information about employees such as competencies, certifications, and evaluations, HRMSs may also provide a solution for managing these data. Many HRMSs contain employee appraisals; orientation checklists; employee competency checklists; development plans; compensation adjustments based on the achievement of personal, unit, or organization goals; and possibly succession plans. The HRMS may also generate reports for TJC.

Unfortunately, little progress has been made in developing an effective or efficient staffing model (Griffiths et al., 2020). However, artificial intelligence (AI) may provide better models to predict needed staffing (Carroll, 2018; Dickerson, 2023). For example, a study by Stonko et al. (2018) presents evidence that AI can predict staffing needs for trauma centers based on the time of year and weather patterns. With advances in technology and analytical methods, future scheduling software will likely include demand forecasting capabilities, which predicts the needs for nurse staffing. Demand forecasting in healthcare is possible because of the repetitive nature of scheduling for surgery or procedures and because admissions for certain illnesses or injuries are more common during certain months of the year. For example, admissions for respiratory infections (e.g., pneumonia, influenza) are more common in the winter months. Demand forecasting can take information from previous winter months to predict the need for nurses in medical units in a particular hospital.

Patient Classification Systems

Patient acuity and staffing are closely related. Patient classification systems can be used to measure actual patient care needs in terms of staffing. Some systems look at patient needs related to daily living activities, treatments, medications, and patient teaching. Another approach assigns time to each task based on hospital-specific, predetermined measures. Some methods use specific nursing diagnoses based on patient dependency.

All patient classification systems now and in the future depend on accurate and timely data input. Some patient classification systems use computer-based data entry and require the nurse to enter characteristics of tasks for use in scoring the patient's acuity. Other systems draw data from nurses' documentation in the computerized patient record, which relieves nurses of the additional step of data entry for patient classification. If nurses delay documentation (regardless of the reason), the patient's acuity is downgraded because the documentation of vital signs, education, dressing changes, and other nursing activities are not present in the record to reflect the patient's true acuity.

Project Management

Much like change/control management, project management is a more recent addition to the job responsibilities of INs found in the HIMSS workforce survey, coming up first in 2020 (HIMSS, 2023). **Project management** is a set of knowledge, skills, tools, and techniques used to achieve successful outcomes (Project Management Institute, n.d.). These outcomes are often defined in terms of time, adherence to budget, and delivering the promised functionality. INs may engage in project management as part of QI initiatives. QI efforts become projects when they affect multiple organizational systems and require cross-departmental collaboration and resources. Project management with QI initiatives often lead to **process improvement**, which are actions taken to identify, analyze, and improve existing processes within an organization. INs will also be heavily involved in project management in the case of new or updated HIT products. As INs are knowledgeable about healthcare and technology, they are key players in HIT projects.

Most project management process models describe five steps: initiating, planning, executing, controlling, and closing (Fig. 11-7). The Project Management Institute publishes the *Project Management Body of Knowledge* (*PMBOK*). The 7th edition of this guide is available for purchase as a softcover or ebook by searching for the title. The PMBOK Guide is an excellent resource for learning more about project management and the systems development life cycle.

Initiating

In the initiating phase, organization members and project planners identify and analyze an organization's mission and vision to determine how a new project (such as a new HIT system) could help

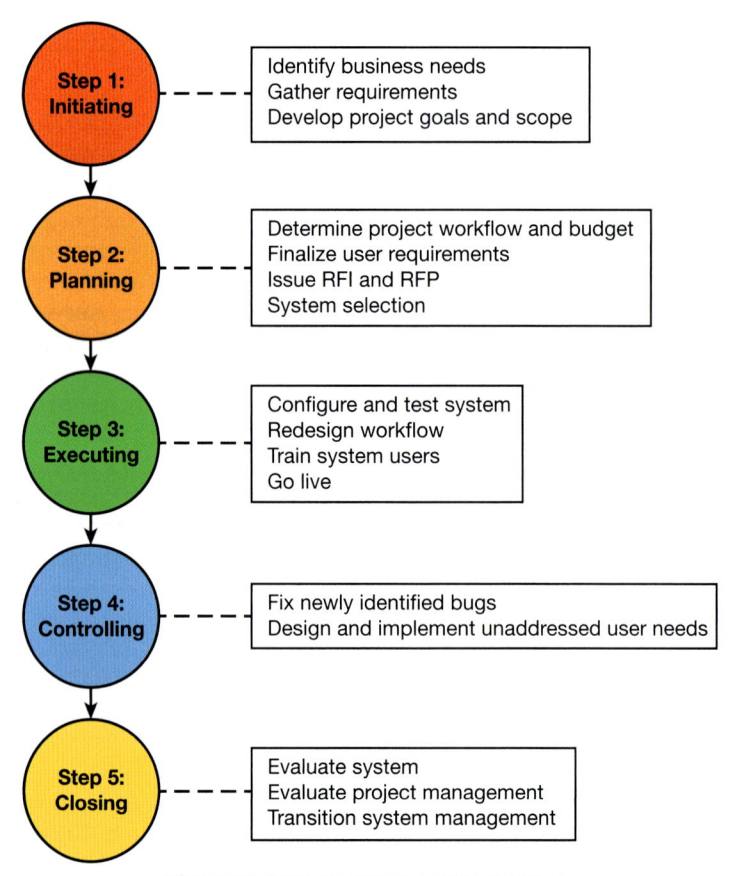

Step 1: Initiating
- Identify business needs
- Gather requirements
- Develop project goals and scope

Step 2: Planning
- Determine project workflow and budget
- Finalize user requirements
- Issue RFI and RFP
- System selection

Step 3: Executing
- Configure and test system
- Redesign workflow
- Train system users
- Go live

Step 4: Controlling
- Fix newly identified bugs
- Design and implement unaddressed user needs

Step 5: Closing
- Evaluate system
- Evaluate project management
- Transition system management

Figure 11-7. Project management steps.

achieve its goals. All stakeholders, from executives to end users, must be a part of the analysis of the vision and mission. Examples of stakeholders include patients, clinicians, managers, executives, payers, and entity or any other person who may use or be affected by the project. INs are prominent stakeholders in projects involving HIT.

After the vision and mission have been analyzed, the next step in initiation is to identify project goals. Poorly defined project goals can result in a failed project. The project goals represent a summary of the functions the project will achieve once it is implemented and fully in use. Similar to patient outcomes, project goals should be specific, measurable, achievable, relevant, and time-bound (SMART). Examples of SMART project goals could be "Prevent patient falls by implementing remote patient monitoring in three units in Hospital A by December 1" or "Improve staff hand hygiene compliance on the oncology unit from 75% to 85% within 2 months."

The next task is to define the **project scope**. The project scope describes the boundaries of a project, functionality, user group(s), and affected departments. The scope may also include a timeline, budget, and additional required resources. Regardless of the size of the project, a clearly defined scope helps all parties involved understand how a project is expected to function, who is involved, and the resources allocated to accomplish the goals. During project implementation, opportunities for additional functionality or goals that could benefit the project's mission can appear. Each new idea requires additional resources and time to accomplish. **Scope creep**, or adding additional unfunded requirements to an existing project, is particularly risky to overall project success and one of the most prevalent causes of project failures (Komal et al., 2020).

Planning

Planning is the second step in project management. This critical phase requires a detailed assessment of the current processes, including workflow analyses and timelines and the implied changes of new processes. **Workflow** is the sequence of steps that need to be completed from the beginning to the end of a process. Engaging staff who perform the work to help map the current workflow is imperative to understand how processes are currently being completed. Effective planning promotes trust and confidence among users and team members.

Financial Considerations

An organization will conduct a financial evaluation of a project. A **cost-benefit analysis** examines the difference between the project's projected expenses and benefits, including health outcomes. Benefits are assigned a monetary value and the net benefit is calculated (benefit minus cost) (CDC, 2021). The HITECH Act passed in 2009 propelled the implementation of EHRs, requiring healthcare facilities to use a certified EHR to receive incentive payments for meaningful use (Gecomo et al., 2020). The HITECH Act tipped the balance of the cost-benefit analysis, rendering not implementing an EHR more expensive to organizations than the considerable cost of implementation and maintenance. By 2020, 96% of all healthcare organizations in the United States were using a certified EHR system (Gecomo et al., 2020).

Return on investment (ROI) is the ratio of net profit over the total cost of the investment. ROI is a major factor to be considered by healthcare agencies when making decisions about which healthcare technology projects to adopt. For healthcare agencies, ROI is not simply determined by the financial benefits. Improving patient care outcomes and managing costs should align with the strategic plans for healthcare agencies. The process of ROI requires scrutiny regarding risks and the associated values. Questions to be considered are "is the risk offset by the potential value?" and "what data are available to support the value?" People involved in budget-making decisions must identify goals and methods for measuring achievement for both tangible and intangible values and risks (Bata & Richardson, 2018).

Healthcare systems increasingly use business models that focus on **tangible assets**, or assets that have physical substance. Examples of tangible assets include a decrease in length of stay, in antiinfective medication costs, in the number of unnecessary medications and tests, and in charges per admission. There is not much variance in tangibles between healthcare settings. However, **intangible assets**, those assets that are not physical, remain critical. Examples of intangible assets include improved decision making, better relationships, improved communication, and user satisfaction. Intangibles may vary among healthcare settings because of the differences in factors, such as organizational culture, physical environments, population served, and staffing. Making a case for intangible assets can be challenging and is an important job of the IN.

Project Requirements

Project requirements represent a detailed list of functions or goals a project must possess to meet an organization's needs. The project team uses these requirements in a variety of ways: (1) finalize the project's scope, budget, and timeline; (2) determine project team membership; (3) negotiate a contract with a vendor; and (4) guide staff for customization or implementation. Requirements are captured by conducting a **needs assessment** that identifies stakeholders' expectations. The needs assessment might include direct observation of current workflow and interviewing department managers and clinicians. A workflow analysis depicts how work is currently accomplished and then describes how the same work might be performed using new or changed processes. The team must differentiate between essential features (needs) and nice-to-have features (wants). Some teams use a rating scale to determine the necessity of features; typically, patient safety features are a higher priority. In project management of HIT, interoperability should be considered during the needs assessment.

The needs assessment lays the groundwork when communicating with potential vendors. A **request for information (RFI)** communicates an organization's interest in purchasing a service or product from a vendor, such as new or enhanced HIT. By providing a detailed list of requirements, vendors can determine if they have the capability to meet the organization's needs. Requirements described in the RFI might include:

- Schedule, design, and budget constraints
- The number of users
- The department(s) that will use the product
- Whether it is a new product or a revised version of an existing product
- In cases of HIT, software and data considerations and the availability of HIT support

The RFI is sent to a list of potential vendors whose products may meet the organization's needs. A matrix, or table, is often used to rate each vendor's response to the RFI and allows for easy comparison across different products. People involved in the rating process should be familiar with the details of the RFI and IT terminology, rendering an IN an optimal choice for this team.

A **request for proposal (RFP)** is a detailed document sent to vendors selected through the RFI process. An RFP asks a vendor to describe how their product specifically meets the organization's requirements and about customization, timeline, and support. A well-written RFP allows the users to compare products effectively. It has three parts—a section that describes the method and deadline for responses, another that describes the organization (e.g., the hospital, primary care office), and the final that describes expectations. Vendor responses to the RFP are reviewed in the same manner as the RFI.

As noted earlier, site visits or interviews with current users are necessary when selecting new HIT. It is important that selection committee members not be overly dependent on vendor advice. Vendors are aiming to sell products and services and may sometimes minimize system weaknesses and overpromise on functionality. Therefore, feedback from actual users is vital. At the end of the planning stage, the vendor and product are selected, and project management moves into the executing phase.

> ### CASE STUDY
>
> In QI studies such as the one in the case study about sepsis screening, the costs of the study itself must be factored into the cost-benefit analysis. These costs include money lost by taking time and energy away from other projects within the organization. Imagine you have an idea for a QI project. How might you justify the time and energy costs of the project to management so that you can get approval to move forward?

Executing

The third stage of project management is execution. This involves adjusting workflow to accommodate the new product or procedure, training the staff involved, and ultimately implementing the product. With HIT projects, this phase involves customizing design once it is received from the vendor, aligning workflow with the design, and preparing end users to interact with the HIT effectively and efficiently. INs are essential for keeping HIT running smoothly. They have the knowledge and communication skills that allow them to use terminology that the healthcare user can understand. They also appreciate the clinician's complex role and recognize potential patient safety issues.

Design and Testing

Once a product is selected, in the case of HIT, the next step is to customize the product to be compatible with user requirements. Typically, the vendor provides a standard product, sometimes known as the product foundation or out-of-the-box functionality. This is like the standard computer that the buyer can customize with additional features. Just as in the customization of a computer, extra features often come at an additional fee.

During the design phase, if applicable, HIT interaction with current system documentation will be developed. Some vendors provide standardized data entry objects or boxes, while others allow unlimited customization by the customer. The decision to build one's own or take the vendor's standard product should be made in the early stages of vendor discovery and selection.

The testing phase will identify and fix any HIT system errors and issues, commonly called bugs. The process of correcting these errors is called debugging. Testing a new HIT system is ongoing and occurs every time the system is upgraded. At a minimum, testing includes features and expected functionality, system hardware and software, and the different phases of use, such as backups, downtime, restarts, data capture and storage, and network communication.

Integration testing ensures interfaces and communication/network functionality work as expected. Technology teams use a set of situations commonly called scenarios or test scripts to test functionality, referred to as **regression testing**. These test scripts are created to depict normal and abnormal events for each functional part of the software and for data integration across interfaces. Clinicians may be involved in devising the features and functionality scenarios and in the actual testing. Often something considered intuitive by the design team may prove confusing for the clinical user.

A test script may not catch every bug; however, each time a new issue is discovered, it should be added to the set of scripts. Over the years, a collection of test scripts can become highly accurate and reduce the issues discovered during implementation. Time invested in testing can save the end user time and lessen frustrations. Delivering a product that works as expected builds end user confidence; testing is a crucial step to meet this aim.

Workflow Redesign

Workflow redesign begins with mapping the current state of the processes being completed and then planning and mapping how the work will be completed in the future with the implementation of a new product (ONC, 2019). Developing a process map of the current state sets the groundwork and understanding of the process. Stakeholders can use process maps to identify the bottlenecks and opportunities for improvement. The Office of the National Coordinator for Health Information Technology (ONC) recommends focusing on critical workflow areas, for example, reviewing workflows of how patients check in and check out, patient transfers, e-prescribing, scheduling, laboratory orders, referral generation and management, and billing (2019). Involving end users is crucial to understanding the current state and planning the future state of the workflow.

Keeping the project's goals and scope in focus is essential in the workflow redesign process to keep the project on track and within budget. When stakeholders start mapping and understanding the complexities of their current processes and consider what is possible in the future, the desire to make additional improvements and expand the project often grows. Changes to scope need to be considered carefully and weighed against the ultimate success of timely implementation.

Preparing End Users

Implementation success depends on how well the clinical users are prepared to work with the new HIT or the changes made to current HIT. Building skills and understanding equipment before implementation is necessary for a smooth transition. Performing a user **skills assessment** identifies users who need additional training and help to develop a plan for training and support of the implementation. Performing a skills assessment may also help identify training resources, such as people who are identified as good super user candidates.

Following the skills assessment, training will be conducted. The trainers may be members of the technology staff, INs, super users, or vendor staff. Training will not only teach staff how to use new HIT but also reinforce new workflows developed during the design process. Trainers should help users learn how to use the new product to support their care roles and should cover security, data accuracy, and how to obtain help. Providing supplemental online tutorials and video clips can also assist clinicians in using HIT successfully. If the skills assessment identifies staff who need training in computer literacy, that should be dealt with in separate learning sessions and target only those with a need. By preparing all users in advance of the implementation, the content can focus on mastering the new system rather than developing elementary computer skills.

Trainers should encourage end users to take responsibility for learning new skills by encouraging questions and seeking feedback on the usefulness of functionality and features. Although showing users where features are located and explaining how they are used is helpful, mastery requires using the HIT within workflow processes; developing several scenarios or simulation case studies that the clinician experiences frequently can enhance user understanding and application of learning. Some organizations also develop self-learning modules that can be accessed from multiple locations, allowing users to learn at their own pace. Trying to cover all training requirements in a single class is tempting but can be overwhelming and lead to restlessness and inattention. The learning plan should include time for frequent breaks, and sessions should not be longer than 8 hours.

Implementation

Implementation or go-live can be a significant milestone depending on the scope of the new product. Many agencies build momentum toward that milestone with preparatory events, presentations, memos, and posters. The event may also include a media release to the local news outlets. Implementation is carefully planned so users have the necessary support, patients are safe, and care processes are interrupted as little as possible.

The success of the go-live is dependent on support system effectiveness. It may be necessary to schedule additional staff for the first few days or weeks, depending on the number of users affected and the level of workflow effect. Initially, 24-hour onsite support may be required, with later support provided by a service desk. Vendor support is important in the initial stages of implementation to troubleshoot unforeseen issues and resolve any problems quickly. The goal should be to have as little disruption in patient care delivery as possible.

The HIT implementation plan should have a contingency plan for a rollback. A rollback refers to backing out of the implementation. Clinicians should not be expected to use HIT that jeopardizes patient care. Rollback issues can be minimized if the HIT is carefully tested before implementation and the users are trained and ready.

Controlling

Controlling is the fourth phase of project management. Even the best technology can have issues. IT staff need time to address the issues discovered once new HIT is in use or after changes have been made. If the project requirement process missed essential workflow steps or requirements, these will be discovered through daily use. INs may be involved in gathering these issues and determining the level of impact and urgency, then IT staff will design and implement the necessary changes.

Closing

Three activities take place in the final closing phase of project management. First, the HIT is evaluated in terms of project goals and requirements. Although evaluation should be a part of every phase of project management, there should be a planned evaluation at least 6 months after implementation. Before that, improvements may be difficult to identify because of issues related to adjusting to new methods of working. If a preevaluation was done before implementation, comparisons are made. Next, the implementation process (e.g., budget and timeline) is evaluated, and lessons learned are documented. Finally, the project team prepares to turn over HIT management to the organization's IT team. As healthcare changes, clinicians may recommend ways that the product should be changed or optimized to better meet the needs of patient populations, adopt new care recommendations, or achieve more efficient workflow practices. In each case, IT staff work with associated staff to assess the request, rate its priority, and determine if it is a minor improvement or if it warrants project status. Established teams and analysts must continually evaluate optimizations, address new initiatives, prepare for software upgrades, and improve the quality of the HIT (Siwicki, 2020).

Leadership

Although leadership was not one of the responsibilities that came up in the HIMSS workforce survey, it is an important skill for INs. It often arises as a component of other responsibilities. For example, system implementation, change/control management, and project management all require strong leadership skills.

Common characteristics of nurse leaders include social intelligence, a commitment to excellence, trustworthiness, empathy, and a willingness to mentor and coach others (Hughes, 2017). Nurse leaders must also be approachable, open-minded, supportive, and empowering, with a clear vision and strategic focus. The ANA defines competencies and skills needed for leadership (ANA, 2018):

- Adaptability: includes flexibility and interpersonal skills
- Integrity and credibility
- Self-awareness: includes self-insight, management, and development
- Strong verbal and written communication skills
- Conflict resolution and negotiation
- Building collaborative relationships: interdisciplinary teamwork
- Business acumen: knowledge and perspective
- Change management
- The courage to take risks
- Influence and power
- Problem-solving with sound judgment
- Vision and strategy: engage in strategic planning

There are many ways to become a nurse leader. Join a professional nursing organization such as the ANA or the National League for Nursing (NLN). Both organizations offer leadership institutes and continuing education that provide training to build leadership skills. The facility in which you work may offer leadership courses, which are often provided through human resources. You can continue your education and become a clinical nurse leader or obtain a master's degree in administrative leadership. If you are an RN, search the internet for continuing education opportunities to improve your leadership skills. In addition, you can express interest in leadership positions in your current place of work, seek out a mentor and ask for constructive criticism from people you admire, become a super user, and participate in unit projects or initiatives. Look for opportunities to engage in interdisciplinary teams to build your communication and conflict resolution skills.

Strategic Planning

An important role for the IN leader is to engage in strategic planning. **Strategic planning** is the process for outlining where a healthcare agency is and where it desires to be in the future. The desired future can be in 3, 5, 10 years, or longer. The strategic planning process identifies resources needed to achieve the future state. Having a strategic plan allows all stakeholders in a healthcare organization to know the path the agency is following and how it will get there. An organization's strategic plan should be a living and breathing document that allows for flexibility (AAMC, n.d.).

Strategic planning should be used for the adoption and implementation of HIT. Healthcare agencies must strategically plan for the right HIT to meet the mission, vision, and goals for the agency (Fitz & Shaikh, 2018). An important part of strategic planning is working with finances. A strategic plan needs to operate within a budget that attempts to predict future costs. Stakeholders must be able to see that the expenditures are offset by patient outcome benefits; they must see an ROI. If the use of HIT is not supported by the institution's strategic plan, it may not be funded.

SUMMARY

- **Informatics nurse job titles.** Informatics nursing is a career choice that has experienced rapid growth with the expanding use of technology in healthcare. The HIMSS Nursing Informatics Workforce Survey revealed the most common career titles include informatics nurse specialist, clinical analyst, manager or director of clinical informatics, nurse educator or instructor, chief nursing informatics officer, and EHR implementation manager.
- **System responsibilities of the informatics nurse.** INs are important to the systems life cycle of healthcare organizations; so many responsibilities of INs are related to systems. System implementation involves selecting and adopting new technology. The IIF can be used to support the adoption of new technology. System optimization and utilization involves designing or updating a system so that it operates as smoothly and efficiently as possible. This is often necessary with EHRs. System development is the process of defining, designing, testing, and implementing new HIT. Examples of the role of the IN in systems development include UIs and communication systems. Change/control management is used to facilitate changes in systems, often using data from unintended consequences that arise. Business continuity plans for continued operation during an unplanned event are necessary.
- **Other responsibilities of the informatics nurse.** QI is the systematic improvement of patient care using a framework of standardized processes and technology to reduce variations in care, achieve predictable results, and improve outcomes. When doing QI, using the PDSA cycle and the Model for Improvement provides guidance and allow for feedback to ensure success. Quality measures for organizations using Medicare and Medicaid are set by the CMS and include the Quality Payment Program, which provides financial incentives to organizations and providers who meet benchmarking goals. TJC provides accreditation to organizations by reviewing quality measures including the NPSGs. QI with staffing can be managed with HRMSs and patient classification systems. Project management involves initiating, planning, executing, controlling, and closing. Leadership responsibilities are important to many other roles. You can learn to be a nurse leader by looking for opportunities on the job, by participating in workshops and leadership institutes, continuing your education, and joining professional nursing organizations. Nurse leaders should be involved in strategic planning to help determine the future state of an organization.

DISCUSSION QUESTIONS AND ACTIVITIES

1. Interview an IN to learn more about their responsibilities. What career description best fits this person? Is this a job you would be interested in doing? Why or why not? Ask the following questions:
   - What is your practice setting?
   - What is your educational background?
   - Are you certified or interested in certification? Why or why not?
   - How long have you been in this role?
   - How satisfied are you with your job?
2. Search a job site for job opportunities for INs and try to find a match to some of the job titles described in this chapter. How much does a nurse in each role make each year? What qualifications are needed?
3. An EHR implementation manager reviews EHR enhancement requests. Think about a request regarding operating room (OR) start times. OR start times should be the time the patient is marked ready for surgery, but some use the anesthesia start time as the start time. Consider how this affects billing since OR time is billed in half-hour increments for anesthesia. If OR start times differ among surgery centers, how are productivity metrics going to be evaluated and compared across campuses?
4. Choose from systems implementation, optimization, utilization, or development and search the internet for an additional example of how the IN engages in this role or give an example from your workplace.

5. Identify a QI nursing project that is needed in your healthcare workplace, or find one on the internet and describe how you would meet the five steps of project management to complete the project.

6. How does your place of work use benchmarking to provide quality outcomes for patients and staff? Give an example of a quality measure and how your workplace compares to others.

7. Search "HCAHPS Care Compare" and review your hospital's outcomes on core measures with three others in your area and two from a different area that have services like your own. What are the next steps for your organization to improve and in which areas?

8. Go to the IHI and locate the QI essentials toolkit. Download one of the tools and fill it out using a QI project you have identified (on the internet, using a library search, or by interviewing a nurse).

9. Identify a nurse leader and describe how their characteristics do or do not match those described in the chapter. Would you consider this leader effective? Why or why not? Give one resource that could help this leader improve.

PRACTICE QUESTIONS

1. Which statement about informatics nursing careers is true?
   a. Nurse educator remains the most common title.
   b. An EHR manager might address tickets or issues reported to the help desk.
   c. A nursing informatics consultant is an executive position.
   d. HIT positions are not expected to grow over the next decade.

2. The space where interactions between humans and HIT occur is known as _____.
   a. throughput
   b. return on investment
   c. big bang
   d. user interface

3. The process of providers entering and sending treatment instructions such as medication, laboratory, and radiology orders via a computer application is known as _____.
   a. computerized provider order entry
   b. clinical decision support system
   c. integrated interface approach
   d. enterprise system integration

4. The project team has identified several opportunities to make additional improvements beyond the project's scope and notified the project manager. The project manager recognizes the request as scope creep. What should they do next?
   a. Inform the project team that the additional requests are outside of the project's scope.
   b. Investigate the request, determining what additional time, funding, and resources would be required for the request.
   c. Ask an analyst if they could make the additional improvements in the project build.
   d. Promise the project team that the additional improvements will be done in the optimization phase.

5. You are leading a team to redesign the specimen collection workflow at your hospital. What should you do first?
   a. Talk about the problems with the current workflow.
   b. Begin brainstorming with the team.
   c. Ask the clinical nurses to describe their ideal workflow.
   d. Map the current workflow.

6. The organization you work for is implementing a new EHR. Which type of conversion involves the least risk?
   a. Big bang
   b. Parallel
   c. Phased
   d. Pilot

REFERENCES

Ahad, A., Tahir, M., Aman Sheikh, M., Ahmed, K. I., Mughees, A., & Numani, A. (2020). Technologies trend towards 5G network for smart health-care using IoT: A review. *Sensors, 20*(14), 4047. https://doi.org/10.3390/s20144047

American Association of Critical Care Nurses. (2022, May 5). *National nurse staffing think tank launched by leading health care organizations develops solutions tool kit to address staffing crisis.* https://www.aacn.org/newsroom/national-nurse-staffing-think-tank-launched-by-leading-health-care-organizations

American Medical Informatics Association (AMIA). (2023). *AMIA 25x5.* https://amia.org/about-amia/amia-25x5

American Nurses Association (ANA). (2015). *Code of ethics for nurses with interpretive statements.* Silver Spring. https://www.nursingworld.org/practice-policy/nursing-excellence/ethics/code-of-ethics-for-nurses/

American Nurses Association (ANA). (2018, July). *Competency model.* ANA leadership. https://www.nursingworld.org/~4a0a2e/globalassets/docs/ce/177626-ana-leadership-booklet-new-final.pdf

American Society for Quality (ASQ). (n.d.b). *Quality improvement associate certification.* Retrieved March 12, 2023 from https://asq.org/quality-press/display-item?item=H1571

Ash, J. S., Sittig, D. F., Dykstra, R., Campbell, E., & Guappone, K. (2009). The unintended consequences of computerized provider order entry: Findings from a mixed methods exploration. *International Journal of Medical Informatics, 78*(Suppl 1), S69–S76. https://doi.org/10.1016/j.ijmedinf.2008.07.015

Association of American Medical Colleges (AAMC). (n.d.). *Strategic planning.* https://www.aamc.org/professional-development/affinity-groups/gip/strategic-planning

Auerbach, D. I., Buerhaus, P. I., Donelan, K., & Staiger, D. O. (2022, April 13). *A worrisome drop in the number of young nurses.* HealthAffairs. https://www.healthaffairs.org/do/10.1377/forefront.20220412.311784/

Bata, S. A., & Richardson, T. (2018). Value of investment as a key driver for prioritization and implementation of healthcare software. *Perspectives in Health Information Management, 15*(Winter), 1g, Online Research Journal https://www.ncbi.nlm.nih.gov/pmc/articles/PMC5869444/

Bhyat, R., Hagens, S., Bryski, K., & Kohlmaier, J. F. (2021). Digital health value realization through active change efforts. *Frontiers in Public Health, 9*(2021), 741424. online. https://doi.org/10.3389/fpubh.2021.741424

Carroll, W. (2018, July 10). Artificial intelligence, nurses and the quadruple aim. *Online Journal of Nursing Informatics (OJNI), 22*(2). https://www.himss.org/resources/artificial-intelligence-nurses-and-quadruple-aim

Centers for Disease Control and Prevention (CDC). (2021, October 20). *Cost-benefit analysis.* U.S. Department of Health and Human Services. Retrieved July 11, 2022, from https://www.cdc.gov/policy/polaris/economics/cost-benefit/index.html

Centers for Medicare and Medicaid Services (CMS). (2018). *Enhancing patient care: Transitioning from the Physician Quality Reporting System (PQRS) to the Merit-based Incentive Payment System (MIPS).* https://www.cms.gov/Medicare/Quality-Initiatives-Patient-Assessment-Instruments/PQRS/Downloads/TransitionResources_Landscape.pdf

Centers for Medicare and Medicaid Services (CMS). (2021). *Quality payment program.* https://www.cms.gov/Medicare/Quality-Payment-Program/Quality-Payment-Program

Centers for Medicare and Medicaid Services (CMS). (2023, September 6). *Quality measurement and quality improvement.* https://www.cms.gov/Medicare/Quality-Initiatives-Patient-Assessment-Instruments/MMS/Quality-Measure-and-Quality-Improvement-

Cullen, L., Hanrahan, K., Edmonds, S. W., Reisinger, H. S., & Wagner, M. (2022). Iowa implementation for sustainability framework. *Implementation Science, 17*(1), 1. https://doi.org/10.1186/s13012-021-01157-5

Dickerson, B. (2023, April 20). *5 ways to use AI and automation to optimize hospital staffing.* https://leantaas.com/blog/5-ways-to-use-ai-and-automation-to-optimize-hospital-staffing/

Drees, J. (2020, February 25). *12 EHR implementations that cost over $100M.* Becker's Healthcare. Retrieved July 11, 2022, from https://www.beckershospitalreview.com/ehrs/12-ehr-implementations-that-cost-over-100m.html

Fitz, T., & Shaikh, M. (2018, October 31). *4 Tactics of effective strategic technology planning for the digital future.* Healthcare Financial Management Association (HFMA). Retrieved July 16, 2022, from https://www.hfma.org/topics/hfm/2018/november/62270.html

Gaines, K. (2022, July 18). *Nursing informatics.* Career Guide Series. Nurse.org. https://nurse.org/resources/nursing-informatics/

Gecomo, J., Klopp, A., & Rouse, M. (2020, March 3). *Implementation of an evidence-based Electronic Health Record (EHR) downtime readiness and recovery plan.* Health Information and Management Systems Society. Retrieved July 11, 2022, from https://www.himss.org/resources/implementation-evidence-based-electronic-health-record-ehr-downtime-readiness-and

Griffiths, P., Saville, C., Ball, J., Jones, J., Pattison, N., & Monks, T., Safer Nursing Care Study Group. (2020, March). Nursing workload, nurse staffing methodologies and tools: A systematic scoping review and discussion. *International Journal of Nursing Studies, 103*, 103487–103506. https://doi.org/10.1016/j.ijnurstu.2019.103487

Healthcare Information and Management Systems Society (HIMSS). (2021). *Electronic Medical Record Adoption Model (EMRAM).* https://www.himss.org/what-we-do-solutions/digital-health-transformation/maturity-models/electronic-medical-record-adoption-model-emram

Healthcare Information and Management Systems Society (HIMSS). (2023). *2022 nursing informatics workforce survey.* https://www.himss.org/sites/hde/files/media/file/2023/04/05/2022-nursing-informatics-workforce-survey.pdf

HealthIT.gov (2021a). *About the ONC health IT certification program.* https://www.healthit.gov/topic/certification-ehrs/about-onc-health-it-certification-program

HealthIT.gov. (n.d.). *Computerized provider order entry: The basics.* Retrieved November 30, 2022 from https://www.healthit.gov/faq/what-computerized-provider-order-entry

Hughes, V. (2017). Standout nurse leaders. What's in the research? *Nursing Management, 48*(9), 16–24. https://doi.org/10.1097/01.NUMA.0000522171.08016.29

Institute for Healthcare Improvement (IHI). (n.d.). *Quality improvement essentials toolkit.* Retrieved March 13, 2023 from https://www.ihi.org/resources/Pages/Tools/Quality-Improvement-Essentials-Toolkit.aspx?PostAuthRed=/resources/_layouts/download.aspx?SourceURL=/resources/Knowledge%20Center%20Assets/Tools%20-%20QualityImprovementEssentialsToolkit_e14261f9-05ff-4a7b-ba25-58c85c4c9e9a/QIToolkit_ParetoChart.pdf

Kangas, C., Iverson, L., & Pierce, D. (2021). Sepsis screening: Combining early warning scores and SIRS criteria. *Clinical Nursing Research, 30*(1), 42–49. https//doi.org/10.1177/1054773818823334

Komal, B., Janjua, U., Anwar, F., Madni, T., Cheema, M., Malik, M., & Shahid, A. (2020). The impact of scope creep on project success: An empirical investigation. *IEEE Access, 8*, 125755–125775. https://doi.org/10.1109/ACCESS.2020.3007098

Langley, G. L., Nolan, K. M., Nolan, T. W., Norman, C. L., & Provost, L. P. (2009). *The improvement guide: A practical approach to enhancing organizational performance* (2nd ed.). Jossey-Bass.

Lockhart, L. (2018). Measuring nursing's impact. *Nursing Made Incredibly Easy, 16*(2). 55. https://doi.org/10.1097/01.NME.0000529956.73785.23

National Association for Healthcare Quality (NAHQ). (n.d.). *Certified professional in healthcare quality*. Retrieved March 13, 2023 from https://nahq.org/individuals/cphq-certification/

National Quality Forum (NQF). (2023a). *About us*. https://www.qualityforum.org/About_NQF/

National Quality Forum (NQF). (2023b, September 14). *NQF to help hospitals better prevent, identify and treat hospital-onset bloodstream infections to improve patient safety*. https://www.qualityforum.org/News_And_Resources/Press_Releases/2023/NQF_to_Help_Hospitals_Better_Prevent,_Identify_and_Treat_Hospital-Onset_Bloodstream_Infections_to_Improve_Patient_Safety.aspx

Office of the National Coordinator for Health Information Technology (ONC). (2019, April 29). *Workflow redesign*. U.S. Department of Health and Human Services. Retrieved July 11, 2022, from https://www.healthit.gov/faq/what-workflow-redesign-why-it-important

Payne, T. H., Corley, S., Cullen, T. A., Gandhi, T. K., Harrington, L., Kuperman, G. J., Mattison, J. E., McCallie, D. P., McDonald, C. J., Tang, P. C., Tierney, W. M., Weaver, C., Weir, C. R., & Zaroukian, M. H. (2015). Report of the AMIA EHR-2020 Task Force on the status and future direction of EHRs. *Journal of the American Medical Informatics Association, 22*(5), 1102–1110.

Project Management Institute. (n.d.). *What is project management?* Retrieved July 11, 2022, from https://www.pmi.org/about/learn-about-pmi/what-is-project-management

Rosseter, R. (2022, October). *Nursing shortage*. AACN. https://www.aacnnursing.org/news-information/fact-sheets/nursing-shortage

Roush, K., Opsahl, A., Parker, K., & Davis, J. (2021). Business continuity planning: An effective strategy during an electronic health record downtime. *Nurse Leader, 19*(5), 525–531. https://doi.org/10.1016/j.mnl.2021.01.003

Scarbrough, H., & Kyratsis, Y. (2022). From spreading to embedding innovation in health care: Implications for theory and practice. *Health Care Management Review, 47*(3), 236–244. https://doi.org/10.1097/HMR.0000000000000323

Siwicki, B. (2020, January 9). Tech optimization: Tips for making EHRs work for your staff and organizational goals. *Healthcare IT News*. Retrieved July 11, 2022, from https://www.healthcareitnews.com/news/tech-optimization-tips-making-ehrs-work-your-staff-and-enable-organizational-goals

Stobierski, T. (2021, April 19). *6 Top careers in healthcare informatics*. https://www.northeastern.edu/graduate/blog/health-informatics-careers/

Stonko, D. P., Dennis, B. M., Betzold, R. D., Peetz, A. B., Gunter, O. L., & Guillamondegui, O. D. (2018). Artificial intelligence can predict daily trauma volume and average acuity. *Journal of Trauma and Acute Care Surgery, 85*(2), 393–397.

Sutton, R. T., Pincock, D., Baumgart, D. C., Sadowski, D. C., Fedorak, R. N., & Kroeker, K. I. (2020). An overview of clinical decision support systems: Benefits, risks, and strategies for success. *npj Digital Medicine, 3*, 17. https://doi.org/10.1038/s41746-020-0221-y

The Joint Commission (TJC). (2023). *National patient safety goals*. https://www.jointcommission.org/standards/national-patient-safety-goals/

U.S. Bureau of Labor & Statistics. (2022). *Computer and information technology occupations*. Occupational Outlook Handbook. https://www.bls.gov/ooh/computer-and-information-technology/home.htm

U.S. Department of Veterans Affairs. (2018). *VA signs contract with Cerner for an electronic health record system*. https://digital.va.gov/ehr-modernization/news-releases/va-signs-contract-with-cerner-for-an-electronic-health-record-system/

U.S. Department of Veterans Affairs. (2020). *VA launches new electronic health record system, reaching milestone in veteran care*. https://www.ehrm.va.gov/news/article/read/va-launches-new-ehr-system-reaching-milestone-in-veteran-care

van Gemert-Pijnen, J. L. (2022). Implementation of health technology: Directions for research and practice. *Frontiers in Digital Health, 4*. 1030194. https://doi.org/10.3389/fdgth.2022.1030194

Wadhwa, R., & Huynh, A. P. (2022, March 9). *The Joint Commission*. StatPearls. https://www.ncbi.nlm.nih.gov/books/NBK557846/

Western Governors University (WGU). (2023). *Healthcare career guides: Clinical informatics specialist career*. https://www.wgu.edu/career-guide/healthcare/clinical-informatics-specialist-career.html

Zenziper Straichman, Y., Kurnik, D., Matok, I., Halkin, H., Markovits, N., Ziv, A., Shamiss, A., & Loebstein, R. (2017). Prescriber response to computerized drug alerts for electronic prescriptions among hospitalized patients. *International Journal of Medical Informatics, 107*, 70–75. https://doi.org/10.1016/j.ijmedinf.2017.08.008

CHAPTER 12

Interoperability at the National and the International Levels

Sally M. Villaseñor and Kristi S. Miller

OBJECTIVES

After studying this chapter, you will be able to:

1. Discuss interoperability and its importance for the efficient exchange of health information.
2. Define the four types of interoperability: foundational, structural, semantic, and organizational.
3. Explain the importance of using standardized terminology for health information exchange (HIE) interoperability.
4. Discuss and give examples of U.S. efforts for promoting interoperable electronic health records.
5. List various international standards organizations and describe how they support global interoperability efforts.
6. Explain how the American Nurses Association Code of Ethics supports the use of interoperable HIEs for improving health on a global scale.
7. Explain how billing terminology standardization is important to reduce the cost of healthcare.
8. Discuss the importance of interoperability in healthcare's future.
9. Relate interoperability to public health and explain how improving the interoperability of HIEs can support public health efforts to predict and control future pandemics.

AACN Essentials for Entry-Level Professional Nursing Education

3.1e Apply an understanding of the public health system and its interfaces with clinical healthcare in addressing population health needs.

3.6a Identify changes in conditions that might indicate a disaster or public health emergency.

5.1c Implement standardized, evidence-based processes for care delivery.

7.3c Participate in evaluating system effectiveness.

8.3e Identify impact of information and communication technology on quality and safety of care.

8.4d Explain the impact of health information exchange, interoperability, and integration on healthcare.

9.1a Apply principles of professional nursing ethics and human rights in patient care and professional situations.

AACN Essentials for Advanced-Level Nursing Education

3.6j Contribute to system-level planning, decision making, and evaluation for disasters and public health emergencies.

7.3g Manage change to sustain system effectiveness.

8.2h Use standardized data to evaluate decision making and outcomes across all systems levels.

8.4g Evaluate the impact of health information exchange, interoperability, and integration to support patient-centered care.

8.5h Assess potential ethical and legal issues associated with the use of information and communication technology.

HIMSS TIGER Competencies

Ethics in health internet technology

Information and communications technology systems applications

Interoperability and integration

Legal issues in health internet technology

Public health informatics

KEY TERMS

Application programming interface (API)

Certified EHR technology (CEHRT)

Foundational interoperability

Health information exchange (HIE)

Interoperability

Mapping

Meaningful use

Open Systems Interconnection (OSI) model

Organizational interoperability

Reference terminology model

Semantic interoperability

Standards

Structural interoperability

Unified Medical Language System (UMLS)

> **CASE STUDY**
>
> One way to control the spread of a disease is to determine who is infected and have them quarantine (stay away from others) until they are no longer able to infect other people. Emergency Use Authorization by the U.S. Food and Drug Administration for COVID-19 laboratory testing rapidly expanded testing opportunities in 2020. However, the ability of healthcare organizations to exchange COVID-19 testing results did not expand, making it difficult to control the spread of the disease. Early in the pandemic, many COVID-19 test results were shared using manual, paper-based results that relied on fax machines, making it difficult to control the spread of the virus (Greene et al., 2021). To streamline the process of conveying test results to providers and patients, healthcare organizations adopted strategies that involved the digital exchange of health information, including patient portals and improved ways for laboratories to communicate, but there remained no national standard for how to transmit COVID-19 test results. This demonstrates the role that interoperability (the ability of healthcare organizations to exchange information) played in the COVID-19 pandemic response and the importance of interoperability for public health. Interoperability is needed to fully and accurately exchange patient data among local, regional, state, and federal healthcare entities.
>
> As you read this chapter, think about strategies for improving interoperability at the local, regional, national, and international levels. What is the role of the informatics nurse in improving interoperability? How can interoperability be used in public health to improve patient outcomes?

Health is an international concern. The COVID-19 pandemic highlighted that the entire world is vulnerable to communicable diseases. To protect the global population, healthcare organizations must be able to exchange information pertaining to contagious diseases with each other at the local, regional, state, national, and international levels. This exchange of information requires healthcare systems to have interoperability.

The purpose of this chapter is to describe the many national and international efforts to make data exchange interoperable. It begins with an overview of interoperability and standards, which serves as a foundation for discussion of the United States' efforts for promoting an interoperable electronic health record (EHR). You will also learn about interoperability at the international level and explore ethical considerations for interoperability.

INTEROPERABILITY AND STANDARDS

Interoperability is the ability to exchange and use information among healthcare systems, including between departments within an organization and between different organizations. In healthcare, interoperability means information systems can transmit and receive information within and across organizational, state, and global boundaries to deliver optimal healthcare to individuals and communities (HIMSS, 2022a). **Standards** refers to the agreement to use a given, formally approved criterion. Together, interoperability and standards allow for the type of health information exchange (HIE) required for the best patient care.

Interoperability can be achieved by adhering to accepted standards for terminology and user interface protocols. Interoperability can also be achieved by using a separate system that supports the exchange of information and allows documents to be read by different operating systems. In healthcare, the consequences of not utilizing standards to promote interoperability can include a drain on financial resources resulting from duplication of tests, the inability to mitigate medical errors because of lack of information, and a decrease in the ability to quickly respond to epidemics and disasters. Interoperability is the technologic solution to a lack of communication among disparate systems.

Imagine a patient arrives in the emergency department requiring surgery. The patient may be transferred to the postanesthesia care unit, the intensive care unit, a surgical floor, and an outside rehabilitation facility and home health agency. In order to provide the best care for this patient, clinical staff in each of these departments and facilities need access to a **health information exchange (HIE)**, which allows doctors, nurses, pharmacists, other healthcare providers, and patients to appropriately access and securely share a patient's vital medical information electronically, thereby improving the speed, quality, safety, and cost of patient care.

Levels of Interoperability

Interoperability occurs in four increasingly complex levels: foundational, structural, semantic, and organizational (HIMSS, 2022a). The levels of interoperability can be related to the data, information, knowledge, and wisdom (DIKW) model (Fig. 12-1).

Foundational interoperability is the lowest and most basic level of interoperability. It refers to the ability of one system to transmit data and another to receive the data without the ability of the receiving system to interpret the data. Systems that have foundational interoperability can send and receive useable data from different systems.

Structural interoperability refers to how the structure or format of the exchanged data is defined by message formats. This process adds meaning and begins the process of transforming data into information. The purpose of structural interoperability is to coordinate work processes. It refers to the uniform format or structure of the exchanged messages. Structural interoperability is necessary to preserve the meaning and purpose of the information. With structural interoperability, data exchanged between information systems allow for interpretation at the data field level.

Semantic interoperability occurs when the information transmitted between systems becomes understandable. In the DIKW model, when information is able to be shared and understood, it contributes to nursing knowledge. At this level, the interpretation and action on messages exchanged by two computers or systems occur without human intervention. The effectiveness of semantic interoperability depends on the interaction between algorithms (rules), the data

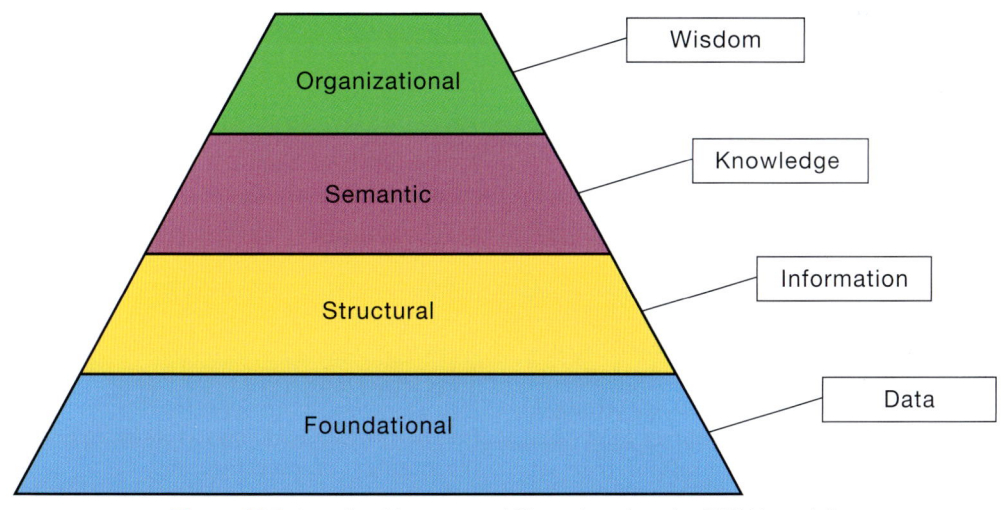

Figure 12-1. Levels of interoperability related to the DIKW model.

used in the message, and the terminology used to designate those data. Semantic operability allows authorized users to receive information from different EHRs to plan and provide safe and effective care. For example, this functionality enables exchange of data from a laboratory system with the pharmacy system. It also enables exchange of data from one healthcare provider with another.

Organizational interoperability facilitates the secure, seamless, and timely use of data both within and between organizations. This includes governance, policy, social, legal, and organizational considerations of entities and individuals that enable shared consent, trust, and integrated end user processes and workflows. Sharing knowledge on a grand scale contributes to healthcare wisdom. In the DIKW model, wisdom refers to the ability to use knowledge that has been created and applied in a variety of systems to improve patient care.

Standards

Interoperability is not possible without standards. A standard is an agreement to use a given protocol, term, or other criterion formally approved by a nationally or internationally recognized professional trade association or governmental body. Standards provide a common language and a common set of expectations that enable interoperability among systems and/or devices (HIMSS, 2022b). Standards are vital in many facets of life. For example, communication requires standards: even in casual communication, differences in language can result in miscommunication. Standardized time is also vital to general functioning. In the mid-19th century, communities could set their own time. In one city, it could be 1 p.m., 30 miles east it could be 1:30 p.m., and another 40 miles northwest it could be 12:30 p.m. Not until railroads arrived did it become necessary to standardize the time (WebExhibits, 2008).

Standards that influence nursing affect the use of equipment and documentation in EHRs. Organizations along with subject-matter experts responsible for setting standards make decisions about what healthcare data should be recorded, how to record it, what terminology to use, and what data should be reported. Organizations that set standards determine terms of interest that describe concepts of importance. For nursing, this means concepts that correctly and succinctly describe assessment findings, interventions, and outcomes of nurse-specific topics, which will ultimately support nursing's unique contributions to patient outcomes. Standardization of data that are dependent on nursing activities can assist in allowing more visibility of the nursing profession in the EHRs and nursing's impact on healthcare outcomes.

As an example, in 2016, the National Pressure Ulcer Advisory Panel (NPUAP) made changes to the terminology and staging system used for the identification and assessment of pressure ulcers and the interventions required to prevent or treat those ulcers. Pressure ulcers are now called pressure injuries, and NPUAP changed its name to National Pressure Injury Advisory Panel (NPIAP).

Upon agreement of standardized terms, standards coding organizations ensure updated terms are included in databases so that related assessments and interventions can be interoperable between disparate systems (NPUAP, 2017). Nurses must have some understanding not only of the process of setting and updating standard terminology but also of the groups involved in setting standards. Box 12-1 displays some of the groups involved in setting standards.

The Office of the National Coordinator for Health Information Technology (ONC) works to promote interoperable HIE at a national level. To create interoperable HIE with EHRs, there are four areas of standardization the U.S. government is focusing on (ONC, 2020):

1. How applications interact with users (e.g., e-prescribing)
2. How systems communicate with each other (e.g., messaging standards)
3. How information is processed and managed (e.g., HIE)
4. How consumer devices integrate with other systems and applications (e.g., tablets)

U.S. EFFORTS FOR PROMOTING INTEROPERABILITY

The U.S. government plays a role in supporting the advancement of interoperability.

Federal agencies purchase, develop, regulate, and fund interoperability technology. In addition,

BOX 12-1 Standard Setting Organizations in Healthcare

American Medical Association (AMA)
American Nurses Association (ANA)
Comité Européen de Normalisation (CEN) or European Committee for Standardization
Healthcare Common Procedure Coding System (HCPCS)
Health Information Exchange (HIE)
Health Information Exchange Organization (HIO)
Health Level Seven (HL7)
International Classification of Disease Version # (ICD-#)
International Electrotechnical Commission (IEC)
International Organization for Standardization (ISO)
Medicare Severity Diagnosis-Related Groups (MS-DRG)
National Center for Health Statistics (NCHS)
National Electronic Disease Surveillance System (NEDSS)
National Electrical Manufacturers Association (NEMA)
National Library of Medicine (NLM)
Outcome and Assessment Information Set (OASIS)
Outcome-Based Quality Improvement (OBQI)
U.S. Office of Management and Budget (OMB)
Office of the National Coordinator (U.S.) for Health Information Technology (ONC)
Open Systems Interconnect (OSI)
Public Health Information Network (PHIN)
Systematized Nomenclature of Medicine—Clinical Terms (SNOMED CT)
World Health Organization (WHO)

they coordinate efforts from public and private sectors to ensure standards are being followed, encourage research and innovation, share best practices, and promote competition. The federal government develops regulations that impact HIE interoperability and provides oversight for its implementation (ONC, 2020).

The Centers for Medicare & Medicaid Services

The Centers for Medicare & Medicaid Services (CMS) promotes interoperability through the Medicare Promoting Interoperability Program (formerly the Medicare and Medicaid EHR Incentive Programs, or Meaningful Use) and the Merit-Based Incentive Payment System (MIPS). In 2020, CMS formalized a rule to promote HIE interoperability.

The Promoting Interoperability Program

CMS established the Medicare Promoting Interoperability Program to encourage healthcare organizations and providers to adopt and demonstrate meaningful use of EHRs and focus on interoperability through adoption of certified EHR technology (CEHRT). **Meaningful use** is the use of aggregated data from EHRs for decision making to improve healthcare delivery. **Certified EHR technology (CEHRT)** is a healthcare information technology (HIT) product that has met or surpassed testing on specific standards and criteria set by CMS. The program provides financial incentives to hospitals who use CEHRT to collect, store, and report on quality measures. The program has largely moved beyond "meaningful use" with an increased focus on interoperability, though the term meaningful use is still used generally to refer to meeting a set of reporting requirements.

Participants in the program are required to report on four scored objectives and measures:

1. Electronic prescribing
2. HIE (e.g., use of EHRs)
3. Provider-to-patient exchange (e.g., use of patient portals)
4. Public health and clinical data exchange

The program is updated with rules that the CMS releases to participants. A ruling in August 2022 gave greater financial incentives to report information electronically about patient illness, injuries, and treatments to public health agencies. Hospitals that use their EHRs rather than faxes and telephone calls to share data with state and local health departments would avoid cuts in payments from Medicare. Public health organizations rely on patient data from hospitals to identify threats to public health and the inequities present in the communities they serve. Before the COVID-19 pandemic, close to 75% of hospitals experienced issues with sending data to health departments, and the data lacked important demographic details (Kan, 2022).

> **CASE STUDY**
>
> Consider how the CMS August 2022 ruling might be a response to the issues encountered in the case study with the interoperability of COVID-19 test results. How might the spread of the COVID-19 virus have been different if incentives to share data electronically had been in place?

Merit-Based Incentive Payment System

The MIPS is a CMS program that determines Medicare payment adjustments related to reported measures and activities. This program grows and changes to meet new demands. For example, in 2022, nurse practitioners and physician assistants became eligible for enrollment. Four performance categories are scored to make up a final MIPS score that determines the payment adjustment:

1. Quality (e.g., readmission rates)
2. Improvement activities (e.g., participation in a low back pain practice improvement project)
3. Promoting interoperability (e.g., completing a security risk analysis, using electronic prescribing, reporting data to public health organizations)
4. Costs (e.g., Medicare spending per beneficiary [patient] and total per capita cost)

Figure 12-2 shows the weight of the four performance categories contributing to the overall MIPS score. The weight of the performance categories can change from year to year, and the benchmark for avoiding financial penalties continues to rise.

Office of the National Coordinator for Health Information Technology

In May 2004, President George W. Bush established the position of National Coordinator for Health Information Technology, who heads the ONC (ONC, 2022). The ONC works with "public and private sectors to develop and implement strategies to advance health IT and information use to achieve high-quality care, lower costs, a healthy population, and engaged individuals" (ONC, 2020a). The ONC connects EHR systems, allowing them to securely share patient information, coordinate care, and improve patient outcomes (ONC, 2019).

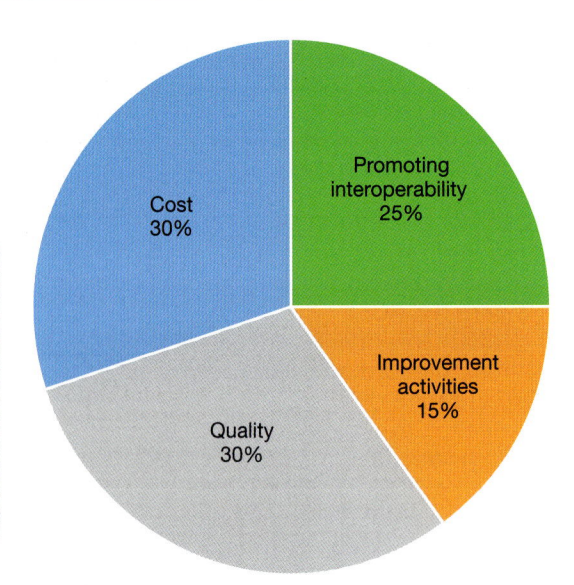

Figure 12-2. The Merit-Based Incentive Payment System (MIPS). (Data from Centers for Medicare & Medicaid Services (CMS). (2023). 2023 Call for cost measures fact sheet. https://mmshub.cms.gov/sites/default/files/2022-Call-for-Cost-Measures-Fact-Sheet.pdf)

The 2020-2025 Federal Health IT Strategic Plan was developed by the ONC in consultation with other federal organizations (ONC, 2020a). To continue advancing HIT interoperability, the 21st Century Cures Act was signed into law on December 13, 2016, to support cost transparency, increase competitive options in medical care, and develop smartphone apps for secure EHR access (FDA, n.d.). The legislation also established the Health Information Technology Advisory Committee (HITAC). The HITAC informs the ONC regarding HIT policies, standards, implementation specifications, and certification criteria relating to the implementation of national and local infrastructure that advances electronic access, exchange, and use of health information (ONC, 2022).

The ONC instituted a regulation (Cures Act Final Rule) in 2020 designed to drive interoperability of HIE by supporting the use of Health Level Seven (HL7) (a set of international standards for transfer of data) standards for **application programming interfaces (APIs)**. APIs enable the real-time connection of phones, computers, and other technologies. Examples include Google Maps, PayPal, ecommerce, and travel booking. Healthcare is one of the only industries in which individuals do not have easy access to electronic information using mobile apps on smartphones (ONC, 2020a). The Cures Act Final Rule also addresses information blocking, a practice that is likely to interfere with the access, exchange, or use of electronic health information.

HIT Adoption Dashboards

The ONC has a dashboard that outlines 18 different measures of office-based physician adoption of HIT (ONC, n.d.b) and 20 different measures for nonfederal acute care hospital adoption (ONC, n.d.a). When interacting with the data, you can choose to view statistics on EHR adoption, interoperability, patient access, and prescribing. Figure 12-3 shows the percentage of physicians who electronically send or receive patient health information with any other provider compared to the percentage of hospitals that electronically send, receive, find, and integrate patient health information from outside providers. As you can see, hospitals are ahead of physician's offices with regard to this measure of interoperability, but with the growth of federal incentive programs, these numbers will continue to increase.

The Centers for Disease Control and Prevention

According to the Centers for Disease Control and Prevention (CDC), "effective interoperability of healthcare data ensures that electronic health information is shared appropriately between healthcare and public health partners in the right format, through the right channel at the right time" (CDC, 2022). Ultimately, the goal of interoperability is to improve public health and patient care.

The CDC supports the public health aspect of the CMS Promoting Interoperability Program by providing reporting objectives for participating hospitals and clinicians. The CDC also provides guidance on implementing data interoperability in the following areas (CDC, 2022):

- Electronic case reporting
- Electronic laboratory reporting (ELR)
- Immunization information systems
- Syndromic surveillance
- Public health registries reporting

The Public Health Information Network (PHIN) is part of the CDC's national effort to increase the ability of public health agencies to electronically use and exchange information by promoting the use of standards (CDC, 2021c). Tools and resources include the PHIN vocabulary access and distribution system, which provides standard vocabularies to the CDC and public health partners; the PHIN messaging system, which is software that allows the secure electronic transport of messages between the CDC and public health information systems; and support for standards and interoperability services.

The National Electronic Disease Surveillance System (NEDSS) is a major component of CDC efforts to support public health (CDC, 2021b). The objective of the NEDSS is to develop and support integrated surveillance systems that can transfer appropriate public health, laboratory, and clinical data efficiently and securely over the internet to allow quick identification and tracking of disease outbreaks.

Unified Medical Language System

The **Unified Medical Language System (UMLS)** is a set of files and software that brings together multiple biomedical languages and standards and makes them uniform in order to have one set of terminology for anatomy, disorders, procedures, tests, drugs, and other biomedical topics. Its purpose is to unify and standardize medical language to lead to effective and interoperable systems, services, and HIE (NLM, 2016). System developers can use the UMLS to ensure that EHRs, software, API, and other HIT will be able to "understand" the meaning of the language of health and biomedicine. The UMLS can also provide search and report functions for less technical users. The UMLS has been used to develop information retrieval systems, facilitate mapping between terminologies,

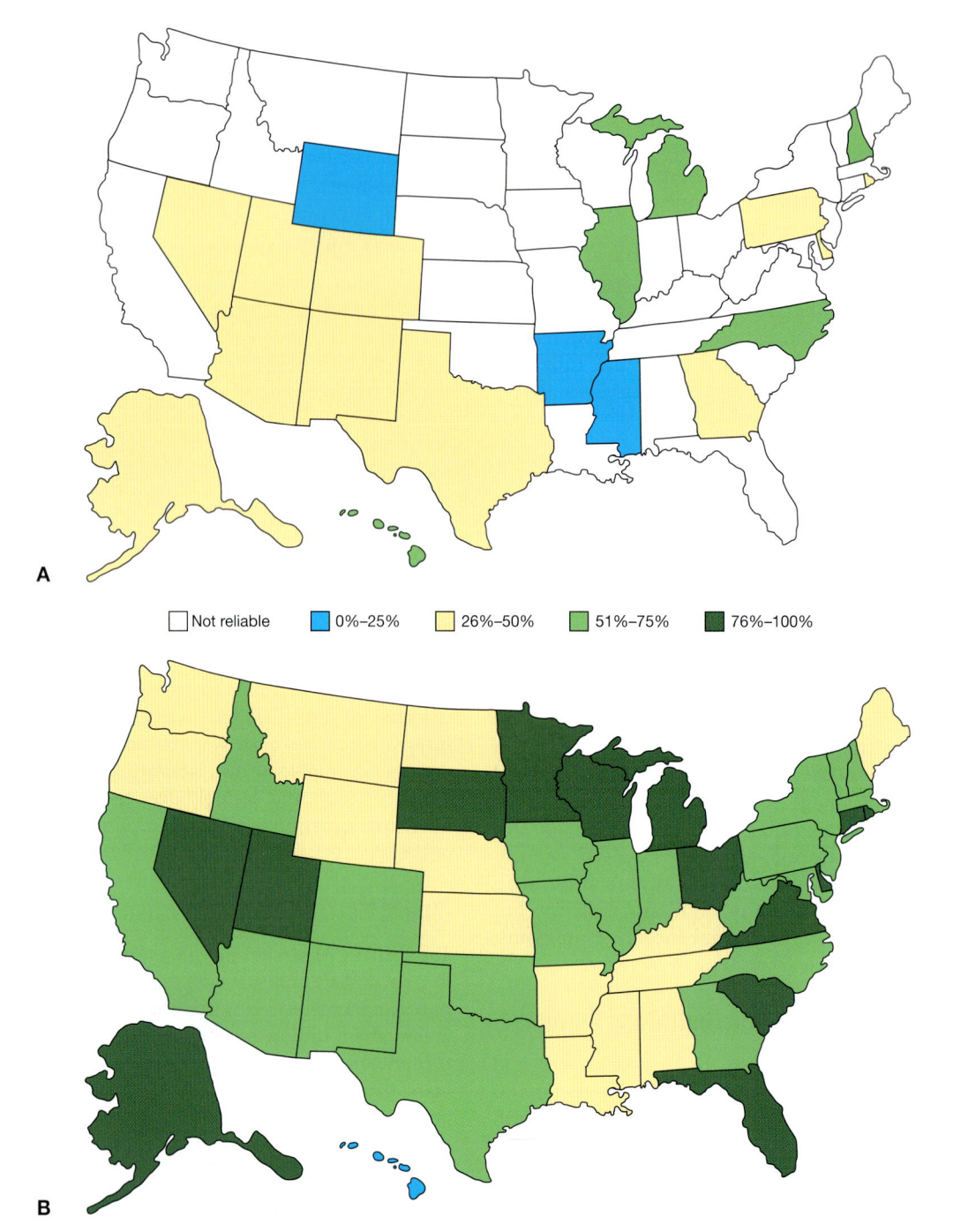

Figure 12-3. Measure of interoperability of physicians **(A)** versus hospitals **(B)**. (**A.** Data from Office of the National Coordinator for Health Information Technology (ONC). (n.d.a). *Non-federal acute care hospital Health IT adoption*. HealthIT.gov. https://www.healthit.gov/data/apps/non-federal-acute-care-hospital-health-it-adoption-and-use. **B.** Data from Office of the National Coordinator for Health Information Technology (ONC). HealthIT.gov. (n.d.b). *Office-based physician Health IT adoption*. https://www.healthit.gov/data/apps/office-based-physician-health-it-adoption)

ETHICAL CONSIDERATIONS FOR INTEROPERABILITY

According to the World Health Organization (WHO) "the highest attainable standard of health is one of the fundamental rights of every human" (WHO, 2022a). In this chapter, you have been asked to consider the importance of interoperability at an international level—a consideration supported by the ANA Nursing Code of Ethics Provision 8, which directs the nurse to collaborate with health professionals and the public to protect human rights, promote health diplomacy, and reduce health disparities. Interpretive Statement 8.1, "Health is a universal right," identifies an obligation for you to advocate for health and human rights at all levels (ANA, 2015). Interpretive statements 8.2 through 8.4 discuss the duty of nurses to engage in collaboration to advance the welfare, health, and safety of all people, promote human rights by affirming human dignity and showing respect for the diversity of the human experience, and advocate for human rights in complex, extreme, or extraordinary practice settings. This means you have a responsibility to be aware of local, regional, national, and international threats to safety and health and an obligation to understand and advocate for the interoperability of HIE to promote all parts of Provision 8. Consider how you can engage in collaborative partnerships that impact legislation, healthcare policies, and relief efforts to relieve disparities and help populations flourish. Consider writing letters to legislators and joining a professional organization that lobbies Congress for equitable healthcare policies.

Provision 9 is also important to consider in this chapter as you find ways to integrate principles of social justice into nursing and health policy. Interpretive Statement 9.4 addresses the role of the nurse in pursuing social justice by trying to influence people in power to address unjust healthcare systems. As you focus on social justice at a global level, consider how interoperability of HIE can be used to control communicable diseases and prevent homelessness, violence, hunger, and human rights violations.

---

and process text to extract concepts, relationships, or knowledge (Amos et al., 2020).

The UMLS consists of three different but related knowledge sources: Metathesaurus defines concepts, Semantic Network provides organization and relationships, and the SPECIALIST Lexicon and Lexical Programs provide resources and tools (Box 12-2).

INTERNATIONAL STANDARDS ORGANIZATIONS

The COVID-19 pandemic was unprecedented in history, and it revealed many of the deficits in public health at a global level. This section will discuss how international organizations are working to promote HIE interoperability that will support public health at a global level. Explore the Ethical Considerations box to learn more about how the American Nurses Association (ANA) Code of Ethics applies to a global perspective of nursing and healthcare.

> **BOX 12-2** Knowledge Sources of the Unified Medical Language System
>
> - *Metathesaurus*: Vocabulary database with over 1 million health-related concepts, their names, and the linkages between them.
> - *Semantic Network*: Provides consistent categorization and relationships of the Metathesaurus concepts, including possible assignment of the categories to the concepts, and defines relationships between the semantic types.
> - *SPECIALIST Lexicon and Lexical Programs*: Contains biomedical words selected for lexical coding. Provides resources and tools needed for the SPECIALIST Natural Language Processing System.
>
> Data from National Library of Medicine (NLM). (2021, March 10). *Unified Medical Language System (UMLS)*. http://www.nlm.nih.gov/research/umls/

Many organizations are involved in developing the standards demanded by the global nature of today's commerce. Two international groups that oversee much of the work involved in developing standards are the International Organization for Standardization (ISO) and the International Electrotechnical Commission (IEC). The IEC sets the standards for the equipment used in hospitals. The ISO sets standards in all other areas, including health.

An international group has member groups that perform work at the national level. There is often collaboration between these groups. For example, the U.S. National Committee of the IEC is an integral member of the American National Standards Institute (ANSI), which is the U.S. member of the ISO.

International Organization for Standardization

Established in 1947, the ISO is a nonprofit group that oversees many international standardization efforts. There is a Central Secretariat in Geneva, Switzerland, that coordinates the system, and it has more than 150 national member groups (ISO, n.d.). Some of its member institutions are part of the governmental structure of their countries, whereas others are from the private sector. The purpose of the ISO is to expedite standardization to facilitate international commerce and to promote cooperation in intellectual, technologic, scientific, and economic activity.

ISO has technical committees in many fields, and each technical committee has working groups with volunteers who do the work. The committee for health informatics is technical committee number 251 (TC 251). In 2014, under TC 251, a working group of volunteers from many nations established a nursing reference terminology model (ISO, 2014). A **reference terminology model** refers to a set of terms based on evidence-based research. Some of the potential uses for this model include facilitating the documentation of nursing problems (diagnoses) and actions (interventions) in electronic information systems. The model also allows for the creation of nursing terminologies in a form that will make **mapping** (matching concepts from one standardized terminology with those having similar meaning from another) among them easier.

The ISO created the **Open Systems Interconnection (OSI) model**, which can be seen in Figure 12-4. The OSI allows HIEs to communicate using standard protocols, providing a way for different computer systems to communicate with each other. It is a universal language for computer networking and is used by systems developers to ensure interoperability. An example of an application layer protocol (Level 7) is the hypertext transfer protocol (HTTP), which was

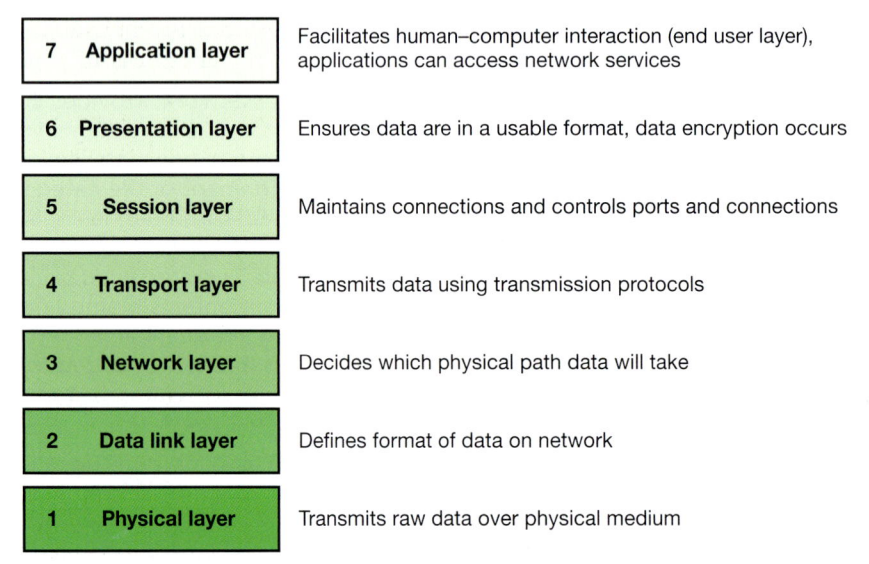

7	Application layer	Facilitates human–computer interaction (end user layer), applications can access network services
6	Presentation layer	Ensures data are in a usable format, data encryption occurs
5	Session layer	Maintains connections and controls ports and connections
4	Transport layer	Transmits data using transmission protocols
3	Network layer	Decides which physical path data will take
2	Data link layer	Defines format of data on network
1	Physical layer	Transmits raw data over physical medium

Figure 12-4. Open Systems Interconnection (OSI) model.

designed for communication between web browsers and web servers, allowing users to communicate data on the web. Level 7 interoperability is crucial due to the international nature of the internet. The lower six levels focus on the physical and logical connections between machines, systems, and applications. An example of a protocol at Level 1 are those used for Bluetooth transmissions, which are short-range local transmissions (Cloudflare, n.d.).

International Electrotechnical Commission

The IEC creates and publishes international standards for all electrical-related technologies (IEC, 2023). These standards serve as the basis for national standards in international contracts, allowing manufacturers to produce consistent and quality products. The objectives of these standards include efficiently meeting the goals of a global market, assessing and improving the quality of products covered by its standards, and contributing to the improvement of human health and safety. In the healthcare field, their standards apply to medical devices with and without software and medical electrical equipment among other things. Think about a patient with a cancerous tumor being treated with radiation therapy. IEC standards apply to the equipment that delivers the radiation, the software that determines where and how much radiation is received, and the devices that monitor how much radiation healthcare workers have been exposed to. There are around 10,000 IEC standards (IEC, 2023).

Health Level Seven

HL7 standards were designed to allow healthcare organizations to participate in HIE consistently and without additional financial expenditures. The term "HL7" refers to the position of their standards in the seven-level OSI model (see Fig. 12-4). The HL7 organization, begun in 1987, is an international community of healthcare subject-matter experts and information scientists based in Ann Arbor, Michigan (HL7, 2022b). It is an all-volunteer, not-for-profit organization that sets standards for functional and semantic interoperability for electronic healthcare data. Its mission is to provide a "comprehensive framework and related standards for the exchange, integration, sharing, and retrieval of electronic healthcare information" (HL7, 2022b). In 2023, 95% of healthcare organizations in the United States adhered to HL7 interface rules and formats. HL7 is the most widely adopted HIE integration standard in the world (Khristich, 2023).

The use of HL7 standard Fast Healthcare Interoperability Resources (FHIR) is encouraged by federal agencies like the Agency for Healthcare Research and Quality, ONC, CMS, CDC, and the National Institutes of Health. FHIR defines how healthcare information can be exchanged among different computer systems regardless of how it is stored. It allows data to be accessed securely, is free to use with no restrictions, and has the support of major vendors like Apple, Microsoft, Google, Cerner, Epic, and most other EHR vendors (ONC, 2020b).

International Classification of Disease

The International Classification of Disease (ICD) is a system healthcare organizations to promote international comparability in the collection, processing, classification, and presentation of mortality (cause of death) statistics. In 17th-century London, John Gaunt began collecting data on causes of death (Chute, 2000). These efforts led to the modern concepts of epidemic and endemic disease patterns; the beginning of the disciplines of population-based epidemiology (the study of the incidence, distribution, and control of disease); and the modern study of data terminologies and classifications.

Not until the 1900s was there agreement in medicine on standardizing causes of death. With the first ICD (Version 1, or ICD-1), the recommendation was for revising the classification every 10 years to ensure that the system remained current with medical practice advances. The Mixed Commission, a group composed of representatives from the International Statistical Institute and the Health Organization of the League of Nations, was responsible for the updates through ICD-5, a version that added morbidity and mortality conditions. The WHO (2022b) took on the responsibility of the ICD-6 in 1946 and has published revisions ever since. It was not until 1968 that the United States adopted the use of ICD codes.

The 43rd World Health Assembly endorsed the ICD-10 version for international use in 1990, and almost immediately, the WHO began development of ICD-11. However, due to excessive costs, coding inconsistencies, political and provider disputes, and healthcare regulations, the United States continued to use ICD-9-Clinical Modification (CM) until 2014 despite the fact that most of the rest of the world used ICD-10 (CDC, 2021a; CMS, 2021a).

The most recent update to ICD-11 was needed because ICD-10 was clinically outdated. ICD-11 ensures semantic interoperability and includes decision support, resource allocation, and reimbursement guidelines (WHO, 2022c). It is a scientifically rigorous product that accurately reflects contemporary health and medical practice and represents a significant upgrade from earlier versions. New features include cluster coding, which creates the ability to link core diagnostic concepts, and ICD-11 is fully electronic, providing access to 17,000 diagnostic categories with over 100,000 medical diagnostic terms (Yes-Him Consulting, 2023). The use of ICD-11 was adopted by the 72nd World Health Assembly in 2019 and came into effect on January 1, 2022 (WHO, 2022b); however, it is unknown when the United States will adopt ICD-11 due to delays similar to those in adopting ICD-10.

The International Statistical Classification of Diseases and Related Health Problems (or the ICD classification of codes) is a detailed listing of known diseases and injuries (WHO, 2022c). Today, nations worldwide use ICD to record mortality and morbidity statistics. Every known disease (or group of related diseases) has a description, a classification, and a unique code. In the United States, the ICD codes are part of the standards required by the Health Insurance Portability and Accountability Act (HIPAA).

In 2020, the COVID-19 pandemic caused an urgent need for updated ICD codes. Emergency use codes for ICD-10 and ICD-11 were instituted for a confirmed diagnosis of COVID-19, COVID-19 as a cause of death, conditions occurring in the context of COVID-19, immunization to prevent COVID-19, and adverse reactions to the vaccine.

CASE STUDY

As discussed in the case study, the COVID-19 pandemic tested the limits of international interoperability and standards. Consider some possible outcomes during the pandemic if the emergency ICD codes had not been instituted.

International Classification of Functioning, Disability, and Health

The International Classification of Functioning, Disability, and Health (ICF) also falls under the auspices of the WHO, which endorsed the ICF at the 54th World Health Assembly in 2001. ICF codes are used to measure health and disability for both individuals and populations (WHO, 2022b). ICF codes focus on the impact of disease on the human experience, including social and environmental factors. Organization of the codes is around body structure, functions, activities of daily living, and participation in life situations. They also contain information on severity and environmental factors. Although not intended as a measurement tool, ICF codes emphasize function rather than disease, and the ICF classification acts to complement ICD-10 to provide information regarding functional status. The ICF codes were designed to be relevant across all cultures, age groups, and sexes, making them useful for heterogeneous populations.

Digital Imaging and Communications in Medicine

Another standards development group that has ties to both national (National Electrical Manufacturers Association) and international groups (IEC) is the Digital Imaging and Communications in Medicine (DICOM) organization. DICOM sets and maintains standards that allow electrical transmission of digital images (DICOM, 2022). Their work makes it possible to exchange medical digital images worldwide. Thus, if you have a magnetic resonance imaging done in London, England, and your doctor is in Chicago,

Illinois, the DICOM standard makes it possible for the doctor to see the image in Chicago just as if it had been done in the local radiology department.

Comité Européen de Normalisation

The Comité Européen de Normalisation (CEN), or the European Committee for Standardization, is a collaboration of standard bodies in Europe. CEN has strong ties to European Union politics, and common European legislation makes approved CEN standards the national standards (CEN, 2022). The standardization of healthcare informatics is the province of the CEN/TC 251. There are several standards relevant to nursing including the PrENV 14032, health informatics system of concepts to support nursing. This standard focuses on the application of nursing terminology within electronic messages and healthcare information systems.

International Health Terminology Standards Development Organization

The International Health Terminology Standards Development Organization (which goes by SNOMED International) is the outgrowth of the joint development of the Systematized Nomenclature of Medicine—Clinical Terms (SNOMED CT) between the National Health Service in the United Kingdom and the College of American Pathologists in the United States (SNOMED International, 2022). SNOMED International continues to work with representatives of countries worldwide to promote more rapid development and worldwide adoption of standard clinical terminology for EHRs.

The Logical Observation Identifiers Names and Codes (LOINC) is a common language (set of identifiers, names, and codes) used for healthcare observations and documentation that enables processing of data entered in EHRs and other databases. LOINC work in conjunction with SNOMED CT. LOINC was initially developed in 1994 as a common terminology for laboratory and clinical observations due to the need to send clinical data electronically from laboratories and other data producers to healthcare organizations (LOINC, 2023).

Development of International Standards

The development of international standards involves a rigorous process. Group members of standard-setting organizations are experts in their fields who become members of a working or technical group of an organization that has been delegated to set a specific standard. Anyone who is an expert in an area and has the time to devote to this endeavor can be a member of a working or technical standard setting group. It is important to have nursing input in the development process to ensure the values of the profession are infused into future standards.

There are four main steps for developing standards:

1. Identify a need.
2. State in operational terms what the standard will accomplish and how.
3. Define terms and specifications for the standard.
4. Test the standard.

Step 3 is the longest and generally involves multiple revisions. Standard development involves a lengthy period of discussion, study of the literature, communication with those outside the group affected by the standard, and research. If the number of parties affected by the new standard is large, the proposed standard is open for public comment. If the comments indicate problems, the group will return to the third step to refine the standard. If there are many changes from the original, the new proposal is open for public comment again. Eventually, members of the group vote on the standard. If they vote in favor, the standard goes to the parent organization for endorsement. If accepted by the parent organization, it then becomes a standard with a prefix indicating the group that set the standard and a number specific to that standard. When the standard needs updates, the approval process repeats itself.

BILLING TERMINOLOGY STANDARDIZATION

In the United States, there is general agreement that healthcare costs are too high. National health spending is projected to grow at a rate of 5.4% per year on average between 2019 and 2028, reaching $6.2 trillion (CMS.gov, 2021b). The American Rescue Plan of 2021 was designed in part to lower healthcare costs for Americans, but other strategies are needed. Standardization of billing terminology is one way to lower the cost of healthcare. When healthcare organizations can compare costs, it allows for a more competitive market.

In the 1980s, diagnosis-related groups and modifications to the ICD codes were used in efforts to standardize government payments for hospital care. Following the lead of the government, many private insurers also adopted them. Efforts to standardize billing for alternative healthcare providers, such as nurse practitioners, led to the Alternative Billing Concepts (ABC) code set. The Patient Protection and Affordable Care Act (ACA), which went into effect in 2010, was designed to curb the growth of healthcare costs as it broadly expanded healthcare coverage. However, the ACA did not reduce the level of healthcare spending, slow spending growth, or decrease premiums and deductibles (Antos & Capretta, 2020).

ICD for Billing

Healthcare providers in the United States transitioned from using ICD-9-CM to ICD-10-CM for billing purposes in 2014, but ICD codes present a one-dimensional view of disease, because they focus only on etiology (the cause of diseases). An example of the failure of ICD-10 codes is that death from medical error is not a diagnostic code. If a patient dies from being given the wrong medication, there is no way to capture that in terms of insurance and billing.

Medicare Severity Diagnosis-Related Groups

The Medicare Severity Diagnosis-Related Groups (MS-DRGs) are sometimes referred as the "daily rate guide." The CMS developed DRGs as a standardized Medicare patient classification system in the early 1980s. Originally intended as a review of the use of hospital resources, DRGs became a system for prospective payment. Under this system, categories of patient groups determined the average consumption of hospital resources. The patient classification category served as the basis for hospital payment. The criteria used for assigning categories included medical diagnosis, surgery, complications, and usually age. Every patient receives a single MS-DRG based on information from the Uniform Hospital Discharge Data Set (CMS, 2023).

There are other DRG systems in use beyond the MS-DRG. For example, the all patient-refined DRG (APR-DRG) represents non-Medicare patients. Other countries, such as England, France, Germany, the Netherlands, and Sweden, developed their own DRG systems based on the U.S. system (Quentin et al., 2013). In some countries with nationalized health systems, DRG codes determine hospital funding.

The Healthcare Common Procedure Coding System

The Healthcare Common Procedure Coding System (HCPCS) is a uniform billing system for Medicare and other insurers (CMS.gov, 2022a). It consists of two levels. Level I uses the current procedural terminology (CPT) numeric coding developed and maintained by the American Medical Association (AMA). Level II uses codes and descriptors for services, supplies, and products not included in CPT codes. Examples of Level II codes include medical equipment, prosthetics, and orthotics. The intent of Level II is to supplement the CPT codes developed by the AMA and keep them current with annual updates.

Outcome and Assessment Information Set

The DRGs are not the only government attempts to contain healthcare costs. Medicare-certified home care agencies must submit an Outcome and Assessment Information Set (OASIS) data set to CMS as a part of the reimbursement procedure. OASIS is a group of data elements that represent a comprehensive assessment for an adult home care patient and the basis for measuring outcomes for Outcome-Based Quality Improvement (OBQI) (CMS.gov, 2016). The items in OASIS were derived from a study to develop a system of home care outcome measures. The Robert Wood Johnson Foundation and CMS funded development of OASIS (CMS, 2022b). The items include sociodemographic and environmental data, support systems, health status, and functional status attributes of adult (nonmaternity) patients. Individual agencies use OASIS data for care planning, demographics, and case mix reports of such patient characteristics as health and functional status at the start of care.

Federal regulations require home healthcare agencies to collect, code, and transmit these data to their state center, which uploads them to CMS. OASIS standardizes what items are collected and what terms are used. Then CMS provides the home health agencies feedback reports based on the OASIS data (CMS, 2022b). Currently, four reports are generated:

1. Agency Patient-Related Characteristics Report
2. Potentially Avoidable Event Report
3. OBQI Report
4. Process Quality Measurement Report

THE IMPORTANCE OF INTEROPERABILITY IN THE FUTURE OF HEALTHCARE

Effective healthcare communication facilitates seamless sharing across systems and standard data formats that can be processed by humans and machines. However, healthcare and clinical data often lack interoperability due to incompatible systems, proprietary software, isolated databases, and antiquated paper records. This slows progress and contributes to a situation in which data are difficult to retrieve, share, and exchange. Four areas where interoperable data and information technology systems are particularly important include big data and artificial intelligence; healthcare communication; health and clinical research; and international cooperation (Lehne et al., 2019). A fast and largely interconnected global data infrastructure with reliable and secure interfaces, international standards for data exchange, and terminologies that define vocabularies for the shared transmission of medical and nursing information would allow worldwide healthcare interoperability to reach its fullest potential in the future.

HL7 holds promise for interoperability by supporting physical and logical connections among machines, systems, and applications, and it integrates terminology, participants, and electronic data exchange structuring (HL7, 2022a). Structuring healthcare data according to international standards will reduce barriers to providing optimal healthcare (Lehne et al., 2019). Interoperability is an example of how improved communication in healthcare can help organizations avoid medical errors and duplication of services while permitting easy retrieval of patient information and a safer, higher-quality patient experience. Interoperability can advance clinical research, especially in epidemiology and public health, with accessible clean data routinely entered by clinicians and nurses in patient care or shared by patients via mHealth apps.

As you read in the case study at the beginning of the chapter, substantial delays in the transfer of COVID-19 test results caused delays in treatment decisions needed for urgent patient management. Greene and colleagues (2021) highlighted the response of New York State to the early COVID-19 pandemic. State and local health departments collaborated with private technology companies to leverage their expertise to deploy COVID-19 laboratory testing solutions. This included setting up ELR services. ELR interfaces are being used increasingly for automated transmission of reportable disease results to public health officials. Although this was a helpful solution in the case of New York, it is still small in scale and would be expensive for smaller laboratories. An HIE is a more centralized and scalable solution. With incentive programs and technologic support available, more laboratories are participating in local, state, or regional HIEs.

SUMMARY

- **Interoperability and standards.** Interoperability is an important feature of HIE that allows healthcare workers to exchange and use information among differing systems, and it has the potential to improve health outcomes, save on costs, and allow for a quick response to a public health crisis. Interoperability is achieved by standardizing terminology and user interfaces. Interoperability occurs in four increasingly complex levels: foundational, structural, semantic, and organizational. A standard is an agreement to use a given protocol, term, or other criterion formally approved by a nationally or internationally recognized professional trade association or governmental body. Changes in standard terminology impact nursing interventions, so nurses have an obligation to be familiar with the process of setting and updating standard terminology.

- **U.S. efforts for promoting interoperability.** Federal agencies purchase, develop, regulate, and fund interoperability technology and coordinate efforts to ensure standards are being followed. The CMS established the Promoting Interoperability Program and the MIPS. The ONC provides a dashboard showing interoperability levels for healthcare organizations and providers. The CDC has developed the PHIN and the NEDSS. The UMLS provides a standardized language system to unify biomedical systems.
- **International standards organizations.** It is crucial for nurses to advocate for global interoperability to address health disparities. There are many international groups and systems developing standards for interoperability including the ISO, which created the OSI model, the IEC, HL7, ICD, ICF, DICOM, CEN, SNOMED International, and LOINC, which works in conjunction with SNOMED CT. Development of international standards is a rigorous process.
- **Billing terminology standardization.** Standards in billing terminology is important to reduce the cost of healthcare. ICD codes can be used for billing, and MS-DRGs are used for prospective payments. The HCPCS is a uniform billing system for Medicare and other insurers, and home care agencies submit OASIS data sets for reimbursement.
- **The importance of interoperability in the future of healthcare.** Global interoperability has the potential to reduce health disparities, prevent medical errors, save costs, improve patient outcomes, anticipate pandemics, and fuel research in promising areas like artificial intelligence and big data. The use of ELR is a small-scale solution to controlling the outbreak of a disease like COVID-19 locally, but HIEs are a solution that can work on a global scale.

DISCUSSION QUESTIONS AND ACTIVITIES

1. Define interoperability in your own words. Search the internet or literature for a healthcare situation in which lack of interoperability could be costly, lead to adverse outcomes, and/or negatively affect quality of care.
2. Explain why standardization in nursing is important for patient outcomes.
3. Discuss safety issues associated with interoperability and system interfaces.
4. What are some positive impacts and benefits of the NEDSS for patients, communities, healthcare providers, and healthcare organizations?
5. Why is the United States lagging behind many countries in adopting ICD-11 codes? Do you think it is important to adopt ICD-11 codes? Why or why not?
6. Discuss three industry standards, initiatives, or networks that support and participate in healthcare interoperability capabilities? How does each that you have identified affect interoperability?

PRACTICE QUESTIONS

1. HIEs function by exchanging data that are translated without human intervention, allowing authorized users to receive information from different EHRs to plan and provide safe and effective care. This is an example of which type of interoperability?
    a. Foundational
    b. Structural
    c. Semantic
    d. Organizational
2. Health Level Seven (HL7) sets standards for functional and semantic interoperability for electronic healthcare data by:
    a. allowing one system to transmit data and another to receive the data without the ability of the receiving system to interpret the data.
    b. providing incentives for organizations to utilize their services.

c. providing a framework for implementing protocols that pass control from the bottom layer up the hierarchy to the top level.

d. developing innovations that speed up the processes for meeting meaningful use and adoption of HIT.

3. Which statement about the ICD is true?

a. The codes are developed by each country to assist with morbidity and mortality classification.

b. These billing codes describe detailed diagnoses.

c. They are used as a classification system for prospective payment.

d. They are used for the measurement of health and disability for both individuals and populations.

REFERENCES

American Nurses Association. (2015). *Code of ethics for nurses.* American Nurses Publishing. https://www.nursingworld.org/practice-policy/nursing-excellence/ethics/code-of-ethics-for-nurses/

Amos, L., Anderson, D., Brody, S., Ripple, A., & Humphreys, B. L. (2020). UMLS users and uses: A current overview. *Journal of the American Medical Informatics Association, 27*(10), 1606–1611. Advance online publication. https://doi.org/10.1093/jamia/ocaa084

Antos, J. R., & Capretta, J. C. (2020). The ACA: Trillions? Yes. A revolution? No. https://www.healthaffairs.org/do/10.1377/forefront.20200406.93812/full/

Centers for Disease Control and Prevention (CDC). (2021a, December 9). *International classification of diseases*, Tenth Revision (ICD-10). https://www.cdc.gov/nchs/icd/icd10.htm

Centers for Disease Control and Prevention (CDC). (2021b, September 24). *National electronic disease surveillance system (NEDSS).* https://www.cdc.gov/nbs/

Centers for Disease Control and Prevention (CDC). (2021c, September 24). *PHIN tools and resources.* http://www.cdc.gov/phin/

Centers for Disease Control and Prevention (CDC). (2022, February 2). *Public health data interoperability.* https://www.cdc.gov/datainteroperability/index.html

Centers for Medicare & Medicaid Services (CMS). (2016, December 27). *OASIS OBQI.* https://edit.cms.gov/Medicare/Quality-Initiatives-Patient-Assessment-Instruments/HomeHealthQualityInits/Downloads/HHQI-OASIS-OBQI.pdf

Centers for Medicare & Medicaid Services (CMS). (2021, December 15). *NHE fact sheet.* https://www.cms.gov/research-statistics-data-and-systems/statistics-trends-and-reports/nationalhealthexpenddata/nhe-fact-sheet.html

Centers for Medicare & Medicaid Services (CMS). (2021, December 21). *ICD-10.* https://www.cms.gov/medicare/coding/icd10

Centers for Medicare & Medicaid Services (CMS). (2022a, May 6). *HCPCS—general information.* http://www.cms.gov/Medicare/Coding/MedHCPCSGenInfo/index.html

Centers for Medicare & Medicaid Services (CMS). (2022b, May 16). *OASIS overview.* https://www.cms.gov/Medicare/Quality-Initiatives-Patient-Assessment-Instruments/HomeHealthQualityInits/OASIS-Data-Sets

Centers for Medicare & Medicaid Services (CMS). (2023, February 7). *MS-DRG classifications and software.* https://www.cms.gov/medicare/medicare-fee-for-service-payment/acuteinpatientpps/ms-drg-classifications-and-software

Chute, C. G. (2000). Clinical classification and terminology: Some history and current observations. *Journal of the American Medical Informatics Association, 7*(3), 298–303. http://www.ncbi.nlm.nih.gov/pmc/articles/PMC61433/?tool=pubmed

Cloudflare. (n.d.). *What is the OSI model?* Retrieved February 23, 2023 from https://www.cloudflare.com/learning/ddos/glossary/open-systems-interconnection-model-osi/

Comité Européen de Normalisation (CEN). (2022). *European Committee for standardization.* https://www.cencenelec.eu/european-standardization/

Digital Imaging and Communications in Medicine (DICOM). (2022). *About DICOM: Overview.* https://www.dicomstandard.org/about-home

Greene, D. N., McClintock, D. S., & Durant, T. J. S. (2021). Interoperability: COVID-19 as an impetus for change. *Clinical Chemistry, 67*(4), 592–595.

Health Level 7 (HL7). (2022a). *HL7—FAQs.* http://www.hl7.org/about/FAQs/

Health Level 7 (HL7). (2022b). *About HL7.* http://www.hl7.org/about/

Healthcare Information and Management Systems Society (HIMSS). (2022a). *What is interoperability?* https://www.himss.org/resources/interoperability-healthcare#Part1

Healthcare Information and Management Systems Society (HIMSS). (2022b). *Interoperability standards.* https://www.himss.org/resources/interoperability-healthcare#Part2

International Electrotechnical Commission (IEC). (2023). *What we do.* https://www.iec.ch/what-we-do

International Organization for Standardization (ISO). (2014, February). *ISO 18104:2014 preview: Health informatics—categorical structures for representation of nursing diagnoses and nursing actions in terminological systems.* https://www.iso.org/standard/59431.html

International Organization for Standardization (ISO). (n.d.). *About us*https://www.iso.org/about-us.html.

Kan, L. (2022, August 31). *Medicare boosts incentives for hospitals to provide data to public health agencies.* The Pew Charitable Trusts. https://www.pewtrusts.org/en/research-and-analysis/articles/2022/08/31/medicare-boosts-incentives-for-hospitals-to-provide-data-to-public-health-agencies

Khristich, S. (2023, January 19). *HL7 integration: How to build interoperability interface for your healthcare systems.* Tateeda. https://tateeda.com/blog/hl7-integration-how-to-build-interoperability-interface-for-your-healthcare-systems

Lehne, M., Sass, J., Essenwanger, A., Schepers, J., & Thun, S. (2019). Why digital medicine depends on interoperability. *NPJ Digital Medicine, 2,* 79. https://doi.org/10.1038/s41746-019-0158-1

LOINC. (2023, February 2). *About LOINC.* https://loinc.org/about/

National Library of Medicine (NLM). (2016, July 29). *UMLS quick start guide.* http://www.nlm.nih.gov/research/umls/new_users/online_learning/OVR_001.html

National Pressure Ulcer Advisory Panel (NPUAP). (2017, January 24). *NPUAP position statement on staging—2017 clarifications.* https://cdn.ymaws.com/npiap.com/resource/resmgr/npuap-position-statement-on-.pdf

Office of the National Coordinator for Health Information Technology (ONC). HealthIT.gov. (2019, October 16). *Health information exchange.* Retrieved from. https://www.healthit.gov/topic/health-it-basics/health-information-exchange

Office of the National Coordinator for Health Information Technology (ONC). HealthIT.gov. (2020a, October). *2020-2025 federal health IT strategic plan.* https://www.healthit.gov/topic/2020-2025-federal-health-it-strategic-plan

Office of the National Coordinator for Health Information Technology (ONC). HealthIT.gov. (2020b, June 3). *How does health information exchange affect your practice.* https://www.healthit.gov/playbook/health-information-exchange/

Office of the National Coordinator for Health Information Technology (ONC). HealthIT.gov. (2022). *About ONC* http://www.healthit.gov/newsroom/about-onc.

Office of the National Coordinator for Health Information Technology (ONC). HealthIT.gov. (n.d.a). *Non-federal acute care hospital Health IT Adoption.* https://www.healthit.gov/data/apps/non-federal-acute-care-hospital-health-it-adoption-and-use

Office of the National Coordinator for Health Information Technology (ONC). HealthIT.gov. (n.d.b). *Office-based physician health IT adoption.* https://www.healthit.gov/data/apps/office-based-physician-health-it-adoption

Quentin, W., Scheller-Kreinsen, D., Blumel, M., Geissler, A., & Busse, R. (2013). Hospital payment based on diagnosis-related groups differs in Europe and holds lessons for the United States. *Health Affairs, 32*(4), 713–723. https://doi.org/10.1377/hlthaff.2012.0876

SNOMED International. (2022). *About us.* https://www.snomed.org/about-us

U.S. Food & Drug Administration (FDA). (n.d.). *21st century Cures act.* Retrieved February 22, 2023 from https://www.fda.gov/regulatory-information/selected-amendments-fdc-act/21st-century-cures-act

WebExhibits. (2008). *Daylight saving time—history, rationale, laws, & dates.* http://www.webexhibits.org/daylightsaving/d.html

World Health Organization (WHO). (2022a, December 10). *Human rights.* https://www.who.int/news-room/fact-sheets/detail/human-rights-and-health

World Health Organization (WHO). (2022b). *International classification of functioning, disability and health (ICF).* http://www.who.int/classifications/icf/en/

World Health Organization (WHO). (2022c). *International statistical classification of diseases and related health problems (ICD).* https://www.who.int/standards/classifications/classification-of-diseases

Yes-Him Consulting. (2023, January 16). *Background & overview of ICD-11 before implementation in 2022.* https://yes-himconsulting.com/icd-11-overview/#:~:text=This%20release%20was%20presented%20at,implementation%20in%20the%20United%20States

CHAPTER 13

Electronic Health Records and Standardized Nursing Terminology

Kristi Miller and Melissa McNeilly

OBJECTIVES

After studying this chapter, you will be able to:

1. Discuss the history and current trends of healthcare records.
2. Differentiate between the different types of electronic records including the electronic medical record, the electronic health record (EHR), and the personal health record.
3. Discuss nursing engagement with EHR development and design including the role of the nurse researcher and the importance of advocacy.
4. Discuss the pros and cons of EHRs and solutions for making EHRs more usable.
5. Explain standardized nursing terminology and the standards that are used today.
6. Explain the ethical obligation of the nurse to advocate for EHRs that support health equity and promote the profession of nursing.

AACN Essentials for Entry-Level Professional Nursing Education

8.1b Identify the basic concepts of electronic health, mobile health, and telehealth systems for enabling patient care.

8.1f Explain the importance of nursing engagement in the planning and selection of healthcare technologies.

8.2e Describe the importance of standardized nursing data to reflect the unique contribution of nursing practice.

8.3d Examine how emerging technologies influence healthcare delivery and clinical decision making.

9.1a Apply principles of professional nursing ethics and human rights in patient care and professional situations.

9.3a Engage in advocacy that promotes the best interest of the individual, community, and profession.

10.3i Recognize the importance of nursing's contributions as leaders in practice and policy issues.

AACN Essentials for Advanced-Level Nursing Education

3.5h Engage in relationship-building activities with stakeholders at any level of influence, including system, local, state, national, and/or global.

3.5i Demonstrate leadership skills to promote advocacy efforts that include principles of social justice, diversity, equity, and inclusion.

8.3g Evaluate the use of information and communication technology to address needs, gaps, and inefficiencies in care.

8.3h Formulate a plan to influence decision-making processes for selecting, implementing, and evaluating support tools.

8.3j Evaluate the potential uses and impact of emerging technologies in health care.

8.4g Evaluate the impact of health information exchange, interoperability, and integration to support patient-centered care.

8.5k Advocate for policies and regulations that support the appropriate use of technologies impacting health care.

9.1h Analyze current policies and practices in the context of an ethical framework.

10.3p Advocate for the promotion of social justice and eradication of structural racism and systematic inequity in nursing and society.

HIMSS TIGER Competencies

Applied computer science

Clinical decision support by Information Technology

Communication

Documentation

Electronic/Mobile Health, telematics, telehealth

Ethics in health internet technology

Information and knowledge management in patient care

Information management research

Interoperability and integration

KEY TERMS

Clinical Care Classification (CCC) system	Nursing Interventions Classification (NIC)	Personal health record (PHR)
Electronic health record (EHR)	Nursing Management Minimum Data Set (NMMDS)	Regional extension center (REC)
Electronic medical record (EMR)	Nursing Minimum Data Set (NMDS)	Social determinants of health (SDoH)
Interface terminology	Nursing Outcomes Classification (NOC)	Standardized nursing terminology (SNT)
Minimum data set		
NANDA International (NANDA-I)	Perioperative Nursing Data Set (PNDS)	

CASE STUDY

In 2017, Serena Williams, one of the most famous tennis players in the history of the sport, almost died from a pulmonary embolism (PE) after giving birth. With a history of blood clots, when she started to feel short of breath, she immediately asked for a computed tomography (CT) scan and a blood thinner. However, it was suggested that she was confused from pain medication and instead of running diagnostics for a PE, the physician performed a leg ultrasound. A CT scan was finally conducted, revealing life-threatening blood clots in her lungs. About 700 people die each year in the United States due to pregnancy- or delivery-related complications, often because their voices are not heard. Furthermore, the risk of pregnancy-related death is three to four times higher for Black people than it is for White people (Salam, 2018), suggesting Black people are experiencing institutionalized racism in healthcare (Dwass, 2022).

Author Jean-Francois and colleagues discuss the potential for electronic health records (EHRs) to reduce racial disparities in maternal morbidity and mortality (2021). The authors propose that integrating data on social determinants of health into EHRs may result in improving the quality of care for people who may bear children and better risk monitoring throughout the continuum of maternity care. **Social determinants of health (SDoH)** are the conditions in the environments where people are born, live, learn, work, play, worship, and age that affect a wide range of health, functioning, and quality-of-life outcomes and risks. Examples of SDoH include quality of housing, transportation, and neighborhoods; racism, discrimination, and violence; education, job opportunities, and income; access to nutritious foods and physical activity opportunities; air and water quality; and language and literacy skills (Healthy People 2030, n.d.).

For example, when income below the poverty threshold was considered an independent risk factor for heart disease and patient income data was integrated into heart disease risk score calculations, hospitals were able to improve their ability to identify at-risk patients for heart disease when compared to traditional calculators (Fiscella et al., 2009). In the same manner, such factors as race, income, and education could be used to identify people at higher risk of maternal complications, which could lead to improved risk monitoring throughout pregnancy and postpartum care to improve the consistency of the quality and safety of maternity care for all people.

As you read this chapter, think about other ways EHRs can be designed and used to improve patient outcomes. How can nurses contribute to EHRs to reduce health disparities?

Nursing documentation is part of everyday nursing life. Record keeping is used to maintain quality and safety standards, improve patient outcomes, and facilitate interprofessional communication. Nurses are taught early in nursing school how to document objectively, keeping in mind that the patient record can be used in a court of law for cases involving medical error, negligence or malpractice. Until federal mandates to use electronic record keeping were activated in 2014, many nurses charted patient information in paper records, and some providers who do not require Medicare or Medicaid reimbursement still use paper record keeping. As healthcare and nursing transition fully to the use of EHRs, nurses can provide input into how EHRs function.

EHRs provide nurses with real-time information about patient status as well as decision support that includes access to information about medications and nursing interventions. Studies have linked the use of EHRs to increased productivity and improved efficiency in nursing. Think about how much time is saved when you do not have to look for a paper chart or look up information about a medication. EHRs can flag critical laboratory values, send medication administration reminders, and improve efficiency by providing templates or "wizards" for faster data entry.

This chapter focuses on electronic record keeping and nursing documentation in healthcare and how informatics nurses can shape technology to improve patient outcomes. In addition, you will learn about standardized terminology used in nursing. There is evidence that the use of standardized terminology in nursing documentation can improve patient outcomes. As you read this chapter, keep in mind that the goal of using EHRs is to improve the quality, safety, and efficiency of healthcare and reduce health disparities. In addition, using EHRs can increase engagement with patients and families by allowing them easy access to their medical records.

HISTORY AND TRENDS OF HEALTHCARE RECORDS

Record keeping in healthcare initially served as a teaching and reference resource. As early as 1600 BC, a papyrus from Egypt was found containing written text about a surgery. Hippocrates wrote many case histories between 460 and 370 BC, which were translated into Arabic in the medieval period. In the 17th century, systematic observations of human anatomy became popular. By the 18th century, Benjamin Rush was keeping detailed casebooks about the practice of bleeding and purging patients, and hospitals in the United States were keeping simple patient records that often consisted only of line items for admission and discharge. In 1808, New York Hospital had case reports that included the history, causes, treatments, and outcomes for patient health issues bound into volumes for preservation. In the 1880s, the use of records as legal documents in insurance and malpractice cases began (Gillum, 2013).

It was not until 1898 that providers began keeping patient records at the bedside as official hospital records. The records were initially chronologic and bound in volumes, making it difficult to retrieve complete records for individuals. To address the issue of scattered, disorganized data, in 1907, Henry Plummer of the Mayo Clinic invented a clinical record-keeping system. Patients were assigned a clinic number and all data for an individual patient was combined into

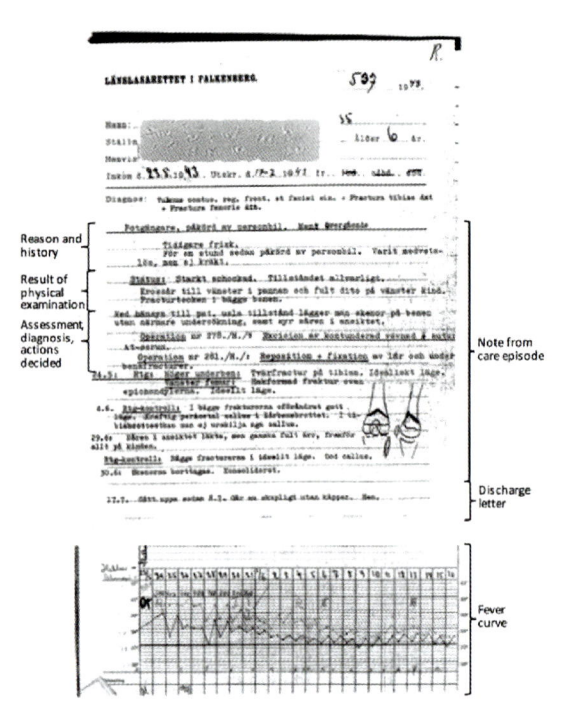

Figure 13-1. Swedish medical record from 1943. (From The history of the patient record and the paper record. *ResearchGate*. https://www.researchgate.net/publication/325122514_The_History_of_the_Patient_Record_and_the_Paper_Record/citation/download. 10.1007/978-3-319-78503-5_2. Image is licensed under CC BY 4.0.)

a single record. These records contained chief complaints, symptoms, and diagnosis, but treatment information was often not included. In 1918, the American College of Surgery launched a program to require hospitals to keep records on all patients, including a summary of care and outcomes, which could be used for quality improvement. Figure 13-1 shows the paper record from 1943 for a 6-year-old child who was hit by a car. The single sheet of paper covers the entire 6 weeks of the stay in the hospital (Dalianis, 2018). Following World War II, rapid improvements in hospital record keeping took place and problem-oriented medical information was introduced in the 1960s (Gillum, 2013).

Using Paper Records

The benefits of using paper include ease of transport and accessibility; a paper record can be used as long as there is a pen; there is no reliance on electricity or technology. A paper record requires no maintenance or downtime. When the electronic health information system is not working, paper records can be a backup method for charting until the system starts working again.

However, paper records have weaknesses. There may only be one copy, and it may be stored in a place that is difficult to access. Illegible handwriting and improper corrections can make paper records difficult to read and sometimes unusable. Paper records can be accidentally or purposefully damaged or destroyed. They are traditionally stamped with the time, leading to errors if they are stamped with the wrong stamp plate. Filing copies of paper records is time-consuming and prone to human error, and they can take up a lot of physical space.

Paper records for patients who require lengthy hospital stays can become large, heavy, and difficult to store on a nursing unit. Retrieving old records for a new admission is often challenging. If the paper record is misfiled, there may be a significant time delay before the paper record is delivered to the nursing unit. Finding information for a patient with multiple readmissions is often overwhelming and may require searches through multiple folders.

Given the relative simplicity of healthcare before the 20th century, detailed record keeping was not viewed as necessary, making paper records sufficient. Most physicians lived and worked in communities and had close ties with their patients. However, in the current healthcare system, care is often delivered by relative strangers who are members of multidisciplinary teams of healthcare professionals. In healthcare facilities today, one patient could include multiple providers, meaning records need to be shared across a variety of practices and have continual updates. Moreover, the cost of care has made documentation and communication among providers essential to the delivery of safe, effective, and continuous care. Documented care is tethered to complex billing and reimbursement systems for healthcare facilities, and care data in paper formats cannot be easily collected, aggregated, and analyzed to improve care outcomes.

Transition to Electronic Records

New computer technology developed in the 1960s and 1970s laid the foundation for the development of the EHR. The Mayo Clinic was one of the first large health systems to use EHRs in the 1960s, and Lockheed developed an electronic system known then as a clinical information system. The University of Utah collaborated with 3M to begin developing Health Evaluation through Logical Processing (HELP), one of the first clinical decision support systems. In 1968, the Computer Stored Ambulatory Record (COSTAR) was put into use at Massachusetts General Hospital. The system had a database that recognized multiple terms for the same disease, allowing users to recognize a given condition across the health system despite variations in terminology at different institutions. In the 1970s, the Department of Veterans Affairs implemented an EHR called VistA (Atherton, 2011).

The Institute of Medicine (IoM) implemented a study of paper record usage in the mid-1980s. The report argued the case for using EHRs as a method of improving patient records (IoM, 1991). By 2004, the need to convert medical records to EHRs was recognized nationally with the creation of the Office of the National Coordinator (ONC) of Health Information Technology (IT). In 2009, EHRs were incorporated into the Health Information Technology for Economic and Clinical Health (HITECH) Act, providing higher payments to providers that used EHRs for relevant purposes and met certain technologic requirements. Health Insurance Portability and Accountability Act (HIPAA) regulations were adjusted to account for electronic protected health information (ePHI) maintained by the EHRs (Atherton, 2011). HIPAA requires that patients be allowed to control access to their medical records (CDC, 2022).

As part of the American Recovery and Reinvestment Act, to maintain Medicaid and Medicare reimbursement levels, healthcare organizations and providers were required to adopt and demonstrate meaningful use of electronic medical records (EMRs) by January 1, 2014 (ONC, 2023a). Providers who did not implement EMR/EHR systems by 2015 were penalized with a 1% reduction in Medicare reimbursements.

There was no mandate at that time for the type or quality of EHR to be adopted, just that it be electronic.

Recall that the concept of meaningful use (the recording and sharing of patient data in digital format) has evolved into providing incentives for using certified EHR technology (CEHRT). The 21st Century Cures Act was signed into law in December of 2016. The Cures Act focuses on the ability to exchange and use electronic health information without special effort on the part of the user, requiring the use of CEHRT that meets international standards. Read Chapter 12 for more information about the Cures Act and interoperability (the ability of systems to share information).

Modern Adoption of EHRs

Figure 13-2 shows the adoption of EHRs and CEHRTs with the newest standards by hospital service type. Although many of these numbers are high, and despite penalties and incentives, only 40% of rehabilitation hospitals and 23% of specialty hospitals were adopters (ONC, 2022). This shows that some hospital service types are having difficulties adopting to new standards.

As of 2019, about 96% of all non-federal acute care hospitals had implemented EHRs. Conversely, only about 72% of physicians in office-based practice had adopted EHRs (ONC, 2022). While this is an improvement over years past, there remains some resistance to replacing paper records with EHRs in some healthcare areas. Some barriers include concerns about patient privacy, cost of purchasing the products, training and workflow, lack of technical training and support, organizational structure and culture, missing or incomplete data, inefficiency, and lack of data standards (Kruse et al., 2018). If organizations do not get adequate support for the adoption of EHRs, adoption can be seen as a burden and an additional expense, rather than as a benefit (Kruse et al., 2018). Chapter 11 goes into more detail about the role of the informatics nurse in promoting the adoption of EHRs.

The rate of adoption of EHR continues to grow in the United States. The use of health information technology (HIT) is improving patient care outcomes, changing how patient care is being delivered, and showing benefits in reducing waste. A systematic review of health information exchange (HIE) and EHRs in long-term care reported that the use of HIE has been shown to decrease both readmissions and adverse events (Kruse et al., 2018). In addition to improving care and outcomes, adopting an appropriate EHR has potential financial benefits. The Centers for Medicare & Medicaid Services (CMS) introduced a guide for healthcare professionals regarding the Medicare EHR Incentive Program, how to qualify for incentives, and the potential for reimbursement penalties for healthcare professionals and organizations that do not participate (CMS, 2022).

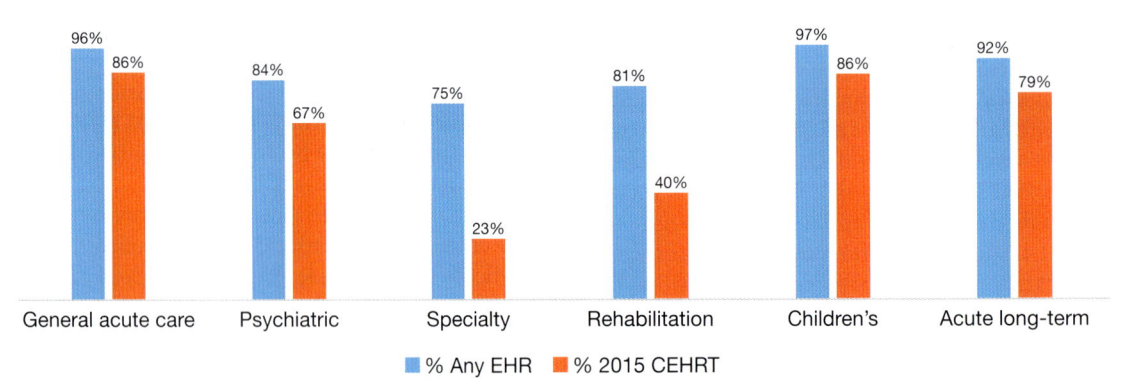

Figure 13-2. Adoption of EHRs and 2015 CEHRTs by hospital service type from 2019 to 2021. (Data from Office of the National Coordinator for Health Information Technology (ONC) (2022 April). Adoption of Electronic Health Records by Hospital Service Type 2019-2021, Health IT Quick Stat #60. *HealthIT.gov*. https://www.healthit.gov/data/quickstats/adoption-electronic-health-records-hospital-service-type-2019-2021)

TYPES OF ELECTRONIC RECORDS

There are many benefits of electronic records, and Box 13-1 lists some of these. But it is important to understand the different types of electronic patient records, which are similar but distinct. The EMR, EHR, and PHR are described in the following sections. The conceptual organization of these electronic records is illustrated in Figure 13-3.

Electronic Medical Records

An **electronic medical record (EMR)** is a digital healthcare record created by healthcare providers or agencies, such as hospitals. An EMR is an electronic version of the traditional paper record used by healthcare providers, and a patient will have one EMR for each different provider or agency. A patient can have many EMRs, for example, one at the health department for immunizations, one at each hospital where care has been provided, and one at each healthcare provider's office.

An EMR is a legal record that describes the care that a patient received during an encounter with the healthcare agency. Instead of hospital visit information being in one or more folders in the medical records department, the EMR is a searchable database. For example, providers could search

---

BOX 13-1 Benefits of Electronic Patient Records

Benefits to Physicians
- Provide evidence-based decision support so providers can more effectively diagnose patients, reduce medical errors, and provide safer care
- Help with monitoring and improving the overall quality of care
- Provide follow-up information after a visit
- Facilitate identifying which patients are due for preventive screening or checkups
- Facilitate organization of information specific to the discipline so that it can be easily located
- Simplify order entry
- Enable safer, more reliable prescribing

Benefits to the Business
- Enhance privacy and security of patient data
- Optimize workflows and increase the number of patients served per day
- Improve documentation and coding for insurance and billing
- Facilitate the process of preparing reports for internal and external entities
- Reduce errors by promoting legible, complete documentation
- Enable providers to improve efficiency and meet their business goals
- Reduce costs through decreased paperwork, improved safety, reduced duplication of testing, and improved health

Benefits to Patients
- Ensure secure sharing of electronic information with patients
- Facilitate individualized treatment anywhere the computer-based patient record is available
- Improve patient and provider interactions and communication, as well as healthcare convenience

Benefits to Data Collection and Analysis
- Allow the ability to track and analyze data over time
- Provide large data banks yielding more valid and precise research

Benefits Specific to EHRs
- Allow the ability to answer questions at local, state, national, and possibly international levels
- Provide one location for all healthcare data
- Ensure secure sharing of electronic information with other clinicians

Benefits Specific to PHRs
- Allow patients to access their records, view medications, and engage in personal health
- Provide the ability to add social health data, such as diet, exercise, or alcohol consumption
- Provide personalized information targeted to patients

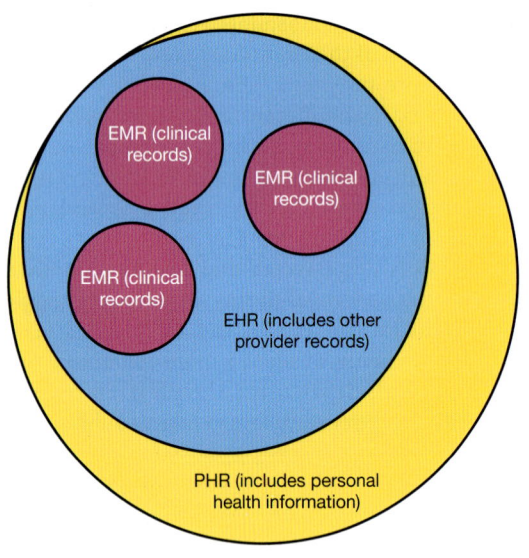

Figure 13-3. Conceptual model of organization of electronic patient records.

for all admissions for treatment of congestive heart failure or all surgeries. The information in the EMR belongs to the patient, but the healthcare provider owns the data. EMR data reside in virtual silos, which are different databases that do not communicate among providers. However, EMRs that meet national standards for interoperability will be able to share health information with the EHR.

See Table 13-1 for an overview of the EMR compared to the EHR.

Electronic Health Records

An **electronic health record (EHR)** is an interoperable electronic healthcare record that contains data from the EMRs of all healthcare providers involved in the patient's care, including care facilities, clinicians, laboratories, and

TABLE 13-1 Comparing Electronic Medical Records and Electronic Health Records

	EMR	EHR
Description	A digital version of a paper chart that contains the medical and treatment history of the patient by a particular provider or agency	A digital record of a patient's overall health including medical and treatment histories, current and previous medications, previous procedures conducted, immunization dates, allergies, radiology images, laboratory test reports, and other vital personal information
Number of providers	One	Multiple
Sharing	Cannot be shared with another healthcare provider	Designed to easily share health information across various healthcare settings
Patient information	Does not move outside the provider's healthcare setting	Allows medical information to move with the patient to various healthcare settings
Use	For diagnosis and treatment	To support medical decision making with various built-in tools
Control	By the provider	By a healthcare organization

Data from Office of the National Coordinator for Health Information Technology (ONC). (n.d.). Frequently asked questions. The office of the National Coordinator for Health Information Technology (ONC). *HealthIT.gov*. Retrieved 11/9/22 from https://www.healthit.gov/faq/what-are-differences-between-electronic-medical-records-electronic-health-records-and-personal

pharmacies involved with the patient's care. EHRs follow patients—to the specialist, the hospital, the nursing home, or even across the country (ONC, n.d.). Interoperability means that the data can be shared electronically among healthcare providers, and each provider can contribute information to the record (CMS, 2022). This is the primary difference between the EHR and EMR (see Table 13-1). EHRs also include evidence-based decision support tools to aid physicians.

Under the EHR model, health information is available from any location where there is internet access and HIE. HIE allows healthcare professionals and patients to access and securely share a patient's medical information electronically. The three key forms of HIE are (Janakiraman et al., 2022):

1. Directed exchange: The ability to send and receive secure information electronically among care providers to support coordinated care
2. Query-based exchange: The ability for providers to find and/or request information on a patient from other providers, often used for unplanned care
3. Consumer-mediated exchange: The ability for patients to aggregate and control the use of their health information among providers

EHRs and the ability to exchange health information electronically improve the quality and safety of care for patients (ONC, n.d.).

Personal Health Records

A **personal health record (PHR)** allows users to maintain and manage their own health information and communicate the information with authorized providers (Sarwal & Gupta, 2021). PHRs share the same characteristics as EHRs, but the patient controls the information. They allow patients to access their healthcare information and even enter data into their own electronic records. There are two main kinds of PHRs: standalone PHRs and tethered or connected PHRs. With a standalone PHR, patients fill in information from their own records, and the information is stored on patients' computers or the internet. In some cases, a standalone PHR can also accept data from external sources, including providers and laboratories. With a standalone PHR, patients could add diet or exercise information to track progress over time. Patients can decide whether to share the information with providers, family members, or anyone else involved in their care.

A tethered, or connected, PHR is linked to a specific healthcare organization's EHR system or to a health plan's information system. With a tethered, social network PHR, patients can access their own records through a secure portal and see their laboratory results, immunization history, and due dates for screenings, plus they can share this information with their family members (Tanhapour et al., 2022). This type of PHR is also known as a patient portal. Common portal communication functions include the ability to make routine appointments, request prescription refills, or receive alerts.

This type of personalization of information has proven successful, especially in the care of patients with chronic diseases such as diabetes and chronic obstructive pulmonary disease. Most patient portals contain some type of decision support using computerized prompts. Some provide secure email messaging features. Using patient portals is one way to meet the needs of consumers who expect personal attention. Consumers desire personalized information individually targeted for them. PHRs and patient portals will further collaborative care—that is, care in which there is a partnership between the patients and their healthcare providers. Healthcare providers and patients can view the PHR together, instead of the healthcare provider only giving orders.

NURSING ENGAGEMENT WITH EHR DEVELOPMENT AND DESIGN

The primary purpose of an EHR is to improve health. Although the EHR may also serve to support billing, reporting, data storage, team communication, or legal documentation, it is crucial to keep the focus on that primary goal. This section considers EHRs from the perspective of an informatics nurse by focusing on development and design considerations.

Complaints About EHRs

Solicited nursing input into problems with EHR usage reveals multiple issues. Challenges associated with EHR use include poor design and usability, complex workflows, duplicate data entry, multiple system logins, difficulty finding patient information, errors in patient records, too many alerts, and poor navigation (Strudwick et al., 2022). Other complaints include the number of clicks it takes to complete a shift, slow speed of use, interference with patient care, high cost, and problems with sharing information among doctors, patients, and other healthcare providers. Another consideration is using the EHR while in the presence of a patient, which may make interactions and communication less personal, leading to lower patient satisfaction. Box 13-2 gives some tips for effectively using the EHR during patient interactions.

Usability is the extent to which an EHR supports clinicians in achieving goals in a satisfying, effective, and efficient manner. Problems with the EHR were identified in all the usability categories: data entry, alerting, interoperability, visual display, availability of information, system automation and defaults, and workflow support (Howe et al., 2018).

> **BOX 13-2 Tips to Avoid Negative Patient Experience While Using EHRs**
>
> - Make apologies for the need to enter information into the EHR before you begin instead of after.
> - Explain you will need to enter important items but that you are still listening.
> - Look up and make eye contact as often as possible.
> - Learn touch typing.
> - Let patients see what you are typing.
> - Do not type continuously.
> - If you can, enter data at the end of a consultation, or write on paper first though this can lead to errors when transcribing information.
> - Do not document during sensitive discussions.
>
> Data from Peckham, C. (2016, August 25). EHR report 2016: Physicians rate top EHRs. *Medscape*. https://www.medscape.com/features/slideshow/public/ehr2016#page=1

Research has shown that poor EHR usability scores are associated with higher rates of nurse burnout. Nurse burnout is associated with poor job performance, high rates of attrition, low patient satisfaction, and poor patient outcomes, including higher mortality rates (Melnick et al., 2021). This research points to the need for nurses to engage with those who design EHRs so that designers can better understand how technology can meet their needs.

EHRs are supposed to improve patient outcomes and reduce error. In a usability and safety analysis of EHRs, the authors found the time to enter a simple order—"Tylenol, 500 mg PO, every 4-6 hours"—took about 1 minute, 14 to 62 mouse clicks, and resulted in a wrong dose or route entered 8% of the time and a wrong rate 30% of the time (Ratwani et al., 2018). In another study, of 9,000 patient safety reports, 36% were attributed to EHR usability issues, and of those events, 19% of events may have resulted in harm (Howe et al., 2018).

EHR Design Problems

In the transition from paper to digital records, the initial design was to replicate the paper chart on a computer screen with the same tabs and dividers. This replication resulted in an EHR that is ill-equipped to handle the demands of modern healthcare. Unfortunately, in the last 30 years of EHR user interface, little has changed with design and functionality, despite major changes in technology.

Vendors of EHRs routinely add more buttons, tabs, and windows to solve problems that arise, resulting in software that is difficult to navigate and is not simple, intuitive, or efficient. Administrators and committees in healthcare organizations often have vendors add mandatory fields and alerts to software that results in a difficult or impossible workflow. People in charge often push users to work with a system that is "good enough" rather than working with providers to improve the system.

Many EHR vendors have a clause in their contracts with organizations that prohibit users from speaking honestly about the system. Screenshots of the systems are often prohibited, making the creation of training modules difficult. It is difficult to troubleshoot or to innovate because so much of what is known about EHRs is proprietary information. There is no process for EHR creators or designers to discuss best practices or learn from the mistakes of others. A gap also persists between the technologies used outside of work compared to what is used at work. Work technology lags due to the cumbersome process of development, innovation, and adoption, whereas consumer products are quick to adopt new technologies (Schmidt, 2019).

Nursing Research on EHRs

Nurse-led research demonstrates the effect nurses can have when they are involved in EHR design and implementation. Lyerla et al. (2022) found that embedding policy and procedure hyperlinks into the EHR improved access and usability. In a study designed to improve discharge timeliness, Younger (2020) used design thinking to develop a patient discharge prototype that was incorporated into the EHR. This prototype led to improved discharge times on a cardiac step-down unit. Cipra (2019) was able to decrease aspiration pneumonia rates in patients who hadn't experienced stroke when an evidence-based aspiration risk assessment tool was adapted to include local hospital findings.

Positive outcomes occur when nurses are engaged in generating ideas for how healthcare organizations can support and optimize the experience of using EHR systems, ensuring solutions are grounded in a nursing perspective (Strudwick et al., 2022).

EHR Solutions

The EHRs with the highest satisfaction ratings have merged healthcare delivery systems and HIT into one department, bringing technology development and implementation together (Schmidt, 2019). Informatics nurses are needed to design EHRs because they have knowledge of technology development and the healthcare field.

Key areas to consider when attempting to improve EHRs are efficiency, safety, how clinicians think, patient care, and user satisfaction (Schmidt, 2019):

- Improve efficiency: Examine ways to improve the interaction of a new user trying to adapt to a system and use it safely and comprehensively. Minimize effect to workflow and quality of care.

- Improve safety: Add alerts about harmful medication interactions, ensure test results are displayed with the dates and times of results, ensure users are properly trained in EHR use, and maintain and update EHRs as needed (The Pew Charitable Trust, 2018). In addition, remove any clauses that prohibit users from comparing notes, testing designs, and sharing best practices.

- Improve how clinicians think: Research how the way information is presented in the EHR can affect the way clinicians think and process information. For example, using checkboxes instead of free text to summarize a patient's story affects a physician's ability to reason, understand, and provide effective care.

- Improve patient care: Improve patient outcomes with EHR design. For example, include more than just alerts to assist physicians; assistance in disease diagnosis and management will go further in improving patient outcomes.

- Improve user satisfaction: Examine how users feel when they use an EHR. For example, if an EHR includes outdated technology, healthcare personnel may conclude their organization does not care about high-quality patient interactions.

Note that assistance with EHRs can be found at a **regional extension center (REC)**, which serves as a resource for EHR implementation. Developed by the ONC, RECs are equipped with personnel who can advise on EHR selection and planning, privacy and security support, meaningful use assistance, and HIE efforts. RECs are in every region of the country. Search for "ONC regional extension center" to locate an REC nearby (ONC, 2023b).

Nursing Advocacy for EHRs

In 2009, the American Nurses Association (ANA) issued a position statement about EHRs recommending that all stakeholders, including nurses and patients, be involved in the design, development, implementation, and evaluation phases of the EHR (ANA, 2009). There are many ways nurses can advocate for more effective EHR design and development. Offer nursing expertise to support decisions about what data can be collected to best support patient care. Volunteer to be a super user and take an active role in the design, implementation, teaching, troubleshooting, and support during the launch of new technology. Propose that staff nurses and nurse executives observe workflow and technology use at the point of care to understand usability issues and barriers to EHR use. This collaboration can facilitate alignment around common goals and support advocacy for interoperable technology. Consider starting a nursing informatics council to ensure nurses are represented on technology implementation teams. An informatics council should include representation from all nursing units to support technology selection, design, testing, and go-live (Hughes et al., 2022).

Getting involved with an organization that works toward EHR innovation and improved design is an excellent way to begin advocating for improved EHRs. Some of these organizations include the following (Schmidt, 2019):

- National Center for Human Factors in Healthcare (run by MedStar Health): Advocacy group for thoughtful, evidence-based EHR design. Their "See What We Mean" group works with the American Medical Association to lobby congress for EHR safety.
- The OpenNotes project: Movement advocating for greater healthcare transparency. They strive to show the beneficial effect of providing patients with full access to their own medical records.
- OpenMRS: Community of healthcare providers working to build an open-source (free) medical record system that is robust, scalable, and user-driven.

BOX 13-3 CASE STUDY

As mentioned in the case study at the beginning of the chapter, changing the design of an EHR to include additional demographic data and data on SDoH could improve quality of care, especially for Black people. Is there a demographic or SDoH that could be included in the EHR at your organization that would improve patient outcomes? How could you advocate for changing the design of your EHR to include these data?

STANDARDIZED TERMINOLOGY IN NURSING

In healthcare, standardized terminology involves using words or multiword expressions to describe symptoms, diagnoses, diseases, treatments, and outcomes that are consistent (or standard) across an organization or across the entire discipline. This chapter covers standardized nursing terminology used in EHRs.

Standardized nursing terminology (SNT) supports the interoperability of EHRs for use by nurses for seamless HIE. Searching for patient data by using the same criteria provides the ability to determine the effect on many patients, not just one. The use of EHRs provides data from nursing practice that can be used to drive improved patient outcomes and the advancement of nursing science when data are harvested from the EHR, aggregated, combined with other data, and studied. These analyses can then be incorporated into the EHR to facilitate practice change and generate more data (Laukvik et al., 2022).

Data analysis can also provide useful information about the effectiveness of nursing interventions, demonstrating how nursing care contributes to outcomes in a way that is measurable. Nurse-sensitive outcomes are patient outcomes based on nursing practice and are influenced by nursing interventions (Veldhuizen et al., 2021). Nurse-sensitive outcomes allow for the measurement of the contributions of nurses in providing inpatient care. Examples include urinary tract infections, pressure injuries, pneumonia, shock, upper gastrointestinal bleeding, and length of stay. Nurse-sensitive outcomes have been used to demonstrate the value of having registered nurses care for patients (Haddad et al., 2022) and to demonstrate the value of mandating nurse-patient ratios (Veldhuizen et al., 2021).

SNT has the potential to contribute to patient care in the following ways:

- Provides coded data entry and retrieval for medical records and for billing
- Enables shared understanding across the continuum of care (e.g., different specialties, clinicians, sites of care, languages, systems)

- Contributes to interoperability among different information systems
- Provides decision support through common links to clinical knowledge bases
- Enables entry to and retrieval from a database or registry
- Enables research reporting and synthesis
- Allows for analysis and aggregation of data
- Creates building blocks for patient safety, quality improvement, and evidence-based practice

In 1989, the ANA Steering Committee on Databases to Support Nursing Practice created a process to recognize terminologies and vocabularies that support nursing practice (ONC, 2017). The ANA currently recognizes specific minimum data sets, interface terminologies, and reference terminologies that support nursing practice (Box 13-3).

BOX 13-3 ANA-Recognized Standard Nursing Terminologies

Minimum Data Sets
Nursing Minimum Data Set (NMDS)
Nursing Management Minimum Data Set (NMMDS)

Interface Terminologies
NANDA International (NANDA-I)
Clinical Care Classification (CCC) System
Nursing Interventions Classification (NIC)
Nursing Outcomes Classification (NOC)
Perioperative Nursing Data Set (PNDS)
Omaha System
International Classification for Nursing Practice (ICNP)

Reference Terminologies
Logical Observation Identifiers Names and Codes (LOINC)
SNOMED Clinical Terms (SNOMED CT)

Data from Office of the National Coordinator for Health Information Technology (ONC). (2017, May 15). Standard nursing terminologies: a landscape analysis. HealthIT.gov. https://www.healthit.gov/sites/default/files/snt_final_05302017.pdf

---

Minimum Data Sets

A **minimum data set** is a list of categories of data, each of which has an agreed-on definition as to what it includes. The categories specify the type of data that meets the essential needs of data users for a specific purpose. ANA recognizes two minimum data sets for nursing terminology: the Nursing Minimum Data Set and the Nursing Management Minimum Data Set.

Nursing Minimum Data Set

The concept of the **Nursing Minimum Data Set (NMDS)** was first discussed at a Nursing Information Systems Conference in 1977 but was not formalized until 1984, when a grant allowed for an NMDS conference in the United States (Freguia et al., 2022). The NMDS has now been established in other countries such as Germany and Sweden. The NMDS has 16 data elements, which include nursing diagnosis, nursing intervention, nursing outcome, nursing intensity, unique individual identifier number, date of birth, sex, race and ethnicity, residence, unique facility identifier, unique health record number, unique health provider identifier, encounter date, discharge date, disposition of client, and expected payer of the bill (Freguia et al., 2022).

Nursing Management Minimum Data Set

The **Nursing Management Minimum Data Set (NMMDS)** was designed to capture data useful to nurse managers, administrators, and healthcare executives, and it complements the NMDS. The NMMDS facilitates data aggregation and improves data accuracy by eliminating terminology variation across technologies and systems (Beale, 2022). The NMMDS allows administrators to pull together information that otherwise resides in different places, such as human resources, scheduling, and billing (Beale, 2022). By providing uniform names, definitions, and coding specifications, the NMMDS facilitates collecting and analyzing to provide information about nursing services at the local, regional, national, and international levels.

Interface Terminologies

Interface terminologies are point-of-care terminologies that include the terms and concepts nurses use to describe and document patient care for individuals, families, and communities (ONC, 2017). This type of SNT serves as a bridge between clinical documentation and the administrative language required in healthcare (terminology used by certain computer programs such as billing and coding languages).

NANDA International

Prior to the use of standardized nursing diagnoses, traditional nursing focused on documentation around medical diagnoses. Today, nurses independently diagnose and treat nursing problems. To accommodate this, in 1982, the North American Nursing Diagnosis Association (NANDA) was established. In 2002, the organization became **NANDA International (NANDA-I)** to reflect their growth outside of North America (NANDA-I, 2023). The purpose of NANDA-I is to ensure that nursing diagnoses, interventions, and outcomes are documented using standardized phrases so the outcomes can be compared across systems. They help "develop, refine and promote terminology that accurately reflects nurses' clinical judgments" (NANDA-I, 2023). NANDA-I provides the basis for most of the other nursing-focused terminologies the ANA recognizes, discussed in the following sections.

Nursing Interventions Classification

The Nursing Interventions Classification (NIC) and Nursing Outcomes Classification (NOC) systems were developed by researchers at the University of Iowa and are part of the Omaha System. NIC was approved by the ANA in 1992, and NOC was approved in 1997 (CNC, 2023). The **NIC** system provides systematic organization of nursing care treatments. The language system was developed to name what nurses do and includes a time estimate of the intervention and the minimum level of training needed to carry it out safely and competently (Rodríguez-Suárez et al., 2022). It is widely used for computerized patient records in healthcare. The classification system includes physiologic and psychosocial interventions, which may be independent or collaborative. The seventh edition of NIC includes 565 research-based interventions (Butcher et al., 2019).

Nursing Outcomes Classification

The **Nursing Outcomes Classification (NOC)** was developed as part of the Omaha System to evaluate the effects of interventions and is designed to complement the NIC standardized language (CNC, 2023). The sixth edition of NIC includes 540 outcomes (Moorhead et al., 2018). Each outcome includes a definition, indicators that can be used to evaluate the related patient status, a target outcome rating, data source, and a Likert scale to identify the patient status. Both NIC and NOC can be used with individuals, families, and communities. They are both mapped to each other and to NANDA-I. Additionally, NIC is mapped to the Omaha System, and NOC is mapped to the Systemized Nomenclature of Medicine Clinical Terminology (SNOMED CT).

Clinical Care Classification

The **Clinical Care Classification (CCC) system** is an interface terminology that was originally designed for home healthcare and was called the Home Health Care Classification System. Now, the CCC is a comprehensive nursing terminology system that includes nursing diagnoses, interventions, and outcomes that can be used in all care settings (McCormick & Newbold, 2022). It includes 21 care components and is designed to determine care costs. The CCC system is used by a variety of U.S. health systems. There is no licensing fee for using CCC, and it is free to download (ONC, 2017).

Perioperative Nursing Data Set

The **Perioperative Nursing Data Set (PNDS)** was developed by the Association of periOperative Registered Nurses (AORN) to standardize the terminology associated with the perioperative experience and support evidence-based practice. The ANA recognized the PNDS in 1999. The goal was to make the patient problems that perioperative nurses manage visible to administrators, financial officers, and healthcare policy makers (AORN, 2022).

Omaha System

The Omaha System was developed between 1975 and 1993 as a federally funded research-based standardized taxonomy available in the public domain. It was designed to enhance practice, documentation, and information management across the continuum of care. The terms are arranged hierarchically from general to specific and it provides structure to document patient needs and strengths, enabling the collection, aggregation, and analysis of clinical data to support quality improvement and communication. The Omaha System was designed to be compatible with computer use from its beginning, and it facilitates interoperability (The Omaha System, 2023).

International Classification for Nursing Practice

The International Council of Nurses (ICN) began developing the International Classification for Nursing Practice (ICNP) in 1990 to classify the nursing phenomena, actions, and outcomes that describe nursing practice (Coenen, 2003). ICPN is a standardized interface terminology that can be used in EHRs to support nursing practice and patient care. The vision of the ICNP is to have nursing data available for use in healthcare information systems worldwide. It appears in the Unified Medical Language System (UMLS) and is a related classification system to the World Health Organization (WHO) family of international classifications. A new release of ICNP is made each year in alignment with SNOMED CT (ICN, 2021).

Reference Terminologies

Reference terminologies are designed to provide a common language that enables clinicians to use terms appropriate for their discipline-specific practices, then map those terms to communicate meaning across systems. Although they are not specific to the nursing discipline, the ANA recognizes two such reference terminologies—Logical Observation Identifiers Names and Codes (LOINC) and SNOMED CT—to use for transmission of nursing data. LOINC has clinical terminology for laboratory tests, measurements, and observations. The Regenstrief Institute created it in 2017, and continues to maintain and distribute it for free (Regenstrief, 2022). The ANA recognized LOINC in 2002.

In 2017, SNOMED International established SNOMED CT, a standardized, multilingual vocabulary of clinical terminology used by physicians and other healthcare providers for the electronic exchange of clinical health information. The National Library of Medicine shares SNOMED CT without charge (Elkheder et al., 2022). It maps to most of the ANA-recognized nursing terminologies, including NIC and NOC. Because of its comprehensiveness, the ability to capture data from all healthcare professionals, and availability, SNOMED CT is an important standard in the EHR and has been approved as a standard for nursing documentation. The ANA recognized SNOMED CT in 1999. SNOMED CT and LOINC are discussed in more detail in Chapter 12.

Clinical pathways are tools used to guide evidence-based healthcare. For example, a total hip replacement clinical pathway includes the workflow expected of all members of the healthcare team and establishes a time frame for evidence-based practice to occur. The pathway provides a standard framework for expectations from the preoperative through the postoperative phase. Clinical pathways have traditionally been paper-based, but clinical pathway digitalization is an emerging research field with the goal of integrating clinical pathways into HIE systems using SNT. Alahmar et al. (2022) engaged in research to introduce automation to clinical pathway standardization using an algorithm that automates the search for SNOMED CT terminology, enabling the location of the proper terms precisely, quickly, and more efficiently.

Nursing Information and Data Set Evaluation Center

In 1995, the ANA established the Nursing Information and Data Set Evaluation Center (NIDSEC) to evaluate vendor implementation of the ANA standardized terminologies in nursing information systems. The NIDSEC's purpose is to evaluate whether the nursing diagnoses are appropriate and outcomes have been improving for patients (Covetus, 2021). The evaluation criteria included clinical content, a clinical data repository (how data are stored and retrieved), and general system characteristics. The ANA encourages nursing system developers to have their systems evaluated against the NIDSEC standards.

Barriers to Implementing Standardized Nursing Terminology

In a study of the integration of nursing knowledge into EHRs, it was reported that although the EHR provides an opportunity to reflect nursing clinical judgment and make nursing care visible, there was a lack of clear alignment among assessment data, NANDA-I, NIC, and NOC in the plan of care (Rossi et al., 2023). There are challenges to incorporating SNT into EHRs. Mapping and maintenance is resource-intensive, and healthcare organizations may have a lack of mapping expertise. Most vendors do not use a single SNT and variability across SNTs renders integration with EHRs difficult. Licensing and copyright fees are a barrier for some terminologies and assessment scales (ONC, 2017).

As discussed earlier, one of the solutions for improving EHRs is through nursing advocacy. The Ethical Considerations box demonstrates that nurses have an ethical duty to advocate for patient-centered EHR interoperability.

ETHICAL CONSIDERATIONS FOR EHR ADVOCACY

The ANA Code of Ethics Provision 9 states that the profession of nursing, collectively through its professional organizations, must articulate nursing values, maintain the integrity of the profession, and integrate principles of social justice into nursing and health policy. Think about the case study at the beginning of the chapter in which integrating data on SDoH into EHRs could result in improved patient outcomes.

Consider Interpretive Statement 9.1, which states that nurses should use a language that evokes the shared meaning of nursing by communicating nursing values to the public (ANA, 2015). Advocating for SNT is also advocating for the profession of nursing by demonstrating to the world what nurses do. Interpretive Statement 9.3 recommends that nurses work to shape healthcare by influencing leaders, legislators, governmental agencies, and other organizations to address SDoH. Actively engaging in the political process by advocating for social justice in nursing and health policy through improvements in EHRs is a way to engage in Interpretive Statement 9.4.

BOX 13-3 CASE STUDY

Read the article discussed in the case study by Jean-Francois et al. (2021). Using what you have learned in this chapter about EHRs and standardized terminology, list some ways the informatics nurse could support Provision 9. How does the ethical concept of justice apply to what you have learned in this chapter?

SUMMARY

- **History and trends of healthcare records.** Patient records have evolved from bedside paper records to EHRs. Although modern adoption of EHRs and CEHRT continues to grow, barriers such as cost, lack of training, decreased productivity, and concerns about privacy keep some healthcare groups from going electronic. Benefits include financial incentives, reduction in readmissions, decreased medical errors, and improved patient access to providers through patient portals. CEHRT is now mandated for use by all providers and organizations using Medicare and Medicaid.
- **Types of electronic records.** Electronic patient records include EMRs, EHRs, and PHRs. EMRs are records created by a single healthcare provider or agency. EHRs are a collection of EMRs from multiple providers and are accessible by all providers. PHRs are similar to EHRs but they allow patients to add their own data and interact with their record.
- **Nursing engagement with EHR development and design.** EHRs were initially designed to replicate paper records, resulting in inefficiencies. Complaints about EHRs include too many clicks needed, slow speed of use, high cost, and information-sharing issues. Poorly designed EHRs can lead to medical errors and nurse burnout. EHR vendors maintain secrecy around their products, making it difficult to compare EHR features when selecting a system. Nursing research demonstrates the effect nurses can have when they are engaged in EHR design and implementation. EHRs can be improved by making them more intuitive, allowing prospective users to

compare notes between vendors, test designs and share best practice, and involving nurses in the design process. Nurses should advocate for patient-centered EHRs. Advocacy organizations are available to make your voice heard.

- **Standardized terminology in nursing.** SNT is important for representing the role of the nurse in HIE of data entered into EHRs. Using standardized terminology promotes interoperability, decision support, research, patient safety, and demonstrates measurable ways nursing care contributes to patient outcomes. The ANA currently recognizes minimum data sets, interface terminologies, and reference terminologies that support nursing practice. Minimum data sets include the NMDS and NMMDS. Interface terminologies include NANDA-I, CCC, NIC, NOC, the PNDS, the Omaha System, and the ICNP. Reference terminologies include LOINC and SNOMED CT. The NIDSEC was established to evaluate vendor implementation of the ANA standardized terminologies in nursing information systems. Nurses have an ethical duty to advocate for patient-centered EHR interoperability by participating in the selection, design, and testing of technology.

DISCUSSION QUESTIONS AND ACTIVITIES

1. What are some advantages and disadvantages of using EHRs? List three solutions for making EHRs more usable.
2. Why is it important to capture what nurses do in EHRs? What can be done with this data?
3. How can data that you collect from an individual patient be used to improve outcomes for other patients? Explain what data you would need to collect to achieve this outcome.
4. Search the library and internet for how nurses are involved in shaping electronic health information. What did you find?
5. Why is it necessary for nursing documentation to use standardized terminology?
6. Investigate whether your healthcare institution EHR uses SNT. How difficult was it to find this information? What SNTs are used in your EHR?
7. List three ways nurses can advocate for the use of SNT in EHRs. Explain how you would advocate for the use of SNT in your healthcare organization.

PRACTICE QUESTIONS

1. A nurse is educating a patient on the purpose of the EMR. Which statement would the nurse include in the patient's education?
    a. "You own and control this information."
    b. "The data in the EMR travel with you to other healthcare facilities."
    c. "You have a right to decide who else looks at your EMR."
    d. "You can use your EMR to schedule follow-up appointments as needed."
2. Nurses may use NANDA-I to provide patient care. How would the nurse use the information from NANDA-I?
    a. To document an event that occurs during the shift
    b. As a protocol when ordering medications
    c. When identifying data to support nursing clinical judgments
    d. When charging a patient for medical supplies used for care
3. What is the main focus of the NMMDS?
    a. To eliminate variations across healthcare areas
    b. To provide a way for managers to charge patients
    c. To allow for a diagnosis to be entered for care
    d. To track patient information in another area

REFERENCES

Alahmar, A., AlMousa, M., & Benlamri, R. (2022). Automated clinical pathway standardization using SNOMED CT- based semantic relatedness. *Digit Health, 8*, 20552076221089796. https://doi.org/10.1177/20552076221089796

American Nurses Association (ANA). (2009, December 11). *Electronic health record*. https://www.nursingworld.org/practice-policy/nursing-excellence/official-position-statements/id/electronic-health-record/

American Nurses Association (ANA). (2015). *Code of ethics for nurses with interpretive statements*. Silver Spring.

https://www.nursingworld.org/practice-policy/nursing-excellence/ethics/code-of-ethics-for-nurses/

Association of periOperative Registered Nurses (AORN). (2022). *Introduction to the perioperative nursing data set*. https://www.aorn.org/education/individuals/continuing-education/online-courses/introduction-to-pnds

Atherton, J. (2011, March). Development of the electronic health record. *AMA Journal of Ethics*. https://journalofethics.ama-assn.org/article/development-electronic-health-record/2011-03

Beale, N. J., & Rajwany, N (2022, January). Implementation of a unique nurse identifier. *Nursing Management, 53*(1), 6–9. https://doi.org/10.1097/01.NUMA.0000805040.87004.37

Butcher, H. K., Bulechek, G. M., Dochterman, J. M., & Wagner, C. M. (2019). *Nursing interventions classification (NIC)* (7th ed.). Elsevier.

Center for Nursing Classification and Clinical Effectiveness (CNC). (2023). *CNC factsheet*. The University of Iowa. https://nursing.uiowa.edu/cncce/facts

Centers for Disease Control and Prevention (CDC). (2022). *Health insurance portability and accountability Act of 1996 (HIPAA)*. Public Health Professionals Gateway. https://www.cdc.gov/phlp/publications/topic/hipaa.html

Centers for Medicare and Medicaid Services (CMS). (2022, October 6). *Promoting interoperability programs*. https://www.cms.gov/regulations-and-guidance/legislation/ehrincentiveprograms#:~:text=In%202011%2C%20CMS%20established%20the,health%20record%20technology%20(CEHRT)

Cipra, E. J. (2019). Implementation of a risk assessment tool to reduce aspiration pneumonia in nonstroke patients. *Clin Nurse Spec, 33*(6), 279–283. https://doi.org/10.1097/NUR.0000000000000484

Coenen, A. (2003). The International Classification for Nursing Practice (ICNP) Programme: Advancing a unifying framework for nursing. *The Online Journal of Issues in Nursing*. https://doi.org/10.3912/OJIN.Vol8No02PPT01

Covetus. (2021). *The importance of NIDSEC (Nursing Information and Data Set Evaluation Center) in healthcare*. https://www.covetus.com/blog/the-importance-of-nidsec-nursing-information-and-data-set-evaluation-center-in-healthcare

Dalianis, H. (2018). *The history of the patient record and the paper record*. ResearchGate. https://www.researchgate.net/publication/325122514_The_History_of_the_Patient_Record_and_the_Paper_Record/citation/download. https://doi.org/10.1007/978-3-319-78503-5_2

Dwass, E. (2022, August 12). Serena Williams saved her own life — but too many women's voices are not heard in medical crises, especially women of color. *MedPage Today*. https://www.medpagetoday.com/popmedicine/popmedicine/100194

Elkheder, M., Gonzalez-Izquierdo, A., Arfeen, M. Q., Kuan, V., Lumbers, T., Denaxas, S., & Shah, A. D. (2022, July). Translating and evaluating historic phenotyping algorithms using SNOMED CT. *Journal of the American Medical Informatics Association*. https://doi.org/10.1093/jamia/ocac158

Fiscella, K., Tancredi, D., & Franks, P. (2009). Adding socioeconomic status to Framingham scoring to reduce disparities in coronary risk assessment. *American Heart Journal, 157*(6), 988–994. https://doi.org/10.1016/j.ahj.2009.03.019

Freguia, F., Danielis, M., Moreale, R., & Palese, A. (2022). Nursing minimum data sets: Findings from an umbrella review. *Health Informatics Journal, 28*(2), 14604582221099826. https://doi.org/10.1177/14604582221099826

Gillum, R. F. (2013). From papyrus to the electronic tablet: A brief history of the clinical medical record with lessons for the digital age. *The American Journal of Medicine, 126*(10), 853–857. https://doi.org/10.1016/j.amjmed.2013.03.024

Haddad, L. M., Annamaraju, P., & Toney-Butler, T. J. (2022, February). Nursing shortage. *National Library of Medicine: National Center of Biotechnology Information*. PMID: 29630227.

HealthyPeople2030. (n.d.). *Social determinants of health*. Office of Disease Prevention and Health Promotion. Retrieved 11/10/22 from https://health.gov/healthypeople/priority-areas/social-determinants-health.

Howe, J. L., Adams, K. T., Hettinger, A. Z., & Ratwani, R. M. (2018). Electronic health record usability issues and potential contribution to patient harm. *JAMA, 319*(12), 1276–1278. https://doi.org/10.1001/jama.2018.1171

Hughes, R., Hooper, V., Kennedy, R., Cummins, M. R., Lake, E. T., & Carrington, J. M. (2022, April 18). Interoperability explained. *American Nurse*. https://www.myamericannurse.com/interoperability-explained-ehr/

Institute of Medicine (IoM). (1991). *Computer-based patient record: An essential technology for health care*. The National Academies Press. https://doi.org/10.17226/18459

International Council of Nurses (ICN). (2021). *International Classification for Nursing Practice (ICNP) technical implementation guide*. https://www.icn.ch/sites/default/files/inline-files/ICNP%20Technical%20Implementation%20Guide_0.pdf

Janakiraman, R., Park, E., Demirezen, E., & Kumar, S. (2022). The effects of health information exchange access on healthcare quality and efficiency: An empirical investigation. *The Institute for Operations Research and the Management Sciences*. https://doi.org/10.1287/mnsc.2022.4378

Jean-Francois, B., Bailey Lash, T., Dagher, R. K., Green Parker, M. C., Han, S. B., & Lewis Johnson, T. (2021). The potential for health information technology tools to reduce racial disparities in maternal morbidity and mortality. *Journal of Women's Health, 30*(2). 274–279. https://www.liebertpub.com/doi/10.1089/jwh.2020.8889

Kruse, C. S., Marquez, G., Nelson, D., & Palomares, O. (2018). The use of health information exchange to augment patient handoff in long-term care: A systematic review. *Applied Clinical Informatics, 9*(4), 752–771. https://doi.org/10.1055/s-0038-1670651

Laukvik, L. B., Lyngstad, M., Rotegård, A. K., Slettebø, Å., & Fossum, M. (2022, April). Content and comprehensiveness in the nursing documentation for residents in long-term dementia care: A retrospective chart review. *BMC Nursing, 21*(1), 84. https://doi.org/10.1186/s12912-022-00863-9

Lyerla, F., Danks, J., Hajdini, H., & Henderson, R. (2022). Embedding policy and procedure hyperlinks into the electronic health record to improve practice, usability, and reduce the risk of litigation. *Journal of PeriAnesthesia Nursing, 37*(6), 778–780. https://doi.org/10.1016/j.jopan.2022.01.008

McCormick, K., & Newbold, S. (2022, May). A tribute to Dr. Virginia K. Saba. *Computers Informatics Nursing, 40*(5), 297–298. https://doi.org/10.1097/CIN.0000000000000935

Melnick, E. R., West, C. P., Nath, B., Cipriano, P. F., Peterson, C., Satele, D. V., Shanafelt, T., & Dyrbye, L. N. (2021). The association between perceived electronic health record usability and professional burnout among US nurses. *Journal of the American Medical Informatics Association, 28*(8), 1632–1641, https://doi.org/10.1093/jamia/ocab059

Moorhead, S., Swanson, E., Johnson, M., & Maas, M. L. (2018). *Nursing outcomes classification: Measurement of health outcomes* (6th ed.). Elsevier.

NANDA International. (2023). *Our story*. https://nanda.org/who-we-are/our-story/

Office of the National Coordinator for Health Information Technology (ONC). (2017, May 15). Standard nursing terminologies: A landscape analysis. *HealthIT.gov*. https://www.healthit.gov/sites/default/files/snt_final_05302017.pdf

Office of the National Coordinator for Health Information Technology (ONC). (2022, April). Adoption of electronic health records by hospital service type 2019-2021, health IT quick Stat #60. *HealthIT.gov*. https://www.healthit.gov/data/quickstats/adoption-electronic-health-records-hospital-service-type-2019-2021

Office of the National Coordinator for Health Information Technology (ONC). (2023a, September 30). Laws, regulation, and policy. *HealthIT.gov*. https://www.healthit.gov/topic/laws-regulation-and-policy

Office of the National Coordinator for Health Information Technology (ONC). (2023b, September 30). Regional extension centers. *HealthIT.gov*. https://www.healthit.gov/topic/regional-extension-centers-recs

Office of the National Coordinator for Health Information Technology (ONC). (n.d.). Frequently asked questions. The office of the National Coordinator for Health Information Technology (ONC). *HealthIT.gov*. Retrieved 11/9/22 from https://www.healthit.gov/faq/what-are-differences-between-electronic-medical-records-electronic-health-records-and-personal.

Ratwani, R. M., Savage, E., Will, A., Arnold, R., Khairat, S., Miller, K., Fairbanks, R. J., Hodgkins, M., & Hettinger, AZ (2018). A usability and safety analysis of electronic health records: A multi-center study. *Journal of the American Medical Informatics Association, 25*(9), 1197–1201. https://doi.org/10.1093/jamia/ocy088

Regenstrief. (2022). Loinc. https://loinc.org/about/

Rodríguez-Suárez, C. A., Rodríguez-Álvaro, M., García-Hernández, A. M., Fernández-Gutiérrez, D. A., Martínez-Alberto, C. E., & Brito-Brito, P. R. (2022, June). Use of the nursing interventions classification and nurses' workloads: A scoping review. *Healthcare, 10*(6), 1141. https://doi.org/10.3390/healthcare10061141

Rossi, L., Butler, S., Coakley, A., & Flanagan, J. (2023). Nursing knowledge captured in electronic health records. *International Journal of Nursing Knowledge, 34*(1), 72–84. https://doi.org/10.1111/2047-3095.12365

Salam, M. (2018, January 11). For Serena Williams, childbirth was a harrowing ordeal. She's not alone. *The New York Times*. https://www.nytimes.com/2018/01/11/sports/tennis/serena-williams-baby-vogue.html

Sarwal, D., & Gupta, V. (2021, October). *Personal health record*. National Library of Medicin: National Center of Biotechnology Information. PMID: 32491689.

Schmidt, G. (2019, March 27). *The role of design in electronic health records: Past, present, & future*. http://www.gregoryschmidt.ca/writing/the-role-of-design-in-ehrs

Strudwick, G, Jeffs, L, Kemp, J, Sequeira, L, Lo, B, Shen, N, Paterson, P, Coombe, N, Yang, L, Ronald, K, Wang, W, Pagliaroli, S, Tajirian, T, Ling, S, & Jankowicz, D. (2022). Identifying and adapting interventions to reduce documentation burden and improve nurses' efficiency in using electronic health record systems (the IDEA study): Protocol for a mixed methods study. *BMC Nursing, 21*(1), 213. https://doi.org/10.1186/s12912-022-00989-w. PMID: 35927701; PMCID: PMC9351241.

Tanhapour, M., Safaei, A. A., & Shakibian, H. (2022, March). Personal health record system based on social network analysis, *Multimedia Tools and Applications, 81*, 27601–27628.

The Omaha System. (2023). *Omaha system overview*. https://www.omahasystem.org/overview

The Pew Charitable Trust. (2018, August 28). *Ways to improve electronic health record safety*. https://www.pewtrusts.org/en/research-and-analysis/reports/2018/08/28/ways-to-improve-electronic-health-record-safety

Veldhuizen, J. D., Bulck, A. O. E., Elissen, A. M. J., Mikkers, M. C., Schuurmans, M. J., & Bleijenberg, N. (2021). Nurse-sensitive outcomes in district nursing care: A delphi study. *Public Library of Science, 16*(5), 1–13. https://doi10.1371/journal.prone.0251546

Younger, S. J. (2020). Advanced practice provider – led strategies to improve patient discharge timeliness. *Nursing Administration Quarterly, 44*(4), 347–356. https://doi.org/10.1097/NAQ.0000000000000435

UNIT V

Using Informatics to Improve Patient Outcomes

Chapter 14	Information Literacy: A Road to Improved Patient Outcomes
Chapter 15	Protecting Patient Privacy and Confidentiality
Chapter 16	Applying Nursing Informatics to Patient Safety

The goal of the Institute for Healthcare Improvement (IHI) is "optimizing health for individuals and populations by simultaneously improving the patient experience of care (including quality and satisfaction), improving the health of the population, and reducing per capita cost of care for the benefit of communities" (IHI, n.d., para. 1). The informatics nurse has an important role in fulfilling this goal by supporting information literacy, protecting patient privacy and confidentiality, and applying informatics to patient safety issues. Recently, health literacy has been explored as a social determinant of health. The informatics nurse can help consumers of healthcare use healthcare information technology (HIT) and the internet to make optimal healthcare decisions. Informatics nurses should possess the information literacy skills to guide patients and families in accessing quality healthcare information. The Health Insurance Portability and Accountability Act (HIPAA) set guidelines to protect patient data, but the increasing risk of cyber attacks on healthcare organizations puts a spotlight on how informatics nurses can help keep that information safe. Finally, patient safety is the top priority of any healthcare professional. In this book, you have learned how important it is to collect data, but it can be difficult to obtain accurate data about medical errors. The informatics nurse must explore other ways to support patient safety. They should advocate for a culture of safety in organizations to make all providers feel secure in reporting problems while adopting HIT that supports patient safety.

Chapter 14, "Information Literacy: A Road to Improved Patient Outcomes," teaches you how to empower consumers to evaluate health information found on the internet. This chapter covers the role of the nurse in improving health information literacy and numeracy, and how information literacy is linked to Healthy People 2030 objectives. The case study reviews research that demonstrated the roles nurses have in health literacy for their patients. Ethics are applied to health literacy and its role in valuing patient preferences and reducing health disparities.

Chapter 15, "Protecting Patient Privacy and Confidentiality," engages the learner in the ethical and legal responsibilities of nurses in protecting patient privacy and confidentiality in the digital era. Consequences of HIPAA violations, best practices for protecting patient data, and methods for authenticating identity are discussed. The case study explores the impact of the theft of a hospital employee's laptop and the importance of encrypting and tracking devices that contain health-related information.

Chapter 16, "Applying Nursing Informatics to Patient Safety," includes a case study about a nurse who was criminally prosecuted for making a medical error that resulted in the death of a patient. This chapter discusses the application of informatics to patient safety principles including medical errors, measuring patient safety, preventing errors, HIT for error prevention, and embracing a culture of safety. This chapter draws from all previous chapters to bring informatics skills and competencies together. Ethical considerations of the nurse's duty to promote a culture of safety, act on questionable practice, advocate for addressing unethical practices, and supporting a hospitable work environment are discussed.

REFERENCE

Institute for Healthcare Improvement (IHI). (n.d.). *Triple aim and population health*. https://www.ihi.org/improvement-areas/triple-aim-population-health

CHAPTER 14

Information Literacy: A Road to Improved Patient Outcomes

Sally M. Villaseñor and Kristi S. Miller

OBJECTIVES

After studying this chapter, you will be able to:

1. Interpret the relationships among information literacy, health literacy, and information technology skills.
2. Analyze the effects of health literacy and health numeracy on patient care and teaching.
3. Describe ways in which literacy issues can be addressed with communication and cultural competence.
4. Analyze the effect of consumer empowerment on healthcare.
5. Describe the approaches to guiding healthcare consumers to high-quality, web-based health information and avoidance of misinformation.

AACN Essentials for Entry-Level Professional Nursing Education

2.8a Assist the individual to engage in self-care management.

2.2e Use evidence-based patient teaching materials, considering health literacy, vision, hearing, and cultural sensitivity.

8.2d Demonstrate the appropriate use of health information literacy assessments and improvement strategies.

8.3a Demonstrate appropriate use of information and communication technologies.

8.5a Identify common risks associated with using information and communication technology.

8.5e Discuss how clinical judgment and critical thinking must prevail in the presence of information and communication technologies.

9.1a Apply principles of professional nursing ethics and human rights in patient care and professional situations.

AACN Essentials for Advanced-Level Nursing Education

2.4g Integrate advanced scientific knowledge to guide decision making. 8.2d: Demonstrate the appropriate use of health information literacy assessments and improvement strategies.

2.8f Develop strategies that promote self-care management.

2.8g Incorporate the use of current and emerging technologies to support self-care management.

8.2g Evaluate the use of communication technology to improve consumer health information literacy.

8.5h Assess potential ethical and legal issues associated with the use of information and communication technology.

HIMSS TIGER Competencies

Electronic/Mobile Health

Ethics in health internet technology

Information and Communication Systems Applications

Information Management Research

Information and Knowledge Management in Patient Care

Quality and Safety Management

Teaching, training, education

KEY TERMS

- Accessibility
- Actionability
- Alt tags
- Braille reader
- Consumer informatics
- Cultural competence
- Cyberchondria
- Flesch Reading Ease
- Flesch–Kincaid Grade Level
- Health literacy
- Health numeracy
- Information literacy
- Information technology skills
- Literacy assessment tools
- Organizational health literacy (OHL)
- Personal health literacy
- Readability
- Screen reader
- Social determinants of health (SDoH)
- Understandability
- Usability

CASE STUDY

A group of researchers conducted a scoping review of the role of nurses in supporting health literacy (Wilandika et al., 2023). A scoping review is a systematic literature review that identifies an emerging body of literature on a given topic and identifies gaps or needs. In their review, the researchers found 13 articles that discussed health literacy related to nursing practice in clinical and community settings, as well as in schools of nursing. They found that nurses act in a supportive role as caregivers, facilitators, and educators to help patients achieve health literacy to improve their health and well-being. Nurses can improve the health literacy skills of their patients by making health information easier to understand, access, utilize, and evaluate. Nurses

> should consider health literacy when planning and delivering healthcare to address imbalances in health equity and improve the quality of care for all patients (Wilandika et al., 2023).
>
> As you read this chapter, think about strategies for assessing and improving information literacy, specifically health literacy, to empower patients and communities. Identify strengths, opportunities, and limitations for each solution. Think about the role of the nurse informaticist in identifying and improving information and health literacy.

Information literacy refers to the awareness that there is need-to-know information and the ability to find it, analyze it for validity and relevance, and interpret it for use. Another definition is "the ability to think critically and make balanced judgements about information we find and use" (CILIP, 2018). One especially important type of information literacy is **health literacy**, which refers to the ability of individuals to locate, analyze, and interpret information specifically related to health and healthcare. Health literacy includes interactive communication between the individual and the health professional as a way of obtaining and understanding health-related information. Health literacy challenges include reading nutrition labels, following discharge instructions, taking prescribed medications, and following immunization schedules. Strong information literacy is needed for strong health literacy, and an individual's level of health literacy can have significant bearing on their health outcomes. Health literacy is recognized as a social determinant of health (SDoH) based on its effect on health outcomes, and the link between poor health outcomes and health literacy is well researched.

In the United States, 88% of adults have health literacy issues, with those older than 65 having the lowest levels of health literacy (Kutner, et al., 2006; Lopez et al., 2022). A report by the Milken Institute found that 42% of people reporting poor health have below-basic knowledge of health literacy (Lopez et al., 2022). Poor health literacy makes it difficult to engage in preventing behaviors and results in poor adherence to recommended interventions and poor self-care. Those with low health literacy are more likely to be admitted for longer hospital stays, be readmitted, and undergo unnecessary visits to the emergency room (Lopez et al., 2022).

Information technology skills, another important aspect of information literacy, relate to skills with information in all its forms: digital, data, visual, written, and verbal. Information technology skills and information literacy overlap with other literacies and are used in everyday life, education, the workplace, and healthcare.

This chapter discusses information literacy and health literacy and how they can be leveraged to improve patient outcomes.

INFORMATION LITERACY IN HEALTHCARE

Nurses play a primary role in patient education. Empowering patients by helping them find reliable sources of information for the management of health conditions, preventative care, and aging is vital to patients' active participation and dialogue with healthcare professionals. To support their patients' health literacy, nurses and others in healthcare need strong information literacy skills themselves. Nurses learn this role in baccalaureate and graduate programs, and it is later reinforced in clinical practice. The emphasis on information literacy across nursing and the healthcare field is increasing.

In addition, health literacy skills are required for generating, using, and translating nursing research. Using information from literature searches changes clinical decisions and clinical practice policies. Literature findings provide information to justify, question, and improve patient care. Synthesis of literature findings, such as those found in the case study, supports positive patient care outcomes and leads to new knowledge, design of solutions, implementation, and evaluation methods. In addition, knowledge from literature findings helps the nurse empower healthcare consumers to become partners in their own care.

Information Literacy Competencies for Nurses

In 2013, the Association of Colleges and Research Libraries (ACRL) approved the Information Literacy Competency Standards for Nursing. They are based on research on the information literacy needs of nursing students preparing to enter the nursing workforce. First published in 2000, these standards provide colleges and universities with tools to position information literacy as an essential learning outcome. These standards address skills needed by nursing students at the associate, baccalaureate, master's, and doctoral levels, as well as for nursing faculty and librarians who support nursing programs. These skills can also be used for continuing education in the nursing profession (ACRL, 2013).

The ACRL standards encourage the use of a common language to discuss information-seeking skills. They can be used to guide librarians and faculty to create learning activities that support the growth of information literacy skills and provide student competencies for curriculum committees. Information Literacy Competency Standards for Nursing include five standards for the information-literate nurse, which are found in Box 14-1 (ACRL, 2013).

Nursing Organizations Promoting Literacy

Several nursing organizations emphasize the importance of information literacy. The American Associations of Colleges of Nursing (AACN) included information literacy in Competency 8.2 of the Essentials. In Subcompetency 8.2d, entry-level students are to use health information literacy assessments and improvement strategies (AACN, 2021) appropriately. In Subcompetency 8.2g, advanced-level nurses should be able to evaluate communication technology used to improve consumer health information literacy (AACN, 2021). The Essentials are used as a roadmap for planning entry- and advanced-level nursing education.

The National League for Nurses (NLN) supports the use of information and healthcare technologies and suggests that faculty should develop their own technologic skills and knowledge and "create clinical experiences for students to assess consumer eHealth literacy and assist patients to translate data for meaningful use" (NLN, 2015). The American Academy of Nursing (AAN) issued a policy brief endorsing health literacy policies, strategies, and initiatives. The brief details multiple recommendations including global use of health literacy universal precautions, collaboration with national healthcare organizations, development of financial incentives for the use of evidence-based models, and advocacy for funding to evaluate health literacy programs in education, practice, and systems of care (Loan et al., 2018). These recommendations align with the AAN's mission to "improve health and achieve health equity by impacting policy through nursing leadership, innovation, and science" (AAN, 2020).

Interprofessional organizations such as the Technology Informatics Guiding Education Reform (TIGER) International Competency Synthesis Project (2020) recognized information and knowledge management as a core competency of clinical nursing, quality management, and coordination of interprofessional care. The Healthcare Information and Management Systems Society (HIMSS) is a global advisor, thought leader, and member-based society committed to reforming the global health ecosystem through the power of information and technology (HIMSS, 2022). The Agency for Healthcare Research and Quality (AHRQ) and the Institute for Healthcare Improvement (IHI) both endorse the use of available resources such as the Health Literacy Universal Precaution Toolkit (Brega et al., 2015). Universal precautions assume that anyone may have difficulty with understanding health information and accessing services. The toolkit provides guidance on improving patient health literacy.

HEALTH LITERACY

The benefit that consumers gain from all the information available today depends not only on its quality and availability but also on the consumer's health literacy. Health literacy includes the capacity to understand instructions on prescription drug bottles, appointment slips, medical education brochures, provider directions, consent forms, and the ability to negotiate complex healthcare systems (NNLM, 2021).

BOX 14-1 Information Literacy Competency Standards for Nursing

Standard 1
The information-literate nurse determines the nature and extent of the information needed by:
- defining and articulating the need for information.
- identifying a variety of types and formats of potential sources for information.
- having a working knowledge of the literature in nursing-related fields and how it is produced.
- considering the costs and benefits of acquiring the needed information.

Standard 2
The information-literate nurse accesses the needed information effectively and efficiently by:
- selecting the most appropriate investigative methods or information retrieval systems for accessing the needed information.
- constructing and implementing efficient and effectively designed search strategies.
- retrieving information online or in person using a variety of methods.
- refining the search strategy if necessary.
- extracting, recording, and managing the information and its sources.

Standard 3
The information-literate nurse critically evaluates the procured information and its sources, and as a result, decides whether to modify the initial query and/or seek additional sources and whether to develop a new research process by:
- summarizing the main ideas to be extracted from the information gathered.
- selecting information by articulating and applying criteria for evaluating both the information and its sources.
- synthesizing main ideas to construct new concepts.
- comparing new knowledge with prior knowledge and determining the value added, contradictions, or other unique characteristics of the information.
- validating understanding and interpretation of the information through discourse with other individuals, subject area experts, and/or practitioners.
- determining whether the initial query should be revised.
- evaluating the procured information and the entire process.

Standard 4
The information-literate nurse uses information effectively to accomplish a specific purpose by:
- applying new and prior information to the planning and creation of a particular product.
- revising the development process for the product.
- communicating the product effectively to others.

Standard 5
The information-literate nurse understands many of the economic, legal, and social issues surrounding the use of information and accesses and uses information ethically and legally by:
- understanding many of the ethical, legal, and socioeconomic issues surrounding information and information technology.
- following laws, regulations, institutional policies, and etiquette related to the access and use of information resources.
- acknowledging the use of information sources in communicating the product or performance.

Adapted from Association of College and Research Libraries (ACRL). (2013). Information literacy competency standards for nursing. https://www.ala.org/acrl/standards/nursing

Healthy People 2030 is a government initiative that sets data-driven national objectives to improve the health and well-being of Americans over the next decade. It includes 358 measurable objectives developed by the U.S. Department of Health and Human Services (HHS) to improve health and well-being in the United States by 2030 (HHS, 2022b), and it plays a role in defining the concept of health literacy on a national level. One of the initiative's overarching goals includes the focus, "Eliminate health disparities, achieve health equity, and attain health literacy to improve the health and well-being of all" (HHS, 2022b). For the development of Healthy People 2030, an independent advisory committee of national health experts updated the 20-year-old definition of health literacy to include definitions of personal health literacy and organizational health literacy.

Personal health literacy is the ability of individuals to find, understand, and use information to make health-related decisions for themselves and others. **Organizational health literacy (OHL)** is the degree to which organizations equitably enable individuals to have personal health literacy (Santana et al., 2021). These definitions emphasize aligning information with a broader systems-level engagement (Parker & Ratzan, 2019). In other words, organizations that pursue OHL make accessing appropriate healthcare easier for patients by making changes to improve communication and help patients find their way around the healthcare system, become engaged in the healthcare process, and manage their own health.

In general, consumers who have good health literacy can manage their health more effectively; however, the global COVID-19 pandemic revealed that low health literacy is a persistent public concern (Paakkari & Okan, 2020). Professionals have a crucial role in advocating for, supporting, and enabling information literacy (CILIP, 2018). Health literacy matters to nurses because it helps support patient participation in preventative care and helps advance personal health goals. Box 14-2 lists skills required for good health literacy.

Health Literacy Movement

The current health literacy movement began when President George H. Bush signed the National Literacy Act in 1991, which addressed reading, writing, and arithmetic, the foundations of functional literacy. President Bush commissioned the U.S. Department of Education to conduct the National Health Literacy Survey in 1992 (U.S. Department of Education, 2002). The survey results demonstrated a significant health literacy concern, with almost one-fifth of the respondents having "very low" health literacy skills. President Bill Clinton addressed health literacy by issuing two executive orders (in 1993 and 1996) that stated regulations must be simple and easy to understand and must use clear language.

In 2004, the Institute of Medicine (IOM) reported that almost half of all Americans had difficulty understanding health information,

---

BOX 14-2 Skills Needed for Health Literacy

Some of the specific health literacy requirements may include:
- Evaluating information for credibility and quality
- Analyzing relative risks and benefits
- Calculating medication dosages (and dosing intervals)
- Interpreting test results
- Locating health information

To accomplish these tasks, individuals may need to be:
- Visually literate (able to understand graphs or other visual information)
- Computer-literate (able to operate a computer)
- Information-literate (able to obtain and apply relevant information)
- Numerically or computationally literate (able to calculate or reason numerically)
- Internet-literate (able to search the internet and evaluate websites)
- Able to articulate their health concerns and describe their symptoms accurately
- Able to ask pertinent questions
- Able to understand spoken medical advice or treatment directions

Data from National Networks of Libraries of Medicine (NNLM). (2021, December 17). An introduction to health literacy. What is health literacy? http://nnlm.gov/outreach/consumer/hlthlit.html

resulting in unnecessary spending of billions of dollars (Nielsen-Bohlman et al., 2004). The IOM concluded that national goals for improving healthcare quality and reducing health disparities would need to include improvements in health literacy. In 2010, President Barack Obama signed the Plain Writing Act, which prompted significant revision of written resources about health information from federal government agencies. This is also when Healthy People changed its overarching goals to include the elimination of health disparities, rather than just reducing them. The Healthy People health literacy workgroup developed the National Action Plan to Improve Health Literacy in 2010 (HHS, 2021).

In Healthy People 2020, the widely cited definition of "personal health literacy" included additional directives to achieve health equity and promote healthy behaviors (HHS, 2021). The definition of health literacy continues to evolve to include the environment surrounding the population of interest. Healthy People 2030 now includes a definition of organizational health literacy, leading to initiatives to train healthcare providers on topics like culturally appropriate care and how to leverage existing community resources (HHS, 2022b). Effective healthcare information must be tailored to the needs of patients and designed to engage their attention (Lopez et al., 2022). See Box 14-3 for a list of Healthy People 2030 objectives related to health literacy. Nursing interventions can directly affect many of these.

Read the Ethical Considerations box later in the chapter about how the American Nurses Association (ANA) Nursing Code of Ethics relates to health literacy.

Health Literacy and Numeracy Surveys

Literacy is an antecedent to health literacy. In 1992, the U.S. Department of Education surveyed over 26,000 adults using the National Adult Literacy Survey (Kirsch et al., 1993). The survey results revealed that 40 to 44 million people had very low literacy skills. To address the literacy issue and improve patient outcomes, the report of the National Work Group on Literacy and Health in 1998 recommended patient education materials be written at no higher than a fifth grade reading level (Wilson, 2009).

> **BOX 14-3** Healthy People 2030 Objectives Related to Health Literacy
>
> - Increase the proportion of adults whose health care provider checked their understanding.
> - Decrease the proportion of adults who report poor communication with their health care provider.
> - Increase the proportion of adults whose health care providers involved them in decisions as much as they wanted.
> - Increase the proportion of people who say their online medical record is easy to understand.
> - Increase the proportion of adults with limited English proficiency who say their providers explain things clearly.
> - Increase the health literacy of the population.
>
> From U.S. Department of Health and Human Services (HHS). (2022). Health Literacy in Healthy People 2030. *Healthypeople.gov*. https://health.gov/healthypeople/priority-areas/health-literacy-healthy-people-2030

Several other national and international surveys followed the 1992 survey. The Adult Literacy and Life Skills (ALL) survey was conducted in 2003 and again in 2006 to 2008. The ALL survey included 19,000 adults 16 years and older, representing those living in their homes and in some prisons from all states, including Washington, D.C. As the first survey to include questions on health literacy, it became a landmark survey. The 2003 ALL survey results showed that adults 65 or older had lower average literacy skills than any other age group; nearly 60% had basic or below basic skills (Kutner et al., 2006).

The most recent literacy survey is the Program for the International Assessment of Adult Competencies (PIAAC) (NCES, n.d.a). This survey was conducted in 39 countries from 2012 to 2017. The survey included literacy and numeracy as well as other cognitive and workplace skills, such as use of information and communications technology. **Health numeracy** is the consumer's ability to interpret and act on numerical information, such as graphical and probabilistic information, needed to make effective health decisions (CDC, 2022). Examples of health numeracy include calculating medication schedules, interpreting laboratory values and food labels, and understanding charts (Stagliano & Wallace, 2013).

On the PIAAC survey of literacy, the United States scored 272, above the international average of 267. On numeracy, the United States scored 257, below the international average of 263 (NCES, n.d.b). It is clear from the results that the United States faces significant challenges with numeracy, a skill necessary to understand decisions related to medical care. A new cycle of the PIAAC survey with updated study instruments started in 2022 with results expected in 2024 before the time of printing of this text.

Factors that Affect Health Literacy

Many factors can influence an individual's health literacy, including socioeconomic status, education, race, ethnicity, age, and disability. On average, adults aged 65 and older have lower health literacy than adults younger than 65. Adults living below the federal poverty threshold have lower health literacy than adults living above the federal poverty threshold. People without insurance or who are publicly insured (e.g., by Medicaid) are also at higher risk of having low health literacy. Almost half of the adults who did not graduate from high school have low health literacy (HHS, 2018).

Some of the greatest disparities in health literacy in the United States occur among non-native English speakers and among underrepresented racial and ethnic groups. The most recent National Assessment of Adult Literacy, performed in 2003, revealed that adults identifying as Hispanic have the lowest average health literacy scores of all groups assessed, followed by Black and then American Indian/Alaska Native adults (Kutner et al., 2006). Discriminatory policies and practices have created limited access to resources and skills needed to obtain, understand, and apply health information. Systemic factors such as low income, limited educational opportunities, racism, mistrust of the healthcare system, and a lack of individualized health information and services are health literacy barriers for these populations.

Social determinants of health (SDoH) are the conditions and the environments in which people are born, live, learn, work, play, worship, and age that affect a wide range of health, functioning, and quality-of-life outcomes and risks. Health literacy is an SDoH due to the effect it has on health outcomes (AHRQ, 2020).

Low health literacy negatively affects the ability of an individual to make health-related decisions. When patients receive health communication materials that do not match their literacy level, patient education is ineffective. Communication barriers between patients and healthcare providers may lead to a variety of negative health outcomes for the patient. For example, a patient who does not fully understand the purpose of a medication or the warning signs that require follow-up with their provider may have poor health outcomes due to not taking the medication as prescribed.

Research has shown that people with low health literacy are more likely to have poor health outcomes in a variety of ways (Kutner et al., 2006). Low health literacy in older adults has been linked to increased reports of pain, limitations of daily activities, poor mental health status, and poor physical function (Kutner et al., 2006). Older adult Medicare beneficiaries with low health literacy have higher medical costs, increased rates of emergency department visits and hospital admissions, and decreased access to healthcare. Also, health literacy is significantly associated with increased mortality and hospital readmission as well as decreased quality of life in patients with cardiovascular diseases (Kanejima et al., 2022).

CASE STUDY

Review the Wilandika (2023) article from the case study. Table 2 in that article summarizes the roles of nurses in health literacy. Knowing the many factors that affect health literacy, what strategies can you find in the article that you could use to help patients make informed medical decisions?

Assessing Health Literacy in Patients

The first part of the nursing process is assessment. Nurses have several reliable and valid **literacy assessment tools** available to assess the health literacy of patients. Examples include the Rapid Estimate of Adult Literacy of Medicine (REALM), the Test of Functional Health Literacy in Adults (TOFHLA), the Newest Vital Sign (NVS), and the Single Item Literacy Screener (SILS) (AHRQ, 2018). Tools appropriate for Spanish-speaking individuals include the Short Assessment of Health Literacy–Spanish and English (SAHL-S&E) and the Short Assessment of Health Literacy for Spanish Adults (SAHLSA-50) (AHRQ, 2018).

A collaboration among Communicate Health, Inc., Boston University, and RTI International funded by the National Institutes of Health's National Library of Medicine created the Health Literacy Tool Shed, a searchable database of health literacy measures that have been published in peer-reviewed journals. This website is a resource to learn about health literacy measurement tools and to find tools that meet each person's needs. There are currently more than 200 tools in this resource, and they can be narrowed down by specific topics, the health literacy domain measured, administration time and mode, and more (Health Literacy Tool Shed, 2024).

The Ethical Considerations box describes the responsibilities of nurses in assessing health literacy in patients.

ETHICAL CONSIDERATIONS FOR HEALTH LITERACY

In Provision one of the ANA Nursing Code of Ethics (2015), the nurse is directed to practice with compassion and respect for the inherent dignity, worth, and unique attributes of every person. Assessing the health literacy of each patient is an ethical obligation because doing so values Interpretive Statement 1.3, which states that patient care is shaped by the patient's preferences, needs, values, and choices. The nurse cannot ask a patient to decide about their care before determining whether they have understood their options. Interpretive Statement 1.4 states patients have a right to self-determination. This directly applies to informed consent and the role of the nurse in ensuring the patient understands what the consent form means for their health outcomes. Self-determination depends on the patient's awareness of their decisions. The ability to comprehend treatment options may be impaired by health literacy level, language proficiency, or educational level. It is important to assess each patient's understanding of treatment options and implications. Health literacy also relates to Provision 8. Interpretive Statement 8.3 directs the nurse to reduce health disparities, which can be done by improving the health literacy of patients. Reflect on your ethical obligations as a nurse to assess and improve the health literacy of your patients. How do you feel about this obligation?

CASE STUDY

In the research covered in the case study, the authors discuss several strategies for assessing health literacy including the importance of cultural competency for nurses, repetition of information, the use of verbal and nonverbal cues by both patient and nurse, and the use of simple language (Wilandika, 2023). Are these strategies emphasized in your education program or place of work? What types of literacy assessments have you observed in healthcare facilities? The next time you are involved in teaching a patient (observing or participating) note how health literacy is assessed.

Addressing Health Literacy Issues

Numerous resources are available to assist healthcare providers in addressing health literacy issues. The federal government has several excellent online resources. For example, the Health Literacy Precautions Toolkit (2020) is available from the AHRQ. The toolkit is a comprehensive file with an array of resources to assist healthcare providers' practices to assess and address the health

BOX 14-4 Health Literacy Resources

- Agency for Healthcare Research and Quality (AHRQ)—Health Literacy Universal Precautions Toolkit
- Centers for Disease Control and Prevention (CDC)—Health Literacy Action Plan
- Institute for Healthcare Improvement (IHI)—Ask Me 3: Good questions for your health
- National Academy of Medicine (NAM) (formerly the Institute of Medicine)—10 Attributes of Health Literate Healthcare Organizations
- National Library of Medicine (NLM)—An Introduction to Health Literacy
- National Institutes of Health (NIH)—Plain Language at NIH
- Pfizer—Health Literacy: Learn to be well
- U.S. Department of Health and Human Services (HHS)—Healthy People 2030

literacy issue. As part of the National Action Plan to Improve Health Literacy, the Centers for Disease Control and Prevention (CDC) has created a health literacy action plan as well (CDC, 2021). Box 14-4 includes examples of health literacy online resources.

No matter the healthcare setting, nurses encounter patients with different levels of health literacy. Good communication skills are essential for supporting patients with the evolution of their health literacy skills. Nurses need to be able to communicate effectively in speaking and writing, make information understandable and actionable, and embody respect for other cultures to ensure successful health outcomes for their patients.

Oral Communication

Oral communication is often the first method of communication between patients and healthcare professionals. However, it is easy for patients to misunderstand medical jargon, negatively affecting health literacy. To help with this and other oral communication issues, healthcare professionals should strive for effective oral communication. Some general rules for effective oral communication include the following:

- Use eye contact.
- Speak slowly and use plain language.
- Limit the communication to three to five things that are essential to know.
- Repeat important information.
- Encourage questions.
- Use pictures, models, or drawings.
- Use the "teach-back" technique, asking the patient to explain the information in their own words.

More tips and scenarios can be found online. For example, the American Medical Association Foundation created a video that can be found on YouTube titled "Health Literacy and Patient Safety: Help Patients Understand," which shows several consumers talking about points of confusion.

Written Communication

The ability to read and understand is an important component of health literacy. Nurses and other healthcare professionals may attempt patient care teaching using printed educational literature or websites that patients and families cannot understand. The Centers for Medicare & Medicaid Services (CMS) offers a toolkit for creating clear and effective written material online (CMS, 2021). The National Institutes of Health (NIH) has a resource to help writers learn to use plain language; it includes recommendations for presenting information and formatting for visual clarity. Search "plain language" on the NIH website.

Several writing strategies improve the **readability,** or the ease with which a reader can successfully decipher, process, and analyze the information. Examples include the following:

- Limit the number of word syllables. For example, use "drugs" instead of "medications."
- Use plain language instead of medical terminologies and jargons.
- Use numbered lists for a step-by-step plan or bullet points to highlight critical points.
- Use graphics with captions to reinforce the meaning of words.
- Restrict the length of the sentences used as much as possible.
- Balance the words with white spaces.

Fortunately, there are several methods to test written information for readability. Microsoft has tools (e.g., Gunning Fog Index, Coleman-Liau Index, SMOG Index). Google offers a free downloadable readability tool called Text Readability Analyzer (TRAY) tool. It gives scores using some common readability indicators (i.e., Flesch Reading Ease, Flesch–Kincaid Grade Level, Gunning Fog Score, Automated Readability Index).

To visualize how readability statistics work, consider a scenario in which you want to refer a patient to a website on heart failure. Searching "heart failure" yields a web page from the Mayo Clinic that you think is valuable. You decide to run readability checks to see if this would be an appropriate reference for your patient (Box 14-5).

As shown in Box 14-5, the text on this web page is difficult to read and best understood by people with at least a high school-level education. However, it is important to understand that website software uses computer algorithms (rules) to provide objective readability data. Before using health education materials, you

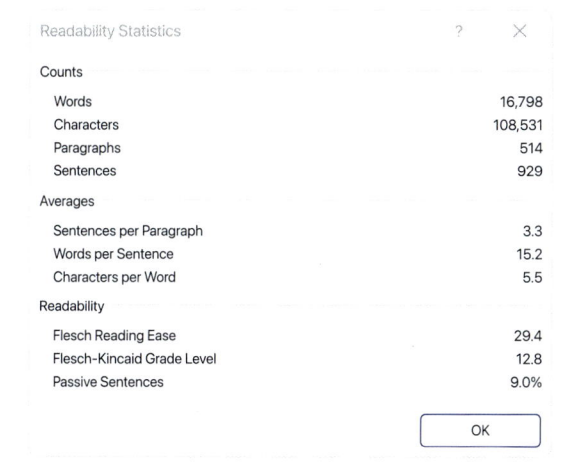

Figure 14-1. Flesch Reading Ease and Flesch–Kincaid Grade Level in Microsoft Word can be found by selecting the Home tab, choosing Editor, and then going to Document stats. A dialogue box will appear showing the readability statistics.

an embedded tool to check document readability using the Flesch Reading Ease and the Flesch–Kincaid Grade Level tests (Fig. 14-1). The **Flesch Reading Ease** calculates a value from a formula using the average sentence length and the average number of syllables per word. The recommended score is between 60 and 70; higher scores correlate with easier readability. The **Flesch–Kincaid Grade Level** test uses the average sentence length and average number of syllables to calculate a U.S. school grade level. It is recommended that patient education resources be written at a sixth-grade level.

Several websites are also available to assess the readability of a document. Grammarly offers free software available for download that reviews spelling, grammar, punctuation, clarity, engagement, and delivery mistakes in English texts, suggesting replacements for the identified errors. It also detects plagiarism. The Grammarly Editor uses a 0-to-100 readability grading scale, in which higher numbers mean easier-to-read documents. In most cases, aim for a score of 60 or higher, which means the document will be easy to read for most people with at least an eighth-grade education. Readable is another website that allows the user to paste text into a window to obtain readability statistics using the Flesch–Kincaid Grade Level or other readability

---

BOX 14-5 Readability of Mayo Clinic Web Page on Heart Failure

Readability scores of the Mayo Clinic page on heart failure (https://www.mayoclinic.org/diseases-conditions/heart-failure/diagnosis-treatment/drc-20373148) include:

Results from Readable
- Grade: A
- Readability Grade Levels
- Flesch–Kincaid Grade Level: 7.6
- Gunning Fog Index: 9.1 (ninth grade)
- Readability Score: Flesch Reading Ease: 59.8 (10th grade)

Results From Grammarly
- Overall score: 90
- Flesch Reading Ease: 62 (eighth to ninth grade)

Results From Google TRAY Readability Tool
- Gunning Fog: 10.4 (10th grade)
- Automated Readability: 10.36 (ninth grade)
- Flesch–Kincaid Reading Ease: 24.55 (graduate)

should use your personal knowledge of your patient to determine whether they would understand the reading material and whether it is appropriate for use.

Understandability and Actionability

Patients need to be able to understand and act using the educational materials that they receive. **Understandability** of education materials is the ability of people from different backgrounds with different levels of health literacy to understand the materials and extract important messages. **Actionability** of educational materials is the ability of people to identify what actions to take based on the information in the material (Zuzelo, 2019). The Patient Education Materials Assessment Tool (PEMAT), which is available on the AHRQ website, is a resource for ensuring educational materials meet the informational need of patients, specifically those with a wide range of literacy abilities and challenges. There are two forms of this tool: PEMAT-P for printable material and for PEMAT-A/V for audio and visual material. Using a valid readability tool in combination with PEMAT is a method to ensure educational materials are readable, understandable, and can be applied correctly and appropriately by patient learners.

Cultural Competence

Simply translating instructions, disease information, and medications for patients with lower levels of literacy or English proficiency is not sufficient. The cultural context of the literacy must be considered as well, including factors such as an individual's age, gender identity, sexual identity, disability, race, ethnicity, and occupation. Culture affects how people communicate, understand, and respond to health information (CDC, 2021). **Cultural competence** is the ability of health organizations and providers to recognize the cultural beliefs, values, attitudes, traditions, language preferences, and health practices of diverse and vulnerable populations and to apply that knowledge to produce a positive health outcome. Competency includes communicating in a manner that is linguistically and culturally appropriate (NIH, 2021).

For many individuals with limited English proficiency (LEP), the communication challenge in English is the primary barrier to accessing health information and services. It is important to have educational materials that are communicated plainly in the learner's primary language, using words, pictures, media, and examples that make the information understandable (HHS, 2021). Figure 14-2 shows one of many brochures from the CDC in a language other than English. Note the combination of pictures, words, and examples.

Providing Patient Information on Healthcare Agency Websites

Most healthcare agencies have websites. The exact contents vary, but they generally provide information about the organization, a map and directions to the agency, a list of the services offered, healthcare information related to their specialties, and other organizational information aimed at marketing. Many healthcare agencies post background information about their providers to aid consumers in selecting someone appropriate, plus forms to request an appointment.

Healthcare agencies may even develop a site that functions more like an extranet where access is restricted to only their patients but the site has no ties to the patients' records or patient portals. Healthcare agencies should have written guidelines for use of the information provided on agency-developed health sites. Agency guidelines are pertinent for extranets that deliver information designed for specific patients. Agency websites must address privacy and security issues, as well as adhere to criteria for all healthcare websites.

Informatics nurses might be asked to participate in the design of their agency's website, or to evaluate the information an existing website contains. Just as with all written communication, think carefully about the target audience. Use web design principles and literacy strategies to achieve the goal. Two important factors that go into designing a website are verifying that the information is accessible to people with disabilities and addressing usability principles.

Accessibility in Web Design

Whether creating a healthcare website or evaluating one, consider that its visitors may have

Chapter 14 Information Literacy: A Road to Improved Patient Outcomes 303

Документ доступний на сайті: https://www.cdc.gov/coronavirus/2019-ncov/if-you-are-sick/steps-when-sick.html

10 КРОКІВ, ЯКІ ВИ МОЖЕТЕ ЗРОБИТИ ВДОМА ДЛЯ ПОДОЛАННЯ ВАШИХ СИМПТОМІВ COVID-19 | COVID-19 |

Якщо у вас ймовірне або підтверджене захворювання на COVID-19

1. **Залишайтеся вдома**, за винятком випадків, коли необхідно звернутися по медичну допомогу.

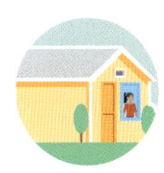

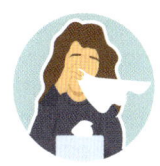

2. Уважно **стежте за своїми симптомами**. При погіршенні симптомів негайно зверніться до свого лікаря.

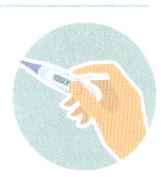

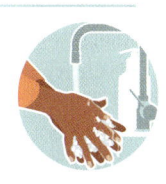

3. **Відпочивайте та підтримуйте водний баланс організму.**

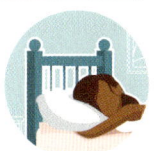

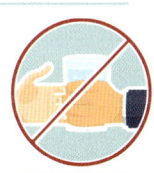

4. Якщо вам призначено прийом у лікаря, **зателефонуйте йому/їй** заздалегідь та повідомте, що ви захворіли або могли захворіти на COVID-19.

5. У випадку невідкладних ситуацій, зателефонуйте до служби 911 і **повідомте черговий персонал** про те, що ви хворієте або можете хворіти на COVID-19.

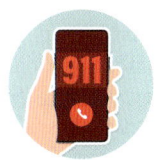

6. **Якщо ви кашляєте або чхаєте, прикривайте свій рот і ніс** серветкою або використовуйте для цього зігнутий лікоть.

7. **Часто мийте руки** водою з милом протягом щонайменше 20 секунд або обробляйте руки засобом для дезінфекції на спиртовій основі, що містить щонайменше 60% спирту.

8. Наскільки можливо, **залишайтесь** у виділеній кімнаті, **окремо від інших людей**, що проживають у вашому домі. Крім того, якщо є декілька ванних кімнат, користуйтеся окремою. Надівайте маску, якщо вам потрібно перебувати поруч з іншими людьми вдома або поза домом.

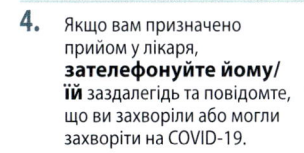

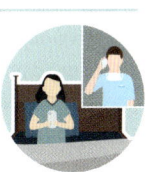

9. **Намагайтеся не користуватися особистими речами** разом з іншими людьми у вашому домі, такими як посуд, рушники й постільні речі.

10. **Обробляйте всі поверхні**, до яких часто торкаються, наприклад прилавки, поверхні столу та дверні ручки. Використовуйте побутові очисні спреї або ганчір'я, відповідно до інструкції з використання на етикетці.

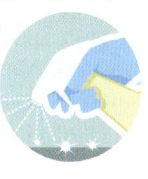

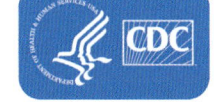

cdc.gov/coronavirus

Figure 14-2. COVID-19 factsheet in Ukrainian language. (From the Centers for Disease Control and Prevention (CDC). (2021, July 26). 10 steps to do at home to treat Covid-19. https://www.cdc.gov/coronavirus/2019-ncov/downloads/10Things-Ukrainian.pdf)

disabilities. Of U.S. adults, 26% have some type of disability. Of those with a disability, 5.9% have trouble hearing, 4.8% have trouble seeing, and 10.8% have cognitive disabilities (CDC, 2020). It is likely that the percentages are even higher in the population of people who access healthcare websites. It is imperative, therefore, that the healthcare website meets standards of **accessibility**, that is, allows individuals with disabilities to access the resource.

The website design should allow for use of a **screen reader** for people with limited sight. A screen reader is a computer feature with speech recognition for those with limited sight; it can translate text to speech. Full-function screen readers are best for those with limited vision. Elementary screen readers are usually bundled with operating systems and can at least help a person with limited vision install a full-function screen reader. Besides translating text to speech, some screen readers can send information to a **Braille reader** placed near or under the keyboard. Users then use their fingers to read the information.

Screen readers have vastly improved from earlier times when they could not interpret tables. Screen readers cannot "read" a graphic or image, so text alternatives called **alt tags** are required. The tag should provide either textual information used by a screen reader in place of the illustration or a link to a site that explains the illustration in text. If there are clickable spots on a graphic, make provisions for finding these links using a screen reader.

There are other disabilities to consider. Around 3% of people with epilepsy have photosensitive epilepsy, in which seizures are triggered by certain rates of flashing lights or contrasting light and dark patterns (Epilepsy Society, 2019). Blinking items on a web page or quick changes from dark to light can cause seizures in people with photosensitive epilepsy and should be avoided. Everyone sees color a little differently, even people who are not colorblind; however, about one in 12 men are colorblind (NEI, 2019). Therefore, when designing a web page, avoid red-green color combinations. People who are hard of hearing will miss any audio on a website. Accessibility for these people is also improved when closed captioning is provided for any resource that is delivered audiovisually.

Usability in Web Design

Usability refers to meeting certain criteria for accessibility. Health websites have many usability problems, particularly for older adults, such as drop-down menus that are not easy to find, too much information on the screen, font size that is too small, lack of instructions for playing video, and navigation problems (Weber et al., 2020). Older adults may also have difficulty using navigation menus and buttons and understanding the meanings of icons when using mobile devices (Li & Luximon, 2020). To avoid usability issues for this population, a sampling of the intended audience should review the website; their feedback will help identify and correct any problems. Although healthcare providers can evaluate the web content, the intended audience should conduct usability testing.

EMPOWERED CONSUMER

Until recently, consumers have not been empowered to make informed decisions about their own healthcare. In the past, consumers did not have the knowledge that healthcare providers do. Healthcare had a culture of paternalism, and there was a perception that patients (consumers) should accept prescribed care without question or consideration of the cost. Even if consumers wanted information about the quality or cost of the care being administered or their own patient records, it was difficult to access. Additionally, in a world in which healthcare consumers were dependent on providers for all their healthcare information needs, patients who questioned orders for care risked being labeled as "difficult" or "noncompliant."

However, the advent of the internet and many key legislative developments granting patients more rights to their health information leveled the playing field. The consumer became able to access much of the same information as the healthcare professional. Today, the internet, social media, and other technology are continually changing the face of the healthcare industry (Land, 2019). Consumers can learn about the quality of care provided by many hospitals and find information about diseases that was previously available only to healthcare professionals. However, the internet empowers consumers to take ownership of their health often without the benefit of advanced education and training to interpret the meaning of the information. Thus, healthcare providers are evolving from simply being care providers to directors of consumer-centric services and consumer-friendly experiences (Land, 2019). To achieve the goal of Healthy People 2030 to "eliminate health disparities, achieve health equity, and attain health literacy" (HHS, 2022b), nurses, healthcare providers, and consumers all need to work together.

Key Legislative Developments

Legislative milestones and federal and private industry efforts paved the way toward the goal of granting individuals access to electronic copies of their health information. Key developments include the 1996 Health Insurance Portability and Accountability Act (HIPAA) Privacy Rule, the Health Information Technology for Economic and Clinical Health Act (HITECH), the federal electronic health records (EHRs) incentive programs, and the 21st Century Cures Act. Related efforts by the HHS and other federal agencies that are currently underway, such as Blue Button, the Office of the National Coordinator (ONC) for Health Information Technology Consumer eHealth Program, and standards and interoperability initiatives, aim to bolster individuals' access to their records (ONC, 2019). In addition, as a part of the 2009 American Recovery and Reinvestment Act, all public and private healthcare providers and other eligible professionals were required to adopt and demonstrate "meaningful use" of electronic medical records to maintain their existing Medicaid and Medicare reimbursement levels (HHS, 2022a). Consequently, the impetus to develop and market patient access to their own healthcare information and the growing field of consumer informatics became top priorities in the United States.

Rise of Consumer Informatics

The easy availability of information on the internet, the push for more cost-effective healthcare, and the desire of many consumers to take more responsibility for their health have resulted in the development of **consumer informatics**, a subspecialty in healthcare informatics. The focus is on empowering consumers through improving health literacy, consumer-friendly language, personal health records, and internet-based strategies and resources (AMIA, 2022). This field is an applied science using concepts from communication, education, behavioral science, and social networking. The design of consumer informatics provides consumers healthcare information, allows consumers to make informed decisions, promotes healthy behaviors and information exchange, and provides social support. Practitioners analyze consumer needs and information use and develop ways to facilitate consumers finding and using health information. They also evaluate the effectiveness of electronic health information and study how this affects public health and the consumer–healthcare provider relationship.

The focus of consumer informatics is on consumers rather than healthcare providers as end users. While some consumer informatics applications may include interaction with healthcare providers, others may not. For example, websites, information kiosks, blood pressure kiosks, eHealth applications, and personal health records all require no interaction with a healthcare provider. The hope is that intelligent informatics applications result in healthcare information that reaches consumers, creating a healthy balance between self-reliance and professional help. Full realization of the potential of consumer informatics depends on the features and breadth of information systems.

Empowering the Healthcare Consumer to Achieve Information Literacy

With the transformation of the healthcare provider–patient relationship from a paternalistic approach in which healthcare providers have all the knowledge to a more participatory approach in which patients take responsibility for their own care, there is an increased need for individuals to have valid health-related information. Health literacy is positively associated with obtaining information from health professionals and the internet (Yamashita et al., 2020). Nurses have a responsibility to ensure consumers have access to useful, up-to-date, relevant information from trusted sources. To reduce health disparities and improve patient outcomes, nurses must advocate for patients to have access to broadband internet and assist patients with searching for resources, using search tools, and evaluating and interpreting information.

Advocacy for Internet Access

Despite increasing internet use, access to the internet is still a limiting factor for many people in the United States. Access to broadband internet is considered an SDoH. According to the Pew Research Center (2022), approximately one quarter of American adults do not have access to broadband internet. This number does not account for the millions of people who have poor or unstable connectivity. Black and Hispanic adults surveyed by the Pew Research Center are twice as likely to have canceled or disconnected their internet service due to financial strain than people identifying as White (2022). Indigenous communities are the least connected when it comes to high-speed internet. Less than half of Indigenous people living on reservations or tribal lands with a computer have access to high-speed internet service compared with 75% to 82% nationally (Early, 2021).

Lack of devices also contributes to a lack of internet access. Adults in rural areas are less likely than adults in urban areas to own traditional or tablet computers and are less likely to have multiple devices or services that enable them to go online. Around a quarter of adults with household incomes below $30,000 a year affirm they do not own a smartphone. About four in 10 adults with lower incomes do not have home broadband services or a desktop or laptop computer. By comparison, each of these technologies is nearly ubiquitous among adults in households earning $100,000 or more a year (Pew Research Center, 2022).

The COVID-19 pandemic exacerbated health disparities related to lack of internet access. Lack of broadband access led to unequal vaccination rates, with Black and Latino individuals receiving the COVID-19 vaccine at significantly lower rates than White individuals (O'Brien, 2021). According to the CDC, many state protocols only allowed those with internet access to register online for vaccinations.

To combat the health disparities related to lack of internet access, nurses should advocate for universal internet access. Joining a political action committee for a national nursing organization such as the ANA can help nurses have a voice with policymakers. The American Library Association (ALA) asserts that broadband access is a human right. You can find out how to advocate for policies and funding that support the Federal Communications Commission's (FCC) Lifeline program to ensure that low-income households have affordable access to the internet and devices to use it (ALA, n.d.). The FCC Lifeline program provides a discount on phone service for qualifying consumers with lower incomes to ensure that all Americans have access (FCC, 2023). You can also call 211 in almost any community and get information about community resources. Finally, patients should be provided with information about where they can access the internet for free (e.g., public libraries).

Finding Effective Internet Resources

According to Clark (2020), 80% of patients use the internet for health-related searches. Of adults born between 1997 and 2012, 45% do not have a primary care physician and 51% of adults born between 1981 and 1996 see a doctor less than once each year (Clark, 2020). The internet is the most likely source of healthcare information for these individuals. The internet is the second most common source from which older adults obtain most of their health information (36%) (Yamashita et al., 2020). In a study by Gordon (2021), 11% of participants said they turn to social media when looking for reliable health information. Nearly one in 10 (9%) also said they use social media to evaluate new treatment options and 7% reported seeking information about medication side effects from social media (Gordon, 2021).

A study in 2019 revealed that 65% of people have used the internet to self-diagnose, but 43% of them became falsely convinced they had a serious disease following self-diagnosis (Kingston, 2019). Of those who engage in self-diagnosis, 84% perceived symptom checkers as a diagnostic tool, saying they provided insights that lead them closer to a diagnosis. Unfortunately, these tools list the correct diagnosis first in only 34% of cases, whereas diagnostic accuracy by a provider is between 85% and 90% (Clark, 2020). The increase in consumers searching for health information on the web has led to **cyberchondria,** a condition in which people become distressed and frightened after repeated and excessive web searches for health information (Starcevic et al., 2020).

The nature of the internet puts a burden on the user to become adept at finding and evaluating sources. There is always concern about the quality of information on the web. Although inaccurate information exists on the web, one can argue that the accuracy of the information is comparable to many traditional sources such as acquaintances, pamphlets, and popular press articles. Rather than criticizing using online resources, it is ideal to guide users to evaluate the quality of online information. If nurses are going to help consumers find and analyze web-based sources, they must develop their own expertise first.

Search tools on the internet fall into three general categories: crawler or spider, human-powered directories, or a combination. Crawler or spider search engines visit each website, "read" each web page and the associated links, and then index or catalogue the information in preparation for a search (Google Developers, 2022). Currently, crawler or spider search engines, such as Google, Yahoo!, and Bing, have widespread use. There are fewer human-driven directories available than electronic crawlers. The Open Directory and Yahoo! Directory are examples. Many search engines are specialized. For example, Find Articles searches print publications, including magazines and select scholarly journals. The Combined Health Information Database (CHID) searches for medical topics.

Once resources are found, they need to be evaluated. The freedom of publication on the internet allows the airing of wide-ranging ideas and opinions, many of which are not in the mainstream. The internet does not have the security of a library in which all material is vetted to a degree. The variety of types of information on the web requires multiple sets of criteria to evaluate information. A rubric that rates the authority of the site, quality, currency, ease of use, privacy, and other resources provides a way to evaluate websites. When finding and evaluating healthcare websites, consumers should determine (Kington et al., 2021; Medical Library Association, 2022):

- Whether the site presents facts or opinions and whether it is science-based and consistent with the best scientific evidence available at the time
- Who is sponsoring the site and whether the site is free of influential bias
- The intended audience
- How often the site is updated
- If the site is transparent and accountable by disclosing its limitations and potential conflicts of interest

An easy method nurses can share with patients for evaluating online information is the CRAAP (Currency, Relevance, Authority, Accuracy and Purpose) test (Box 14-6).

Healthcare providers can guide patients to trusted websites for web-based health information and teach them how to evaluate websites themselves. Nurses should counsel patients to ask for assistance when searching the web for healthcare information. Certification from an authority, such as the Health on the Net (HON) Foundation, an international nonprofit organization, mitigates the need for personal evaluation of the site. The HON Foundation provides a website online for professionals, patients, and individuals to use (HON Health on the Net Foundation, 2020). The foundation also provides a downloadable tool to assist users in finding certified health information websites using the Chrome and Firefox browsers.

Talking to Patients About Misinformation

Science and healthcare are constantly evolving, and the rapid development of information technology has had a great effect on healthcare (Qi et al., 2021). It is easy for people who use the internet and social media to generate and share content; therefore, rapid dissemination of health misinformation is possible (Parker & Ratzan, 2019). This is a challenge, as it places healthcare providers in a position of advocating for the best available science and evidence. Therefore, one of the facets of information literacy is the ability to identify misinformation and communicate that with patients. Healthcare professionals have the responsibility to convey truthful information to patients, peers, and communities and have essential roles

> **BOX 14-6** CRAAP Test for Evaluating Information Sources From the Internet
>
> **Currency**
> How recent is the information?
> How recently has the website been updated?
> Is it current enough for your topic?
>
> **Relevance**
> What kind of information is included in the resource?
> Does the information relate to your topic or answer your question?
>
> **Authority**
> Who is the creator or author?
> What are the credentials? Can you find any information about the author's background?
> Who is the publisher or sponsor?
> Are they reputable?
> What is the publisher's interest (if any) in this information?
> Are there advertisements on the website? If so, are they clearly marked?
>
> **Accuracy**
> Is the information supported by evidence?
> Does the author list information sources or references?
> Can you verify any of the information in another source or from personal knowledge?
> Are there spelling, grammar, or typographical errors?
>
> **Purpose/Point of View**
> Is this fact or opinion?
> Is it biased? Does the author seem to be trying to push an agenda or particular side?
> Is the creator or author trying to sell you something? If so, is it clearly stated?
>
> Data from Lewis, A. B. (2018). "What Does Bad Information Look Like? Using the CRAAP Test for Evaluating Substandard Resources." Issues in science and technology librarianship (1092-1206), (88).

in helping patients obtain reliable, evidence-based health information (Wu & McCormick, 2018). Health outcomes can be improved by combating misinformation and disseminating evidence-based, relevant information (Kyabaggu et al., 2022).

Even with thorough evaluation of online information, patients may arrive for an office visit with online information that is inaccurate or new to the healthcare provider. Conflicts can arise if the patient does not trust the provider. When a patient presents inaccurate or new information they have obtained on their own, consider accessing the website with the patient. Websites with personal accounts of a disease may have inaccurate information. Use evaluation criteria to assess the website. If no web address is available, attempt to duplicate the search. Even if you are unsuccessful, you have demonstrated to the patient that you respect them and are interested in their well-being.

Nurses can help debunk healthcare misinformation by acknowledging what is known and what is not known. As a nurse, you can influence how patients are affected by any information they receive from any source by answering their questions and clarifying misunderstandings. Always keep in mind that a self-diagnosis or other information that is new to you may be accurate. If the information is from a reliable source and contradicts your understanding, acknowledge it. You may discover that the patient has unanswered questions, is frightened, needs more understanding of the underlying disease, or just needs more information. You can direct your patients to a resource or symptom checker by recommending trustworthy sites. In many cases, especially if the information is suspect, working with the patient might take patience and tact, but it is vital in providing care.

Motivational interviewing (MI) is a technique that can be used to help patients acknowledge when they have mixed feelings about their situations and become collaborative, active participants in changing their opinions or behaviors. MI can be used to counsel patients about misinformation (Hall et al., 2012). Training for using MI can be found online, but to get started, use the acronym RULE: *r*esist the defensive reflex; *u*nderstand the patient's own motivations; *l*isten with empathy; and *e*mpower the patient. RULE can be used to approach a situation with both objectivity and emotional intelligence.

More details about identifying and combatting misinformation can be found in Chapter 4.

> **CASE STUDY**
>
> Review the research from the case study, in which 13 articles were identified that discuss health literacy related to nursing practice (Wilandika, 2023). How many of these articles discuss empowering the consumer? Are there strategies or interventions that appeal to you or that you have used successfully with patients? Be sure you have a plan in place for how to respond when a patient or colleague engages with or shares misinformation.

SUMMARY

- **Information literacy in the healthcare profession.** Nurses must be information-literate to solve problems in healthcare. Information competency standards for nurses are available to guide nursing education in academia and healthcare settings. Numerous organizations support and promote information and health literacy, including the AACN, NLN, AAN, HIMSS, AHRQ, and the TIGER project.
- **Health literacy.** Healthy People 2030 defines personal and organizational health literacy to support the role of the healthcare professional in advocating for, supporting, and enabling information literacy to improve patient outcomes. The health literacy movement is focused on reducing health disparities, achieving health equity, and improving healthcare quality. Despite the efforts of healthcare professionals, health literacy and numeracy remain low in the United States. Many factors can influence an individual's health literacy, including socioeconomic status, education, race, ethnicity, age, disability, and native language. The effect of low health literacy is such that it is now considered an SDoH. There are many literacy assessment tools for assessing the health literacy of patients and the levels of educational materials. Oral and written communication should match the health literacy level of patients. It is also important to embody cultural competency when educating patients. Website creators, especially those of healthcare organizations, should address accessibility and usability, ensuring content can be accessed by people with disabilities or low understanding of technology.
- **Empowered consumer.** A history of paternalism in healthcare has hampered efforts to engage patients in self-care. Legislative milestones have supported consumer involvement with their healthcare including access to electronic copies of health information. Consumer informatics is a subspecialty that focuses on empowering consumers through improving health literacy. Most Americans use the internet to obtain healthcare information. Nurses have a responsibility to educate patients to evaluate information found on the internet for veracity. The HON Foundation and the CRAAP test are both useful for determining the reliability of information found online. Nurses must keep an open mind and anticipate the need to support patients with assessing and using online information.

DISCUSSION QUESTIONS AND ACTIVITIES

1. The nursing student has been assigned to assess the health literacy of their community. What populations are at risk for low health literacy? What are some risk factors for low health literacy? Who is responsible for improving the health literacy of the community? How can healthcare providers assist patients with low health literacy?

2. Imagine you are a nurse working to discharge an older patient with a new diagnosis of congestive heart failure. The patient does not speak English and has an eighth-grade education. How will you ensure the discharge information you provide this family is understood?

3. Google a common health problem such as asthma and perform a readability analysis of the top three websites you find. Report your findings. What sites are the most readable for patients? Is the information useful for teaching a patient with low health literacy?

4. You are designing a web page about ways to limit dietary sodium. What resources would you use to ensure the readability score is at the fifth-grade level, and that the web page is accessible to your clinic population of older adult patients?

5. How could you advocate for increased high-speed internet access for individuals? What arguments would you present? Identify specific ways to advocate and any legislation that is being put forward.

6. Evaluate a health website using the CRAAP method. What are the strengths and limitations of the website? Discuss your findings.

PRACTICE QUESTIONS

1. Which statement by the nurse indicates an understanding of health information literacy?
   a. "Most Americans have a high level of health literacy."
   b. "The American Library Association created the Information Literacy Competency Standards in 2013."
   c. "The AACN includes information literacy in Competency 8.2 of the Essentials."
   d. "The Health Literacy Universal Precaution Toolkit is used to target only those with low health literacy."

2. You are providing education for a patient about COVID-19 vaccinations. The patient is hesitant, stating they saw a post online saying the COVID vaccines can mutate DNA. This statement indicates a primary need for education in which area?
   a. Misinformation
   b. Readability
   c. Cyberchondria
   d. Actionability

3. Methods to improve the readability of patient education pamphlet include which strategy?
   a. Use of medical terminologies and jargons
   b. Use of all available space for text
   c. Numbered lists for a step-by-step plan
   d. Graphics without captions to reinforce the meaning of words

REFERENCES

Agency for Healthcare Research and Quality (AHRQ). (2018, November). *Health literacy measurement tools (Revised)*. https://www.ahrq.gov/health-literacy/research/tools/index.html

Agency for Healthcare Research and Quality (AHRQ). (2020, September). *Health literacy universal precautions toolkit*. http://www.ahrq.gov/professionals/quality-patient-safety/quality-resources/tools/literacy-toolkit/index.html

American Academy of Nursing (AAN). (2020). *2021-2024 strategic plan*. https://www.aannet.org/about/strategic-plan-2021-2024

American Association of Colleges of Nursing (AACN). (2021, April 6). *The Essentials: Core competencies for professional nursing education*. https://www.aacnnursing.org/Portals/42/AcademicNursing/pdf/Essentials-2021.pdf

American Library Association (ALA). (n.d.). *Broadband: Summary of positions*. https://www.ala.org/advocacy/broadband

American Medical Informatics Association (AMIA). (2022). *Informatics: Research and practice. What is informatics?* https://amia.org/about-amia/why-informatics/informatics-research-and-practice

American Nurses Association (ANA). (2015). *Code of ethics for nurses*. American Nurses Publishing. https://www.nursingworld.org/practice-policy/nursing-excellence/ethics/code-of-ethics-for-nurses/

Association of College and Research Libraries (ACRL). (2013). *Information literacy competency standards for nursing*. https://www.ala.org/acrl/standards/nursing

Brega, A. G., Barnard, J., Mabachi, N. M., Weiss, B. D., DeWalt, D. A., Brach, C., & West, D. R. (2015). *Health literacy universal precautions toolkit*, 2nd ed. AHRQ Publication No. 15-0023-EF http://www.ahrq.gov/professionals/quality-patient-safety/quality-resources/tools/literacy-toolkit/index.html. Agency for Healthcare Research and Quality.

Centers for Disease Control and Prevention (CDC). (2020, September 16). *Disability impacts all of us*. https://www.cdc.gov/ncbddd/disabilityandhealth/infographic-disability-impacts-all.html

Centers for Disease Control and Prevention (CDC). (2021, December 9). *Culture & health literacy*. https://www.cdc.gov/healthliteracy/culture.html

Centers for Disease Control and Prevention (CDC). (2022, June 10). *Understanding literacy and numeracy*. https://www.cdc.gov/healthliteracy/learn/understandingliteracy.html

Centers for Medicare and Medicaid Services (CMS). (2021, December 1). *Toolkit for making written material clear and effective*. http://www.cms.gov/Outreach-and-Education/Outreach/WrittenMaterialsToolkit/index.html

CILIP. (2018). *Information literacy (re) defined*. https://infolit.org.uk/ILdefinitionCILIP2018.pdf

Clark, M. (2020, December 10). 37 Self diagnosis statistics: Don't do it yourself. *Etactics*. https://etactics.com/blog/self-diagnosis-statistics

Early, J., & Hernandez, A (2021). Digital disenfranchisement and COVID-19: Broadband internet access as a social determinant of health. *Health Promotion Practice, 22*(5), 605–610.

Epilepsy Society. (2019). *Photosensitive epilepsy*. https://epilepsysociety.org.uk/about-epilepsy/epileptic-seizures/seizure-triggers/photosensitive-epilepsy

Federal Communications Commission (FCC). (2023). *Lifeline program for low-income consumers*. https://www.fcc.gov/general/lifeline-program-low-income-consumers

Google Developers. (2022, May 26). *In-depth guide to how Google search works*. https://developers.google.com/search/docs/advanced/guidelines/how-search-works

Gordon, D. (2021, October 6). 1 in 10 Americans turn to social media for health information, new survey shows. *Forbes*. https://www.forbes.com/sites/debgordon/2021/10/06/1-in-10-americans-turn-to-social-media-for-health-information-new-survey-shows/?sh=6fec493b3d93

Hall, K., Gibbie, T., & Lubman, D. I. (2012). Motivational interviewing techniques - facilitating behaviour change in the general practice setting. *Australian Family Physician, 41*(9), 660–667. PMID: 22962639.

Health Literacy Tool Shed. (2024). *Find measures*. https://healthliteracy.bu.edu/all

Health on the Net Foundation. (2020). The 8 principles of the HONcode certification of websites. https://www.hon.ch/en/certification/social-networks.html

Healthcare Information and Management Systems Society (HIMSS). (2022). *Who we are*. https://www.himss.org/who-we-are

Kanejima, Y., Shimogai, T., Kitamura, M., Ishihara, K., & Izawa, K. P. (2022). Impact of health literacy in patients with cardiovascular diseases: A systematic review and meta-analysis. *Patient Education and Counseling, 105*(7), 1793–1800. https://doi-org.uscupstate.idm.oclc.org/10.1016/j.pec.2021.11.021

Kingston, H. (2019, December 31). *LetsGetChecked survey reveals need for better thyroid health awareness*. https://www.letsgetchecked.com/articles/letsgetchecked-survey-reveals-need-for-better-thyroid-health-awareness/

Kington, R. S., Arnesen, S., Chou, W-Y. S., Curry, S. J., Lazer, D., & Villarruel, A. M. (2021). Identifying credible sources of health information in social media: Principles and attributes. *National Academy of Medicine*. https://doi.org/10.31478/202107a

Kirsch, I. S., Jungeblut, A. Jenkins, L., & Kolstad, A. (1993). *Adult literacy in America: A first look at the findings of the National Adult Literacy Survey*. http://nces.ed.gov/pubsearch/pubsinfo.asp?pubid=93275

Kutner, M., Greenberg, E., Jin, Y., & Paulsen, C. (2006). *The health literacy of America's adults: Results from the 2003 National Assessment of Adult Literacy*. US Department of Education, National Center for Education Statistics. https://eric.ed.gov/?id=ED493284

Kyabaggu, R., Marshall, D., Ebuwei, P., & Ikenyei, U. (2022). Health literacy, equity, and communication in the COVID-19 era of misinformation: Emergence of health information professionals in infodemic management. *JMIR Infodemiology, 2*(1), e35014. https://doi.org/10.2196/35014

Land, T. (2019). Healthcare's present and future: Consumer centered, consumer driven. *Frontiers of Health Services Management, 36*(2), 1–2. https://doi.org/10.1097/HAP.0000000000000074

Li, Q., & Luximon, Y. (2020). Older adults' use of mobile device: Usability challenges while navigating various interfaces. *Behaviour & Information Technology, 39*(8), 837–861. https://doi.org/10.1080/0144929X.2019.1622786

Loan, L. A., Parnell, T. A., Stichler, J. F., Boyle, D. K., Allen, P., VanFosson, C. A., & Barton, A. J. (2018 January-February). Call for action: Nurses must play a critical role to enhance health literacy. *Nursing Outlook, 66*(1), 97–100. https://doi.org/10.1016/j.outlook.2017.11.003

Lopez, C., Kim, B., & Sacks, K. (2022). *Health literacy in the United States: Enhancing assessments and reducing disparities*. Milken Institute. https://milkeninstitute.org/sites/default/files/2022-05/Health_Literacy_United_States_Final_Report.pdf

Medical Library Association. (2022). *For health consumers and patients: Find good health information*. http://www.mlanet.org/resources/userguide.html

National Center for Education Statistics (NCES). (n.d.a). Program for the International Assessment of Adult Competencies (PIAAC). *Data collection schedule and plans*. https://nces.ed.gov/surveys/piaac/schedule.asp

National Center for Education Statistics (NCES). (n.d.b). Program for the International Assessment of Adult Competencies (PIAAC). *U.S. PIAAC results in international context*. https://nces.ed.gov/surveys/piaac/results/summary.aspx

National Eye Institute (NEI). (2019, July 3). *Color blindness*. https://www.nei.nih.gov/learn-about-eye-health/eye-conditions-and-diseases/color-blindness

National Institutes of Health (NIH). (2021, July 7). *Cultural respect*. https://www.nih.gov/institutes-nih/nih-office-director/office-communications-public-liaison/clear-communication/cultural-respect

National League for Nursing (NLN). (2015). *A vision for the changing faculty role: Preparing students for the technological world of health care*. https://www.nln.org/docs/default-source/uploadedfiles/about/nln-vision-series-position-statements/nlnvision-8.pdf?sfvrsn=1219df0d_0

National Networks of Libraries of Medicine (NNLM). (2021, December 17). *An introduction to health literacy. What is health literacy?* http://nnlm.gov/outreach/consumer/hlthlit.html

Nielsen-Bohlman, L., Panzer, A. M., Kindig, D. A., & Institute of Medicine, Committee on Health Literacy. (2004). *Health literacy: A prescription to end confusion*. National Academies Press. http://www.nap.edu/openbook.php?record_id=10883&page=1

O'Brien, S. A. (2021, February 4). *Covid-19 vaccine rollout puts a spotlight on unequal internet access*. https://www.cnn.com/2021/02/04/tech/vaccine-internet-digital-divide/index.html

Office of the National Coordinator for Health Information Technology (ONC). (2019). Blue button. *HealthIT.gov*. https://www.healthit.gov/topic/health-it-initiatives/blue-button

Paakkari, L., & Okan, O. (2020). COVID-19: Health literacy is an underestimated problem. *Lancet Public Health, 5*(5), 249–250. https://doi.org/10.1016/S2468-2667(20)30086-4

Parker, R. M., & Ratzan, S. (2019). Re-enforce, not re-define health literacy—Moving forward with health literacy 2.0. *Journal of Health Communication, 24*(12), 923–925. https://doi.org/10.1080/10810730.2019.1691292

Pew Research Center. (2022). *Digital divide*. https://www.pewresearch.org/topic/internet-technology/technology-policy-issues/digital-divide/

Qi, S., Hua, F., Xu, S., Zhou, Z., & Liu, F. (2021). Trends of global health literacy research (1995-2020): Analysis of mapping knowledge domains based on citation data mining. *PLoS One, 16*(8), e0254988. https://doi.org/10.1371/journal.pone.0254988

Santana, S., Brach, C., Harris, L., Ochiai, E., Blakey, C., Bevington, F., Kleinman, D., & Pronk, N. (2021). Updating health literacy for Healthy People 2030: Defining its importance for a new decade in public health. *Journal of Public Health Management and Practice, 27*(Suppl. 6), S258–S264. https://doi.org/10.1097/PHH.0000000000001324

Stagliano, V., & Wallace, L. S. (2013). Brief health literacy screening items predict newest vital sign scores. *Journal of the American Board of Family Medicine, 26*(5), 558–565. https://doi.org10.3122/jabfm.2013.05.130096

Starcevic, V., Berle, D., & Arnáez, S. (2020). Recent insights into cyberchondria. *Current Psychiatry Reports, 22*(11), 56. https://doi.org/10.1007/s11920-020-01179-8

Technology Informatics Guiding Education Reform (TIGER). (2020). *TIGER international competency synthesis project global health informatics: Competency recommendation frameworks*. https://www.himss.org/resources/global-health-informatics-competency-recommendation-frameworks

U.S. Department of Education. (2002, April). Adult literacy in America: A first look at the findings of the National Adult Literacy Survey. NCES 1993-275. http://nces.ed.gov/pubs93/93275.pdf.

U.S. Department of Health and Human Services (HHS). (2018, September). Health literacy. *Healthypeople.gov*. https://www.healthypeople.gov/2020/topics-objectives/topic/social-determinants-health/interventions-resources/health-literacy

U.S. Department of Health and Human Services (HHS). (2021, October 6). *HHS continues to improve access for LEP individuals*. https://www.hhs.gov/civil-rights/for-individuals/special-topics/limited-english-proficiency/hhs-continues-to-improve-access-for-lep-individuals/index.html

U.S. Department of Health and Human Services (HHS). (2022a, March 23). *American recovery and Reinvestment Act of 2009*. https://www.acf.hhs.gov/occ/resource/pi-2009-03

U.S. Department of Health and Human Services (HHS). (2022b). Health literacy in healthy people 2030. *Healthypeople.gov*. https://health.gov/healthypeople/priority-areas/health-literacy-healthy-people-2030

Weber, K. K., Koh, D. D., Stone, L. L., & Lac, A. A. (2020). Savvy seniors: A content analysis of the usability of older adult resource websites. *Innovation in Aging, 4*(Suppl. 1), 413. https://doi.org/10.1093/geroni/igaa057.1330

Wilandika, A., Pandin, M. G. R., & Yusuf, A. (2023). The roles of nurses in supporting health literacy: A scoping review. *Frontiers in Public Health, 11*, 1022803. https://doi.org/10.3389/fpubh.2023.1022803

Wilson, M. (2009). Readability and patient education materials used for low-income populations. *Clinical Nurse Specialist, 23*(1), 33–42; quiz 41–42. https://doi.org/10.1097/01.NUR.0000343079.50214.31

Wu, J. T., & McCormick, J. B. (2018). Why health professionals should speak out against false beliefs on the internet. *AMA Journal of Ethics, 20*(11), E1052–E1058. https://doi.org/10.1001/amajethics.2018.1052

Yamashita, T., Bardo, A. R., Liu, D., & Cummins, P. A. (2020). Literacy, numeracy, and health information seeking among middle-aged and older adults in the United States. *Journal of Aging and Health, 32*(1), 33–41. https://doi.org/10.1177/0898264318800918

Zuzelo, P. (2019). Understandability and actionability. Using the PEMAT to benefit health literacy. *Holistic Nursing Practice, 33*(3), 191–193. https://doi.org/10.1097/HNP.0000000000000327

CHAPTER 15

Protecting Patient Privacy and Confidentiality

Kristi Miller, Janna Lock, and Allison Devine

OBJECTIVES

After studying this chapter, you will be able to:

1. Discuss how the American Nurses Association Nursing Code of Ethics applies to the protection of patient privacy and confidentiality.
2. Explain how you can protect patient privacy and confidentiality.
3. Identify legal issues surrounding the protection of personal health information, including the Health Insurance Portability and Accountability Act (HIPAA).
4. Explain the consequences of HIPAA violations and how to avoid them.
5. Discuss principles of data security and how to prevent a security breach.

AACN Essentials for Entry-Level Professional Nursing Education

1.2e Demonstrate ethical decision making.
3.1i Identify ethical principles to protect the health and safety of diverse populations.
8.5a Identify common risks associated with using information and communication technology.
8.5c Comply with legal and regulatory requirements while using communication and information technologies.
8.5d Educate patients on their rights to access, review, and correct personal data and medical records.
9.1a Apply principles of professional nursing ethics and human rights in patient care and professional situations.

AACN Essentials for Advanced-Level Nursing Education

8.5g Apply risk mitigation and security strategies to reduce misuse of information and communication technology.
8.5h Assess potential ethical and legal issues associated with the use of information and communication technology.
8.5j Promote patient engagement with their personal health data.

8.5l Analyze the impact of federal and state policies and regulation on health data and technology in care settings.

9.1i Model ethical behaviors in practice and leadership roles.

HIMSS TIGER Competencies

Consumer health informatics

Data protection and security

Ethics in health internet technology

Information and knowledge management in patient care

Internet technology risk management

Legal issues in health internet technology

Public health informatics

KEY TERMS

Audit trail
Authentication
Automatic logout
Biometric
Confidentiality
Data security
Data breach
Firewall
Health Insurance Portability and Accountability Act (HIPAA)
HIPAA Privacy Rule
Login
Privacy
Privacy Rights Clearinghouse
Protected health information (PHI)
Risk assessment
Security breach
Single sign-on
Two-factor authentication (2FA)
Universal patient identifier (UPI)
White hat hackers

CASE STUDY

Since electronic health records (EHRs) were first used in 1992, there has been concern over protection of patient health information. Stealing paper records is not difficult on a small scale, but thieves would need a large truck to steal 20,431 paper records. However, stealing a laptop that contains that same number of EHRs would not require any heavy physical lifting.

In February 2017, a laptop was stolen from the vehicle of an employee of Lifespan, part of the Rhode Island health system. The employee's work emails may have been stored in a file on the device's hard drive, which gave the thieves access to names, medical record numbers, demographic information, partial addresses, and prescribed medications for 20,431 patients. A U.S. Department of Health and Human Services (HHS) Office for Civil Rights (OCR) investigation found that Lifespan had not implemented encryption of all devices used for work purposes, nor did it sufficiently track or inventory all devices that might contain patient health information. The hospital system was ordered to pay $1,040,000 and put a corrective action plan in place to settle the violation (Miliard, 2020).

Security breaches can happen to any institution without proper security features in place. As you read this chapter, think about what you can do as a nurse to protect the privacy and confidentiality of patient health information.

The proper protection of patient information is a major concern for all healthcare team members, and informatics plays a key role in protecting patient privacy and confidentiality. Rapid technology development and implementation require healthcare professionals and organizations to stay current to keep patients safe. Healthcare personnel with access to protected patient information have an obligation to abide by professional, ethical, and legal standards when handling that information. This chapter addresses the responsibilities of nurses in terms of informatics in protecting patient privacy and confidentiality in the digital era.

PRIVACY AND CONFIDENTIALITY

The words "privacy" and "confidentiality" are often used interchangeably. When discussing healthcare information, **privacy** applies to individuals. It is the right of patients to control what happens to their health information. Patients have the right to control who has access to their health information and to disclose or not disclose that information to others. They also control the circumstances, the timing, and the extent to which information may be disclosed. It is the role of the nurse to safeguard that right to privacy not just for patients but for their families and communities. **Confidentiality** applies to information; it is an agreement to maintain the secrecy of sensitive information or documents. It is the duty of authorized care providers to maintain all patient health information as secret, except to other care providers who need access to that information and to others that the patient has consented to allow access. Box 15-1 provides a brief overview of how to maintain privacy and confidentiality.

As technology evolves at a staggering rate, providing protection has become more challenging. Healthcare professionals are being asked to balance the risks associated with patient autonomy and the greater good. Laws and regulations vary by state, and misconceptions about what they can and cannot do for patient privacy persist. Nurses are advocates for patient privacy and for policies and practices that protect the confidentiality of patient information.

Nurses must also support an environment that protects confidentiality and for the development of policies that protect personal and clinical health information at all levels. The Ethical Considerations box discusses how the American Nurses Association (ANA) Nursing Code of Ethics applies to privacy and confidentiality.

ETHICAL CONSIDERATIONS FOR PATIENT PRIVACY AND CONFIDENTIALITY

Provision three of the ANA Code of Ethics (2015) states, "The nurse promotes, advocates for, and protects the rights, health, and safety of the patient." Interpretive Statement 3.1 calls on nurses to protect the privacy and confidentiality of patients. The need for healthcare does not justify unwanted, unnecessary, or unwarranted intrusion into a person's health information. Privacy also falls under the ethical concept of patient autonomy, a person's right to make decisions about their lives without interference from others. Maintaining confidentiality demonstrates respect for others. Think about how you will respond to situations where patient privacy or confidentiality is being compromised. Having a plan for what to do if patient privacy or confidentiality is breached is important. Practicing what you will say before it happens will help you embody the values of the Code of Ethics with professionalism and empathy while keeping the patient at the center of care.

Ensuring Patient Privacy

Safeguarding the privacy of patients is one of the primary ethical responsibilities of nurses. In nursing school, one of the first topics taught is to facilitate patient privacy. Closing doors, drawing curtains around hospital beds, and draping patients with blankets while bathing protect privacy and dignity. Home visits might need to be timed to ensure the privacy the patient desires and needs. Sensitive matters should be discussed with patients when they are alone, and permission should be obtained before having those discussions with others are around. When gathering patient data, there will be

> **BOX 15-1** How to Maintain Privacy and Confidentiality
>
> 1. Follow workplace security and privacy policies to protect confidential patient health information.
> 2. Be compliant with HIPAA rules and regulations.
> 3. Understand the definition of PHI, when, how, and with whom it can be shared. Examples of PHI covered by HIPAA include:
>   - Demographic information
>   - Health conditions, including diagnoses and test results
>   - Clinical data, such as lab results, diagnostic test results, procedures, and medications
>   - Billing and payment information
>   - Photographs
> 4. Keep all PHI out of the public's eye.
> 5. Discard PHI appropriately in accordance with your workplace privacy policy.
> 6. Consult your HIPAA privacy officer regarding suspicious activities.

many topics patients wish to keep private, and patients have every right to expect the nurse to maintain this privacy.

Patient privacy also needs to be considered when interviewing a patient. The environment should be such that the interview cannot be overheard. Additionally, only pertinent health information required to render care should be gathered. Another item to be considered is the placement of technology on which charting is done. Ideally, screens should not be visible to anyone except the person charting. The nurse must log off before leaving the area; otherwise, anyone who approaches the screen will be able to access private information.

In addition to these actions, nurses also need to be familiar with institutional policies on privacy; the requirements of the Health Insurance Portability and Accountability Act (HIPAA), discussed later; and the laws, rules, and regulations for the use and protection of electronic health information.

Regulating Patient Privacy

Each state defines **protected health information (PHI)** differently and has different standards for if, when, and how victims of HIPAA violations are notified. PHI is any information about health status, provision of healthcare, or payment for healthcare that is created or collected by a covered entity and can be linked to a specific individual. The **Privacy Rights Clearinghouse**, which maintains an online record of all types of security breaches, has information on laws, reports, and advocacy, including data breach notification rules, in each state. In 2002, California became the first state to recognize the need to alert residents when their data were exposed in security incidents. In 2018, the last two states, South Dakota and Alabama, enacted data breach notification statutes to protect their residents (Privacy Rights Clearinghouse, 2023).

Regulatory agencies such as state boards of nursing, the Centers for Medicare & Medicaid (CMS), and The Joint Commission provide patient privacy rules for individuals and organizations to follow. A person or agency caught not following a rule may be penalized. The penalty for breaking a rule might be a fine but could also involve temporary or permanent loss of privileges.

Protecting Confidentiality

Many nurses spend full days with patients and their information, reviewing records, recording health histories, administering medications, and providing interventions. Being constantly surrounded by this information makes it vital to understand how to maintain confidentiality.

Confidentiality of private information located in digitized records starts with the users. Confidentiality is a balancing act. Properly securing healthcare records can make accessing them more difficult and time-consuming. Users must understand the need for protecting information but also tailor their behaviors to guarantee this protection. To prevent unauthorized users from accessing patient information, login information cannot be written down and left out and screens with patient data exposed cannot be left unattended. This may be inconvenient, but confidentiality is more important than convenience.

Authentication

The potential for health records to end up in the wrong hands has always been a concern for healthcare providers, but the conversion from paper to EHRs has brought into focus how facilities keep patients' health records confidential. Electronic records bring the potential for a massive number of health records to be breached. Unauthorized entrance to a healthcare system gives a cyber criminal easy access to a huge number of records. The first line of defense is an authentication process to prevent unauthorized access or entrance to the system. **Authentication** is the process of verifying a person's identity to prevent unauthorized access to healthcare records.

Login Name and Passwords

Anyone who has ever used a network in a healthcare agency or a secure site on the web becomes familiar with login names (user identifications) and passwords. Most systems today rely on a login name and a password for authentication. A **login** is a name the user enters to be able to use the systems and applications that the device can access. Various systems of designating login names are used, such as the first initial and last name, many of which are easy to guess and generally remain the same throughout the network.

Because logins can be easy to guess, the rules for passwords are often more stringent and vary from agency to agency. The best passwords are difficult for unauthorized users to guess or to figure out by trying various combinations until the correct one is found. Using a combination of uppercase and lowercase letters, numbers, and special characters is the most secure. Institutions and workplaces may have policies on how often to change passwords. These policies are based on the premise that after a given length of time, one's password has likely been compromised, either purposely or accidentally. Additionally, most systems prohibit users from reusing a password.

Organizations must balance the benefit of time-restricted passwords with the pitfalls of forcing a change too frequently. Frequent changes can result in users writing the password down and pasting it somewhere visible. Not changing frequently enough leaves users open to having the security of their account breached. More information about how to protect devices and personal information can be found in Chapter 3.

Network administrators may face difficulties regarding logins and passwords. For example, they need to be able to provide temporary logins and passwords to short-term system users, such as temporary staff and nursing students. There must be a network policy for closing the accounts of both temporary users and other workers who leave their positions because unused accounts are in danger of being hacked. Network administrators also must deal with regulatory pressure, security threats, and the cost of help desks. Password problems are among the top day-to-day issues encountered at information technology (IT) help desks.

Two-Factor Authentication

Two-factor authentication (2FA) requires two methods of identification to access an account. 2FA is an extra layer of security used to ensure that persons trying to gain access are who they say they are. First, a user enters their login and password. Then, instead of immediately gaining access, they are required to provide another piece of information (Fig. 15-1). This second factor typically comes from one of the following categories (TwilioAuthy, n.d.):

- Something the user knows: A personal identification number (PIN), a second password, or answers to "secret questions"
- Something the user has: A credit card, a code sent to a smartphone, or a small hardware token
- Something the user is: A biometric pattern of a fingerprint, an iris scan, or a voice print

Hardware tokens, the oldest form of 2FA, are small, similar to a key fob, and produce a numeric code every 30 seconds. When a user tries to access an account, they enter the displayed 2FA code into the site. Other versions of hardware tokens automatically transfer the 2FA code when plugged into a computer. These fobs are expensive and are easy to lose, leading to the development of other 2FA methods.

Text message and voice-based 2FA sends a code directly to the user's phone. After receiving

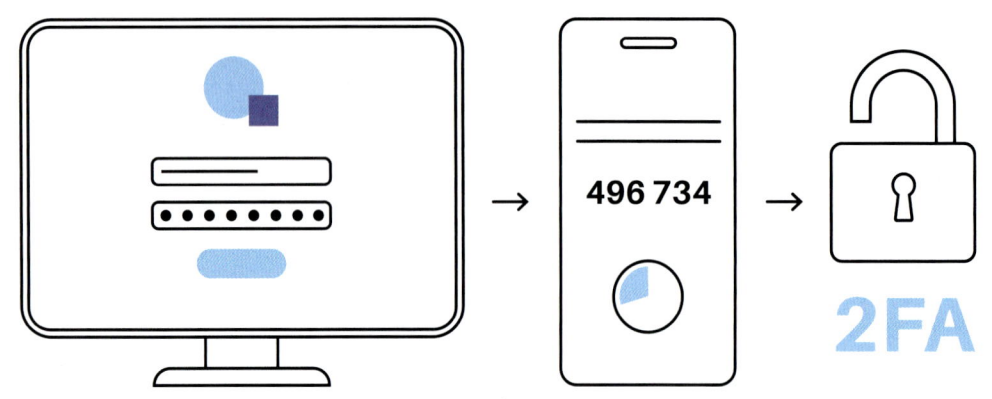

Figure 15-1. Two-factor authentication. (Shutterstock/Pikovit.)

a username and password, the site either texts or calls the user with a unique one-time passcode (OTP). The user then enters the OTP back into the application. Voice-based 2FA is more frequently used in places where smartphones are expensive or where cell service is poor. Text message and voice-based 2FA are the least secure ways to authenticate users.

Software tokens are the most popular form of 2FA. The user installs a free 2FA app available for mobile, wearables, or desktop platforms. A software-generated time-based OTP (TOTP, or "soft token") is generated. After entering a username and password, the user enters the code shown on the app. Soft tokens are typically valid for less than a minute, making them less vulnerable to hackers.

Push notifications for 2FA utilize websites and apps to tell the user that an authentication attempt is taking place. The device owner views the details and approves or denies access with a single touch. Push notification eliminates the opportunity for phishing or unauthorized access, but it only works with internet and with devices that can use the software.

Biometric 2FA is authentication in which a person's identity is confirmed with fingerprints, retina patterns, facial recognition, handwriting, and voice recognition (Fig. 15-2). Ambient noise, pulse, typing patterns, and vocal prints are also being explored (TwilioAuthy, n.d.). Biometric authentication is gaining in popularity because it does not rely on human memory and thus is more secure (nothing ever needs to be written down). In essence, you are your own password with biometrics.

Automatic Logout

Between the times that users log in and out, they are responsible for anything that is done from their account. When a nurse leaves a screen unattended with patient data exposed, the patient's confidentiality is breached. Any unauthorized person can access patient health information and can make entries into the system under the nurse's name. Just as you lock your car or your home, develop the habit of logging off before leaving your workstation.

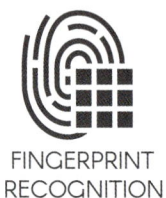

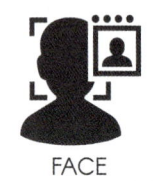

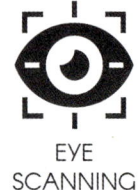

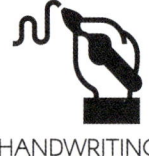

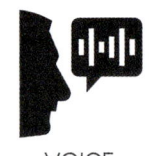

FINGERPRINT RECOGNITION | FACE AUTHENTICATION | EYE SCANNING | HANDWRITING RECOGNITION | VOICE AUTHENTICATION

Figure 15-2. Types of biometric authentication. (Shutterstock/FishCoolish.)

Knowing emergencies often arise that involve calling a nurse away from the screen, most systems time out after a given length of time with no input activity. **Automatic logout** is a built-in safety feature for clinical information systems in which the information system automatically logs the user out after a designated period. Your organization's designated HIPAA security official is often involved in deciding how long the interval is before a user is automatically logged out. If the interval is too short, it can become annoying to users who must go through the entire login process repeatedly. If the interval is too long, it could allow someone else to perform unauthorized activities. Finding the best interval is a necessary balancing act to protecting confidentiality.

Single Sign-On

Use of different logins for every clinical application can be problematic. Having multiple passwords that expire on a regular basis creates the same problem as having passwords expire too frequently—users may write down the passwords to remember them, leaving them accessible to unauthorized users. Each login requires authentication and forces the busy professional to wait before completing a transaction. **Single sign-on** (SSO) allows a user to access multiple clinical applications with only one login and password for authentication. This is more efficient, improves workflow, and prevents accidental breaches of security and confidentiality. A disadvantage is that if an SSO is compromised, all applications and services linked to it may also be at risk. Because of this, an additional authentication factor should be considered for applications that require a secure network.

> **CASE STUDY**
>
> Think about the case study in which a stolen laptop was used to gain access to patient information. How could the strategies for protecting patient confidentiality have prevented this data breach?

HEALTH INSURANCE PORTABILITY AND ACCOUNTABILITY ACT

The 1996 **Health Insurance Portability and Accountability Act (HIPAA)** has affected the entire healthcare industry, including healthcare information technology (HIT). The purpose of the law was to improve the effectiveness and efficiency of healthcare. It was also designed to prevent medical fraud by standardizing the electronic exchange of financial and administrative data. HIPAA and its subsequent modifications address the protection of health information exchanged electronically. The law addressed several areas pertaining to healthcare information, including simplifying healthcare claims, providing standards for healthcare data transmission, and ensuring the security of healthcare information (HHS, 2021).

HIPAA security standards call for a "technology-neutral" method for the transmission of data among healthcare organizations. "Technology-neutral" means that any system can import and read the data. This is like the use of rich text format (RTF), which permits most word processors to read documents created by other word processors. In this way, healthcare organizations are not forced to use outdated technology to comply with HIPAA standards.

HIPAA Privacy Rule

If you have visited a healthcare provider in the United States, then you have signed a HIPAA form. The **HIPAA Privacy Rule** requires that an individual provide signed authorization to a covered entity before the entity may use or disclose certain protected health information (Fig. 15-3). The HIPAA Privacy Rule applies to healthcare providers that conduct standard healthcare transactions electronically; healthcare clearinghouses; or health plans (HHS, 2021). Once the HIPAA form has been signed, these healthcare entities may use or disclose PHI (e.g., imaging, laboratory and pathology reports, diagnoses, other medical information) without the patient's further authorization for treatment purposes. A HIPAA authorization form gives covered entities permission to use PHI for purposes other than treatment, payment, or healthcare operations. Those other purposes would be stated on the form.

HIPAA AUTHORIZATION FOR USE OR DISCLOSURE OF HEALTH INFORMATION

Date: _____, 20____

I. **THE PATIENT.** This form is for use when such authorization is required and complies with the Health Insurance Portability and Accountability Act of 1996 (HIPAA) Privacy Standards.

      Patient's Name: _____
      Date of Birth: _____, 20____
      Social Security Number: _____-____=____

II. **AUTHORIZATION.** I authorize _____ ("Authorized Party") to use or disclose the following: (check one)

    ☐ - All of my medical-related information.
    ☐ - My medical information ONLY related to: _____.
    ☐ - My medical-related information from _____, 20____ to _____, 20____.
    ☐ - Other: _____.

Hereinafter known as the "Medical Records."

III. **DISCLOSURE.** The Authorized Party has my authorization to disclose Medical Records to: (check one)

    ☐ - Any party that is approved by Authorized Party.
    ☐ - ONLY the following party:
        Name: _____
        Address: _____
        Phone: (____) ____-_____ Fax: (____) ____-_____
        E-Mail: _____

IV. **PURPOSE.** The reason for this authorization is: (check one)

    ☐ - **General Purpose.** At my request (general).

    ☐ - **To Receive Payment.** To allow the Authorized Party to communicate with me for marketing purposes when they receive payment from a third party.

    ☐ - **To Sell Medical Records.** To allow the Authorized Party to sell my Medical Records. I understand that the Authorized Party will receive compensation for the disclosure of my Medical Records and will stop any future sales if I revoke this authorization.

    ☐ - **Other.** _____.

Figure 15-3. Sample HIPAA authorization form.

Universal Patient Identifier

HIPAA calls for the use of unique identifying numbers for all healthcare providers, employers, health plans, and patients. Providers have national provider identifiers (NPIs), and employers use employer identification numbers (EINs). These numbers are used in all HIPAA standard transactions (CMS, 2022).

However, a **universal patient identifier (UPI)**, a single medical identification number assigned to each patient in the United States, has not been established. Much like a Social Security number (SSN), a UPI would be unique to each person or entity and used only with regard to health information. The primary benefit for the UPI would be to accurately match patients with their medical records no matter where they sought care. The Joint Commission publishes a list of patient safety goals every year, and "identify patients correctly" has been on the list for several years (The Joint Commission, 2024). Mismatched patient records and duplicate patient records would be remedied with UPIs. UPIs would save lives, cut costs, and enable easier public health research (Alder, 2023a).

However, there is currently a ban on the use of federal funding for the development of UPIs. The biggest political argument against the UPI is that the government would become involved in individual healthcare. Some people believe that a UPI would open people up to governmental involvement in medical decisions, unauthorized medical research, and higher risks of medical data theft (Alder, 2023a; Frieden, 2023). This topic has created much debate, and nurses and nursing students may find it a valuable avenue to engage in political advocacy.

HITECH Act and HIPAA Protection

The Health Information Technology for Economic and Clinical Health (HITECH) Act went into effect in 2009 as part of the American Recovery and Reinvestment Act. The HITECH Act magnified HIPAA to promote the implementation of EHRs and support technology in the United States. It strengthened the privacy and security portions of HIPAA, increased the financial penalties for healthcare organizations that did not comply with HIPAA, and forced business associates of healthcare organizations to comply with HIPAA (Alder, 2024).

In 2013, the HITECH Act Interim Final Rule defined unsecured PHI and the term "security breach" (HHS, 2017). A **security breach** is any incident that results in unauthorized access to computer data, applications, networks, or devices. The HITECH Act required agencies to ensure that private health information is secure and to prevent a breach or unauthorized access or disclosure of the information.

HIPAA Violations

A HIPAA violation occurs when an organization or individual fails to comply with one or more of the provisions of the HIPAA Privacy, Security, or Breach Notification Rules. An example of this is found in the case study when the healthcare organization, Lifespan, neglected to provide encryption or adequate tracking for devices, resulting in a security breach. Some other examples of organizational and individual HIPAA violations can be found in Box 15-2.

Common types of HIPAA violations include:

- Looking at healthcare records without permission or authorization
- Not performing an organization-wide risk analysis
- Failure to address security risks
- Denying patients access to their health records
- Failure to enter into a HIPAA-Compliant Business Associate Agreement
- Insufficient PHI-access control measures
- Failing to use encryption or equivalent security to safeguard electronic PHI
- Exceeding the 60-day deadline for notifying individuals of breaches
- Unauthorized PHI disclosures
- Improper disposal of PHI

HIPAA violations may be deliberate or unintentional. An example of an unintentional HIPAA violation is when an employee of the IT department is allowed to view PHI when working to resolve technologic issues with PHI storage or retrieval. An

BOX 15-2 Examples of HIPAA Violations

Organizational HIPAA Violations
- Certain cyber criminals gained access to a health insurance provider's computer system with a phishing email that installed malware. They accessed the PHI of 10.5 million individuals, and the breach went undetected for 9 months. HHS OCR investigated and fined the company $6.85 million.
- The Federal Bureau of Investigation discovered that anyone could access the server for a medical imaging company and view the PHI of over 300,000 individuals with a simple search. The company failed to notify the affected individuals until 147 days after the discovery. The company was fined $3 million and ordered to adopt a corrective action plan.
- A local public agency in Los Angeles County that provides health coverage to residents with lower incomes was identified on social media when members discovered they could access the PHI of other patients. This was due to a manual processing error and affected around 500 individuals. Later, the agency reported a data breach themselves to the OCR that was due to a mailing error that affected almost 1,500 patients. They were fined $1.3 million for multiple violations and a lack of risk analysis and appropriate security measures.
- In response to a negative review online by a patient, a dental practice posted PHI about the patient including full name and treatment recommendations, plus derogatory comments about the patient. HHS OCR determined this was impermissible disclosure of PHI. After refusing to remove the post online and not cooperating with the investigation or responding to a subpoena, the dental practice was fined $50,000 for willful violation and neglect with no correction.
- An employee at a New York medical center stole data from more than 12,000 patients and sold it to an identity theft ring. The HHS OCR found that the medical center had failed to perform a risk assessment to identify the potential risks and vulnerabilities to the electronic PHI. The medical center settled the investigation and had to pay a $4.75 million penalty.
- The Associated Press published an article about a nonprofit medical center and its response to COVID-19. The HHS OCR opened an investigation when they saw that the article included information and photographs about several patients. The medical center had not obtained authorizations from the patients to be included in the article, and it faced an $80,000 fine and agreed to adopt a corrective action plan.

Individual HIPAA Violations
- After a cardiothoracic surgeon was terminated from a hospital, he illegally accessed the medical records system over 300 times. He viewed the PHI of his former immediate supervisor and coworkers as well as that of several celebrities. The physician pled guilty and was sentenced to 4 months in jail along with a $2,000 fine.
- A patient at a large hospital signed a release form requesting that his PHI be sent to a post office box. Instead, the hospital faxed the document to the patient's employer. Based on his medical status, the patient was asked to quit his job and lost his health benefits. He filed a lawsuit for $2.5 million in damages. The hospital did not attempt to compensate the patient but did agree to review its policies and procedures.

(Continued)

- After pop star Britney Spears was hospitalized for psychiatric issues, 6 doctors and 13 employees at the medical center accessed her records. None of these individuals had a legitimate medical reason to view her PHI. At the same hospital, celebrities Farah Fawcett and Maria Shriver also had their data exposed to unauthorized personnel, with some of the information sold to tabloids. Numerous physicians and employees were suspended or terminated in these cases, and the hospital was fined $865,500.

Data from Alder, S. (2011, July 8). UCLA hospitals receives $865K HIPAA fine for failing to protect celebrity medical records. *The HIPAA Journal*. https://www.hipaajournal.com/ucla-hospitals-receives-865k-hipaa-fine-failing-protect-celebrity-medical-records/; HIPAA Security Suite. (2019, September 25). *HIPAA Horror Stories: 5 True HIPAA Violation Cases*. https://hipaasecuritysuite.com/hipaa-horror-stories-5-true-hipaa-violation-cases/; SecureFrame. (2022, January 13). *HIPAA Violations: Examples, Penalties +5 Cases to Learn*. https://secureframe.com/blog/hipaa-violations; The HIPAA Journal. (2024). *HIPAA violation cases*. https://www.hipaajournal.com/hipaa-violation-cases/.

example of a deliberate violation is when breach notification letters are not sent to patients within 60 days or there is a failure to perform an organization-wide risk assessment. Financial penalties for unintentional HIPAA violations are lower than those for willful HIPAA violations. If an organization commits a willful violation of HIPAA laws, the maximum fines apply.

The goal of financial penalties is to prevent violation of HIPAA laws while ensuring organizations are held accountable for their actions (or lack of them) related to the protection of patient privacy and the confidentiality of health data. Penalties for HIPAA violations can be issued by the HHS OCR and state attorneys general. Organizations are required to adopt corrective action plans to bring policies and procedures up to HIPAA standards and may incur financial penalties. Penalties for HIPAA violations apply to healthcare providers, health plans, and healthcare clearinghouses.

Ignorance of HIPAA regulations is no excuse for violating them. Each organization is responsible for ensuring that the HIPAA rules are understood and followed. HIPAA requires that each agency assign a HIPAA officer the responsibility for overseeing efforts to secure electronic data. This person must be proficient in IT, auditing, agency policies and practices, ethics, state and federal regulations, and consumer issues. This ensures organizations cannot claim ignorance of HIPAA regulations.

Your employer should have a process for reporting HIPAA violations if you witness one. When in doubt, report the violation to your supervisor, manager, or departmental head. If that is not an option, reach out to your HIPAA officer.

Penalties for HIPAA Violations

Penalties can potentially be issued for all organizational HIPAA violations. However, HHS OCR tries to use nonpunitive measures when possible. Cases are typically resolved through voluntary compliance, issuing technical guidance, or accepting a plan to address the violations and change policies and procedures to prevent future violations. Factors that are considered when determining penalties include prior history, financial condition, level of harm, how long the violation was allowed to persist, how many people were affected, and the type of data exposed. The willingness of the organization to assist with the investigation is also considered (HIPAA Journal, 2024). Financial penalties for HIPAA violations are reserved for the most serious violations. The four violation categories and the financial penalty for each are outlined in Table 15-1.

Individual HIPAA violations can be identified in various ways. The employer may identify them during a required HIPAA risk assessment, the HHS OCR may find them during a HIPAA audit, or the patient(s) who were victimized may report it. If an individual breaks HIPAA rules, the employer may deal with it internally. Punishment may include termination, license suspension, or criminal charges (Alder, 2023b). The consequences for individuals breaking HIPAA rules

TABLE 15-1 2024 HIPAA Financial Penalty Structure for Organizations[a]

Penalty Tier	Minimum Penalty per Violation	Maximum Penalty per Violation	Maximum Annual Penalty Amount
Tier 1: Lack of knowledge	$137	$68,928	$2,067,813
Tier 2: Reasonable cause	$1,379	$68,928	$2,067,813
Tier 3: Willful neglect	$13,785	$68,928	$2,067,813
Tier 4: Willful neglect (not corrected within 30 days)	$68,928	$2,067,813	$2,067,813

[a]Dollar amounts are adjusted for inflation. Last updated in January 2024.
Data from HIPAA Journal. (2024). *What are the penalties for HIPAA violations?* https://www.hipaajournal.com/what-are-the-penalties-for-hipaa-violations-7096/

depend on the severity of the violation and other factors:

- The nature of the violation
- Whether there was knowledge that HIPAA rules were being violated
- Whether action was taken to correct the violation
- Whether there was malicious intent or the violation was for personal gain
- The amount of harm caused by the violation
- The number of people affected by the violation

Civil penalties for HIPAA violations can range from $100 to $25,000 per violation. Criminal penalties can be severe. Fines for willful violations of HIPAA range from $50,000 to $250,000 (Alder, 2023b). Restitution may need to be made to the victims. A jail term is likely for a criminal HIPAA violation. Criminal violations related to negligence can result in a prison term of up to 1 year. Obtaining PHI under false pretenses carries a maximum prison term of 5 years. Knowingly violating HIPAA with malicious intent or for personal gain can result in a prison term of up to 10 years. A 2-year jail term for aggravated identity theft is mandatory.

If an individual can make a case that a HIPAA violation occurred due to a lack of training, the employer is held liable for failing to provide training. Employers are required to document HIPAA training attendance, content, and timing.

> **CASE STUDY**
>
> In the case study, Lifespan received a financial penalty and was ordered to put a corrective action plan into place. Contact your HIPAA security officer to find out if your institution or facility has ever had to pay a HIPAA fine. Did the financial penalty affect the functioning of the institution? Have any of your colleagues ever been involved in a HIPAA violation or have they heard of a nurse who was involved? What penalties were assessed?

Limitations of HIPAA Protection

HIPAA is so prevalent that some have come to mistakenly believe that all health records are private and confidential. For example, in the case of *Beard v. City of Chicago*, a paramedic from the city's fire department took a medical leave of absence. The fire department had copies of all employees' medical records. They read Beard's medical records and discovered that she was being treated for depression and subsequently terminated her. The plaintiff pleaded that her HIPAA rights had been violated, but the court ruled that HIPAA was not applicable because the fire department did not fall into any one of the three categories that HIPAA covers; it was not a fee-for-service healthcare provider, a health plan, or a healthcare clearinghouse (Beard v. City of Chicago, 2004).

HIPAA has been criticized for not protecting all private health information. The HITECH Act serves to bridge the limitations of HIPAA. However, if the health information does not fall under HIPAA or the HITECH Act, the information is not protected. Examples include patient health records stored at their homes, on their personal devices, or those kept on file at a health club.

DATA SECURITY

Nurses, as well as all healthcare providers and technical staff, need to understand and follow the principles of data security. **Data security** involves protecting data in three ways: ensuring the accuracy of the data, protecting the data from unauthorized eyes, and managing data loss.

Protecting Data Accuracy

Accuracy of data can be improved with methods that check data during input, such as using standardized terms and phrases (covered in more detail in Chapter 13). However, when incorrect entries are made, even if they are corrected within the predetermined time limit, a record of all the entries is kept within an audit trail. An **audit trail** is a chronologic record detailing electronic transactions that is commonly used with clinical information systems to monitor appropriate access and use of information. It provides a list of who accessed the system, the date, the time, and the activity. The existence of the audit trail encourages users to input data as accurately as possible.

Protecting Data From Unauthorized Internal Access

Unauthorized access to data within an organization is minimized by assigning appropriate levels of access and performing periodic record access audits. Who has access to what information differs from agency to agency and is usually determined by necessity and ease of use. Access to patient records is needed when patients are cared for by multiple providers or are transferred from one department to another. Whenever a patient record is accessed, an audit trail reveals which individual worker accessed which record at what time and where, so documenting the reason for accessing records is important for protection from legal action. Audit trails must be routinely examined to determine if breaches of security are occurring and may be closely scrutinized after the discovery of a medical error.

Audit trails can identify the user who accessed the record by username, the internet protocol (IP) address, the pages accessed, and the length of time of the access. Audit trails assisted in identifying the employees in a famous breach that occurred in 2008 when University of California Los Angeles Medical Center fired 13 employees and suspended six others for looking at the medical record of the celebrity Britney Spears (Ornstein, 2008). Organizational regulations vary for access to patient records. Many institutions provide access only to records of patients on the unit where the healthcare worker is stationed and index the employees by job description. Other institutions provide no limits, giving individuals the responsibility to limit themselves to looking only at patient records necessary to perform their duties. Limiting access too severely can prohibit holistic care and put patients in jeopardy if access is needed in an emergent situation.

Protecting Data From Unauthorized External Access

Most healthcare institutions are connected to and use the internet. Preventing outsiders from accessing institutional information has become a major responsibility of IT departments. One of the first lines of defense for protecting against unauthorized access is a firewall. A **firewall** is a computer network system that blocks incoming and outgoing data using a set of rules. It operates in one of two ways; it examines all messages entering and leaving a system and blocks those that do not meet specific criteria, or it allows or denies messages based on whether the destination port is acceptable. Firewalls require constant maintenance.

To ensure a system is safe from prying eyes, some agencies hire **white hat hackers** who attempt to penetrate their information systems. A hacker or cyber criminal is an individual or team of people who use technology to commit malicious activities on digital systems or networks with the intention of stealing sensitive company information or personal data and generating profit. White hat hackers have the skills to be cyber criminals but are ethically opposed to security abuse. Their job is to identify security weaknesses, allowing the IT department to devise protection for any security breaches found.

Systems also need protection from outsiders who gain physical entrance to the agency. The first line of defense against this type of breach includes staff education on the importance of data security. Staff should be encouraged to expect identification from unfamiliar persons and to refuse access to anyone without recognized authorization. Chapter 4 goes into detail about the ways cyber criminals attempt to achieve security breaches and how to protect patient data.

Protection From Data Loss

Data loss is a major concern for healthcare organizations. Examples of circumstances that can cause data loss and affect continuity of care include disasters such as the September 11, 2001 attacks, Hurricanes Katrina in 2005 and Sandy in 2012, and the tornadoes that destroyed St. John's Medical Center in Missouri in 2011 (Adler & Bauer, 2016) and Moore Medical Center in Oklahoma in 2013 (Brumfield, 2014). Security breaches by cyber criminals can also cause data loss. As medical information is increasingly electronic, the physical loss of paper medical records becomes less of a concern. However, electronic medical data are still at risk for loss or damage.

To provide protection, data must be routinely backed up and stored offsite in a secure location. Backup systems should be periodically examined to ensure data integrity and confirm that the reinstallation of data into the system goes smoothly. A disaster recovery plan needs to be devised and tested in conjunction with key people in the agency to ensure adequate protection. One of the first tasks in planning for disaster recovery is to perform a risk analysis. This analysis determines vulnerabilities and appropriate control measures. Identification of system weaknesses can prevent data loss due to disaster. A disaster plan should be tested at least twice a year.

Data Security Breaches

As stated earlier, a security breach results in information being accessed without authorization. Typically, it occurs when an intruder bypasses security mechanisms. A security breach is the break-in, whereas a **data breach** is defined as the cyber criminal getting away with the information. As seen in Chapter 4, cyber criminals may attempt security breaches using phishing tactics, which can trick employees into revealing private login information (DNI, n.d.). All phishing scams should be reported to the Anti-Phishing Working Group.

Security breaches can happen with paper records as well. Examples include the overturning of a truck carrying paper records; someone tampering with postal mail; or the theft or loss of patient paper files, devices, or drives. Cyber criminals often receive media attention because so much can be stolen relatively invisibly and quickly, but data breaches involving paper records can be just as damaging. A data security breach is unlawful and can result in fines, imprisonment, or both.

Prevalence of Breaches

According to the Identity Theft Resource Center (ITRC, 2024), there were more data compromises reported in the United States in 2023 than in any year since the first state data breach notice law became effective in 2003. The overall number of data compromises (3,205) went up by 77% over 2022, though the number of victims continued to decrease (down by 16% in 2023 compared to the previous year) as identity criminals focus more on specific data types rather than mass data acquisition. Figure 15-4 shows the trend over the past decade for the number of compromises and victims.

The ramifications for those affected by data breaches are potentially devastating if the criminals use it maliciously for personal gain. Healthcare was the industry with the greatest number of data compromises in each of the past 5 years with 25% of the total compromises in 2023 (ITRC, 2024), giving credence to concerns that we must work harder to protect the private and confidential information of healthcare consumers. The role of the informatics nurse in data protection is more important than ever.

Number of Data Compromises

Number of Victims

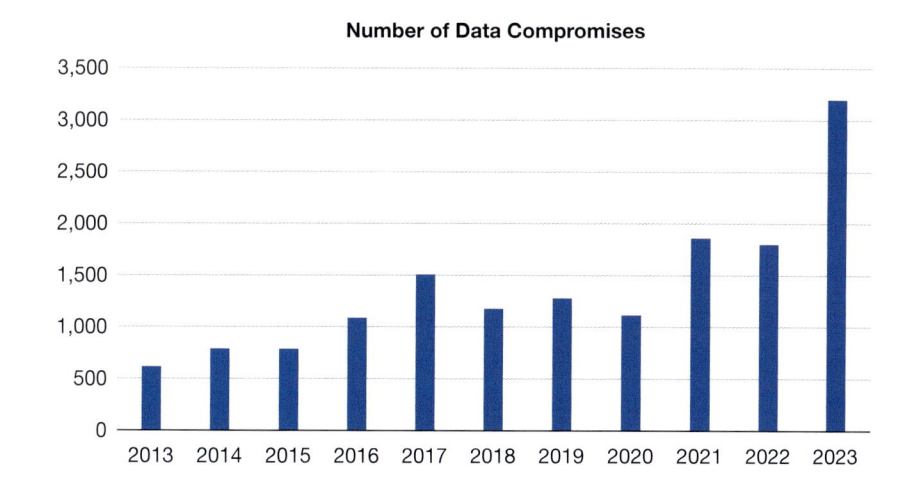

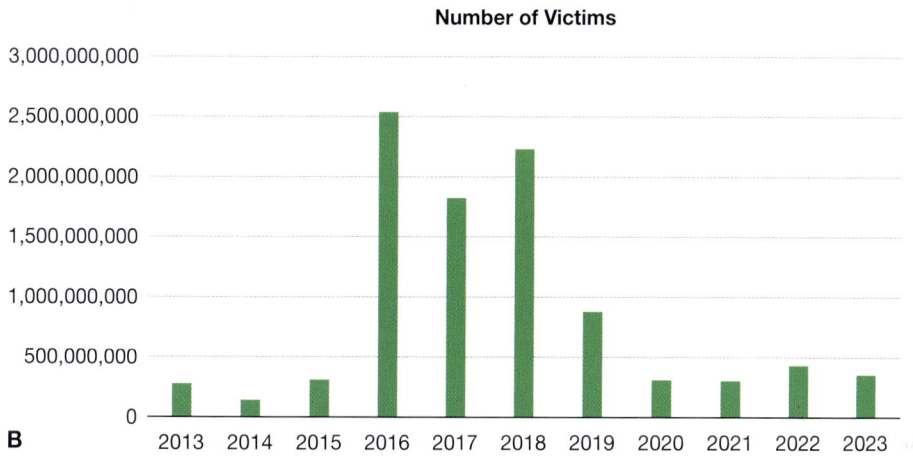

Figure 15-4. Compromise trends from 2013 to 2023 showing the number of data compromises **(A)** and the number of victims **(B)**. (Data from Identity Theft Resource Center (ITRC). (2024, January). 2023 data breach report. https://www.idtheftcenter.org/wp-content/uploads/2024/01/ITRC_2023-Annual-Data-Breach-Report.pdf.)

Prevention of Breaches

The prevention of data security breaches is paramount, and actions must be proactive. Methods for proactive prevention of security breaches include risk assessments, employee training, and data encryption and data loss prevention software. The HIPAA Security Rule requires that covered entities and their business associates conduct a risk assessment of their healthcare organization. A **risk assessment** helps an organization ensure it is compliant with HIPAA's administrative, physical, and technical safeguards. A risk assessment also helps reveal areas where an organization's PHI could be at risk (HHS, 2022). The Security Risk Assessment Tool from the Office of the National Coordinator for Health Information Technology (ONC) suggests components of risk assessments include (ONC, n.d.):

- Reviewing policies and procedures
- Analyzing system vulnerabilities
- Taking inventory of personally identifiable information and personal health information
- Reviewing pertinent regulations
- Monitoring employee compliance
- Tracking external threats

Privacy and security training with employees must include more than an understanding of HIPAA. Employees must understand how system logins, secure access, and data encryption work. Healthcare institutions need to have a plan in place to prevent the loss of portable devices and drives and provide training on this to all employees.

Data encryption is a method of protecting vulnerable data that requires a password to decode and read files or drives. A common misconception is that data sent from a secure email server are automatically protected by encryption. Rather, encryption software must be in place. Encryption software is available without a fee, but the IT department should be consulted regarding the selection of appropriate encryption software. Users can encrypt an entire hard drive or individual folders and files if necessary. Encryption software requirements differ from agency to agency, but best practice is to encrypt all portable healthcare agency devices.

Data loss prevention software can be used to track and locate lost or stolen devices. Loss prevention software is proprietary and may require a subscription fee for use. After a device is determined lost or stolen, the owner contacts the software company and the police. When the device next connects to the internet, the locator software sends a message to the recovery team, which works with the local police to find the missing device. If the device locator software includes data security features, all data can be deleted remotely from the missing device. If the located software package includes geolocation software, the physical location of the device can be identified using WiFi or global positioning system technology.

All users of mobile devices must take a proactive stance to protect electronic health information. Inattention to data security can cause devastating results for healthcare consumers whose personal information has been stolen. Thinking back to the case study, if the healthcare organization Lifespan had completed a risk assessment or some of the other strategies mentioned hereinbefore, it might have prevented cyber criminals from accessing PHI from a stolen employee laptop.

SUMMARY

- **Privacy and confidentiality.** Ensuring patient privacy and confidentiality is a primary ethical and legal duty of nurses. To protect privacy and confidentiality, be familiar with your institution's policies, state and national laws, and the ANA's ethical guidelines. There are multiple ways to authenticate the identity of anyone trying to access patient information including the use of a login name and password, 2FA, and biometric authentication. Other ways to protect confidentiality include using password policies, automatic logouts, and avoiding SSO.

- **HIPAA.** HIPAA was passed in 1996 to protect the privacy and confidentiality of patient health information. The law requires each healthcare agency have a designated HIPAA officer to enforce the HIPAA Privacy Rule with signed authorization for disclosure of PHI. HIPAA also requires the use of a universal identification numbers. In 2009, the HITECH Act was passed to better protect electronic records. The term "security breach" was included in a later ruling. HIPAA violations occur when organizations or individuals fail to comply with HIPAA rules. Nurses need to be familiar with the many ways HIPAA violations can occur. Fines for accidental violations are lower than those for willful violations. Financial penalties can be issued for organizational HIPAA violations, though cases are usually resolved through voluntary resolution of the issue that may include technical changes. If an individual violates HIPAA laws, depending on the severity of the violation, they could face fines, termination, suspension of their nursing license, or criminal charges. Not all medical records are private and confidential.

- **Data security.** Data security involves ensuring data accuracy, protecting data from unauthorized internal or external damage, and preventing data loss. An audit trail is used to monitor appropriate access to information. A firewall blocks incoming and outgoing data using a set of rules. White hat hackers are useful for determining data security weaknesses that are vulnerable to cyber criminals. Disaster recovery plans can prevent data loss. A security breach occurs when data are accessed without authorization, whereas a data breach occurs when cyber criminal takes the information. Risk assessment, data encryption, and use of data loss software are strategies to prevent security breaches.

DISCUSSION QUESTIONS AND ACTIVITIES

1. Explore the Privacy Rights Clearinghouse. Discuss at least three recent health information breaches and identify strategies to prevent those breaches. What are the current privacy regulations in your state?
2. Discuss the strengths and weaknesses of HIPAA and the HITECH Act. Contact the HIPAA officer at your institution and ask what is being done to protect patient privacy and confidentiality.
3. Identify three strategies used to protect patient health information. Search the internet and look for a recent technologic advance in data protection and describe it.
4. Discuss the methods for ensuring privacy and confidentiality of PHI in a local clinical setting. Identify the penalties the agency uses for employees that breach confidentiality and security policies.
5. How does a strong password help protect health information in electronic records? What other strategies can be used to protect access?
6. Imagine a colleague asks you to chart something for them using their employee login. How would you respond? What would you do if you discovered that you have accidentally looked at the PHI of a patient for whom you are not directly caring?

PRACTICE QUESTIONS

1. Which strategy for protecting confidentiality requires entering another piece of information after you have entered your username and password?
   a. Single sign-on
   b. Audit trails
   c. Automatic logout
   d. Two-factor authentication

2. Which strategies can be used to ensure patient privacy? Select all that apply.
   a. Using biometrics for access to patient records
   b. Discussing sensitive matters with patients when they are alone
   c. Logging off of your computer when you leave your workstation
   d. All the above

3. The HIPAA Privacy Rule includes which requirement?
   a. A signed authorization to disclose PHI
   b. A designated HIPAA officer
   c. Dedicated privacy laws
   d. An annual risk assessment

REFERENCES

Adler, E., & Bauer, L. (2016, May 11). Joplin tornado of 2011: In St. John's medical center, heroism in the face of horror. *The Kansas City Star*. Retrieved from http://www.kansascity.com/news/local/article64775907.html

Alder, S. (2023a, February 24). *Time to stop blocking a national patient identifier system*. HIPAA Journal. https://www.hipaajournal.com/time-to-stop-blocking-a-national-patient-identifier-system/

Alder, S. (2023b, February 22). *What happens if you break HIPAA rules?* HIPAA Journal. https://www.hipaajournal.com/what-happens-if-you-break-hipaa-rules/

Alder, S. (2024). What is the HITECH act? *HIPAA Journal*. https://www.hipaajournal.com/what-is-the-hitech-act/

American Nurses Association [ANA]. (2015). *Code of ethics for nurses* (2nd ed.). Silver Spring. http://nursingworld.org/MainMenuCategories/EthicsStandards/CodeofEthicsforNurses.aspx

Beard v. City of Chicago, 299 F. Supp. 2d 872 C.F.R. (N.D. Ill, 2004).

Brumfield, B. (2014, May 20). *Moore, Oklahoma, looks back on tornado that killed 24 one year ago*. CNN. Retrieved from https://www.cnn.com/2014/05/20/us/oklahoma-moore-tornado-anniversary/index.html

Centers for Medicare Medicaid (CMS). (2022, April 25). *Unique identifiers overview*. https://www.cms.gov/priorities/key-initiatives/burden-reduction/administrative-simplification/unique-identifiers

Da Na Ia. (n.d.) *Counterintelligence tips: Spear phishing and common cyber attacks*. https://www.dni.gov/files/NCSC/documents/campaign/Counterintelligence_Tips_Spearphishing.pdf

Frieden, J. (2023, January 25). Unique patient identifier funding once again barred by congress. *MedPage Today*. https://www.medpagetoday.com/practicemanagement/informationtechnology/102812

HIPAA Journal. (2024). *What are the penalties for HIPAA violations?* https://www.hipaajournal.com/what-are-the-penalties-for-hipaa-violations-7096/

Identity Theft Resource Center (ITRC). (2024, January). *2023 data breach report*. https://www.idtheftcenter.org/wp-content/uploads/2024/01/ITRC_2023-Annual-Data-Breach-Report.pdf

Miliard, M. (2020, July 28). *Unencrypted stolen laptop costs lifespan more than $1M*. https://www.healthcareitnews.com/news/unencrypted-stolen-laptop-costs-lifespan-more-1-million

Ornstein, C. (2008, March 15). *Hospital to punish snooping on spears*. Retrieved from http://articles.latimes.com/2008/mar/15/local/me-britney15

Privacy Rights Clearinghouse. (2023, January 27). *Data breaches*. https://privacyrights.org/resources/data-breach-notification-united-states-and-territories

The Joint Commission. (2024). *2024 hospital national patient safety goals*. https://www.jointcommission.org/standards_information/npsgs.aspx

The Office of the National Coordinator for Health Information Technology (ONC). (n.d.). *Security risk assessment tool*. https://www.healthit.gov/topic/privacy-security-and-hipaa/security-risk-assessment-tool

TwilioAuthy. (n.d.). *What is two-factor authentication (2FA)?* Retrieved September 29, 2022 from https://authy.com/what-is-2fa/

U.S. Department of Health and Human Services (HHS). (2021, May 17). *HIPAA for professionals*. https://www.hhs.gov/hipaa/for-professionals/index.html

U.S. Department of Health and Human Services (HHS) (2017, June 16). *HITECH act enforcement interim final rule*. https://www.hhs.gov/hipaa/for-professionals/special-topics/hitech-act-enforcement-interim-final-rule/index.html

U.S. Department of Health and Human Services (HHS). (2022, October 20). *The security rule*. https://www.hhs.gov/hipaa/for-professionals/security/index.html

CHAPTER 16

Applying Nursing Informatics to Patient Safety

Kristi Miller

OBJECTIVES

After studying this chapter, you will be able to:

1. Define the term "medical error," and discuss the types, causes, and costs of medical errors.
2. Explain why measuring patient safety is difficult and give examples of ways medical errors and medication errors can be measured.
3. Discuss strategies for preventing errors including the steps involved in a root cause analysis.
4. Discuss healthcare information technology used for medication error prevention.
5. Explain the role of a culture of safety and high reliability organizations in reducing patient harm.
6. Identify ways to measure a culture of safety in healthcare organizations and schools of nursing.
7. Identify patient safety resources and how they can support patient safety efforts.

AACN Essentials for Entry-Level Professional Nursing Education

2.5d Incorporate evidence-based intervention to improve outcomes and safety.
3.1i Identify ethical principles to protect the health and safety of diverse populations.
5.1a Recognize nursing's essential role in improving healthcare quality and safety.
5.1b Identify sources and applications of national safety and quality standards to guide nursing practice.
5.2a Describe the factors that create a culture of safety.
5.2b Articulate the nurse's role within an interprofessional team in promoting safety and preventing errors and near misses.
5.2c Examine basic safety design principles to reduce risk of harm.
5.2d Assume accountability for reporting unsafe conditions, near misses, and errors to reduce harm.

5.2e Describe processes used in understanding the causes of error.
5.2f Use national patient safety resources, initiatives, and regulations at the point of care.
6.2e Apply principles of team leadership and management performance to improve quality and assure safety.
8.3e Identify impact of information and communication technology on quality and safety of care.

AACN Essentials for Advanced-Level Nursing Education
2.5i Prioritize risk mitigation strategies to prevent or reduce adverse outcomes
2.5j Develop evidence-based interventions to improve outcomes and safety.
5.1j Use national safety resources to lead team-based change initiatives.
5.2g Evaluate the alignment of system data and comparative patient safety benchmarks.
5.2h Lead analysis of actual errors, near misses, and potential situations that would impact safety.
5.2i Design evidence-based interventions to mitigate risk.
5.3f Foster a just culture reflecting civility and respect.
5.3g Create a safe and transparent culture for reporting incidents.

HIMSS TIGER Competencies
Change/stakeholder management
Communication
Consumer health informatics
Data analytics
Documentation
Electronic/Mobile Health, telematics, telehealth
Ethics in health internet technology
Information and communications technology systems applications
Information and knowledge management in patient care
Internet technology risk management
Legal issues in health internet technology
Quality and safety management
Teaching, training, education

KEY TERMS

Barcode medication administration (BCMA)	Culture of safety	National Patient Safety Goals (NPSGs)
Clinical decision support system (CDSS)	High reliability organizations (HROs)	Root cause analysis (RCA)
Computerized provider order entry (CPOE)	Medical error	Sentinel event
	Medication error	Smart infusion pumps

CASE STUDY

During a busy shift at Vanderbilt University Medical Center (VUMC), nurse RaDonda Vaught accidentally administered the paralytic vecuronium to a patient instead of the calming sedative midazolam (which has the brand name Versed). The vecuronium caused the patient to stop breathing, leaving her with brain damage before the error was discovered. The nurse admitted the mistake, saying she was training someone on how to use the automated dispensing cabinet and was distracted. Although she took responsibility for her part in the error, she said the hospital was also partially responsible, describing problems with information flow between the electronic health record (EHR), the electronic medication cabinet, and the pharmacy. It was revealed that nurses and other staff commonly bypassed safety features in the electronic medication cabinet. In addition, analysis of the error revealed that after administering the drug, the patient was not monitored. Vaught lost her nursing license and was convicted of criminally negligent homicide and abuse of an impaired adult. She was sentenced to 3 years of probation, fined $3,000, and billed for more than $30,000 in legal expenses (Beres, 2022).

In 2023, Vaught appealed to reinstate her license, arguing that the flaws in VUMC's automated medication dispensing system contributed to the patient's death (Fiore, 2023). Her appeal was denied. In response to the error, VUMC revised their policy to require continuous monitoring of any patients given a high-alert medication such as vecuronium. All staff responsible for administering medications are now required to complete education through Vanderbilt's online education system (Kelman, 2022b). VUMC has thus far received no punishment for the fatal error (Kelman, 2022a). Vaught committed to working with others on a bill to give nurses possible immunity from criminal prosecution for mistakes.

What is the role of the informatics nurse (IN) in preventing errors like this from happening? What tools, strategies, and technology could be used to protect patients, nurses, and other healthcare professionals from making medical errors?

In 2000, the Institute of Medicine (IOM) published a report on patient safety in healthcare called *To Err Is Human* (IOM Committee on Quality of Health Care in America, 2000). This was one of the first instances of Americans being made aware of the large number of patients dying each year due to medical error. The authors called for the development and testing of new technologies to reduce medical errors. Since that report, there has been progress in the use of healthcare information technology (HIT) to support patient safety; however, there is difficulty in determining the effect of HIT on patient safety due to issues with measuring medical errors. Other challenges include discovering the causes of errors or providing consistent, workable solutions (Rodziewicz et al., 2023). In 2016, the death toll from medical errors was reported to be more than 400,000 per year, placing medical error as the third leading cause of death (Makary & Daniel, 2016), but this number has been disputed by many experts due to the difficulties encountered with measuring harm from medical error (Shojania & Dixon-Woods, 2017).

Patient safety is paramount to the field of nursing. In this book, you have learned about many situations in which the IN can support patient safety. For example, Chapter 3 discussed the use of cloud computing to protect patient safety. Chapter 7 focused on how to find research on reducing patient falls. Chapter 8 outlined data collection and Chapter 9 discussed analyzing data for improved patient outcomes. Chapter 10 discussed how to professionally share findings to add to nursing knowledge about patient safety issues. INs can improve patient safety through research, leadership, advocacy, and education. This chapter is about the role of the IN in supporting patient safety efforts. As you read this chapter, think about what you have learned in previous chapters and consider how informatics can be used to measure medical errors and what the IN can do with data to support patient safety.

MEDICAL ERRORS

As you learned in Chapter 13, standardization of terms is an important step in improving patient outcomes. However, there is no standard definition of the term "medical error" that has been agreed on at the national or international levels. A leading researcher in the field of human error defined it as the "failure of a planned sequence of mental or physical activities to achieve its intended outcome when these failures cannot be attributed to chance" (Reason, 1990). An expert on patient safety defined medical error as an "unintended act (either omission or commission) or an act that does not achieve its intended outcome" (Leape, 1994). In summary, we might define **medical error** as a preventable adverse effect of medical care. A **sentinel event** is the most serious type of error and is defined as a patient safety event that results in death, permanent harm, or severe temporary harm (TJC, 2024b).

It is important to pay attention to situations with hazards (factors that could cause harm) or risks (the likelihood that harm may be caused) to prevent errors before they occur. In the case study, having a high-risk medication such as vecuronium in the medication cart presents a hazard. A near miss is when a patient could have been harmed by an error but was not because of chance, prevention, or mitigation. In the case study, if at any point RaDonda Vaught had noticed she had the wrong medication and had not administered it, that would have been considered a near miss. You will learn in this chapter how reporting and analyzing near misses, hazards, and risky situations can prevent medical errors.

Types of Errors

Because a universal definition of "medical error" has not been clearly established, finding a ranked list of the most common medical errors is difficult (Rodziewicz et al., 2023). The most common type of medical error is generally believed to be medication errors (TJC, 2021). Other common medical errors include healthcare-associated infections, injuries from falls, obstetric adverse events, pressure injuries, surgical site infections, venous thromboses (blood clots), wrong site/wrong procedure surgeries, and incorrect diagnoses (Carver et al., 2021). Box 16-1 lists some general categories of medical errors.

The Joint Commission (TJC) conducts a yearly analysis of reported sentinel events to improve

---

BOX 16-1 Types of Medical Errors

Diagnostic Errors
Error in diagnosis
Delay in diagnosis
Failure to use indicated tests
Use of outdated tests or therapies
Failure to act on diagnostic results

Treatment Errors
Incorrect performance of operation or procedure
Error in treatment administration
Use of incorrect dose or dosage method
Delay in treatment
Use of inappropriate care

Preventative Errors
Failure to give prophylactic treatment
Failure in monitoring or follow-up

Other Errors
Failure of communication
Failure of equipment
Failure of other systems

Adapted from Institute of Medicine (US) Committee on Quality of Health Care in America. (2000). In L. T. Kohn, J. M. Corrigan, & M. S. Donaldson, (Eds.). *To err is human: Building a safer health system*. National Academies Press (US). http://www.ncbi.nlm.nih.gov/books/NBK225182/

patient safety. However, sentinel events are voluntarily reported, so this analysis likely represents only a small fraction of those that occur. In 2023, the 10 most common reported sentinel events are (TJC, 2024b):

1. Falls—48%
2. Wrong surgery—8%
3. Unintended retention of foreign object—8%
4. Assault/rape/sexual assault/homicide—8%
5. Delay in treatment—6%
6. Suicide—5%
7. Fire/burns—4%
8. Medication management—2%
9. Perinatal event—2%
10. Self-harm—2%

Falls have been the leading sentinel event since 2018 (TJC, 2023b).

Medication Errors

Medication errors are a leading cause of harm to patients with an estimated annual cost of $42 billion in the United States (WHO, 2022). A **medication error** is an error of commission or omission during any part of the process beginning when a clinician prescribes a medication and ending when the patient receives the medication (AHRQ, 2019a). An adverse drug event (ADE) is the harm the patient experiences because of exposure to a medication, but it is not always due to error or poor care (e.g., allergic reactions, predictable side effects). A preventable ADE results from a medication error that reaches the patient and causes harm. A potential ADE is a medication error that reaches the patient and does not cause harm.

Despite error reduction interventions that are discussed later in the chapter, medication errors are common. In a review of 91 direct observation studies, errors occurred for 8% to 25% of medications administered (MacDowell et al., 2021). Nurses spend a great deal of time administering medications, but few studies have documented either the type or frequency of errors that involve nurses or nursing students. A systematic review of the incidences, causes, and consequences of ADEs found that there is a great deal of diversity in the methods and other factors for measuring the incidence of ADEs (Wolfe et al., 2018). In a study of nursing students, medication errors accounted for almost 60% of error and near miss data collected (Silvestre & Spector, 2023).

Wrong dose accounted for the most errors, followed by use of an incorrect procedure, wrong route, incorrect dilution, and wrong medication. Nursing students were more likely to make errors later in their programs when they were working independently and with higher-acuity patients. About half of the errors occurred in patients older than 56 years, and more than half occurred with female patients (Silvestre & Spector, 2023). Many medication errors occur with pediatric patients due to complexities of weight-based dosing. Intravenous medications had an especially high error rate of between 48% and 53% (MacDowell et al., 2021).

Causes of Medical Errors

Despite knowing the types of medical errors that occur, finding the reasons for these errors and identifying consistent solutions is challenging (Rodziewicz et al., 2023). In one study, the most identified causes of medication errors included not checking the patient's identity or allergy status and not following the rights of medication administration (Silvestre & Spector, 2023). Other causes include poor communication, poorly coordinated care, fragmented insurance networks, human error resulting from overwork and burnout, manufacturing error, equipment failure, diagnostic error, poor design of buildings that can result in patient falls, a lack of familiarity with systems or equipment, variation in physician practice, and incivility.

Some errors are blameworthy events that should be dealt with by disciplinary policies and procedures; these are not the focus of this chapter. What is important is that healthcare organizations have a clear policy for determining if an error was blameworthy. Many state boards of nursing have evaluation tools. For example, the North Carolina Board of Nursing (NCBON) has developed a complaint evaluation tool to assist with making decisions about the consequences for nursing errors. The tool evaluates nursing behavior in five categories:

1. General nursing practice
2. Understanding/level of experience
3. Internal policies and standards
4. Decisions or choices made by the nurse
5. Ethics/credibility and accountability

Each of these criteria is evaluated on a point system. Zero points are given for human error, between 1 and three points for at-risk behavior, and 4 and five points for reckless behavior (NCBON, 2023). As an example, a nurse with prior counseling for a single related issue within the past 12 months would get two points, and a nurse with prior written counseling for the same practice issue within 12 months would be considered reckless and get four points. The higher the total number of points on the tool, the more likely it is to be reported to the state board of nursing. Points are taken away for mitigating factors such as communication breakdown, lack of resources, interruptions, working extra shifts, staffing issues, or insufficient orientation and are added for aggravating factors such as knowingly creating a risk for more than one patient, threatening or bullying behavior, or taking advantage of a leadership position.

Electronic Health Record Systems

Errors can occur in many ways when working with EHR systems. In the implementation phase, users working with a new system may have inadequate training. Users may create new pathways that bypass safety features, resulting in errors. During transition from one system to another, safety features may be disabled to allow access to two different systems. Duplication of data, missing data, or gaps in data can occur. In later phases, bugs and failures can occur, such as with the problems seen in the case study. The electronic medication cart was unable to communicate with the EHR, which caused the staff who were using it to bypass important safety features. Bypassing safety features saves time but can result in medical error. The IN can prevent errors from EHR use by designing education around the importance of using safety features, advocating for IT fixes, ensuring a culture of safety, and communicating with end users to discover problems as they arise. Staff who know they would be heard without punishment are more likely to share their concerns.

Incivility

Workplace incivility is "low-intensity deviant behavior with ambiguous intent to harm the target, in violation of workplace norms for mutual respect. Uncivil behaviors are characteristically rude and discourteous, displaying a lack of regard for others" (bib_andersson_and_pearson_1999Andersson & Pearson, 1999). Examples include phone use during meetings, gossip, eye rolling, rude comments, impatience with questions, and heavy sighing. Researchers have demonstrated that civility, teamwork, and engagement are vital for the success of healthcare organizations (Lewis, 2023). Experiencing incivility has been linked to negative cognitive effects including reduced ability to concentrate or pay attention (Porath et al., 2015). Incivility has been associated with medical errors, complications, mortality, compromised patient safety, and lower quality of care (Lewis, 2023). In one survey, researchers found that 81% of physicians and 52% of nurses demonstrated incivility and that the participants linked incivility to adverse outcomes, job dissatisfaction, and an increase in errors (Maddineshat et al., 2016).

Most data on incivility are collected from surveys and questionnaires (Lewis, 2023), meaning it is voluntary and self-reported and thus unlikely representative of the true nature of healthcare environments. The IN can play an important role in dealing with incivility by identifying and measuring the effects of incivility on patient safety using techniques such as observation. As you learned in Chapter 8, collecting various types of data can support improved decision making and inform evidence-based practice (EBP).

Cost of Medical Errors

The exact financial cost of medical errors is not known. As previously stated, the World Health Organization (WHO) estimated the annual cost of medication errors to be $42 billion in the United States (WHO, 2022). Another report found that medical errors account for between $4 and $20 billion per year in the United States and are associated with increased morbidity and mortality, prolonged hospitalizations, and higher costs of care (Rodziewicz et al., 2023). The effect of making errors on healthcare providers is also an important "cost" to consider. Making an error can be devastating to both the personal and professional lives of nurses who are exposed to criticism and reproach from their supervisors. Some nurses are unable to continue their profession or find another job because of embarrassment or shame. Nurses who continue to practice may fear making new mistakes and have decreased confidence in their own abilities.

In the case study, the cost to the patient was the loss of her life. Her family suffered the cost of losing a beloved family member. The cost to the nurse was both emotional and financial. She had to pay thousands of dollars in legal fees, lost her job and her nursing license, and now her name will forever be associated with this mistake due to news and social media coverage (Kelman, 2022b). In this situation, the hospital has not yet had to pay; however, often healthcare organizations are sued by victims of medical error for damages. These costs can result in millions of dollars in legal fees.

MEASURING PATIENT SAFETY

One of the difficulties of discussing patient safety is the concept of measurement. Before you can set out to change something, you must decide how to measure the current situation and measure improvement. The measurement of patient safety is complicated and an area in which the IN can play a useful role. There is no single validated method for measuring the overall safety of care in a given healthcare setting. The IN might choose to gather data on what resources an organization has in place to improve safety, such as EHRs or protocols for implementing a response team after a serious adverse event has occurred. An IN might also measure adherence to safety standards such as the number of surgical patients who have a complete postoperative checklist or the number of patients who are rated as being at a high fall risk who have fall prevention measures in place. The prevalence or incidence of adverse events is another measurement that can support quality improvement projects.

Measures that may be helpful include missed nursing care (the frequency with which required care elements are not completed); medication reconciliation (the number of patients for whom a complete medication history was documented on admission); or use of the Leapfrog Hospital Survey, which evaluates hospitals based on their use of patient safety practices such as computerized provider order entry (CPOE). Table 16-1 shows examples of safety measurement strategies.

Counting Medical Errors

In Chapter 12, you learned about the use of the International Classification of Diseases (ICD) billing codes as a form of standardized terminology to support billing. These codes were first used in 1949 when there was little understanding that medical error could result in patient death. Thus, medical error as a cause of death is not covered by the ICD. National mortality statistics are calculated using billing codes, so medical error has been excluded from national health statistics (Makary & Daniel, 2016). Research funding and public health priorities are informed by the rankings of causes of death, so medical error does not get the same level of attention as other causes such as cancer and heart disease. Other barriers to measuring medical errors include unclear definitions of what constitutes an error. A lack of standardized nomenclature and overlapping definitions hinders data analysis, synthesis, and evaluation (Rodziewicz et al., 2023).

Voluntary Error Reporting

The Patient Safety and Quality Improvement Act (PSQIA) of 2005 established a voluntary reporting system to ensure data would be gathered on patient safety and healthcare quality issues. The PSQIA provides federal confidentiality protection for patient safety information and established penalties for violations of confidentiality. Voluntary error reporting (VER) by healthcare providers is the primary way healthcare organizations identify system hazards and patient safety events, but it has been estimated that 50% to 96% of errors go unreported (Woo & Avery, 2021). Organizations should understand the limitations of VER and use additional methods to explore errors. Box 16-2 lists tips for increasing error reporting and decreasing patient harm.

TABLE 16-1 Examples of Safety Measurement Strategies

Measurement Strategy	Advantages	Disadvantages
Retrospective chart review	Contains rich and detailed clinical information Considered the "gold standard" Can improve efficiency of this strategy by using a trigger tool or software tool to identify charts	Costly and labor-intensive Data quality variable due to incomplete clinical information Retrospective review only
Voluntary error reporting system	Useful for internal quality improvement Highlights adverse events perceived as important by providers	Voluntary reporting captures only a fraction of adverse events Retrospective review only
Automated surveillance	Can be retrospective or prospective Standardized protocols help identify patients at high risk for adverse events	Electronic data required to run automated surveillance High proportion of triggered cases are false positives
Administrative/claims data	Low-cost and readily available Can track events over time and across large populations	Lack of detailed clinical data Variability and inaccuracy of coding (ICD-9-CM vs. ICD-10-CM) across and within systems High proportion of false positives and false negatives
Patient reports	Capture errors not easily recognized by other methods Provide data from patient perspective	Measurement tools are still in development Voluntary reporting captures only a fraction of adverse events Retrospective review only

Adapted from Wachter, R. M. (2012). *Understanding patient safety*, 2nd ed. McGraw-Hill Professional. ISBN: 9780071765787.

The Agency for Healthcare Research and Quality (AHRQ) certifies and publishes a list of patient safety organizations (PSOs) (OCR, 2022). The primary activities of PSOs are to collect and analyze voluntarily reported data from healthcare providers and conduct activities to improve patient safety and healthcare quality (AHRQ, n.d.). The AHRQ lists the steps needed for an organization to become a certified PSO, and each PSO must have a workforce that is trained in analyzing patient safety events. Hospitals, clinicians, and other healthcare professionals confidentially report information to PSOs for the aggregation and analysis of patient safety events.

BOX 16-2 Best Practices to Encourage Error Reporting

Build trustworthiness by...
- Demonstrating a passion for safety and the prevention of patient harm and acknowledging the high-risk nature of healthcare and human fallibility.
- Ensuring confidentiality for reporters, individuals involved in errors, and patients.
- Being visible in work areas, being available for discussions about patient safety, and sharing responsibility for errors.
- Including patient safety in the organization's mission, vision, values, and strategic goals.

Create an open and fair culture of learning by...
- Being fair and equitable in response to an adverse patient safety event and using disciplinary actions only for reckless conduct or acts that knowingly or purposely cause harm.
- Discussing hazards, close calls, adverse events, lessons learned, and risk-reduction strategies, encouraging error reporting, and using external data to make proactive system changes.

Provide clarity by...
- Providing staff with clear definitions and examples of the types of errors, close calls, and hazards that should be reported.
- Covering the error-reporting process (with examples) during orientation for all providers and staff.

Simplify error reporting by...
- Ensuring providers and staff have formal and informal pathways for reporting hazards, close calls, and errors.
- Using a simple reporting system that requires minimal training.
- Testing the reporting systems for clarity and ease of use, and making modifications as needed before or after implementation.

Maintaining credibility and utility by...
- Developing guidelines to identify and prioritize events for which RCA is appropriate and useful.
- Establishing pathways for sharing the lessons learned from error analysis.
- Fixing system vulnerabilities and supporting system enhancements suggested by staff.
- Empowering staff to correct safety hazards using appropriate communication with leadership.
- Consistently providing feedback to staff regarding the actions planned and taken to prevent errors.
- Establishing interdisciplinary pathways for sharing of error stories and error-reduction strategies.
- Ensuring actions taken have been successful in reducing risk, error, and/or patient harm.
- Encouraging external reporting to PSOs and addressing problems at the regulatory, standards, and industry levels.

Reward patient safety efforts by...
- Establishing pathways for thanking and rewarding staff who report errors or hazards and for patient care units for demonstrating measurable improvements in patient safety.
- Celebrating results and actions taken by the organization based on the information received in reports.

Remove bias by...
- Not overreacting to a singular event with unwarranted disciplinary sanctions even when a patient is harmed.
- Establishing that the severity of harm from an error does not determine whether it is addressed by leadership.
- Giving attention to repetitive patient safety problems, even if patients have not yet been harmed.

(Continued)

> **BOX 16-2** Best Practices to Encourage Error Reporting *(Continued)*
>
> **Reinforce a culture of safety by...**
> - Assigning new providers and staff to a mentor to assist with the error-reporting process.
> - Requiring new providers and staff to practice reporting at least one safety hazard during their orientation period.
> - Including participation in error, close call, and hazard reporting as core elements in all staff members' job descriptions and performance evaluations.
>
> Adapted from Institute for Safe Medication Practices (ISMP). (2021, August 25). Pump up the volume: Tips for increasing error reporting and decreasing patient harm. https://www.ismp.org/resources/pump-volume-tips-increasing-error-reporting-and-decreasing-patient-harm

The PSQIA created and maintains the Network of Patient Safety Databases (NPSD) to provide an interactive, evidence-based resource for healthcare providers, PSOs, and other healthcare organizations (AHRQ, 2020). The NPSD contains nonidentifiable data submitted by PSOs, which allows users to identify and track patient safety concerns to mitigate patient safety risks and reduce harm. The NPSD uses dashboards and charts to make data easy to understand. NPSD data are available to the public through the AHRQ's annual National Healthcare Quality and Disparities Report (NHQDR). These reports give an overview of the state of healthcare in the United States. They include national and state data in categories such as effectiveness of care, patient safety, birth-related complications, healthcare-associated infections, medication information, and more.

TJC requires that healthcare organizations have an incident reporting system (IRS) that healthcare providers can use for VER. To encourage VER, healthcare IRS software should be easy for staff to use, requiring minimal training. IRS should also be customizable, interoperable (with the EHR, pharmacy, and other ancillary services), have a centralized portal with real-time reporting capable of conversion to multiple file formats, and be automatically routed to concerned units, stakeholders, and leadership. An IRS should be compliant with the Health Insurance Portability and Accountability Act (HIPAA) (see Chapter 15), be outcome-focused, and have postimplementation vendor support. It should also increase VER. In one example, an emergency department introduced a mobile messaging application-based IRS for hospital-issued smartphones to encourage voluntary reporting. The application resulted in a 12-fold increase in incident reporting with a large increase in satisfaction rates by end users (Siddiqui et al., 2021). Brainstorming and implementing innovative approaches such as this are good ways for the IN to be involved in voluntary reporting initiatives.

Nursing students are also able to participate in VER. The National Council of State Boards of Nursing has created a national data repository for reporting errors and near misses in schools of nursing using the Safe Student Reporting tool, which collects program-specific data using an anonymous online platform. This tool is different from other voluntary reporting tools that only collect medication errors made by nursing students in that it also allows for reporting other errors and near misses (e.g., falls, needlestick injuries) (Silvestre & Spector, 2023).

While increasing the volume of error reporting is vital, it is important not to use error reporting as a measure of success. Error rates are inaccurate because they are based on voluntary reporting in an environment in which staff may be afraid to report an error. Strengthening the safety culture of an organization should naturally result in an increase in error reporting. Instead of using error reporting as a measure of improvement, consider measuring the number of system changes implemented because of error reporting. It is important for healthcare organizations to conduct in-depth analyses of reported errors to demonstrate to the staff that their efforts and concerns matter and to ensure outcomes result in systemic changes rather than just increasing education. Organizations should report data to external reporting systems such as the NPSD for large-scale tracking and trend analysis. In addition, it is important to share system changes with staff; organizations should be transparent about errors without identifying individuals. When staff have input into process changes and feel their concerns are heard and acted on, they are more likely to report hazards and errors. Sharing information about errors gives everyone the chance to learn from them.

Reporting Medication Errors

Medication errors, near misses, and hazards involving nurses or other healthcare professionals should also be reported using IRSs. Knowing the types of medications involved, the time of day errors occur, and what type of error (e.g., wrong dose, route, medication, person, and time) can help with the design of interventions that specifically address the needs of healthcare organizations. Medication errors and near misses can also be reported to TJC, the Food and Drug Administration (FDA), and the Institute for Safe Medication Practices (ISMP). The ISMP, in conjunction with the National Coordinating Council for Medication Error Reporting and Prevention (NCC MERP), provides links for consumers and healthcare practitioners to report medication errors (NCC MERP, n.d.). They facilitate the analysis of the reported errors using a system-based approach to create actionable change (Fig. 16-1). This error reporting analysis has resulted in practice changes such as (ISMP, 2022b):

- Using a weekly dosage regimen for oral methotrexate in electronic systems when medication orders are entered
- Dispensing vincristine and other vinca alkaloids in a mini bag of a compatible solution and not in a syringe
- Weighing each patient on admission and during each outpatient or emergency department encounters to avoid reliance on stated, estimated, or historical weight

The ISMP does not calculate or release statistics about common causes, types of adverse events, or certain other factors from the error reports because most medication errors are not discovered and/or not reported. The incidents that are reported to ISMP represent an even smaller fraction of errors reported in all ways. Because this sample is small and nonrandom, scientifically valid incidence rates or other statistics cannot be accurately calculated.

The lack of information on medication errors at the national and international levels for both nurses and nursing students is an opportunity for the IN. Sharing data about medication error types, locations in agencies, level of staff involved, products involved, and factors contributing to error allows for analysis that can lead to strong interventions to prevent future error. INs can be instrumental in establishing systems to better enable medication error reporting, and in establishing solutions to prevent these errors.

Other Ways to Measure Errors

Since so few errors are reported voluntarily, it is important to use other methods to collect data to

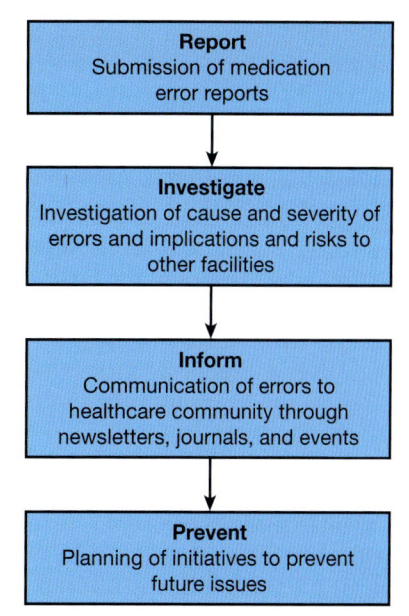

Figure 16-1. How the ISMP turns medication error reports into action plans. (Data from Institute for Safe Medication Practices (ISMP). (2024). What we do with your reports. https://www.ismp.org/error-reporting/what-we-do-your-report)

better understand the causes of errors. Methods include chart review, direct observation, patient safety indicators, and trigger tools. However, there is a great deal of variability in these other methods so no measuring tool is likely to provide a complete picture of medical errors.

When choosing a method, the IN should consider that chart review and direct observation of medication administration are expensive and time-consuming. The Institute for Healthcare Improvement (IHI) Global Trigger Tool for Measuring Adverse Events uses chart review of triggers such as sudden transfer to another unit; abnormal laboratory results, procedure, or treatment complications; and medication-related triggers such as abrupt medication stops, the use of reversal agents (such as naloxone), or prescribing diphenhydramine to signal an error may have occurred. IHI offers training and a list of triggers to identify potential errors. The global trigger tool provides instructions and forms for collecting the data needed to track three measures (Griffin & Resar, 2009):

1. Adverse events per 1,000 patient days
2. Adverse events per 100 admissions
3. Percent of admissions with an adverse event

One study used the Global Trigger Tool to retrospectively study a random sample of 2,341 admissions from 10 hospitals in North Carolina over a period of 5 years (Landrigan et al., 2010). They chose North Carolina because hospitals in the state demonstrated a high level of engagement in patient safety efforts, including a 96% rate of hospital enrollment in a national patient safety campaign (compared to 78% in other states). The researchers found that there was no reduction in preventable harm over the 5-year period during which the study was conducted, suggesting further efforts are needed to ensure safety interventions are effective.

Other ways to measure error include creating a strategic plan such as the California Medication Error Reduction Plan framework, using hospital standardized mortality ratios, measuring AHRQ patient safety indicators, and asking patients to report errors (ISMP, 2022a). You can proactively identify risks using the ISMP Medication Safety Self-Assessment tool to assist your organization with identifying opportunities to reduce harm before a patient safety event occurs (ISMP, 2023).

Whatever measures are used, error rates should not be used to compare one organization to another due to differences in culture, definition, patient populations, and the types of reporting and detection systems. Variations in what constitutes an error and the threshold to report an error also exist (ISMP, 2021).

PREVENTING ERRORS

Despite the best intentions of healthcare workers, medical errors continue to occur. In fact, medical errors have caused the general public to consider the American healthcare system only "moderately safe" (Carver et al., 2021). One of the most important ways to prevent a repetitive error is to analyze the error and put prevention interventions in place. An organization committed to patient safety may designate a patient safety officer who ensures there is a plan for analyzing errors when they occur. Although reporting sentinel events to TJC is voluntary, TJC does require that accredited institutions have a comprehensive process in place for the systematic analysis of sentinel events.

Systems Approach

British psychologist James Reason pioneered the systems approach to preventing errors. His analysis of errors in aviation and nuclear power revealed that safety failures are usually caused by multiple, small errors in environments with underlying system flaws (AHRQ, 2019c). He introduced the Swiss cheese model to describe the phenomenon (Fig. 16-2). In this model, errors are the result of flawed systems (the holes in the cheese are the flaws). When the flaws align in multiple systems, hazards can get through the holes, resulting in a safety failure. Regarding medical errors, the goal of the systems approach is to identify these holes to shrink them or create enough overlap with other systems so they never line up in the future. Reason also asserted that human error is inevitable. Despite best efforts, everyone makes mistakes. The systems approach attempts to catch human errors before they happen, a more realistic goal than creating flawless healthcare providers.

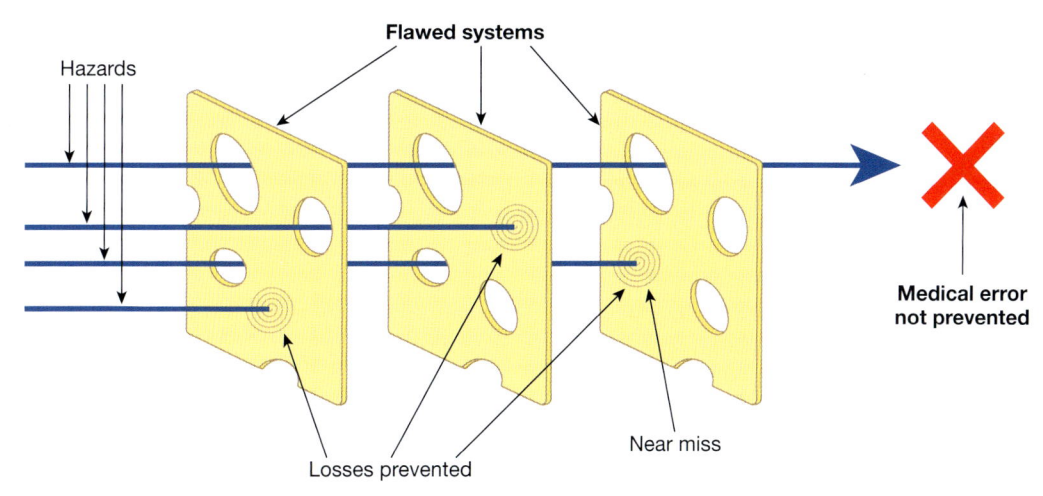

Figure 16-2. Swiss cheese model of medical errors.

The system approach describes errors as either active or latent. In healthcare, active errors involve frontline workers such as nurses and occur at the point of contact between a human and a larger system. They can also be described as "sharp-end" errors, which come from the idea of a surgeon holding a scalpel that is in contact with a patient, an example of the human side of healthcare errors. An active error occurred when RaDonda Vaught withdrew the wrong medication from the electronic dispensing machine and gave it to the patient. Latent errors are failures of an organization or design that allow active errors to cause harm. These are also described as "blunt end" errors, referring to the many layers of the healthcare system not in direct contact with patients but that can influence how easy it is to make (or not make) an error. Examples of latent errors from the case study include the failure of the electronic dispensing machine to communicate with the EHR or pharmacy, the ability of nurses to easily bypass safety features, and the lack of a hospital policy requiring that patients be monitored after receiving a medication.

Latent factors are frequently present in many healthcare organizations. For example, hierarchies in healthcare organizations cause both real and perceived power imbalances, which can prevent someone low in the hierarchy from speaking up in high-risk situations. Imagine a new nurse double-checking a medication dose. Even if a new nurse is concerned about an incorrect dose, they might not feel confident questioning the supervising nurse who has many years of nursing experience. Other common latent factors include the pressure to see patients quickly to keep costs low, technologic problems with HIT, overly complicated workflows, faulty equipment, poor communication, or lack of knowledge or ability. Figure 16-3 shows how latent factors can contribute to an error.

Root Cause Analysis

Root cause analysis (RCA) is one of the most utilized tools for analyzing error (Singh et al., 2023). RCA focuses on analyzing systemic factors instead of on blaming individuals and guides implementation of interventions that will decrease the likelihood of similar events happening in the future (AHRQ, 2019b). An RCA answers a series of "why" questions (called the "five whys") to find the root cause of a problem (Fig. 16-4). The IHI has also developed an updated method called RCA squared (RCA^2) that focuses on the importance of preventing future harm by taking action (IHI, 2015). This section focuses on the traditional RCA methodology.

An actual error or the potential for an error to occur triggers an RCA. TJC requires that an RCA be started within 72 hours of an error and be completed within 30 to 45 days to ensure that those involved do not forget what happened and

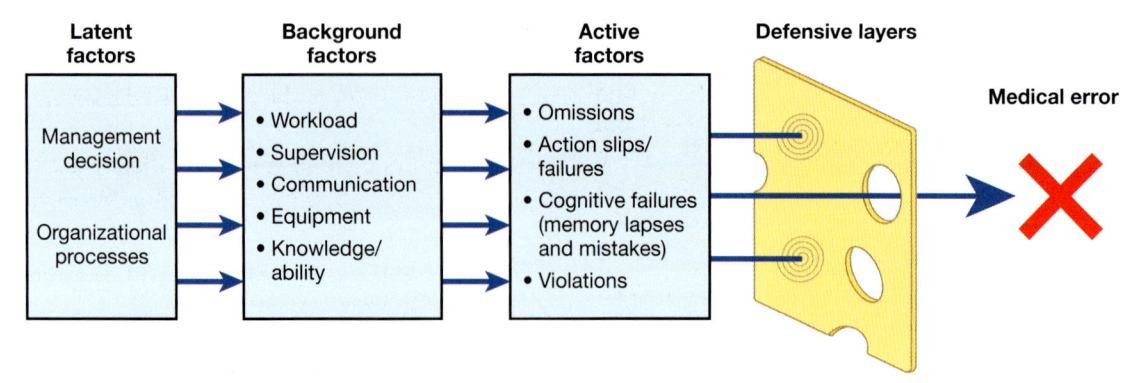

Figure 16-3. Effect of latent and active factors on occurrence of medical errors.

that interventions can be identified as soon as possible to prevent additional errors from occurring. RCA begins with a timeline for the error followed by a problem statement and a causal tree. An action plan is developed from the causal tree that includes at least one strong intervention that, when implemented, will help prevent the error from happening again.

Consider the case of unexpected hypoglycemia in a critically ill patient (Bates, 2002). The 68-year-old patient had cardiac bypass and was much improved after a difficult postoperative course. However, on the morning of her planned transfer out of the intensive care unit, she had a grand mal seizure. She had no history of seizure and was not on any antiseizure medications. The team drew blood and took her for a computed tomography (CT) scan to rule out stroke or cerebral hemorrhage. While in transit, the lab paged the physician to report her serum glucose level was undetectable. Despite multiple infusions of glucose, she never woke and died 3 days later. In the investigation that followed, it was found that her intravenous (IV) line had been flushed with insulin, not the prescribed heparin.

After a sentinel event such as this, the PSO or other staff trained in the use of RCA interviews all parties involved in the error to gather information and create a timeline. People involved in the error are then invited to an interprofessional work session that can include the patient, family member, or a patient advocate in addition to pharmacy personnel, physicians, nurses, administrative personnel, and others. The facilitator begins the session by explaining that the purpose of the work is to focus on problems, not on people. Using the timeline, the team comes up with a problem statement designed to stimulate conversation about why the error occurred. The goal is to use the problem statement to work through the "five whys" until root causes of error are discovered.

It is important to choose a problem statement that leads to a comprehensive discussion of all possible "whys." A problem statement that is too narrow prevents discovery of important causes, but

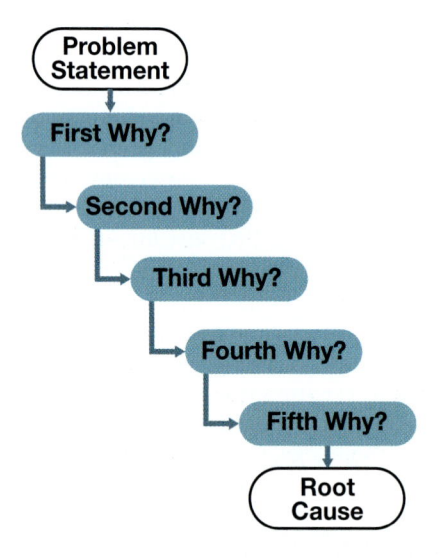

Figure 16-4. Exploring a problem through root cause analysis. (Shutterstock/Master_shifu.)

one that is too wide may result in waste of time. A problem statement focused on an individual does not yield strong interventions. The goal is to find interventions that prevent someone else from repeating the mistake, not punishing the person who made the error. There are many options for problem statements for the death of this patient:

- The patient died (too wide).
- The nurse gave the wrong medication (focuses on individual culpability).
- Serum glucose was 0 (too narrow).
- Discovery of unexpected hypoglycemia was delayed (a good choice).

Once a problem statement has been chosen, the facilitator asks, "why did this happen?" The U.S. Department of Veterans Affairs (VA) National Center for Patient Safety has tools for asking triggering questions, as well as guidance on how to use the "five whys." Some guidelines for exploring the "five whys" and getting to the root cause of a problem include (VA, 2021):

- Clearly show the cause-and-effect relationship.
- Use specific and accurate descriptors.
- Human error must have a preceding cause.
- Violations of procedure are not root causes.
- Failure to act is only causal if there is a duty to act.

Some members of the team may have preconceived ideas for why the error occurred. It is ideal for participants to become prepared, but encourage them to keep an open mind during the brainstorming process. Brainstorming can yield surprising causes team members may not have thought of. As discussion of the problem continues, new ideas may arise. One technique recommended for RCA is to write every idea on sticky notes on a board or wall to facilitate changes while keeping all ideas visible. No ideas are removed, but they may be moved to a holding area in case they are found to be of use later. Figure 16-5 shows how sticky notes can be arranged for an RCA and how the notes would be transferred into a flow chart diagram.

The next step is to identify interventions. A successful RCA yields a positive response to the question, "If these interventions had been in place at the time of the error, would it have been prevented?" The interventions put into place after the death of this patient included:

- Insulin was added to the automated dispensing device.
- Staff were educated to keep medications secure.
- Nurses were reminded to keep medication carts locked.
- The use of multidose vials of insulin and heparin was discontinued.
- Policy was changed to use saline flushes to restore patency of arterial lines.
- The interdisciplinary team would examine how to expedite the delivery of medications to patients.

TJC requires strong interventions be identified for sentinel events. Strong interventions, such as discontinuing the use of multidose vials, may require great effort and expense to implement, but after implementation require little effort. Weak interventions, such as educating staff, are easy to implement but require continued effort to maintain. Table 16-2 shows examples of interventions ranked from weak to strong. TJC also requires that an RCA action plan include evidence that organizational leadership and key stakeholders are involved, findings are thoroughly explained, relevant literature is considered, and that the RCA has internal accuracy and consistency with no contradictions or unanswered questions (Singh et al., 2023).

Due to the large amount of data available from RCAs, analysis of aggregated data is an opportunity for the IN to explore medical error prevention on a deeper level. Aggregate review RCA functions to address improvements to patient safety processes rather than focusing on a single event (VA, 2021). VA facilities have been conducting RCAs for several decades and therefore have great amounts of data for analysis. For example, approximately 100 acute and long-term VA facilities contributed data for the analysis of the results of 176 RCAs for patient falls. After the implementation of RCA action plans, 34.4% of the facilities reported reduced falls and 38.9% reported reduced injuries from falls. Specific interventions included environmental assessments and toileting interventions (Mills et al., 2005).

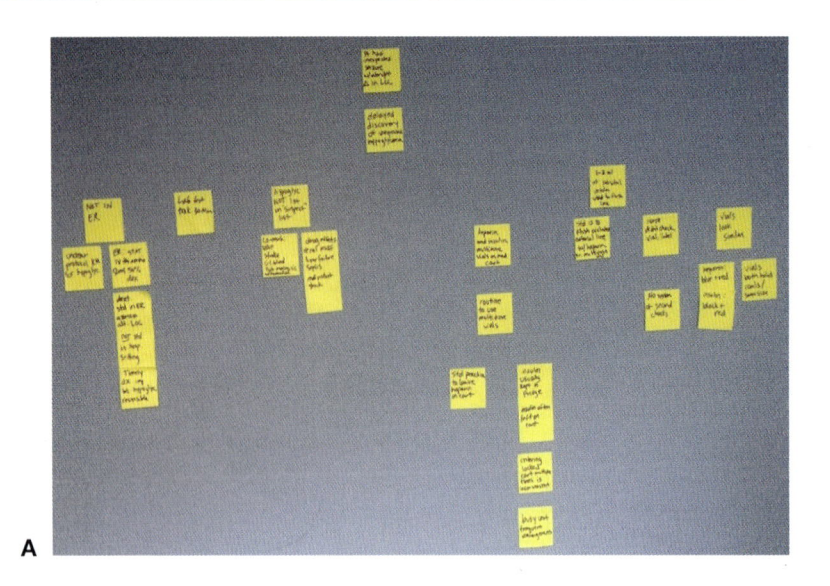

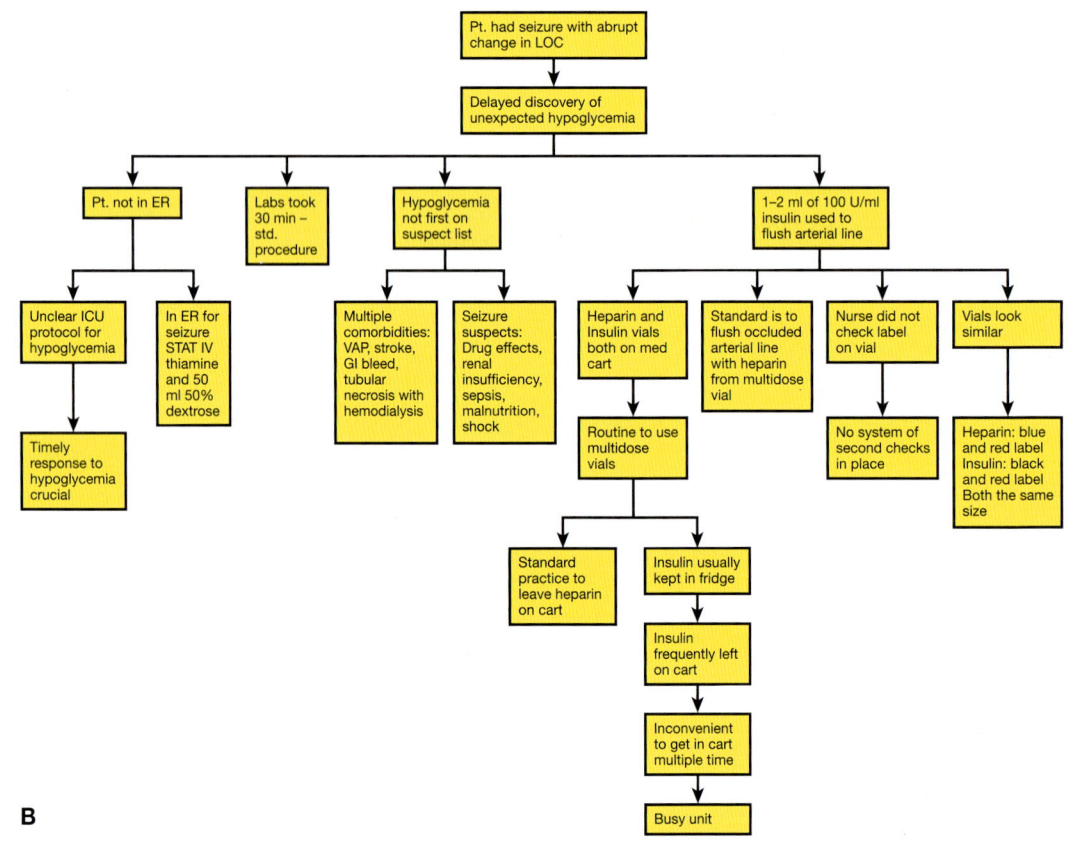

Figure 16-5. Use of sticky notes for root cause analysis (A) to generate a flowchart (B).

TABLE 16-2 Continuum of Strength of Actions

Strength of Actions	Examples of Actions
Stronger Actions *Remove dependence on the human to "get it right" (physical, permanent)*	Physical/architectural changes (replacing revolving doors with sliding doors to reduce falls) New device with usability testing before purchase (test outpatient glucose meters, select best for population) Forcing functions (all passwords must be eight characters, eliminate universal adaptors) Simplify or remove unnecessary steps Standardize equipment or process (same pump used throughout the hospital system) Involving leadership (morning safety rounds by leadership) High reliability training (simulation, competency evaluation)
Intermediate Actions *Reduce reliance on the human to "get it right"*	Increased staffing/decreased workload Software enhancements (computer alerts for drug-drug interactions) Eliminate or reduce distractions (dedicated medication nurse) Checklists (near computer showing steps necessary to login) Enhanced documentation (highlight medication name and dose on IV bags) Redundancy (Independent double check by two nurses) Simulation training (practice patient communication in simulated or lab environment with after action critique and debrief) Eliminate look-alike and sound-alike medications Standardize communication tools
Weaker Actions *Rely solely on the human to "get it right" (support/clarify processes)*	Double check (one person calculates dosage, another person reviews calculation) Warnings and labels (caution sign reminding all computer users to maintain strong, unique passwords for system accounts, audible alarms) New procedure/memorandum/policy (remember to store medications in authorized places) Training (in-service demonstration of clean-bag technique) Additional study/analysis (interdisciplinary team to study needed changes)

There are challenges associated with conducting RCA. The time it takes can be costly. Each RCA requires 20 to 90 person hours to complete. There is often no power to enforce the interventions discovered by the team. Therefore, when conducting an RCA, it is important to ensure a deep evaluation of the error, keep the focus on systemic issues and not on disciplining a person, look for multiple solutions that might be effective, and beware of

> **CASE STUDY**
>
> Read about the events leading up to the administration of vecuronium by RaDonda Vaught. Use the five whys to determine the root causes of the error. See how many latent or background factors you can identify.

choosing the easiest solution that will not prevent the problem from recurring.

Health Information Technology for Medication Error Prevention

Implementing HIT can improve patient safety by reducing the possibility of human error on the part of healthcare providers. HIT can help reduce medication errors and improve compliance to practice guidelines (Alotaibi & Federico, 2017). Box 16-3 lists strategies to prevent ADEs, many of which involve the use of HIT.

Computerized Provider Order Entry and Clinical Decision Support Systems

Computerized provider order entry (CPOE) is the process of using computer support to enter provider orders. CPOE was first developed to improve the safety of medication orders. Some CPOE systems prompt the provider about patient allergies, drug-drug or drug-lab interactions, and interventions based on EBP recommendations. Modern systems allow providers to order lab tests, procedures, referrals, and consultations. CPOE is often integrated with a **clinical decision support system (CDSS)** (Chapters 9 and 11), a system that enhances medical decision making by matching patient data to existing clinical knowledge and then presenting patient-specific assessments or recommendations to the clinician. CDSS serves as an error prevention tool by providing drug administration guidelines for route, dosing, and frequency. In a meta-analysis of CPOE with CDSS, a significant reduction in medication errors and adverse drug reactions was observed (Alotaibi & Federico, 2017). However, the use of CPOE without CDSS does not appear to reduce medication errors.

CDSS improves the ability of healthcare professionals to make decisions about patient care with evidence-based clinical knowledge and patient

---

BOX 16-3 Strategies to Prevent Adverse Drug Events at Different Stages

Prescribing
- Adhere to conservative prescribing principles to avoid unnecessary medications.
- Use CPOE, especially when paired with CDSSs.[a]
- Perform medication reconciliation during transitions in care.

Transcribing
Use CPOE to eliminate handwriting errors.[a]

Dispensing
- Involve clinical pharmacists to oversee the medication dispensing process.
- Use uppercase lettering and other strategies to minimize confusion between look-alike and/or sound-alike medications.
- Use ADCs for high-risk medications.[a]

Administration
- Adhere to the "five rights" of medication safety (right medication in the right dose at the right time by the right route to the right patient).
- Use BCMA to ensure medications are given to the correct patient.[a]
- Minimize interruptions to allow nurses to administer medications safely.
- Use smart infusion pumps for IV infusions.[a]
- Use multicompartment medication devices for patients taking multiple medications in ambulatory or long-term care settings.[a]
- Improve patient comprehension of administration instructions through patient education and revised medication labels.

[a]Highlighted examples involve healthcare information technology, emphasizing the importance of this in preventing adverse drug events.
Adapted from Agency for Healthcare Research and Quality (AHRQ). (2019a, September 7). Medication errors and adverse drug events. https://psnet.ahrq.gov/primers/primer/23/medication-errors-and-adverse-drug-events.

information. There is also evidence that the use of CDSS improves the quality of care and patient safety, but the IN should be aware that results vary with different system designs and implementation methods. A systematic review, found that the use of reminders for physicians led to improvements in medication and laboratory ordering and clinical outcomes (Shojania et al., 2009). However, up to 33% of CDSS alerts were ignored in a study of 18,115 drug alerts (Shah et al., 2006). Another study found that providers were more likely to use the CDSS when it demanded justification for the reason for overriding CDSS advice (Alotaibi & Federico, 2017).

Automated Dispensing Cabinets

An automated dispensing cabinet (ADC) is a computerized medicine cabinet used in healthcare settings to store and dispense medications near the point of care (Fig. 16-6). ACDs were introduced in the 1980s to control medication inventory, minimize workload for the pharmacy, and track medication dispensing and billing. A controlled trial on the effect of ADCs on patient safety found that the use of ADCs resulted in a 28% reduction in the rate of medication errors in a hospital critical care unit (Chapuis et al., 2010). However, the ADCs did not reduce errors that resulted in patient harm. Another study compared hospital units using ADCs to ones using more traditional methods. It showed a significantly lower error rate, fewer interruptions per hour, and faster preparation times on the ADC units (Jumeau et al., 2023).

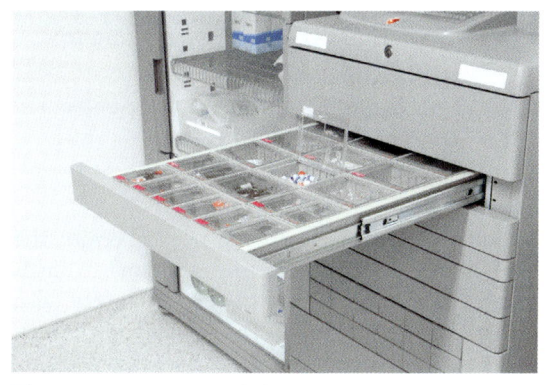

Figure 16-6. Automated dispensing cabinet. (Shutterstock/Healthy Definition.)

Although ADCs can significantly lower medication errors, they cannot eliminate human errors, so diligence is still required when working with these systems (Tu et al., 2023).

In a recent analysis of the RaDonda Vaught case, pharmacists suggested several features could be incorporated into the ADC to prevent the error from recurring. They recommended that access to neuromuscular blocking agents (NMBAs) such as vecuronium should be eliminated outside of perioperative areas where they are routinely used. It was also suggested that the override function on ADCs be limited only to cases and medications that require immediate removal, that any override should be verified by the pharmacy, and that data on the frequency and type of medication overrides be collected (Ro & Holcomb, 2022). The ISMP recommends the entry of a minimum of the first five letters of the medication name. RaDonda Vaught reported typing in "VE" when looking for Versed and taking the first medication listed (which was vecuronium). NMBAs should also be accompanied by prominent warning labels indicating respiratory paralysis and need for ventilation not only on the medication, but also in the ADC pocket drawers and lids where they will be clearly visible on opening. In addition, barcode scanning should be implemented for all areas.

Barcode Medication Administration

Barcode medication administration (BCMA) is a form of mobile healthcare technology that integrates electronic medication administration records with barcode technology (Chapters 5 and 11). With BCMA, each drug is labeled with a unique barcode. When a patient is prescribed a medication, it appears in their electronic medical record, which the nurse uses to remove medications from the ADC. The patient is also identified with a unique barcode on their wristband. The administration of each drug involves scanning the patient's wristband and the medication to ensure the "five rights" are being followed: the right medication is being given to the right patient in the right dose by the right route at the right time.

BCMA may reduce medication administration errors by upward of 50% to 80% (Alotaibi & Federico, 2017; Owens et al., 2020). BCMA has been found to reduce errors related to wrong time, wrong dose, wrong medication, and wrong route (Shah et al., 2016). When BCMA is combined with CPOEs, CDSSs, and ADCs, this is called closed loop medication administration. In this process, the entire medication administration cycle (prescribing, processing, dispensing, and administering) is electronic and is as automated as possible. Adhering to a closed-loop medication administration can further reduce medication errors (Shermock et al., 2023). BCMA and other medication automation are unlikely to eliminate medication errors entirely, but it does go a long way toward making medication administration safer for patients.

Smart Infusion Pumps

Smart infusion pumps enable the automatic delivery of IV fluids and medications within the bounds of preset parameters (Fig. 16-7). They were first introduced into healthcare in the early 2000s to reduce medication errors associated with IV administration. The pumps have drug libraries and dose error reduction systems (DERSs) that include limits and safeguards to prevent errors. Smart infusion pumps allow the user to choose the desired medication from an approved list and input the required patient information (e.g., patient identification, weight, age), after which the pump calculates the infusion rate. The DERS alerts the user if the calculated rate exceeds normally acceptable dosing limits. Limits can be hard (cannot be overridden at the pump) or soft (a warning is provided, but the user can still start the infusion after acknowledging the limits).

Compared to traditional gravity methods of IV administration, the use of smart infusion pumps has been shown to reduce the incidence of ADEs and medication administration errors, even more so when they are combined with electronic prescribing and BCMA (Jani et al., 2021). Hard limits are more effective than soft limits; overriding dose error alerts and bypassing drug libraries and DERS completely are common causes of IV pump error. Commonly reported IV administrating errors with smart infusion pumps include medication not being dispensed, the wrong pump rate, or an incorrect drug or dose (Giuliano, 2018). Although smart infusion pumps reduce IV errors, there has been a call for updating smart pump technology to address the large number of errors that continue to occur.

Read the Ethical Considerations box to understand how the American Nurses Association (ANA) Code of Ethics applies to patient safety.

> ### CASE STUDY
> Implementation of HIT can cause additional time and work for nurses, resulting in workarounds. Workarounds are actions nurses take to deliver care and accomplish work, despite those actions deviating from protocol and policy. What HIT is used in your place of work to protect patient safety? Do nurses report satisfaction with these preventative measures? What workarounds have nurses developed to save time? Have there been any errors due to the use of these workarounds?

CULTURE OF SAFETY

To address the high number of medical errors, the IOM has urged healthcare organizations to institute a culture of safety. A **culture of safety** (also known as a just culture) is the combination of attitudes and behaviors toward patient safety that are conveyed when walking into a health facility (ECRI, 2019). "The single greatest impediment to error

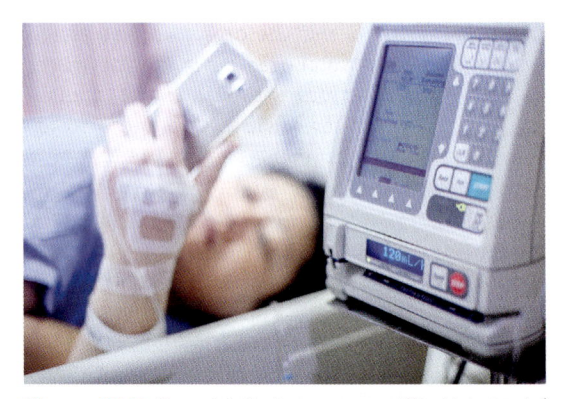

Figure 16-7. Smart infusion pumps. (Shutterstock/koonsiri boonak.)

ETHICAL CONSIDERATIONS FOR PATIENT SAFETY

Provision three of the ANA Code of Ethics (2015) states that the nurse promotes, advocates for, and protects the rights, health, and safety of the patient. Several principles of this provision apply to patient safety. Principle 3.3 covers performance standards and review mechanisms. Nurses must have the knowledge, skills, and disposition to perform professional responsibilities that require preparation beyond the basic academic programs. This is in full recognition of the relationship of nurse competencies, performance standards, review mechanisms, and educational preparation to patient safety and care outcomes. Principle 3.4 is about professional responsibility in promoting a culture of safety. Nurses must participate in the development, implementation, and review of and adherence to policies that promote patient health and safety, reduce errors and waste, and establish and sustain a culture of safety. Errors and near misses must be reported to the facility and to the patient, and system factors that contributed to the errors must be addressed. Principle 3.5 discusses protection of patient health and safety by acting on questionable practice. Nurses must act in all instances of incompetent, unethical, illegal, or impaired practice and follow the chain of command until the issue is corrected.

Interpretive Statement 4.1 speaks to the authority, accountability, and responsibility of the nurse. Nurses are always accountable for their own actions. Interpretive Statement 4.2 discusses accountability for nursing judgments, decisions, and actions. When considering patient safety, veracity or truth telling and nondeception apply to the importance of disclosing errors with the patient and the community. Nonmaleficence (not inflicting harm) is the duty of all healthcare workers. Interpretive Statement 6.3 states that nurses must participate in interprofessional workplace advocacy to address unethical practice, continue to express concerns about these practices, and resign after repeated unsuccessful attempts to change unjust practice to preserve integrity or risk being complicit. Interpretive Statement 1.5 covers the relationship the nurse has with colleagues and others, including unlicensed personnel. The nurse has a duty to create a culture of respect to ensure safe, quality patient care. This includes engaging in a hospitable work environment by dedicating oneself to civil interactions.

prevention...is that we punish people for making mistakes" (Leape, 1994). Healthcare has perpetuated a culture of shame and blame in which those at the point of error are held accountable. In a culture of safety, errors are reported without fear of negative consequences and are examined to discover both individual and systemic contributing factors with the goal of putting interventions in place that will prevent future error (Berry et al., 2020). Box 16-4 lists tenets of a safety culture. Also refer back to Box 16-2. Many of the methods to encourage error reporting are also qualities of a culture of safety.

A culture of safety is found in **high reliability organizations (HROs)**, which are organizations that have fewer than normal accidents. There are five principles of HROs that are responsible for the "mindfulness" that prevents error when faced with unexpected situations: preoccupation with failure, reluctance to simplify, sensitivity to operations, commitment to resilience, and deference to expertise.

HROs minimize adverse events by committing to safety at all levels, from leadership to bedside staff. A culture of safety acknowledges the high-risk nature of the organization's activities, promotes a blame-free environment where staff can report errors without fear of punishment, and encourages collaboration and discourages hierarchies. Improving the culture of safety within healthcare is essential to reducing errors. Low safety culture scores are linked to increased error rates, and adoption of specific safety culture measures has been associated with lower error rates (Berry et al., 2020). Although hospitals routinely survey safety culture, none have been reported to achieve the level of a culture of safety found in HROs. Poor teamwork and communication, a culture of low expectations, and authority

> **BOX 16-4** Tenets of a Culture of Safety
>
> - Apply transparent, nonpunitive approach to reporting, and learn from errors and unsafe conditions.
> - Use transparent processes for distinguishing human or system errors from blameworthy actions.
> - Involve leadership to model behaviors and eliminate intimidating behaviors.
> - Implement and enforce policies that support a culture of safety and the reporting of errors and unsafe conditions.
> - Recognize and celebrate members who report errors and unsafe conditions and who have safety improvement suggestions.
> - Use a validated tool to establish baseline and measure safety culture.
> - Analyze safety culture survey results to find opportunities for quality and safety improvement.
> - Analyze safety assessments to develop and implement improvement initiatives at a unit level.
> - Integrate safety culture training into projects and processes.
> - Assess system strengths and weaknesses and prioritize improvements.
> - Perform organizational safety culture assessment periodically to review progress and sustain improvement.
>
> Adapted from The Joint Commission (TJC). (2017). 11 tenets of safety culture. https://www.jointcommission.org/-/media/tjc/documents/resources/patient-safety-topics/sentinel-event/sentinel_events_11_tenets_of_a_safety_culture_infographic_2018pdf.pdf

differentials such as those found between physicians and nurses all contribute to a failure to achieve a culture of safety.

In a seminal report, Leape et al. (2009) described the culture of healthcare as hierarchical, lacking in teamwork, and focused on individual blame. Despite the adoption of just culture principles that include shared accountability and non-punitive responses to error, employees continue to report unfair treatment related to medical error in healthcare organizations (Paradiso & Sweeney, 2019). How we educate nurses may play a role in this climate. Schools of nursing have historically dealt with student errors with discipline or penalties (Walker et al., 2020). Students report being afraid to speak up and are reluctant to report errors (Walker et al., 2019). Adoption of a culture of safety during a program of study affects the overall culture of healthcare. This improves patient safety by ensuring members of healthcare professions have taken on the norms, values, and practices of a culture of safety. A transformation in the education of healthcare workers is essential to creating and maintaining a culture of safety in healthcare.

Participating in RCA may help dispel a culture of blame and foster a culture of safety. The American Association of Colleges of Nursing (AACN) Essentials recommend that processes used in understanding causes of error, such as RCAs, be included in entry-level professional nursing education (AACN, 2021). The Quality and Safety Education for Nurses (QSEN) competencies, which have been incorporated in the AACN Essentials, included the recommendation that nursing students engage in RCA rather than blaming when errors or near misses occur (Cronenwett et al., 2007). Teaching nursing students about RCA and involving them in simulated RCA experiences should be used as an instructional strategy to prevent student medication error. However, there are few published educational strategies about how to teach RCA (Miller et al., 2016). This may be an avenue for exploration for INs.

INs should embrace a culture of safety and provide the leadership necessary to adopt the principles of HROs. The IN can advocate for making safety a top priority in strategic planning. INs should help create and review patient safety policies and procedures, be aware of safety trends, collect patient safety data on a regular basis, and support quality improvement projects that include patient safety.

> **CASE STUDY**
>
> Recall from the case study that even though RaDonda Vaught admitted her part in the medical error, she ultimately lost her nursing license and was convicted of criminally negligent homicide. Thinking about the outcome of her situation, if you were involved in a medication error, what would be your course of action?

Measuring Safety Culture

A good way to measure patient safety is to assess the commitment of an organization to adopting a culture of safety. The IN can affect patient safety by engaging in research and EBP projects (Chapter 7) on this topic using valid and reliable survey instruments. Several patient safety organizations have developed survey instruments for use in healthcare organizations. In addition, surveys to measure safety culture in schools of nursing have also been recently developed.

Surveys for Healthcare Organizations

The AHRQ released the Survey of Patient Safety (SOPS) in 2004. This survey is regularly updated and given to healthcare providers and other staff and includes topics such as teamwork; staffing and work pace; organizational learning and continuous improvement; response to error; leadership support for patient safety; communication about error; communication openness; reporting patient safety events; hospital management support for patient safety; and handoffs and information exchange. In addition, the survey collects data on the number of events reported and the patient safety rating (AHRQ, 2023b). The AHRQ provides SOPS geared toward hospitals (Hospital Survey of Patient Safety Culture, or HSOPSC), medical offices, nursing homes, community pharmacies, and ambulatory surgery centers. These surveys are publicly available in the United States for download and use, though international users should contact the AHRQ for permission to use the surveys outside the United States. Users of the surveys can submit their data to the AHRQ and receive a customized feedback report that compares their results with the database. Researchers may request access to the data sets through the AHRQ (AHRQ, 2023b).

The Safety Attitudes Questionnaire (SAQ) was developed in 2006 by researchers with funding from the Robert Wood Johnson Foundation and the AHRQ and is a reliable and valid tool for measuring a culture of safety. The SAQ maintains a high level of continuity with its predecessor, the Flight Management Attitudes Questionnaire, a traditional human factors survey with a 20-year history in aviation (Sexton et al., 2006). Positive SAQ scores have been correlated with fewer medication errors, shorter lengths of stay, and fewer adverse outcomes (Nordén-Hägg et al., 2010). The SAQ covers four themes: safety climate, teamwork climate, stress recognition, and organizational climate. The SAQ elicits caregiver attitudes using six factor climate scales: teamwork, safety, job satisfaction, perceptions of management, working conditions, and stress recognition. When used in preintervention/postintervention methodology, the SAQ factors have demonstrated sensitivity to quality improvement interventions, demonstrating that safety climate can be targeted and improved. The SAQ has been adapted for use in intensive care units, operating rooms, general inpatient settings, and ambulatory clinics. The survey is available for public use by contacting the study authors (UTHealth Houston, n.d.).

Another tool is the Just Culture Assessment Tool (JCAT). The JCAT was developed to distinguish between overall patient safety culture and the presence of a just culture in healthcare organizations (Logroño et al., 2023). The JCAT is a valid and reliable tool that measures aspects of just culture for patient safety.

Surveys for Schools of Nursing

The Just Culture Assessment Tool for Nursing Education (JCAT-NE) was developed from the JCAT to measure safety culture in schools of nursing (Walker et al., 2019). The JCAT-NE was found to be a valid and reliable measure of just culture. The researchers used the JCAT-NE to assess prelicensure nursing students' perceptions of just culture in 15 schools of nursing (SONs). Most participants (78%) reported that their SON has a safety reporting system, 15.4% had been involved in a safety event, and 12% had submitted an error report (Walker et al., 2020). Low scores were reported for ease of use for safety reporting systems, being given time to prepare a report, and faculty encouragement of reporting.

A recent study by some of the same researchers used the JCAT-NE and the JCAT to compare the experiences of subjects at two points in time: when they were nursing students during their last semester of nursing school and once they had graduated and were working as registered nurses for 6 to 12 months (Walker et al., 2024). They found that JCAT-NE and JCAT scores at these two points in time were not statistically different, a positive result suggesting students are using the knowledge and attitudes about just culture learned during their education when they move into practice. This newer study also found that 85% of students had a safety reporting system in their SON, an improvement over the previous 78%. This increase is likely the result of the expanding inclusion of safety education in nursing programs. Of concern, however, is that scores decreased significantly for openness of communication, continuous improvement process, and fear of reporting for the registered nurses who had moved to practice, suggesting that not all healthcare organizations create a culture that promotes error reporting (Walker et al., 2024).

Using tools such as the SAQ would allow nursing schools to measure the effectiveness of interventions among cohorts as well as to provide researchers with a common language to communicate about student attitudes about safety culture and knowledge of safe medication administration. A research study tested whether engaging nursing students in RCA about a medication error would affect their attitudes about safety culture as measured by the SAQ (Miller, 2022). It was found that education about RCA is associated with a positive change in safety culture attitudes, meaning the use of RCA as an educational intervention in prelicensure nursing education has the potential to improve safety culture in schools of nursing.

The School of Nursing Culture of Safety Survey (SON-COSS) is another example of a survey that was adapted to nursing schools from an existing professional survey: the AHRQ HSOPSC (Hershey, 2017). The SON-COSS has 42 five-point Likert items to assess 10 dimensions of patient safety as well as two questions not covered by the dimensions (patient safety grade and number of events reported); demographic questions; and one question with a free text box. The SON-COSS was found to maintain its reliability and validity for use in prelicensure nursing students. After further revision, the SON-COSS (renamed SON-COSS-R) was given to members of the National Student Nurses Association. Although most students gave their schools a patient safety grade of "very good" or "excellent" (92.8%), 85.6% reported that they had never reported an error. These results are comparable to the JCAT-NE result in which only 12% of students had submitted an error report (Walker et al., 2020). This result implies students do not understand the value of reporting errors, which is a hallmark component of a culture of safety (Miller, 2021).

Patient Safety Organizations

There are numerous patient safety organizations with resources and guidelines to help hospitals with error prevention efforts. The WHO connects nations, healthcare providers, and organizations to promote health. The WHO has a patient safety page on its website with world health statistics including a mortality database, an international data dashboard for COVID-19, and a database for health inequalities. They also provide access to data collection tools, resources for emergencies and disasters, fact sheets on global health topics, and a newsroom that reports on global safety issues. The WHO created a Global Patient Safety Action Plan for 2021 to 2030 that provides a framework for countries to develop national action plans on patient safety (WHO, 2021). To address medication errors, they launched the Medication Without Harm campaign in 2017 to increase awareness of medication use and safety with a call for action of "KNOW. CHECK. ASK." (WHO, 2022). September 17 was declared World Patient Safety Day and focused on medications without harm (WHO, n.d.).

ECRI (originally founded as the Emergency Care Research Institute) is an international, independent, nonprofit organization that helps healthcare organizations improve quality, reduce costs, and achieve better patient outcomes. ECRI conducts independent medical device evaluations and is designated as an EBP center by the AHRQ (ECRI, 2019). The ISMP is a nonprofit organization devoted to preventing medication errors. It publishes newsletters with real-time error information and hosts the only national voluntary medication error reporting program (ISMP, n.d.a). In 2020, ECRI and ISMP formally affiliated to become one of the largest federally certified PSOs in the world (ISMP, n.d.a).

The AHRQ is the federal agency charged with improving the safety and quality of healthcare for all Americans. It supports research efforts, creates materials to teach and train healthcare professionals, and generates benchmarks and data used by policymakers and providers. AHRQ patient safety resources include patient safety email updates, surveys on patient safety culture, toolkits for eliminating hospital-acquired infections, health literacy tools, and the Patient Safety Network (PSNet), which features a collection of tools, continuing education, news, and resources on patient safety (AHRQ, 2023a). A useful feature of PSNet is a weekly highlight of the latest patient safety literature, news, and expert commentary.

TJC is an accrediting body for healthcare organizations and programs. They offer patient safety resources for "do not use" abbreviations, "look-alike sound-alike" drugs, advancing effective communication, and improving patient and worker safety. Patient safety topics include zero harm, healthcare worker safety, workplace violence prevention, and emergency management. Each year, TJC gathers data about emerging patient safety issues and creates a list of **National Patient Safety Goals (NPSGs)** for various programs including hospitals, ambulatory care, assisted living, home care, and office-based surgery centers for the following year. The 2024 NPSGs for hospitals include (TJC, 2024a):

- Identifying patients correctly
- Improving staff communication
- Using medicines safely
- Using alarms safely
- Preventing infection
- Identifying patient safety risks
- Improving healthcare equity
- Preventing mistakes in surgery

They also have a link for reporting a patient safety concern or complaint. Sentinel events are reported to TJC, which publishes a sentinel event alert newsletter that identifies specific types of events and high-risk conditions, describing common causes and steps to reduce risk. TJC works with accredited organizations to manage sentinel events and prevent them from happening. Sentinel Event Alert 66 is about eliminating disparities for pregnant patients and references the life-threatening complications experienced by Serena Williams that have been covered in more detail in Chapter 13 (TJC, 2023).

The IOM, founded in 1970, was integral in alerting the public about the hazards facing patients through their publication *To Err is Human* (IOM [U.S.] Committee on Quality of Health Care in America, 2000). The IOM was renamed the National Academy of Medicine (NAM) in 2015 and is one of the three academies that make up the National Academies of Sciences, Engineering, and Medicine (the National Academies). These private, nonprofit institutions work outside of the government to provide objective perspectives on science, technology, and health (NAM, n.d.). In 2022, they issued a statement on the conviction of RaDonda Vaught that urged healthcare organizations and lawmakers to understand that medical errors are most often caused by system failures. Although individuals have accountability for errors, the errors are usually the result of problems with system safeguards. Organizations have a duty to engage in system-level changes that make it simple for individuals to "do the right thing" as well as establish protective interventions that prevent harm to patients despite individual error (NAM, 2022).

In 2017, two of the most prominent healthcare safety organizations, the IHI, and the National Patient Safety Foundation (NPSF) combined forces under the IHI. The IHI has a triple aim: improving patient care quality and patient satisfaction; improving the health of populations; and reducing the cost of healthcare. The IHI has a patient safety essentials toolkit that includes the situation, background, assessment, recommendation (SBAR) technique for improving communication among healthcare professionals, action hierarchy (a component of RCA^2 that can help with identifying the strongest actions), a daily huddle agenda, and Failure Modes and Effects Analysis (FMEA), a systematic, proactive method for identifying potential risks and their effects (IHI, n.d.c).

Certification in Patient Safety

Professionals who demonstrate a high level of proficiency in the core standards of patient safety can earn the Certified Professional in Patient Safety (CPPS) credential from the IHI. Certification is a computer-based examination over five patient safety domains: culture; leadership; patient safety risks and solutions' measuring and improving performance; and systems thinking and design/human factors. A baccalaureate degree and 3 years of experience in a healthcare setting or an associate degree plus 5 years of experience are needed to take the exam. Since 2012, more than 6,000 healthcare professionals have earned the CPPS credential (IHI, n.d.b). Online review courses and self-assessments are offered through the IHI.

SUMMARY

- **Medical errors.** A medical error is an unintended healthcare outcome caused by a defect in the delivery of care to a patient. Healthcare errors may be errors of commission (doing the wrong thing), omission (not doing the right thing), or execution (doing the right thing incorrectly). Combined with sentinel events, near misses, and hazards, there is a financial and emotional cost. It is important to explore systemic causes of error to improve patient safety, such as the use of EHRs and incivility. Medication error is the most common type of error. Because nurses are so involved in medication administration, they are often involved in errors.
- **Measuring patient safety.** Patient safety is difficult to measure due to a lack of standardized measures, definitions, and outcomes. Measuring medical errors is complicated further because most errors are voluntarily reported. VER data should be gathered through IRSs, aggregated at the national level, and shared with stakeholders. Medication errors should be reported through IRSs and to national organizations such as the ISMP. Measurements should include data from a variety of sources including VER, direct observations, trigger tools, and chart review. Error rate should not be used as a measure of success.
- **Preventing errors.** Preventing errors is one of the most important goals of any healthcare organization. The systems approach suggests errors occur because of flawed systems. RCA is one method used to analyze errors. The process starts with a problem statement and results in at least one strong intervention. HIT for medication error prevention includes CPOE with CDSSs, ADCs, BCMA, and smart infusion pumps.
- **Culture of safety.** A culture of safety is the combination of attitudes and behaviors toward patient safety that are conveyed by a healthcare organization. A culture of safety is found in HROs that have utilized safety principles to reduce harm from accidents. Measuring safety culture is a good way to measure success with patient safety efforts. Surveys can be conducted in healthcare organizations and in schools of nursing using a wide variety of instruments. Patient safety resources include the WHO, ECRI, the AHRQ, TJC, the NAM, and the IHI, the last of which provides for certification in patient safety.

DISCUSSION QUESTIONS AND ACTIVITIES

1. Compare and contrast medical errors, sentinel events, near misses, and hazards, and give an example of each.
2. Search the internet for a publicized case of medical error other than the RaDonda Vaught case, and identify three systemic causes for the error. What were the legal, emotional, financial, and physical consequences of the error for the patient, the nurse, and the healthcare organization where the error occurred?
3. Explain the difficulties with measuring errors. What are some ways to measure errors? How does your facility measure errors?
4. Explore the process for handling medical errors at your place of work. Is your organization a patient safety organization? Why or why not? How are incidents reported? Are they shared with staff? Are data shared with a national organization? If so, which one?

5. Explore the NPSD (AHRQ, 2020). Create a graph and explain the results.
6. Interview a nurse about medical error and ask:
   - Have you ever made an error? If so, describe it.
   - How did it make you feel?
   - What do you think caused the error?
   - What were the consequences of the error for you, the patient, and the organization?
   - Was an RCA performed? Did anything change after the error was made?
7. Explore the RaDonda Vaught case by reading the Kelman article (2022b). Use what you have learned about RCA to create a timeline, answer the five whys, and identify strong interventions that could prevent this error from happening again.
8. What HIT is used at your place of work? Is it used correctly? Explore some reasons for misuse, workarounds, and overrides.
9. Does your place of work have a culture of safety? Is there a survey used at your school or healthcare organization to measure a culture of safety? If not, identify one person you could talk to about its importance. What is their role and opinion about a culture of safety?
10. Identify a patient safety organization that interests you. What resources are available for the IN? What is the most useful feature of the site?
11. Discuss the role of the IN in patient safety.

PRACTICE QUESTIONS

1. Which patient safety term is defined as an act of commission or omission that could have harmed the patient but did not cause harm because of chance, prevention, or mitigation?
   a. Medical error
   b. Sentinel event
   c. Hazard
   d. Near miss
2. The nurse is designing a quality improvement project to reduce sentinel events. Reducing which event would have the greatest effect on the number of reported sentinel events?
   a. Patient falls
   b. Incivility
   c. Medication error
   d. Firing nurses who make mistakes
3. Which statement by the nurse indicates an understanding of how to measure patient safety?
   a. "The most valid measurement of patient safety is the rate of error."
   b. "The ICD-10 billing codes for cause of death can be used to identify medical error."
   c. "Voluntary error reporting is the primary way healthcare organizations identify safety events."
   d. "PSOs are responsible for maintaining incident reporting systems in hospitals."
4. What is the correct order of the steps of RCA?
   a. Ask the "five whys"
   b. Create a timeline
   c. Have the team create a problem statement
   d. Create an action plan with a strong intervention
5. Which is not a best practice in a culture of safety?
   a. Transparent error reporting
   b. Disciplining nurses who are involved in medication errors that cause harm
   c. Leaders admitting when they make mistakes
   d. Organizational preoccupation with failure

REFERENCES

Agency for Healthcare Research and Quality (AHRQ). (2019a, September 7). *Medication errors and adverse drug events*. https://psnet.ahrq.gov/primers/primer/23/medication-errors-and-adverse-drug-events

Agency for Healthcare Research and Quality (AHRQ). (2019b, September). *Root cause analysis*. https://psnet.ahrq.gov/primer/root-cause-analysis

Agency for Healthcare Research and Quality (AHRQ). (2020, August). *What is the Network of Patient Safety Databases (NPSD)?* https://www.ahrq.gov/npsd/what-is-npsd/index.html

Agency for Healthcare Research and Quality (AHRQ). (2023a, January). *Quality and patient safety resources*. https://www.ahrq.gov/patient-safety/resources/index.html

Agency for Healthcare Research and Quality (AHRQ). (2023b, January). *SOPS databases*. https://www.ahrq.gov/sops/databases/index.html

Agency for Healthcare Research and Quality (AHRQ). (n.d.). *Patient Safety Organization (PSO) program*. https://pso.ahrq.gov/

Agency for Healthcare Research and Quality (AHRQ), Patient Safety Network (PSNet). (2019c, September 7). *Systems approach*. https://psnet.ahrq.gov/primer/systems-approach

Alotaibi, Y. K., & Federico, F. (2017). The impact of health information technology on patient safety. *Saudi Medical Journal, 38*(12), 1173–1180. https://doi.org/10.15537/smj.2017.12.20631

American Association of Colleges of Nursing (AACN). (2021, April 6). *The new AACN essentials*. https://www.aacnnursing.org/Education-Resources/AACN-Essentials

American Nurses Association. (2015). *Code of ethics for nurses*. American Nurses Publishing. https://www.nursingworld.org/practice-policy/nursing-excellence/ethics/code-of-ethics-for-nurses/

Andersson, L. M., & Pearson, C. M. (1999). Tit for tat? The spiraling effect of incivility in the workplace. *Academy of Management Review, 24*(3), 452–471.

Bates, D. W. (2002). Unexpected hypoglycemia in a critically ill patient. *Annals of Internal Medicine, 137*(2), 110–116. https://doi.org/10.7326/0003-4819-137-2-200207160-00009

Beres, N. (2022, May 23). Supporters help pay fines former VUMC nurse RaDonda Vaught owed to state. https://www.newschannel5.com/news/supporters-help-pay-fines-former-vandy-nurse-radonda-vaught-owed-to-state

Berry, J. C., Davis, J. T., Bartman, T., Hafer, C. C., Lieb, L. M., Khan, N., & Brilli, R. J. (2020). Improved safety culture and teamwork climate are associated with decreases in patient harm and hospital mortality across a hospital system. *Journal of Patient Safety, 16*(2), 130–136. https://doi.org/10.1097/PTS.0000000000000251

Carver, N., Gupta, V., & Hipskind, J. E. (2021). Medical error. In *StatPearls*. StatPearls Publishing. http://www.ncbi.nlm.nih.gov/books/NBK430763/

Chapuis, C., Roustit, M., Bal, G., Schwebel, C., Pansu, P., David-Tchouda, S., Foroni, L., Calop, J., Timsit, J.-F., Allenet, B., Bosson, J.-L., & Bedouch, P. (2010). Automated drug dispensing system reduces medication errors in an intensive care setting. *Critical Care Medicine, 38*(12), 2275–2281. https://doi.org/10.1097/CCM.0b013e3181f8569b

Cronenwett, L., Sherwood, G., Barnsteiner, J., Disch, J., Johnson, J., Mitchell, P., Sullivan, D. T., & Warren, J. (2007). Quality and safety education for nurses. *Nursing Outlook, 55*(3), 122–131. https://doi.org/10.1016/j.outlook.2007.02.006

Ecri. (2019, June 14). *Culture of safety: An overview*. https://www.ecri.org/components/HRC/Pages/RiskQual21.aspx

Fiore, K. (2023, December 5). RaDonda Vaught loses appeal to get her nursing license back. *Medpage Today*. https://www.medpagetoday.com/special-reports/features/107672

Giuliano, K. K. (2018). Intravenous smart pumps: Usability issues, intravenous medication administration error, and patient safety. *Critical Care Nursing Clinics of North America, 30*(2), 215–224.

Griffin, FA, & Resar, RK. (2009). *IHI global trigger tool for measuring adverse events* (2nd ed.). IHI Innovation Series white paper. Institute for Healthcare Improvement. https://www.ihi.org/resources/white-papers/ihi-global-trigger-tool-measuring-adverse-events#downloads. Institute for Healthcare Improvement.

Hershey, K. (2017). *Pre-Licensure nursing students' perceptions of safety culture in schools of nursing*. Electronic Theses and Dissertations. East Tennessee State University. Paper 3317. https://dc.etsu.edu/etd/3317/

Institute for Healthcare Improvement (IHI). (2015). *RCA2: Improving root cause analyses and actions to prevent harm*. National Patient Safety Foundation. https://www.ihi.org/resources/tools/rca2-improving-root-cause-analyses-and-actions-prevent-harm#downloads

Institute for Healthcare Improvement (IHI). (n.d.b). *Certified Professional in Patient Safety (CPPS)*. https://www.ihi.org/education/cpps

Institute for Healthcare Improvement (IHI). (n.d.c). *Patient safety essentials toolkit*. Retrieved March 30, 2023. https://www.ihi.org/resources/Pages/Tools/Patient-Safety-Essentials-Toolkit.aspx

Institute for Safe Medication Practices (ISMP). (2021, August 25). *Pump up the volume: Tips for increasing error reporting and decreasing patient harm*. https://www.ismp.org/resources/pump-volume-tips-increasing-error-reporting-and-decreasing-patient-harm

Institute for Safe Medication Practices (ISMP). (2022a, November 2). *California medication error reduction plan: Time for regulators and accreditors to adopt similar initiatives*. https://www.ismp.org/resources/alifornia-medication-error-reduction-plan-time-regulators-and-accreditors-adopt-similar

Institute for Safe Medication Practices (ISMP). (2022b). *ISMP targeted medication safety best practices for hospitals*. https://www.ismp.org/guidelines/best-practices-hospitals

Institute for Safe Medication Practices (ISMP). (n.d.a). *About us*. Retrieved April 5, 2023. https://www.ismp.org/about

Institute of Medicine (IOM) (US) Committee on Quality of Health Care in America. (2000). In Kohn, L. T., Corrigan, J. M., & Donaldson, M. S., (Eds.). *To err is human: Building a safer health system*. National Academies Press (US). http://www.ncbi.nlm.nih.gov/books/NBK225182/

Jani, Y. H., Chumbley, G. M., Furniss, D., Blandford, A., & Franklin, B. (2021) The potential role of smart infusion devices in preventing or contributing to medication administration errors: A descriptive study of 2 data sets. *Journal of Patient Safety, 17*(8), e1894–e1900. https://doi.org/10.1097%2FPTS.0000000000000751

Jumeau, M., Francois, O., & Bonnabry, P. (2023). Impact of automated dispensing cabinets on dispensing errors, interruptions and pillbox preparation time. *European Journal of Hospital Pharmacy: Science and Practice, 30*(4), 237–241. https://doi.org/10.1136/ejhpharm-2021-002849

Kelman, B. (2022a, March 24). In Nurse's trial, investigator says hospital bears 'heavy' responsibility for patient death. *KFF Health News*. https://kffhealthnews.org/news/article/radonda-vaught-fatal-drug-error-vanderbilt-hospital-responsibility/

Kelman, B. (2022b, March 27). The RaDonda Vaught trial has ended. In This timeline will help with the confusing case. *The Nashville Tennessean*. https://www.tennessean.com/story/news/health/2020/03/03/vanderbilt-nurse-radonda-vaught-arrested-reckless-homicide-vecuronium-error/4826562002/

Landrigan, C. P., Parry, G. J., Bones, C. B., Hackbarth, A. D., Goldmann, D. A., & Sharek, P. J. (2010). Temporal trends in rates of patient harm resulting from medical care. *New England Journal of Medicine, 363*(22), 2124–2134. https://doi.org/10.1056/NEJMsa1004404

Leape, L. L. (1994). Error in medicine. *JAMA, 272*(23), 1851–1857.

Leape, L., Berwick, D., Clancy, C., Conway, J., Gluck, P., Guest, J., Lawrence, D., Morath, J., O'Leary, D., O'Neill, P., Pinakiewicz, D, Isaac, T, & Lucian Leape Institute at the National Patient Safety Foundation, (2009). Transforming healthcare: A safety imperative. *Quality & Safety in Health Care, 18*(6), 424–428. https://doi.org/10.1136/qshc.2009.036954

Lewis, C. (2023). The impact of interprofessional incivility on medical performance, service and patient care: A systematic review. *Future Healthcare Journal, 10*(1), 69–77. https://doi.org/10.7861/fhj.2022-0092

Logroño, K. J., Al-Lenjawi, B. A., Singh, K., & Alomari, A. (2023). Assessment of nurse's perceived just culture: A cross-sectional study. *BMC Nursing, 22*(1), 348 (2023). https://doi.org/10.1186/s12912-023-01478-4

MacDowell, P., Cabri, A., & Davis, M. (2021, March 12). Medication administration errors. PSNet. *Agency for Healthcare Research and Quality.* https://psnet.ahrq.gov/primer/medication-administration-errors

Maddineshat, M., Rosenstein, A. H., Akaberi, A., & Tabatabaeichehr, M. (2016). Disruptive behaviors in an emergency department: The perspective of physicians and nurses. *Journal of Caring Sciences, 5*(3), 241–249. https://doi.org/10.15171/jcs.2016.026

Makary, M. A., & Daniel, M. (2016). Medical error—the third leading cause of death in the US. *BMJ, 353*, i2139. https://doi.org/10.1136/bmj.i2139

Miller, K. S. (2021, September 23). *Creating a culture of safety in schools of nursing.* In *National league for nursing education summit.* National Harbor.

Miller, K. S. (2022). Comparing the effects of traditional education and root-cause analysis on nursing students' attitudes about safety culture and knowledge of safe medication administration practices: An experimental study. *Nurse Educator, 47*(3), 139–144. https://doi.org/10.1097/NNE.0000000000001126

Miller, K., Haddad, L., & Phillips, K. (2016). Educational strategies for reducing medication errors committed by student nurses: A literature review. *International Journal of Health Sciences Education, 3*(1). https://dc.etsu.edu/ijhse/vol3/iss1/2

Mills, P. D., Neily, J., Luan, D., Stalhandske, E., & Weeks, W. B. (2005). Using aggregate root cause analysis to reduce falls and related injuries. *Joint Commission Journal on Quality and Patient Safety, 31*(1), 21–31. https://doi.org/10.1016/S1553-7250(05)31004-X

National Academy of Medicine (NAM). (2022, April 19). *NAM statement on the importance of ensuring a systems-based approach to patient safety and quality.* https://nam.edu/nam-statement-on-the-importance-of-ensuring-a-systems-based-approach-to-patient-safety-and-quality/

National Academy of Medicine (NAM). (n.d.). *About.* Retrieved April 20, 2023. https://nam.edu/about-the-nam/

National Coordinating Council for Medication Error Reporting and Prevention (NCC MERP). (n.d.). *Home page.* Retrieved April 19, 2023. http://www.nccmerp.org/

Nordén-Hägg, A., Sexton, J. B., Kälvemark-Sporrong, S., Ring, L, & Kettis-Lindblad, A. (2010). Assessing safety culture in pharmacies: The psychometric validation of the Safety Attitudes Questionnaire (SAQ) in a national sample of community pharmacies in Sweden. *BMC Clinical Pharmacology, 10*, 8, 8–8. https://doi.org/10.1186/1472-6904-10-8

North Carolina Board of Nursing (NCBON). (2023, February 3). *Complaint evaluation tool.* https://www.ncbon.com/discipline-compliance-employer-complaint-complaint-evaluation-tool-cet

Office for Civil Rights (OCR). (2022, December 23). *Patient safety and quality improvement act of 2005 statute and rule.* https://www.hhs.gov/hipaa/for-professionals/patient-safety/statute-and-rule/index.html

Owens, K., Palmore, M., Penoyer, D., & Viers, P. (2020). The effect of implementing bar-code medication administration in an emergency department on medication administration errors and nursing satisfaction. *Journal of Emergency Nursing, 46*(6), 884–891. https://doi.org/10.1016/j.jen.2020.07.004

Paradiso, L., & Sweeney, N. (2019). Just culture: It's more than policy. *Nursing Management, 50*(6), 38–45. https://journals.lww.com/nursingmanagement/fulltext/2019/06000/just_culture__it_s_more_than_policy.9.aspx

Porath, C. L., Gerbasi, A., & Schorch, S. L. (2015). The effects of civility on advice, leadership, and performance. *Journal of Applied Psychology, 100*(5), 1527–1541. https://doi.org/10.1037/apl0000016

Reason, J. (1990). *Human error.* Cambridge University Press.

Ro, M., & Holcomb, E. (2022, June 27). More lessons learned from RaDonda Vaught case. *Pharmacy Practice News.* https://www.pharmacypracticenews.com/Operations-and-Management/Article/06-22/More-Lessons-Learned-From-RaDonda-Vaught-Case/67213?ses=ogst

Rodziewicz, T. L., Houseman, B., & Hipskind, J. E. (2023). *Medical error reduction and prevention.* In *StatPearls.* StatPearls Publishing. http://www.ncbi.nlm.nih.gov/books/NBK499956/

Sexton, J. B., Helmreich, R. L., Neilands, T. B., Rowan, K., Vella, K., Boyden, J., Roberts, P. R., & Thomas, E. J. (2006). The Safety Attitudes Questionnaire: Psychometric properties, benchmarking data, and emerging research. *BMC Health Services Research, 6*(1), 44. https://doi.org/10.1186/1472-6963-6-44

Shah, K., Lo, C., Babich, M., Tsao, N. W., & Bansback, N. J. (2016). Bar code medication administration technology: A systematic review of impact on patient safety when used with computerized prescriber order entry and automated dispensing devices. *The Canadian Journal of Hospital Pharmacy, 69*(5), 394–402.

Shah, N. R., Seger, A. C., Seger, D. L., Fiskio, J. M., Kuperman, G. J., Blumenfeld, B., Recklet, E. G., Bates, D. W., & Gandhi, T. K. (2006). Improving acceptance of computerized prescribing alerts in ambulatory care. *Journal of the American Medical Informatics Association: JAMIA, 13*(1), 5–11. https://doi.org/10.1197/jamia.M1868

Shermock, S. B., Shermock, K. M., & Schepel, L. L. (2023). Closed-loop medication management with an electronic health record system in U.S. and Finnish hospitals. *International Journal of Environmental Research and Public Health, 20*(17), 6680.

Shojania, K. G., & Dixon-Woods, M. (2017). Estimating deaths due to medical error: The ongoing controversy and why it matters. *BMJ Quality & Safety, 26*(5), 423–428.

Shojania, K. G., Jennings, A., Mayhew, A., Ramsay, C. R., Eccles, M. P., & Grimshaw, J. (2009). The effects of on-screen, point of care computer reminders on processes and outcomes of care. *The Cochrane Database of Systematic Reviews, 2009*(3), CD001096. https://doi.org/10.1002/14651858.CD001096.pub2

Siddiqui, S., Marin, J., Kupsky, G., Quan, T., Frasure, S. E., Sikka, N., & Pourmand, A. (2021). A novel approach to establish and enhance event reporting systems among resident physicians. *AEM Education and Training, 5*(3), e10554, https://doi.org/10.1002/aet2.10554

Silvestre, JH, & Spector, N. (2023). Nursing student errors and near misses: Three years of data. *Journal of Nursing Education, 62*(1), 12–19. https://doi.org/10.3928/01484834-20221109-05

Singh, G., Patel, R. H., & Boster, J. (2023). *Root cause analysis and medical error prevention*. In *StatPearls*. StatPearls Publishing. http://www.ncbi.nlm.nih.gov/books/NBK570638/

The Joint Commission (TJC). (2021, April 14). *Sentinel event alert*. https://www.jointcommission.org/-/media/tjc/documents/resources/patient-safety-topics/sentinel-event/sea-39-ped-med-errors-rev-final-4-14-21.pdf

The Joint Commission (TJC). (2023, January 17). *Sentinel Event Alert 66: Eliminating disparities for pregnant patients*. https://www.jointcommission.org/-/media/tjc/newsletters/sea-66-maternal-mm-and-he-1-13-23-final.pdf

The Joint Commission (TJC). (2024a). *2024 National Patient Safety Goals*. https://www.jointcommission.org/standards/national-patient-safety-goals/

The Joint Commission (TJC). (2024b). *Sentinel event data 2023 annual review*. https://www.jointcommission.org/-/media/tjc/documents/resources/patient-safety-topics/sentinel-event/2024/2024_sentinel-event-_annual-review_published-2024.pdf

The University of Texas Health Science Center at Houston (UTHealth Houston) Center for Healthcare Quality and Safety. (n.d.). Safety Attitudes and Safety Climate Questionnaire. *UTHealth Houston*. Retrieved April 16, 2023https://www.uth.edu/chqs/safety-survey.

Tu, H-N., Shan, T-H., Wu, Y-C., Shen, P-H., Wu, T-Y., Lin, W-L., Yang-Kao, Y-H., & Cheng, C-L. (2023). Reducing medication errors by adopting automatic dispensing cabinets in critical care units. *Journal of Medical Systems, 47*(1), 52. https://doi.org/10.1007/s10916-023-01953-0

U.S. Department of Veterans Affairs (VA) Veterans Health Affairs (VHA). (2021, February 5). *Guide to performing a root cause analysis: A companion slide set for field education*. VHA National Center for Patient Safety. https://www.patientsafety.va.gov/docs/RCA-Guidebook_02052021.pdf

Walker, D., Altmiller, G., Barkell, N., Hromadik, L., & Toothaker, R. (2019). Development and validation of the Just Culture Assessment Tool for Nursing Education. *Nurse Educator, 44*(5), 261–264. https://doi.org/10.1097/NNE.0000000000000705

Walker, D., Altmiller, G., Hromadik, L., Barkell, N., Barker, N., Boyd, T., Compton, M., Cook, P., Curia, M., Hays, D., Flexner, R, Jordan, J, Jowell, V, Kaulback, M, Magpantay-Monroe, E, Rudolph, B, Toothaker, R, Vottero, B, & Wallace, S (2020). Nursing students' perceptions of just culture in nursing programs: A multisite study. *Nurse Educator, 45*(3), 133–138. https://doi.org/10.1097/NNE.0000000000000739

Walker, D., Hromadik, L, Baker, M, & McQuiston, L. (2024). Just culture: Nursing students transition to practice—a longitudinal study. *Nurse Educator, 49*(1), 1–7. https://doi.org/10.1097/NNE.0000000000001486

Wolfe, D., Yazdi, F., Kanji, S., Burry, L., Beck, A., Butler, C., Esmaeilisaraji, L., Hamel, C., Hersi, M., Skidmore, B., , Moher, D, & Hutton, B (2018). Incidence, causes, and consequences of preventable adverse drug reactions occurring in inpatients: A systematic review of systematic reviews. *PLoS ONE, 13*(10), e0205426. https://doi.org/10.1371/journal.pone.0205426

Woo, M. W. J., & Avery, M. J. (2021). Nurses' experiences in voluntary error reporting: An integrative literature review. *International Journal of Nursing Sciences, 8*(4), 453–469. https://doi.org/10.1016/j.ijnss.2021.07.004

World Health Organization (WHO). (2021, August 3). *Global patient safety action plan 2021-2030: Towards eliminating avoidable harm in health care*. https://iris.who.int/bitstream/handle/10665/343477/9789240032705-eng.pdf?sequence=1

World Health Organization (WHO). (2022, September 17). *Medication without harm*. https://www.who.int/initiatives/medication-without-harm

World Health Organization (WHO). (n.d.). *Patient safety*. Retrieved March 30, 2023. https://www.who.int/teams/integrated-health-services/patient-safety.

APPENDIX A

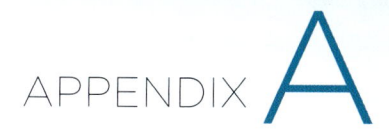

Creating a Database With Microsoft Access

Kristi Miller

A database is a tool for collecting and organizing information. Database software for home and small businesses is designed to handle smaller volumes of data and numbers of users as compared to industry databases. Individuals commonly use Microsoft Access, and it is likely you will use this software in nursing school or when working on projects. This appendix will briefly describe how to create and use a database in Microsoft Access. Some common database terminology is seen in Box A-1.

Using Access, you can:

- Add new data to a database, such as a new patient.
- Edit existing data in the database, such as changing the current status of the patient.
- Delete information, perhaps if a patient is discharged.
- Organize and view the data in different ways.
- Share the data with others via reports, email messages, an intranet, or the internet.

Microsoft Access allows creation of databases that contain tables, forms, queries, and reports. This makes it possible to use a piece of data many times, even though it has only been entered once (Microsoft 365 Support, n.d.).

CREATING AND USING A DATABASE

To build skills creating and using Microsoft Access, we will walk through a scenario to build a database from scratch. In this scenario, you decide to do a pilot study in which you ask students about self-care activities before and after they view a learning module on self-care. You might use paper and pencil to sketch out ideas for a database to collect and manage the data.

The first step is to open Microsoft Access. Much like in Microsoft Excel, database templates are available (Fig. A-1). For this scenario, select a blank database from the template options. A blank database is shown in Figure A-2.

Tables

A database table is similar in appearance to a spreadsheet in that data are stored in rows and columns. As a result, it is usually easy to import a spreadsheet into a database table. One database can contain more than one table. For example, a patient health record that uses three tables is not three databases but instead one database that contains three tables. The main difference between storing data in a spreadsheet and storing it in a database is in how the data are organized.

BOX A-1 Database Terminology

Atomic level data
Data that cannot be reduced; for example, for patient name, atomic level data would be the first name in one field, and the last name in a second field (first and last name together are not atomic level data)

Field
Smallest structure in a database; multiple fields make up a single record; fields are within a column in a spreadsheet (see Fig. A-2)

Form
A user interface in which you can enter and edit your data; act like surveys and are used to collect data that can be added to a database

Lookup table
A list of allowable entries for a field that is linked to that field

Normalization
Organizing data into tables within a database to eliminate redundancies

Primary key
A unique piece of data that identifies a record within a table; will be used in multiple tables to connect the record across tables; an example would be an assigned employee or student ID that is unique to each person

Query
Used to ask questions of one or more related tables or other queries; in a relational database it is the search function; output looks identical to a table but provides a custom view of the data; one of the characteristics that make databases powerful

Record
All information about a single "member" of a table; records are made up of multiple fields; make up a row in a spreadsheet (see Fig. A-2)

Report
Provides data organized to fulfil a user need, used to print information in a table or from a query

Sort
Rearranging the records in a table based on the data in a field or fields in a table; the simplest is a primary sort (sorted based on one field), but sorts can be done in any number of fields

Table
A collection of related information consisting of records (see Fig. A-2); each record is made up of fields; multiple tables may make up a single database

To get the most use out of a database, the data need to be organized into tables so that redundancies do not occur, a process called normalization. For example, if you are storing information about patients, each patient should only need to be entered once in a table that is set up just to hold patient data. Data about medications will be stored in its own table, and data about staffing will be stored in another table. Part of normalization involves ensuring each field contains atomic level data. For blood pressure, when the systolic and diastolic pressures are in one field, the data are not at the atomic level; they would need to be split into a systolic field and a diastolic field. A combination of first and last names in one field is not at the atomic level.

Each row in a table is referred to as a record. Records are where the individual pieces of

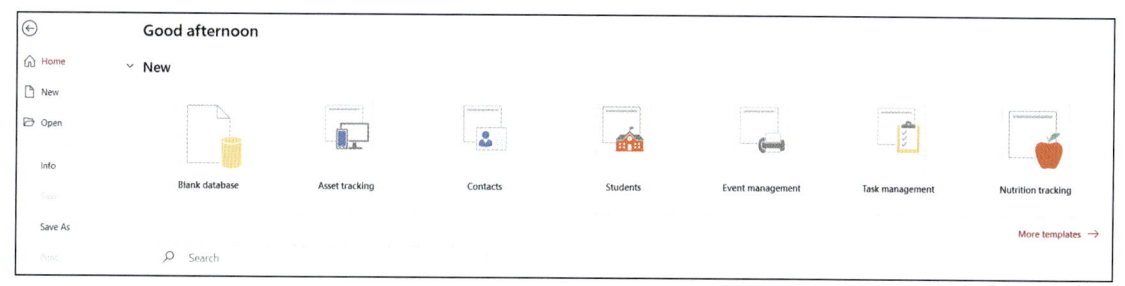

Appendix A Creating a Database With Microsoft Access

Figure A-1. Templates available in Microsoft Access.

information are stored. Each record consists of one or more fields. Fields correspond to the columns in the table. For example, you might have a table named "Patients" where each record (row) contains information about a different patient, and each field (column) contains a different type of information about the patient (e.g., first name, last name, address). Fields must be designated as a certain data type, whether it is text, date or time, number, etc.

Another way to describe records and fields is to visualize a library's old-style card catalogue. Each card in the cabinet corresponds to a record in the database. Each piece of information on an individual card (author, title, and so on) corresponds to a field in the database.

Each table includes a field identified as the primary key, the unique identifier of a record in a table. One column of fields will be identified as the primary key data. The primary key might be a unique identifying number used for each patient. That unique data will be used in multiple tables to connect a single record (patient) throughout multiple tables.

For the blank database you created, Table 1 will contain participant information. To name this table, select the "View" button, and you will be prompted to name the table (Fig. A-3). Once named, you can toggle back and forth between the design view and datasheet view (Fig. A-4), using whichever view is easiest for you when designing your table. The datasheet view (see Fig. A-3)

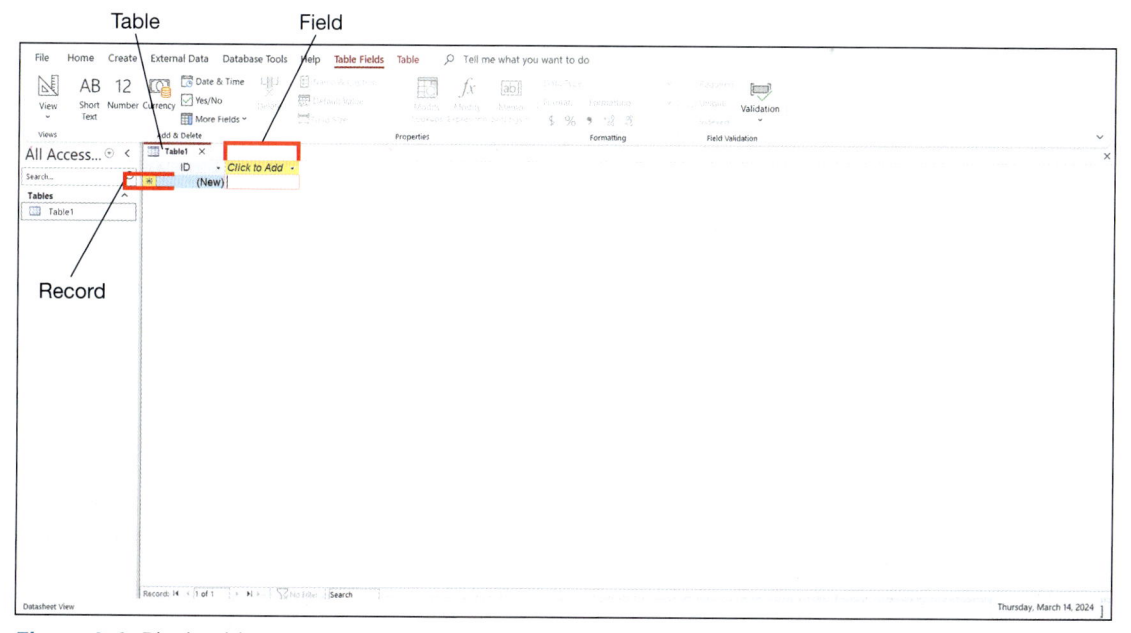

Figure A-2. Blank table.

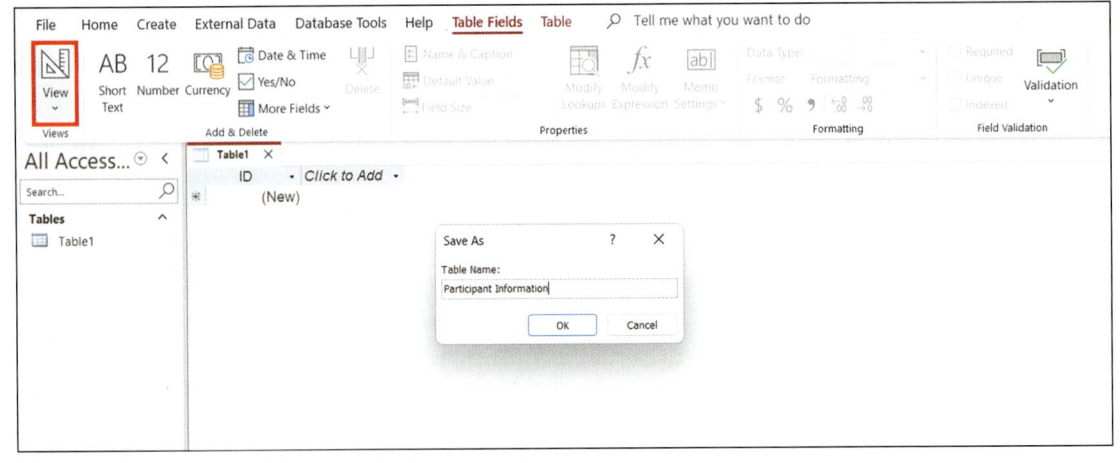

364 **Appendix A** Creating a Database With Microsoft Access

Figure A-3. Naming a table, shown in datasheet view.

displays all the values of calculation fields and their records. In the design view (see Fig. A-4), the tables can be created and modified. In the design view, you can see that the first field (named "ID" by default) is marked as the primary key.

Now you will add fields for participant ID, highest degree earned, type of school, semester in school, and employment. Right click on the heading of the first column, and select "Rename field" and change it to "Participant ID." For the other fields, click on "Click to Add" to get a drop-down menu, where you will select "Lookup & Relationship" for the type of field (Fig. A-5). This type of field will provide you with a list of options. In the box that pops up, select "I will type the values that I want". You will add the values or options you want for your lookup table,

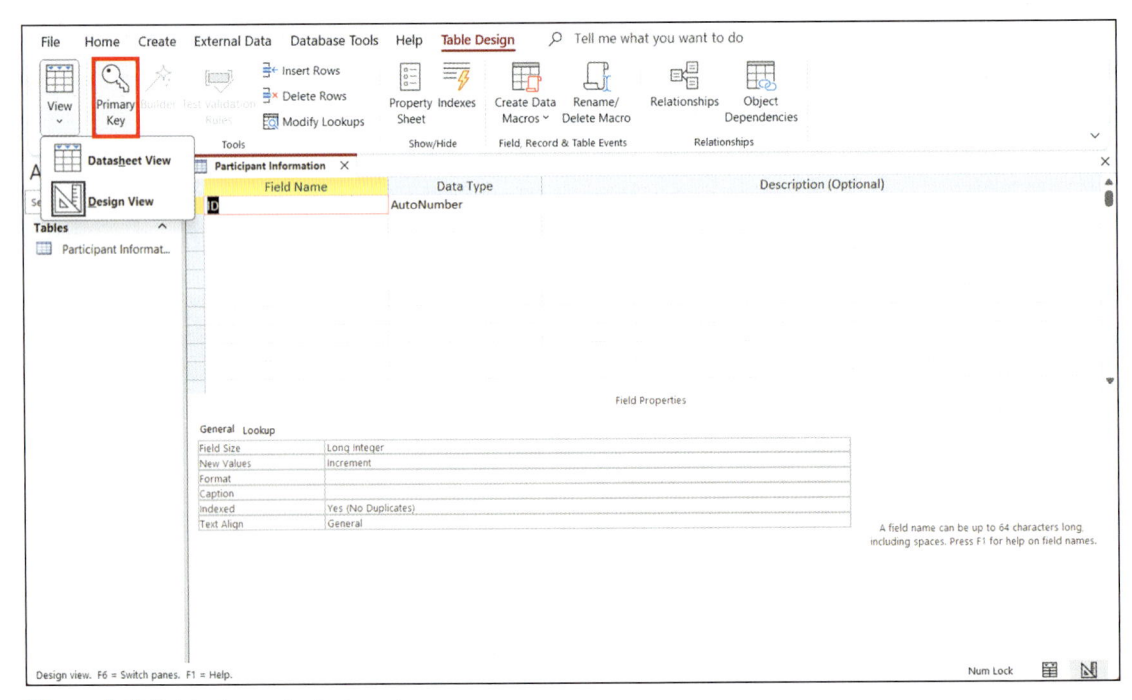

Figure A-4. Table shown in design view.

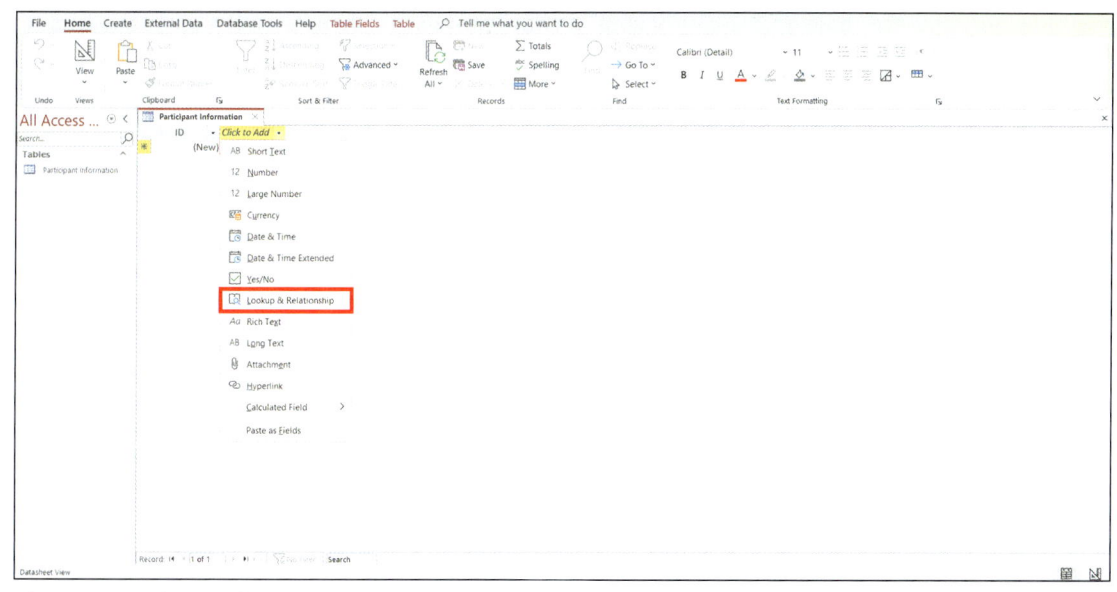

Appendix A Creating a Database With Microsoft Access   **365**

Figure A-5. Adding a field using Lookup & Relationship type.

and then give the field a title. Create the following options in the next four column fields:
- Highest degree: High School, Associate Degree, Baccalaureate Degree, Other (Fig. A-6)
- Type of school: ADN, BSN, RN-BSN, MSN, Other
- Semester in nursing school: 1, 2, 3, 4
- Employment: Not employed, Part-time, PRN/As needed, Full-time

Figure A-7 shows what the participant table looks like after the fields have been created and some data have been gathered.

To create a second table, go to the "Create" tab, and select "Table" from the menu bar. Name this new table "Self-Care Activities." Rename the first field "Activity ID," and it will again be the primary key. Create new fields as with the first table, but

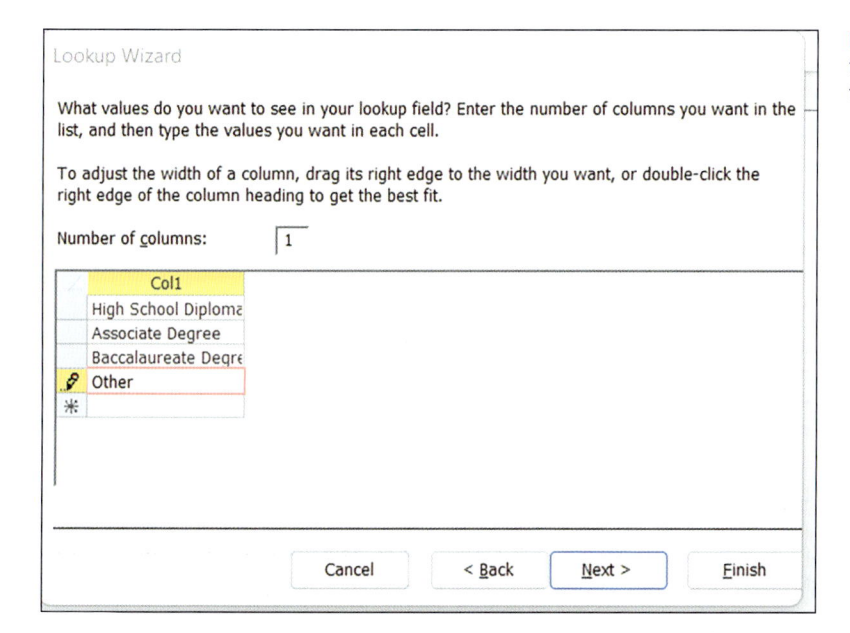

Figure A-6. Adding options to a Lookup & Relationship type field.

this time, you will use "Lookup & Relationship" only in the "Activities" and "Average time spent" fields (make sure to select "I will type the values that I want" in the box that pops up). For the other fields, select the different field types from the drop-down menu that are listed below in parentheses:

- Participant ID: (Number)
- Module viewed? (Yes/No)
- Activities: Relaxation (yoga, meditation), Hang with friends, Exercise (run, bike), Spa (hair, nails), Shop, Clean, Listen to music, Other
- Number of times per week: (Number)
- Average time spent: 0 to 15 minutes; 16 to 30 minutes; 31 to 60 minutes; more than 60 minutes
- How do you feel afterward? (Short text)

Figure A-8 shows a comparison between the design view (A) and datasheet view (B). The primary key, "Activity ID" is labeled.

To link the participant ID field in both tables, go to the "Database Tools" tab and select the "Relationships" button in the menu bar. Under the "Add Tables" row to the right, drag each table to the center of the screen, called the graphical user interface (GUI). Then, from the participant information table, drag the "Participant ID" field over to the "Self-care activities" table. A dialogue box will pop up; click "create" to relate the two fields (Fig. A-9).

Relating the two fields signals to the database that these two fields are the same field across the two tables. This is how Access knows these two tables are related to each other. Click "Close" and then "Save" (Fig. A-10).

Forms

To add data to your tables, you can add data yourself or you can import external data into your database using the "External data" tab. You can also create a form, which acts like a survey that individuals can fill out to collect data. Forms allow you to create a user interface in which participants can enter and edit data. Forms often contain command buttons and other controls that perform various tasks. You can create a database without using forms by simply editing your data in the table datasheets. However, most database users prefer to use forms for viewing, entering, and editing data in the tables.

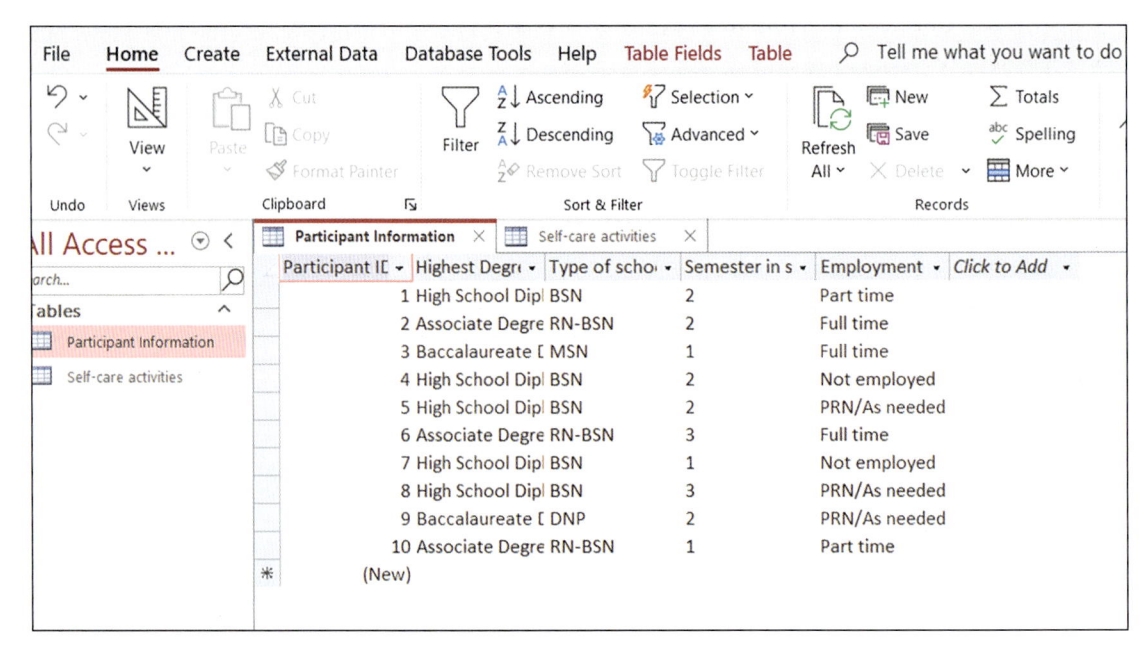

Figure A-7. Table with fields added and data entered.

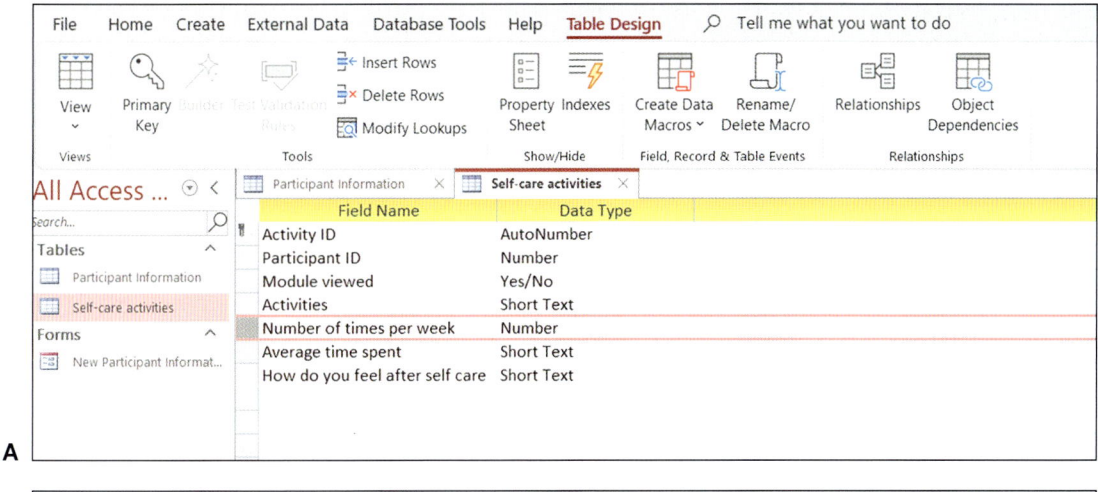

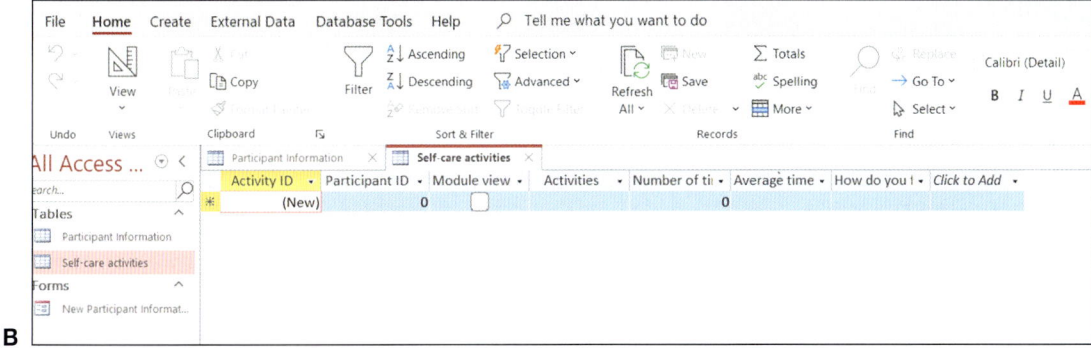

Appendix A   Creating a Database With Microsoft Access   367

Figure A-8. Self-care activities table. **A.** Design view. **B.** Datasheet view.

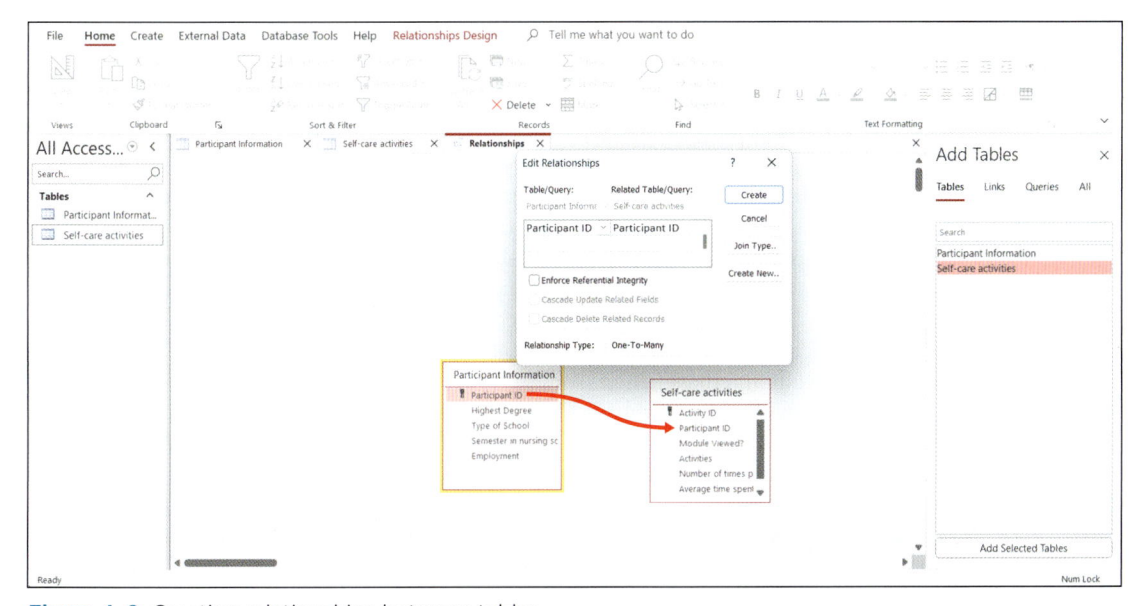

Figure A-9. Creating relationships between tables.

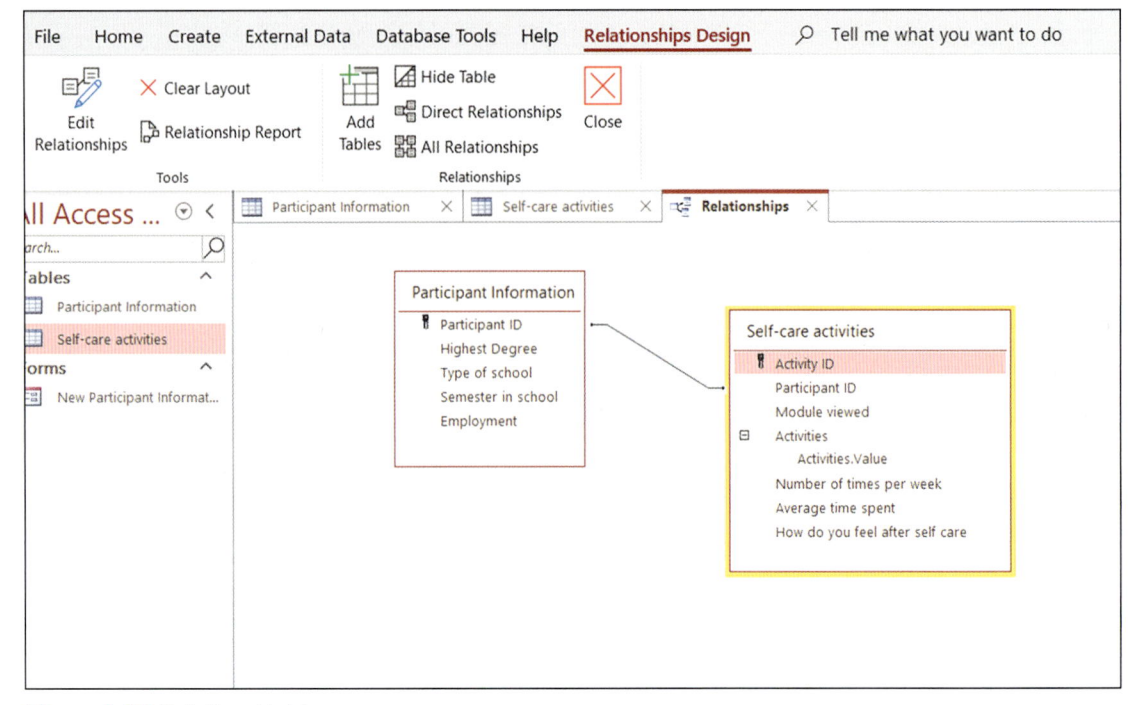

Figure A-10. Relational tables.

You can program command buttons to determine which data appear on the form, open other forms or reports, or perform a variety of other tasks. For example, you might have a form named "Intake Form" in which you work with patient intake data. The intake form might have a button that opens a medication history form where you can enter a new medication for that patient.

Forms also allow you to control how other users interact with the data in the database. For example, you can create a form that shows only certain fields and allows only certain operations to be performed. This helps protect data and to ensure that the data are entered properly.

Create a form in the "Participant Information" table. Go into that table in your database; then select the "Create" tab and push the "Form" button. This will show you the information for each participant (Fig. A-11). You can use the tools in the "Forms Layout Design" tab at the top to customize your form, add a logo, and design. You can add new records in form view as well. When you are done formatting the form, you can close it and name it. A good name for this form would be "New Participant Information."

Queries

A query is used to ask questions of one or more related tables or other queries. The output of a query looks identical to a table, but it provides a custom view of the data. Queries are one of the characteristics that make databases powerful. The ability to create information from the data in a database is limited only by the ingenuity of the query creator. Querying is a powerful and important tool in all electronic databases, not just relational ones.

With the progression from paper to electronic library catalogues as well as web search tools, most of us have had experience with some type of database searching. You have probably searched the web or needed references on a specific subject and used an electronic bibliographic catalogue to find them. When you enter keywords for a search, you are creating a query. When you click the "Search"

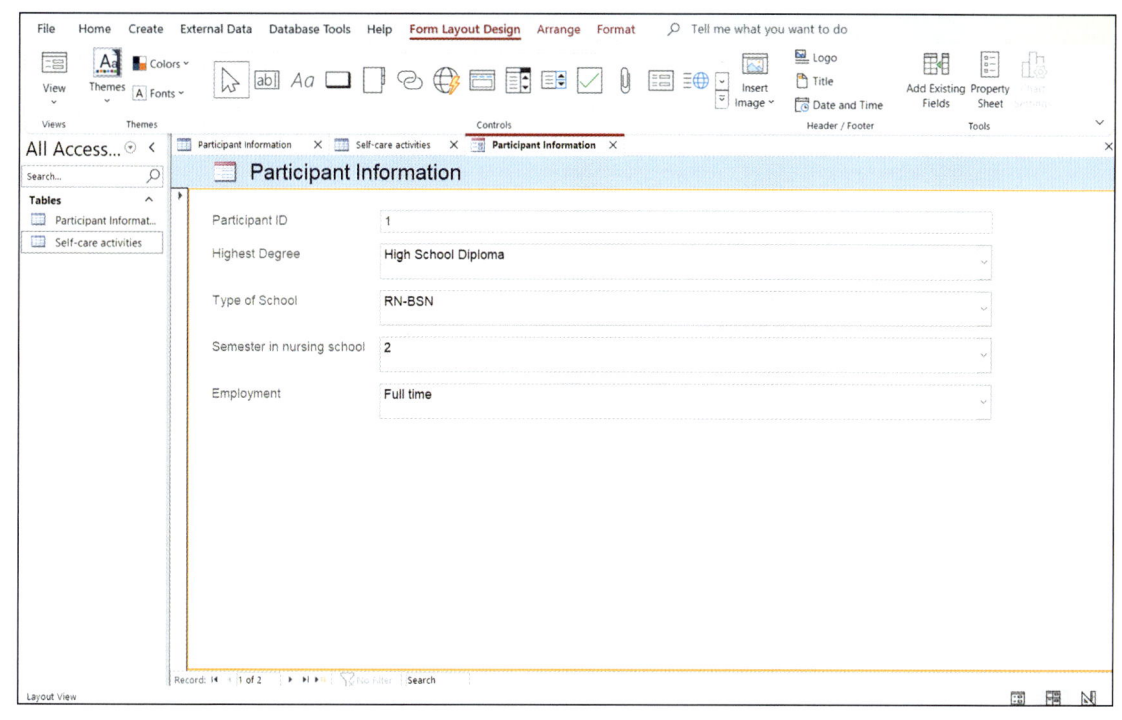

Appendix A Creating a Database With Microsoft Access   369

Figure A-11. Creating a form.

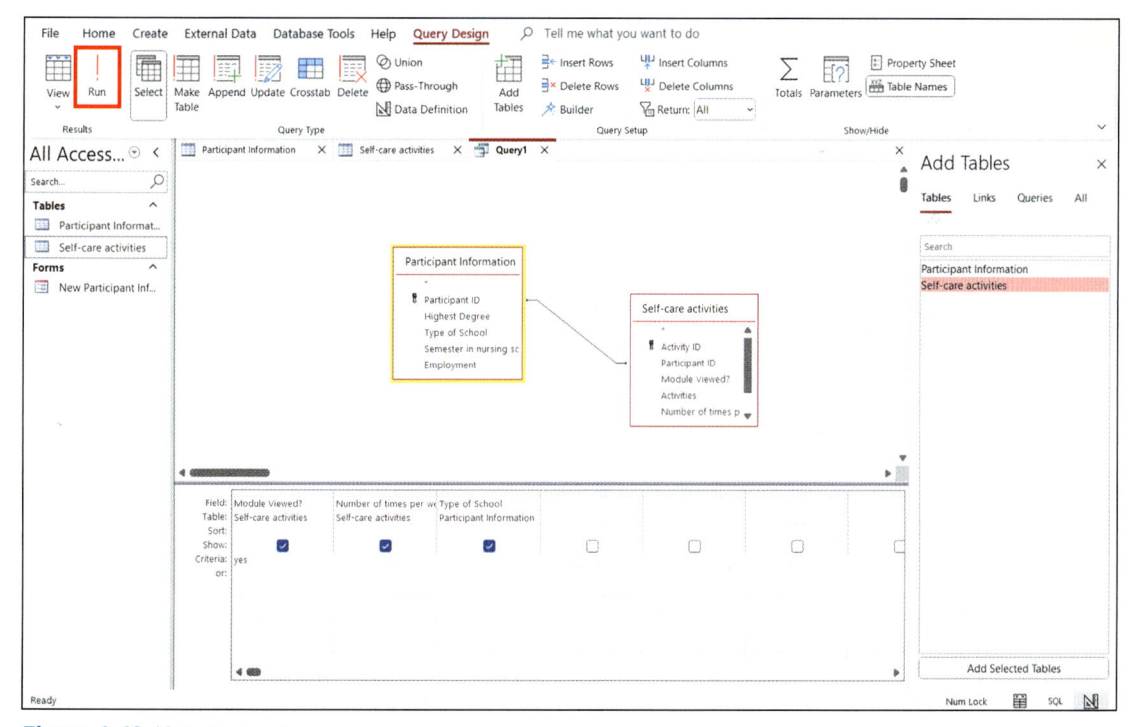

Figure A-12. How to create a query.

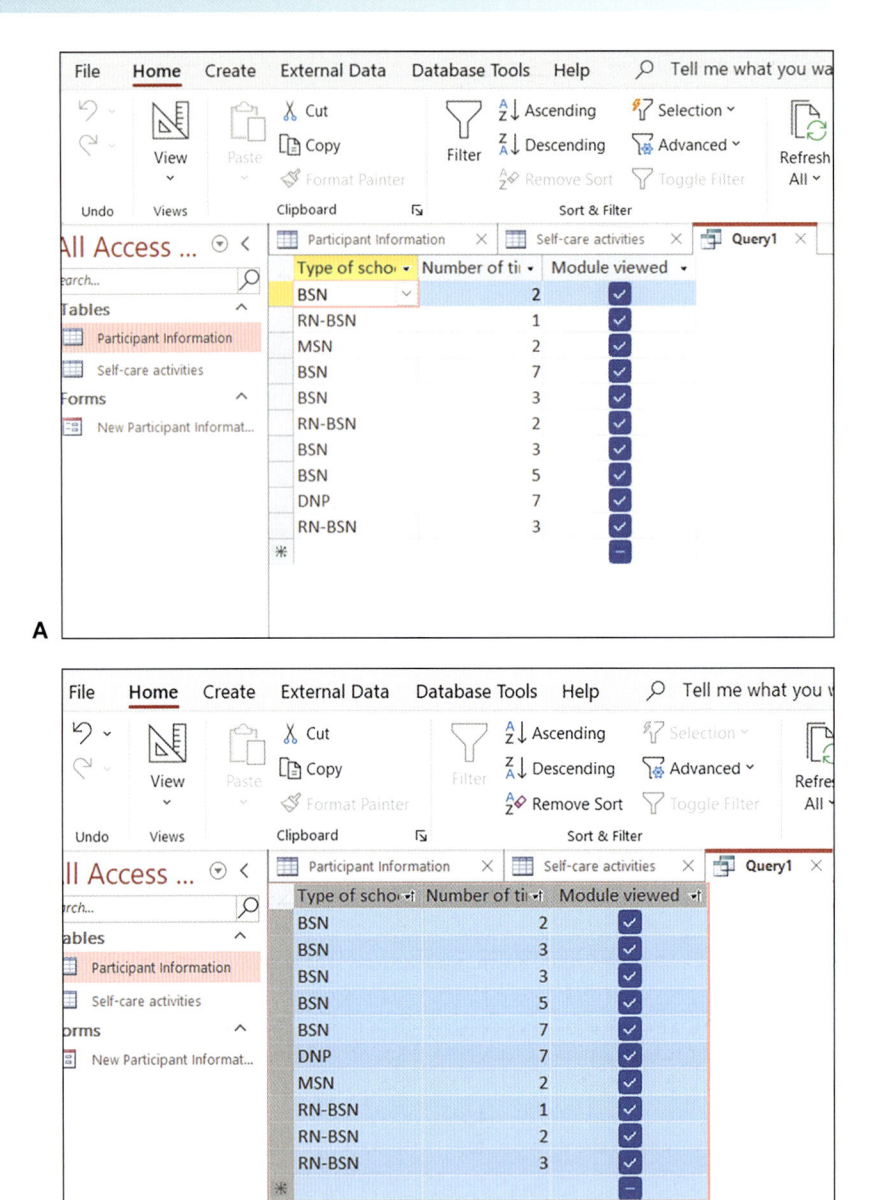

Figure A-13. Results of a query **(A)** and then sorted by type of school **(B)**.

button, the search tool looks for records that meet the criteria in the query.

To design a query for your database, go to the "Create" tab and click on "Query Design" in the menu bar. As you did when you created a relationship between tables, drag each of the tables to the GUI.

You want to know if the type of school program a student is enrolled in has an impact on the number of times per week a student engages in self-care for those who viewed the learning module. Select those three fields between the two tables (double click on the field and it will populate the field in the query box at the bottom of

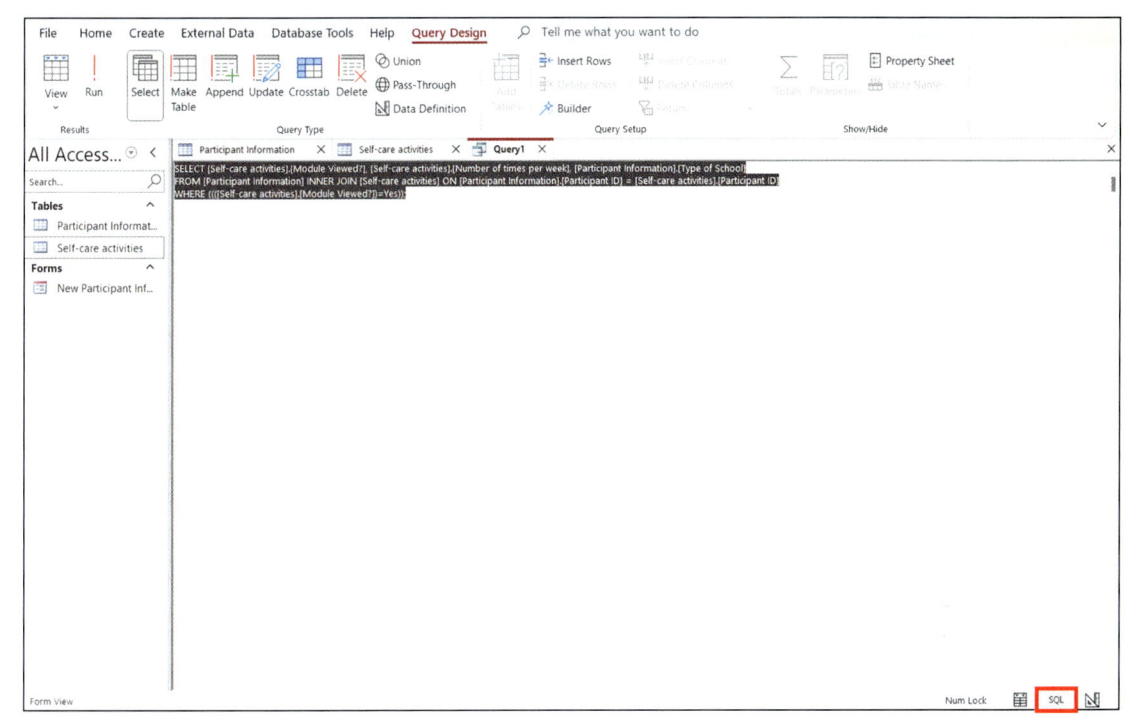

Figure A-14. How to view SQL.

the screen) (Fig. A-12). Limit the query to show only students who have watched the module by typing "yes" under "Module viewed" and in the "Criteria record" (row). Click on the "Run" button and you will see the results (Fig. A-13A). To better understand the results, you can sort by "Type of Program" to arrange the data in that way (Fig. A-13B). You can save the query and view it at any time. It will update as new data are added.

If you want to see the structured query language (SQL) for this query, select the box in the bottom right corner (Fig. A-14).

Reports

Reports are what you use to format, summarize, and present data. A report usually answers a specific question, such as "How many students are engaged in exercise as a self-care activity?" or "What characteristics make it more likely that a student will engage in self-care?" Each report can be formatted to present the information in the most readable way possible.

Reports may include charts (graphs) as well as calculations on data. Reports should be designed in such a way that the information will be easy for the person who needs the report to understand. Reports can be formatted for printing, but they can also be viewed on the screen, exported to another program, or sent as an attachment to an email message. Reports can present information from more than one table as well as from queries. When you run a report after constructing it and saving it, it displays all data that are currently in the associated tables. In other words, the report has a dynamic display of the most recent data. Reports provide a way to analyze data, so it is important to take your time creating a well-designed report.

Just as you did with query, go to the "Create" tab, and then select "Report" from the menu bar. Sort the report by frequency of self-care activities and then print it out or copy it into a poster or presentation to share your data with others (Fig. A-15).

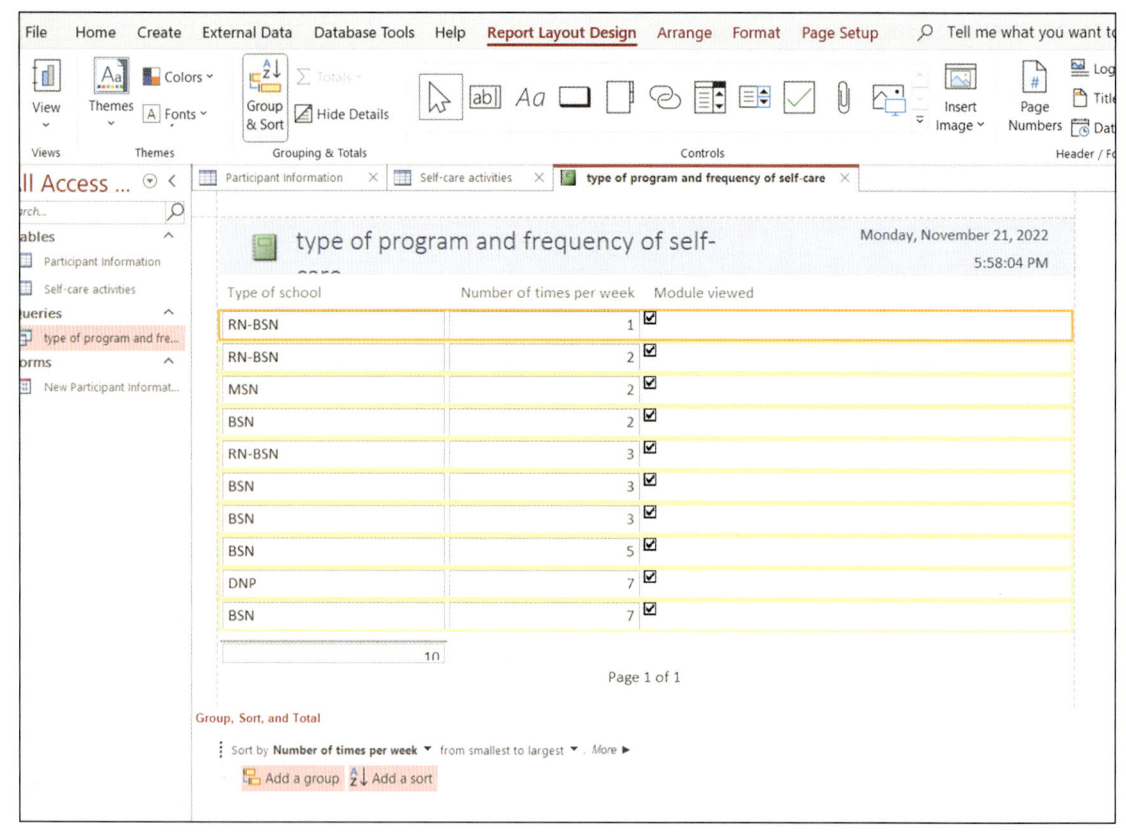

Figure A-15. Creating a report.

Sorting

You can apply many of the spreadsheet functions, such as formula construction, sorting, and data formatting, to retrieve information stored in a database. Sorting is one of the most important features. When you enter data into a database, you create a record. The records are often not entered in the order in which you need to view. Like spreadsheets or word processing tables, sorting is just rearranging the records in a table based on the data in a field or fields in a table. The simplest sort is a primary sort; that is, the records are resorted based on one field. An example would be reordering records in a database based on last name to produce a table.

Most database software is not limited to sorting on just one field. For example, in Microsoft Access, you can create primary, secondary, tertiary, and even further levels of sorts, each built on the groupings provided by the sort one level above it. In a tertiary sort, the records will first be sorted in a primary sort so that those that have similarities in the sort field are listed together. Then, another sorting is done on another field on records in each group created from the primary sort (the secondary sort); finally, a tertiary sort can be performed on another field of each group from the secondary sort. For example, a primary sort is performed on all patients in a hospital by the type of surgery; then, the records are reordered within each type of surgery in a secondary sort so that those from the same unit within each type of surgery are together. For a tertiary sort, the records are further reordered so that the records on a given unit for each type of surgery are reordered by the primary surgeon. This type of grouping is most useful in producing reports that need to look at a given characteristic within various groups.

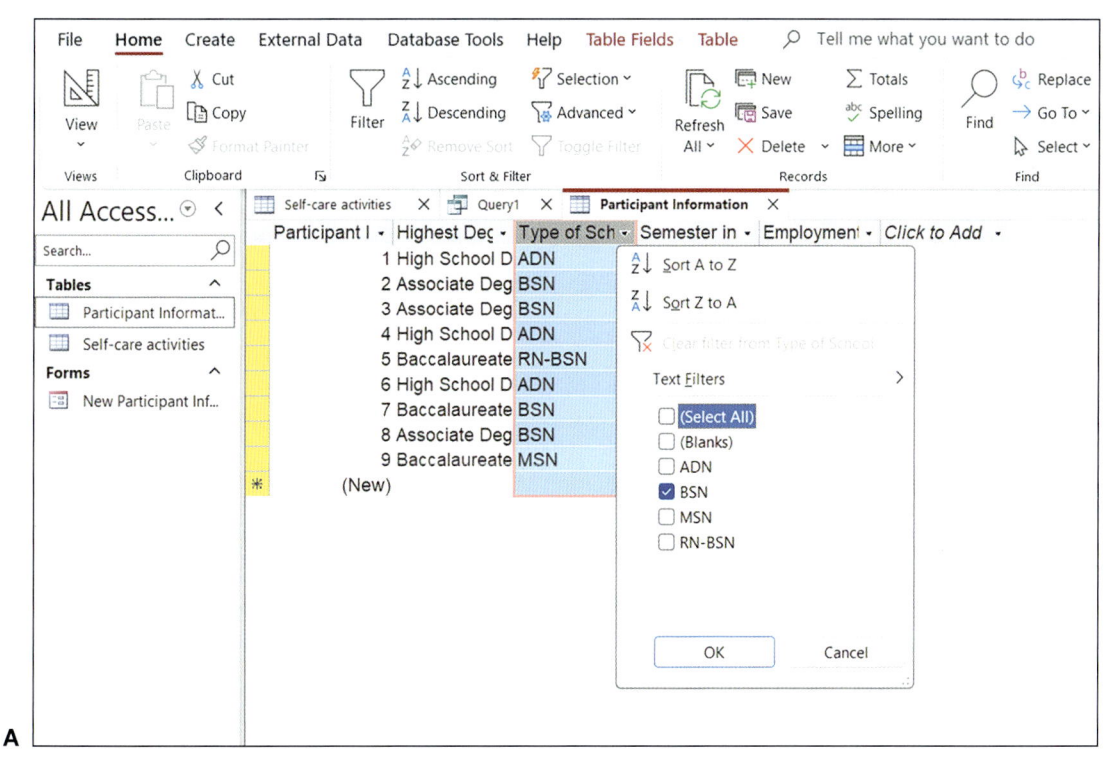

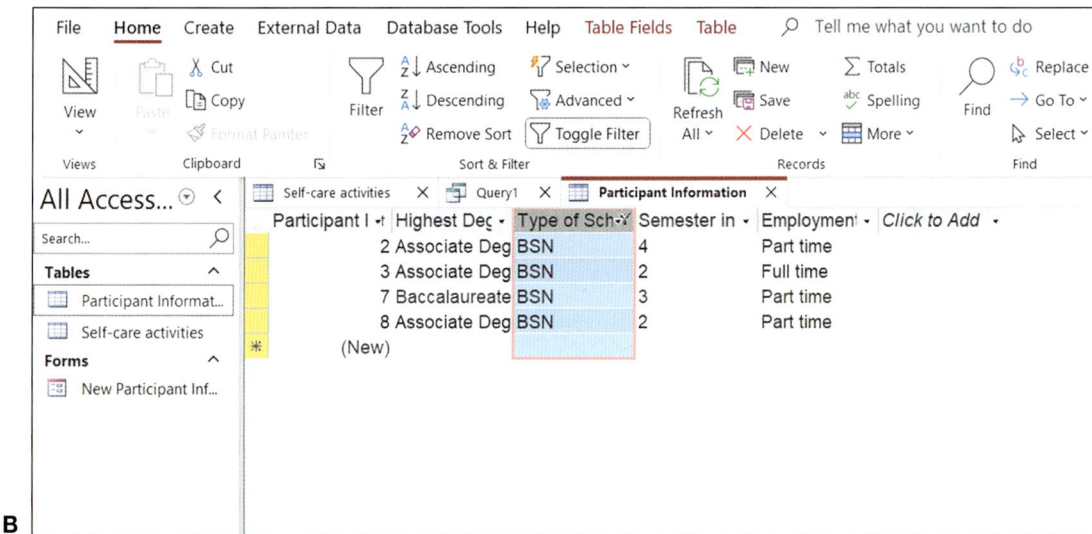

Appendix A Creating a Database With Microsoft Access 373

Figure A-16. How to sort data **(A)**, and then the result of the sort **(B)**.

To perform a sort, go into a table and select the drop-down arrow next to the name of the field (Fig. A-16A). This will allow you to sort alphabetically or filter so that your sort includes or excludes specific entries. If you sort the Type of school column using "BSN" and push "OK," it will show just the reports with BSN (Fig. A-16B). You can sort other columns from that screen, for example, by selecting only "3" or "4" under Semester in Nursing school to further limit your sort.

If you want to learn more about manipulation of data such as how to use formulas or format your data in Access, use your search engine to find an online tutorial that will show you how to achieve your goals.

REFERENCE

Microsoft 365 Support. (n.d.). *Create a database in Access*. Retrieved November 20, 2022 from https://support.microsoft.com/en-us/office/create-a-database-in-access-f200d95b-e429-4acc-98c1-b883d4e9fc0a

APPENDIX B

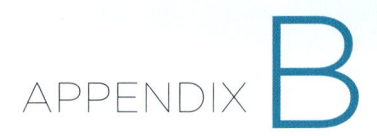

Mastering Spreadsheet Software to Assess Quality Outcomes

Jean Mellum and Kristi Miller

Before computers, a spreadsheet was a physical book full of large sheets of paper with rows and columns (Fig. B-1). They were mainly used to keep track of money, and data were manually entered using a pen or pencil. The first digital spreadsheet was developed in 1979 as the personal computer was beginning to be more widely used (Mattessich, n.d.). Today, spreadsheets are electronic tools for information management. Digital spreadsheets are created using software programs that allow you to organize, sort, and analyze data. A spreadsheet is an electronic depiction of a chart that organizes alphanumeric data in rows and columns. Memos, notes, dates, or narrative comments can also be stored within a spreadsheet. Spreadsheet software is commonly used by consumers and organizations to manage numerical data. In healthcare settings, spreadsheets are valuable because they can store multiple types of data about multiple patients, such as address and phone number, diagnoses, and dates of office visits.

Remarkably, the first spreadsheet design was so functional that it has not changed much over the years. Rather, features have been added, such as charts and menu bars, to make it easier for entering data and using formulas for making calculations. Spreadsheet programs are designed to be intuitive. Functions and menu bars in spreadsheet applications share similarities with other software programs used in healthcare and office settings. Learning one software program such as Microsoft Word for creating a text document is transferable to using a spreadsheet program such as Microsoft Excel.

At the first glance, a spreadsheet may look like a table, and they can be used to create tables that can then be imported into other programs. However, they are much more powerful than simple tables because they can be used for sorting, analyzing, and manipulating data. Furthermore, data sets can be copied from spreadsheets and inserted into other programs. For instance, a nurse researcher may enter data on participants into a spreadsheet and upload the data into another software program for advanced statistical analysis. Any time you need to analyze numbers, an electronic spreadsheet is a good choice.

SPREADSHEETS IN NURSING

Spreadsheet skills are invaluable to all nurses. Spreadsheets allow you to store, retrieve, analyze, and sort data and information to meet a variety of nursing needs. Case management nurses use spreadsheets to organize patient lists and pertinent patient-level data including dates of services. Public health nurses may use spreadsheets to manage data for disease outbreaks in a local area, across a state, or on a global scale. Nurses in an office setting can capture postal and email addresses for use with office management software. Nurses engaging in research use spreadsheets to collect, organize, and analyze data that can be used to improve patient outcomes.

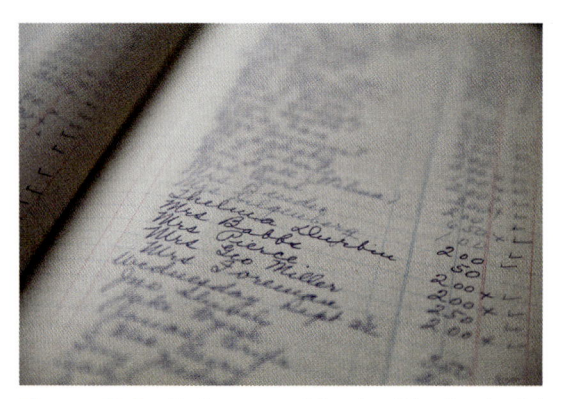

Figure B-1. Early spreadsheet. (Shutterstock/Charlotte Lake.)

Across the healthcare system, nurses use spreadsheets for quality tracking and assessing nursing interventions and patient outcomes. Quality improvement teams can examine data around adverse drug events, sepsis, stroke, ventilator-acquired pneumonia, and bloodstream infections in an effort to develop quality improvement programs and analyze their results. Medication errors, patient falls, hospital-acquired infections, length of stay, clinical outcomes, and other nursing concerns are frequently analyzed through spreadsheet software. Spreadsheets are also used for administrative functions such as staff scheduling, time, and attendance records, calculating nursing hours per patient day for staffing decisions, budget analysis, and Failure Mode Event Analysis. In academic settings, spreadsheets are used to analyze student responses to test questions, rank candidates for nursing program admission decisions, calculate course grades and grade point averages, and prepare research data for statistical analysis.

As you learn about what they can do, you will see even more ways to use your spreadsheet knowledge to manage electronic patient and healthcare data. Spreadsheets allow nurses to calculate changes in data or trend data and examine what changes are happening over time. Or when looking at medication management, spreadsheets provide data to examine nurses' administration of narcotics and which nurses are administering the most narcotics to patients. Spreadsheet technology provides a tool for supporting documentation of care and serves as a record for communicating pertinent information to support team communication. A spreadsheet serves as a standardized format for storing, organizing, and retrieving information across all systems levels.

Like other office software, learning new spreadsheet skills is a lifelong journey. Although there are a few changes in the basic functionality of spreadsheet software, emerging vendors and new versions of software provide novel features for data manipulation, analysis, and display. Remember that spreadsheet competencies include knowledge about what the spreadsheet can do for nursing and nurses.

The purpose of this appendix is to provide an overview of spreadsheet features useful in the nursing setting, but there are many resources to use when developing your spreadsheet competencies including free online tutorials with easy-to-follow videos. Some examples of learning resources include:

- LinkedIn Learning may be offered by college libraries and many public libraries. To access LinkedIn Learning from a library website, check with the library information desk.
- Microsoft Training
- Google Drive Support
- Goodwill Community Foundation
- YouTube videos ranging in length from a few minutes to 1 hour if you wish to do additional training on your own

Spreadsheets for Evidence-Based Practice

A spreadsheet is a valuable tool for collecting evidence-based sources for a literature review. For instance, your spreadsheet could have headings that include the title, authors, type of study, sample size, and other features collected from the references used in your project. By using a spreadsheet for a literature review, it is easy to manipulate data and then copy and paste the table into a Word document or PowerPoint presentation. The table can be reformatted to the purpose at hand.

From the spreadsheet, you can sort and categorize the data and information by author's last name or type of study, for example. Data for a literature review is easier to manipulate and organize using

Appendix B Mastering Spreadsheet Software to Assess Quality Outcomes

	A	B	C	D	E	F	G	H	I
1	Author, year		Conceptual		Sample	Methodology	Instrument	Results	
2	Adhikari (2013)		none		Senior BSN students (n=21) in the UK	Qualitative Action research, ethnography - a multidisciplinary approach to medication safety: focus groups, interviews	none	Students report limited pharmacology knowledge and confidence, 5-rights are taught, Recommend increased use of multidisciplinary teamwork	
3	Dolansky (2010)		none		A junior BSN student in the US	Qualitative Case study of student using Root Cause Analysis (RCA)	N/A	Factors identified: environmental, personal, unit communication and culture and education	
4	Lin (2013)		none		BSN students (n=34) in Taiwan	Qualitative Semi structured interviews about learning experiences in pediatric medication management	N/A	8 themes revealed. To decrease anxiety and increase competence, instructors should provide self-directed learning activities and resources and provide a secure environment to discuss medication errors	
5	Reid-Searl (2008)		Grounded Theory		Senior BSN students (n=28) in Australia; theoretical sampling	Qualitative Interviews about importance of supervision in medication administration	N/A	Students report making increased errors when there is a lack of supervision by an RN	
6	Vaismoradi (2014)		none		2nd, 3rd, 4th semester BSN students (n=24) in Iran	Qualitative Focus groups, content analysis of causes of medication errors	N/A	Under-developed caring skills in medication management and unfinished learning of safe medication management. Program left them vulnerable to drug errors.	
7	Valdez (2013)		Eindhoven model		Junior & Senior BSN students (n=329), Iran	Structural equation modeling of factors affecting medication errors	survey developed by author, valid and reliable	Five factor dimensions. Poor adherence to the five rights is an important mediator between all 5 factors and medication errors. Developed a model to explain how student nurses make med errors	

Figure B-2. Using a spreadsheet for research.

a spreadsheet rather than when using a table in a word processor document. Figure B-2 is an example of a spreadsheet used to organize research data for a publication on how to teach nursing students about medication administration safety (Miller et al., 2016). This spreadsheet can be used to sort the research data by author but also by conceptual framework or instrument if needed.

CREATING AND USING A SPREADSHEET

Before you start entering and analyzing data, familiarize yourself with basic spreadsheet terminology, which can be found in Box B-1. Figure B-3 shows a sample of a single worksheet pointing out some of the major features. Box B-2 provides principles and tips for creating spreadsheets.

To help learn the basics of spreadsheets, you can practice with data sets available on the internet. Search for "CORGIS data set project" for samples. From there you can select CSV to view raw data sets for various topics. You can download and open these on your computer. There are several popular spreadsheet software programs, but the examples presented here are from Microsoft Excel. The CSV files from CORGIS open in Microsoft Excel but can be used with other software programs. Open one of these data sets on your computer as you read this appendix, and practice the functions discussed.

Templates

To get started using spreadsheets, use one of the templates available for the spreadsheet software. A template provides a pattern of content for software applications. Spreadsheet software often includes predesigned templates, either with the program or as a download from an associated website. It may be easier to modify a template than to build a spreadsheet from scratch, or a template may give you ideas about how you would like to arrange your own data in a spreadsheet. You can save spreadsheets as template files for reuse. For more information on the use of spreadsheet templates, check the software "Help" menu. Figure B-4 shows some of the templates available through Microsoft Excel.

Worksheet

A workbook is a file that contains one or more worksheets (also known as spreadsheets or sheets). A worksheet is an individual data table within a workbook that allows for data organization in columns and rows. Worksheets are like a placeholder for data tables and are incorporated into the workbook file to represent different aspects of the data. If you were arranging health and wellness data, you may have a worksheet for the whole group of patients then a worksheet for groups based on sex.

BOX B-1 Spreadsheet Terminologies

Active cell
The cell in use and where data are inserted are outlined by a color and/or darker border; in the sample spreadsheet (see Fig. B-3), the active cell is D21, which represents the total population of the state of Maine.

Alphanumeric data
Data or character that is either a letter or a number

Cell
A box on the spreadsheet that represents data; the intersection of data associated with the specific row and the column

Cell address
The "coordinates" of a cell represented by a letter (associated with the column) and a number (represents the row); the cell address for the active cell is D21 and is shown below the menu bar in the mid-upper left side of the spreadsheet (see Fig. B-3)

Cell range
A group of contiguous cells in a spreadsheet (e.g., B11:D13); users can name ranges of cells and use this name in commands instead of the cell location to create formulas.

Column
Organized vertically on the spreadsheet and automatically labeled using a letter; include categories of data such as data collected for each patient. In the sample spreadsheet (Fig B-3), column A lists the states, and column B shows the death rates from cancer

Conditional formatting
Formatting that allows the user to highlight cells with certain values or conditions to make cells easy to identify; changes the appearance of a cell or cell range based on a condition or criteria

Formula
A mathematical equation that provides instructions to the computer for processing the data; formulas provide a way to calculate data

Freeze
A function that allows the user to keep one part of a spreadsheet visible while scrolling to another area on the spreadsheet; freezing the headings on columns is helpful to keep column headers at the top of the page while scrolling down a long list of data

Row
Organized horizontally on spreadsheet and automatically labeled using a number; data in each row represents data unique to that row. Row 1 often lists the headers for each column with Row 2 starting the data; in the sample spreadsheet (see Fig. B-3), the rows represent data collected from each U.S. state. \

Spreadsheet
An electronic tool for information management commonly used in the care of patients, communities, and populations; multiple spreadsheets (also called sheets or worksheets) may make up a single workbook

Workbook
An electronic file that contains one or more spreadsheets (also known as sheets or worksheets)

Worksheet
Also called a spreadsheet or sheet; an individual data table within a workbook that allows for data organization; multiple worksheets may make up a single workbook; in the sample spreadsheet (see Fig. B-3), the worksheet tab indicates the worksheet the user is on at the bottom; additional sheets can be added using the plus sign to the right of the tab

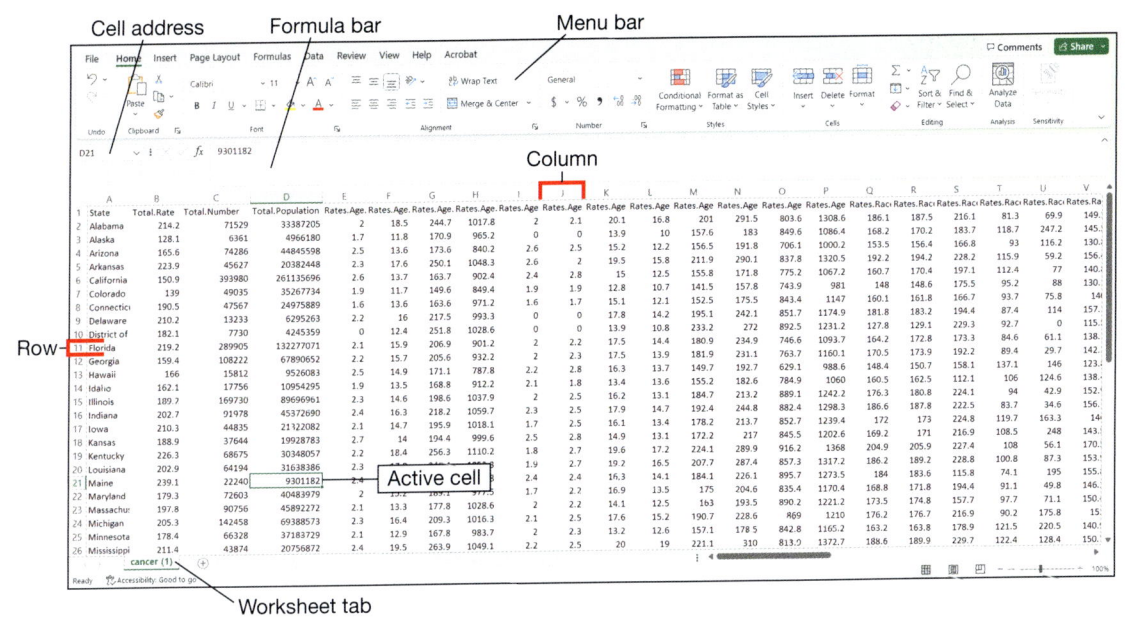

Appendix B Mastering Spreadsheet Software to Assess Quality Outcomes   379

Figure B-3. Sample spreadsheet showing common spreadsheet features.

BOX B-2 Tips for Creating and Using Spreadsheets

- Begin the spreadsheet development process with a clear purpose and carefully thought-out design.
- Draft the spreadsheet on a piece of paper first and name the column headers.
- Save an original copy of your data before doing any work or formatting; then, if data are lost or compromised, you will always have the original data set.
- Use conditional formatting tools to assist users in interpreting data.
- Use charts to assist users in interpreting aggregate data.
- Use formulas rather than entering precalculated numbers into cells to avoid data entry errors. Check, recheck, and validate each formula and formula output.
- Write out and analyze complex formulas prior to entering them into cells.
- Keep the spreadsheet size as small as possible. A worksheet with hundreds of columns may be more manageable if it is broken down into several worksheets.
- The "undo" button can be used to eliminate the previous action if mistakes are made. When you see that you have made a mistake, it is best to undo it immediately.
- Use cell protection to prevent users from inadvertently changing a formula or data.
- If the spreadsheet is critical, there should be explicit guidelines, rules, and testing policies for developers.
- Be a smart consumer of spreadsheet information by scrutinizing the quality of the spreadsheet data; do not assume that it is correct.
- If using spreadsheet with text, be concise with the use of words. If necessary, use the "wrap text" function to incorporate the words in the column and wrap the text inside the cell to fit the column width.

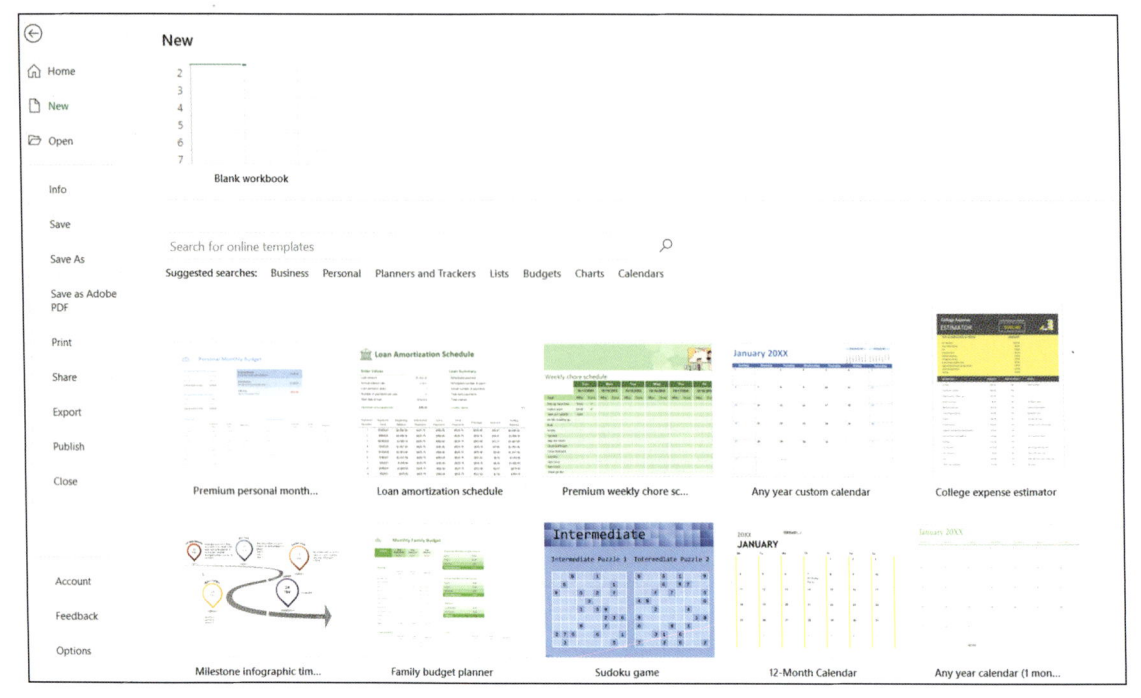

Figure B-4. Templates.

Sheets are named to find data reports in the workbook easily. The worksheet tab is at the bottom of the screen in the Excel file and shows the name of the sheet (see Fig. B-3). The default name is "Sheet 1," but this can easily be changed to a more useful name by right clicking on the tab and then selecting "Rename." Sheet names differentiate the sheets and help you remember the contents of the sheet. A new worksheet can be added to a file by clicking the plus sign beside the worksheet tab.

Microsoft Excel has tabs each of which reveal a different menu bar (see Fig. B-3). The menu bar in the worksheet provides easy access to tools for organizing, manipulating, and formatting data.

Sorting and Filtering

Data in a spreadsheet can be sorted from low to high or high to low to see the progression of data. Open a spreadsheet from CORGIS, and highlight or select all the data in the worksheet. In the menu bar under the data tab, select "Sort" and a window will open. Check the box next to "My data has headers," and then sort by one of the column headers. After clicking "OK," it will sort the entire sheet based on the data in the column header you selected. For example, Figure B-5 shows cancer death rate data from CORGIS (Kafura, 2019). Sorting the data by "Types. Breast.Total." and from the smallest to the largest reorders the rows so that the states are listed in order based on the death rate from breast cancer. With a quick glance, you can now see that the state with the lowest death rate from breast cancer is Utah. Note that if you only highlight one column and perform the "sort" function, that column is sorted, but the rest of the data remain static. You must highlight the entire spreadsheet when sorting to ensure that all data are sorted together.

Excel allows you to use the filter function to search for data that contain an exact phrase, number, date, and more. Again, using the cancer death rate data from CORGIS, you can select "Filter" in the menu bar under the data tab. You will see that each column header now has a drop-down arrow next to it. To find out how

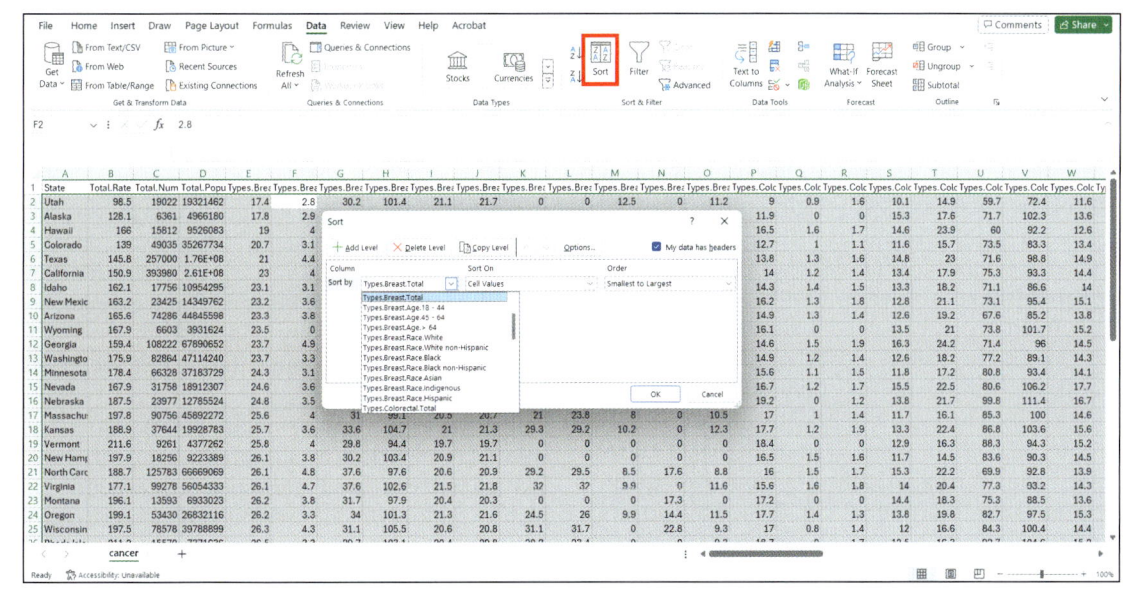

Appendix B Mastering Spreadsheet Software to Assess Quality Outcomes 381

Figure B-5. Sorting.

many states have a breast cancer death rate of 0 for individuals identifying as Hispanic, select the drop-down arrow for column "Types.Breast. Race.Hispanic", and select "0" (or type "0" in the search box) (Fig. B-6). Be sure to use the quotation marks around the zero; if you do not, you will also get any results that contain a "0." Click "OK," and you will see that 14 states had zero people identifying as Hispanic die from breast cancer. This function is also useful if you want to find the data for a particular row. In these data, filtering for a specific state temporarily removes data from all other states from view. Try using the filter function for your state.

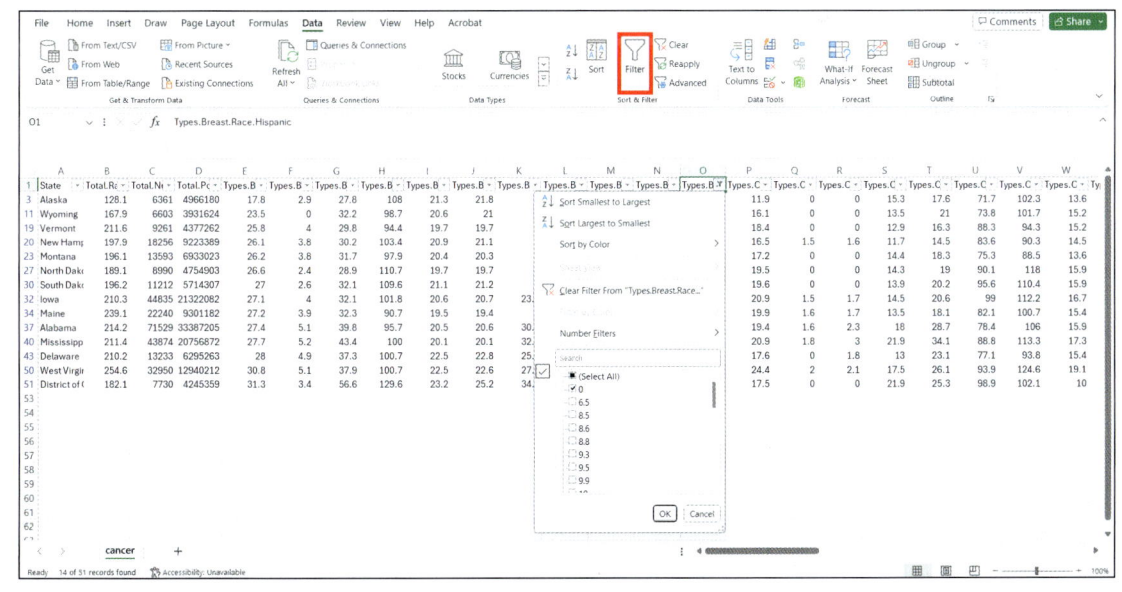

Figure B-6. Filtering.

Formulas

A spreadsheet formula is a mathematical equation that provides instructions to the computer for processing the data and is used in spreadsheet calculations. In Excel, the formula bar is in the upper part of the screen and to the right of the active cell box (see Fig. B-3). Formulas make it easy to solve problems without manual calculations.

Spreadsheet software has many formulas built in that you can use by simply selecting a button. In the cancer death rate spreadsheet, highlight the data in Column C ("Total. Number"), which shows the total number of people who died from cancer in each state. Select the "Autosum" button from the menu bar under the "Formulas" tab. Figure B-7 shows how the formula bar populates with a formula that adds all the data in Column C. Press the "enter" button, and the total will appear under the data: 4014910. This tells you the total number of deaths from cancer in the United States represented in this data set.

Creating Formulas

For more complicated or specialized calculations, formulas can be created within Excel. To create a formula, select a cell where you want the answer to appear. In the cell, or in the formula bar, type an equal sign (=), which indicates the start of a formula. Next, select a cell that provides data for the calculation, or type the cell address (letter and number combination) in the formula bar. Then insert an operator such as + for addition or – for subtraction. Select another cell (or type the cell address). After you hit "enter," the answer appears. Errors can creep into a spreadsheet when entering formulas into cells, so it is generally recommended that you use the point-and-click method for selecting cells, rather than entering cell addresses manually.

The principles and symbols of formula calculation are identical in all spreadsheet software. The characters used for specific calculations, such as multiplying or dividing, are not necessarily the same as used on paper. An asterisk (*) is used to denote multiplication. If you use "x," the computer is unable to distinguish the character "x" from a multiplication symbol. A computer formula for the multiplication of "5 times 50" is "5*50." The forward slash (/) denotes division. To use the computer to divide 10 by 5, the formula is "10/5."

In the cancer death rate spreadsheet, the death rate (number of deaths per 100,000 people) has already been calculated in Column B. However,

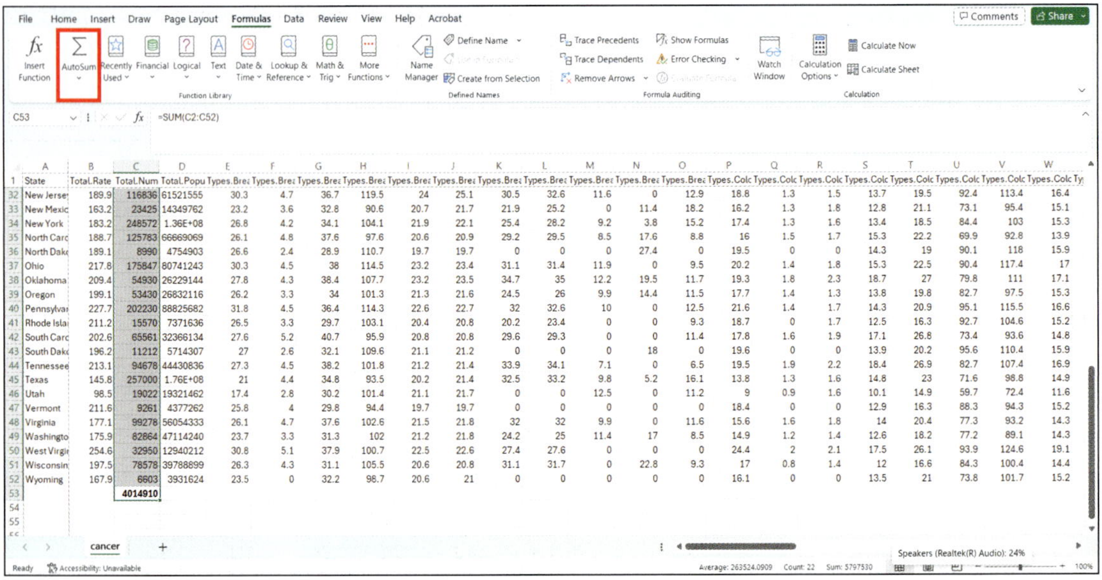

Figure B-7. Autosum.

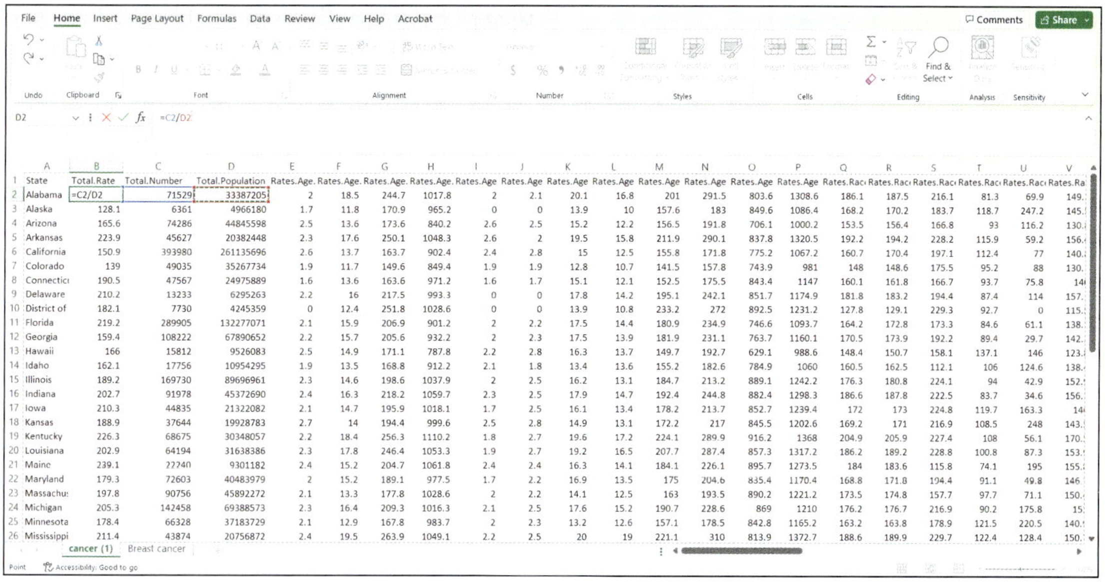

Appendix B   Mastering Spreadsheet Software to Assess Quality Outcomes   383

Figure B-8. Creating formulas for calculations.

try the calculation yourself using a formula: In the cancer sheet tab, select Cell B2, and delete the death rate for Alabama (214.2).

1. Type = in Cell B2
2. Select Cell C2
3. Type /
4. Select Cell D2
5. Hit "enter"

The result 0.0021424 should appear (Fig. B-8).

To obtain the rate originally calculated (which is several orders of magnitude above this result), you need to multiply your answer by 100,000. To do this, go back to Cell B2 and add *100000 to your formula. Hit "enter" and you will see the number 214.24075 appear. To round to one decimal place, make B2 your active cell by clicking on it. Then go to the "Home" tab and select the decrease decimal symbol until you only have one decimal place to the right of the decimal (Fig. B-9). You should now see the answer: 214.2.

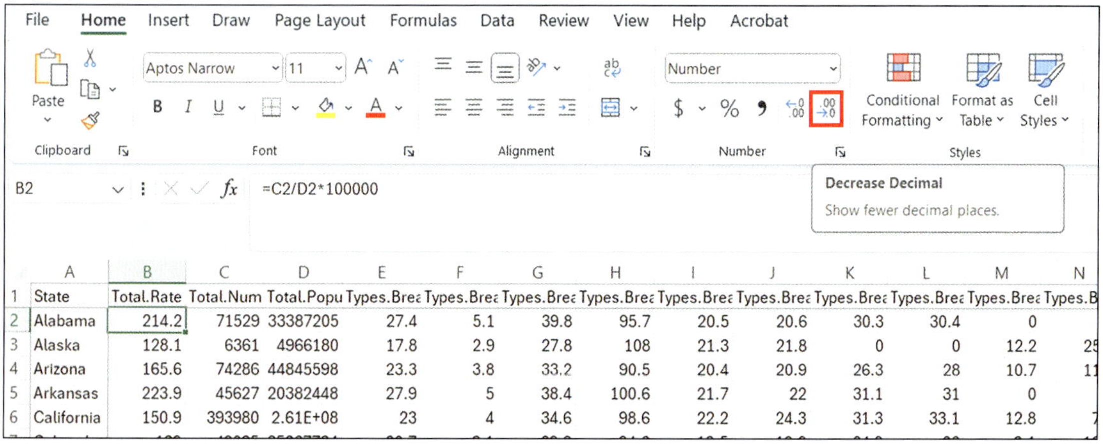

Figure B-9. Decreasing decimal.

Order of Mathematical Operations

When performing arithmetic, computers follow the order of operations for mathematics. Three factors determine the order to perform mathematical procedures:

1. The kind of computation required
2. Nesting, or the placement of an expression within parentheses
3. Left-to-right placement of the expressions in the command

The left-to-right placement is important regarding multiplication and division (which are equal) and addition and subtraction (which are equal). They are performed in left-to-right order.

The computer performs operations using algebraic protocols and can be memorized using the following pneumonic:

- *P*lease (parentheses)
- *E*xcuse (exponents)
- *M*y (multiplication)
- *D*ear (division)
- *A*unt (addition)
- *S*ally (subtraction)

Additional tutorials for using formulas are available from Microsoft and on YouTube.

Formatting Cells

The appearance of cells in a spreadsheet can be adjusted by formatting the cells. Much like in word processing programs, the menu bar under the "Home" tab includes sections for font and alignment. Select a cell to make it active, or highlight a group of cells, columns, or rows, and then make font and alignment choices in the menu bar. Alternately, right click on the highlighted cell(s) and select "Format Cells." The menu box that pops up has alignment, font, border, and fill tabs (Fig. B-10).

Formatting Textual Data

Some formatting is specifically useful when the data within cells are text. For example, if cells contain a lot of text, a good formatting option is to wrap text. By wrapping text, the words take the shape of the cell, even if the words overflow the cell boundary. The cell height (and thus row height) may grow to accommodate the text, but it keeps the text from running outside of cells. The wrap text button is on the menu bar under the "Home" tab (see Fig. B-10).

You may want to merge cells within a spreadsheet to create a different heading. Select the cells you want to merge into one and choose the "Merge & Center" button on the menu bar under the "Home" tab (see Fig B-10). Merging cells is a good way to add headings above just certain columns.

Another useful text formatting option is "Text to Columns." Consider a spreadsheet with the names and addresses for all employees on a nursing unit. Both first and last names are included together in the cells of the first column. This makes it impossible to sort by last name because the first name is listed first. You can use the "Text to Columns" feature to separate the names. Insert a blank column next to the column that you want to change. If the name includes a middle name or initial, insert two blank columns. In the menu bar under the "Data" tab, choose the "Text to Columns" button and follow the set of suggestions in Excel to make the changes. This tool is useful for analyzing data that have been extracted from a hospital information system. Data imported from other information systems may have complex data inserted into cells in ways that do not fit your needs. "Text to Columns" can help you reformat the data in a way that works for you.

Formatting Numerical Data

Spreadsheet software provides several ways to format cells with numerical data. For numbers, the cell defaults to the format that matches the type of data entered, which is called "general." However, depending on what type of numbers they are, you can format them in different ways. Spreadsheet software allows formatting of numerical data as rounded or decimal numbers, currency, accounting, date, time, percentage, fraction, scientific (exponents), text, special, and custom. Numbers with value that would be used in a calculation, for example, added, subtracted, multiplied, or divided, should be formatted to match their value (e.g., money, time, percentage). Numbers with no numerical value that are not used in calculations

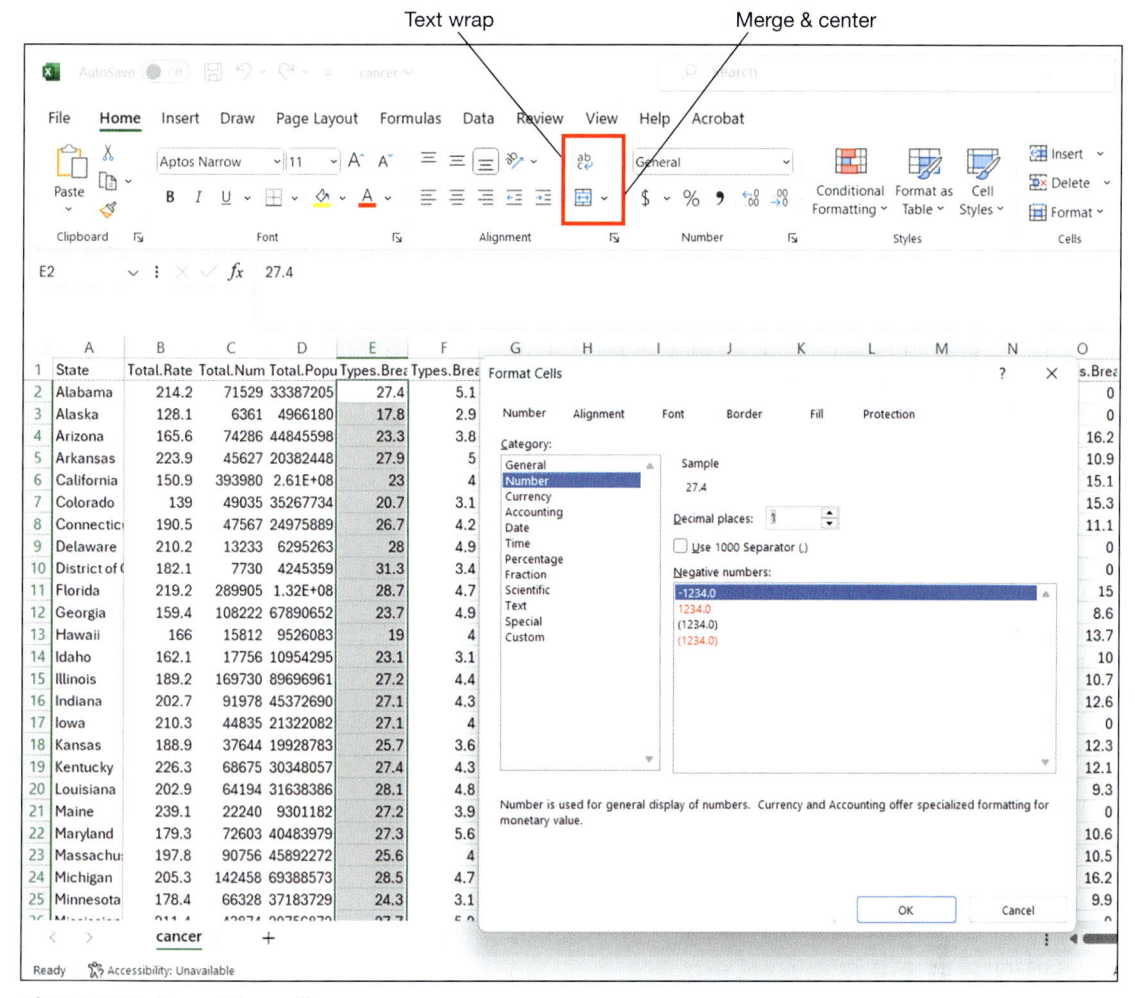

Figure B-10. Formatting cells.

such as admission numbers, zip codes, social security numbers, and telephone numbers should be formatted as text since they represent an object, person, or place.

To format a cell data type, right click on a cell or on a group of highlighted cells and select "Format Cells." In Figure B-10, the highlighted column is formatted as a number with one decimal place.

Since you can use date and time for calculations, format them as numbers. If you enter a date such as 3/12 (with no parentheses) into a cell, the spreadsheet automatically displays the data as a date defaulting to the current year. To enter a time, enter it using a colon, for example, 4 a.m. or 2 p.m.. If you want to change the way that the date or time is displayed, in the "Format Cells" menu, select one of the various types under the "Date" or "Time" options. Spreadsheet software also allows you to enter a date and time together in a single cell. These date and time combinations are useful in nursing when calculating a time difference for an event that begins one day and ends the next. For example, a patient may be admitted to the emergency department (ED) on 1/2/2024 at 10 p.m. and discharged on 1/3/2024 at 1:25 a.m. When you enter a formula to calculate the difference between these times, the calculation appears as an unformatted number. In the example, the result is 0.14236111111. To get the decimal number to display as a time difference, format the cell

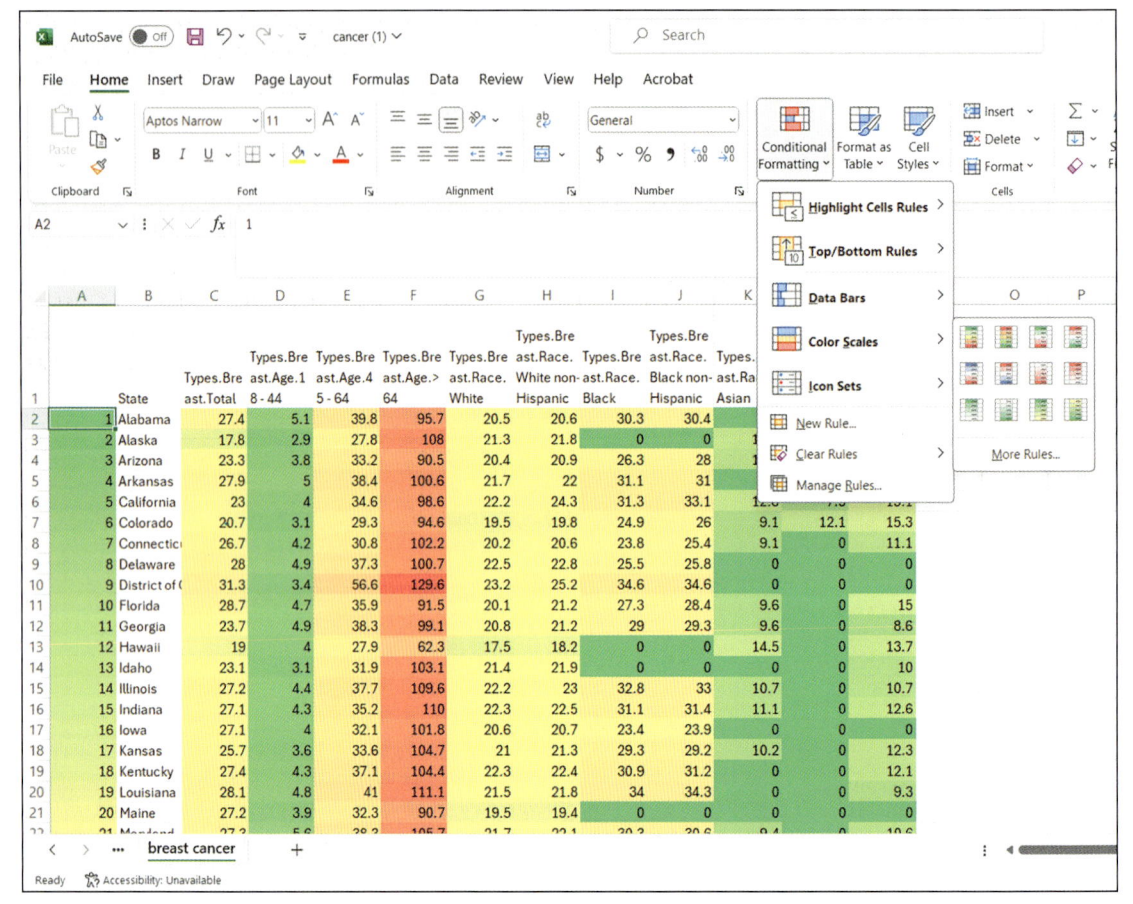

Figure B-11. Conditional formatting.

Figure B-12. Freezing column headers.

as short time, meaning only hours and minutes. The reformatted cell displays 3:25.

Conditional Formatting

Conditional formatting makes it easy to highlight cells with certain values or criteria to make them easy to identify. You can use conditional formatting to highlight cells that contain values that meet a certain condition, or you can format a whole cell range and vary the exact format as the value of each cell varies. For instance, in a spreadsheet associated with patient falls, falls with injuries can be highlighted with one background color in the cells, and the falls without injuries can be a different color, therefore making the distinction in the spreadsheet easy to find.

As an example from the cancer death rate data, let us look at just the breast cancer data. Using the "Conditional Formatting" button, you can apply a red-yellow-green color scale (Fig. B-11). You can also select "New Rule" to define the rules of the conditional formatting. If there is a list of consecutive numbers (such as Column A in Fig. B-11), you can see how the color scale changes as

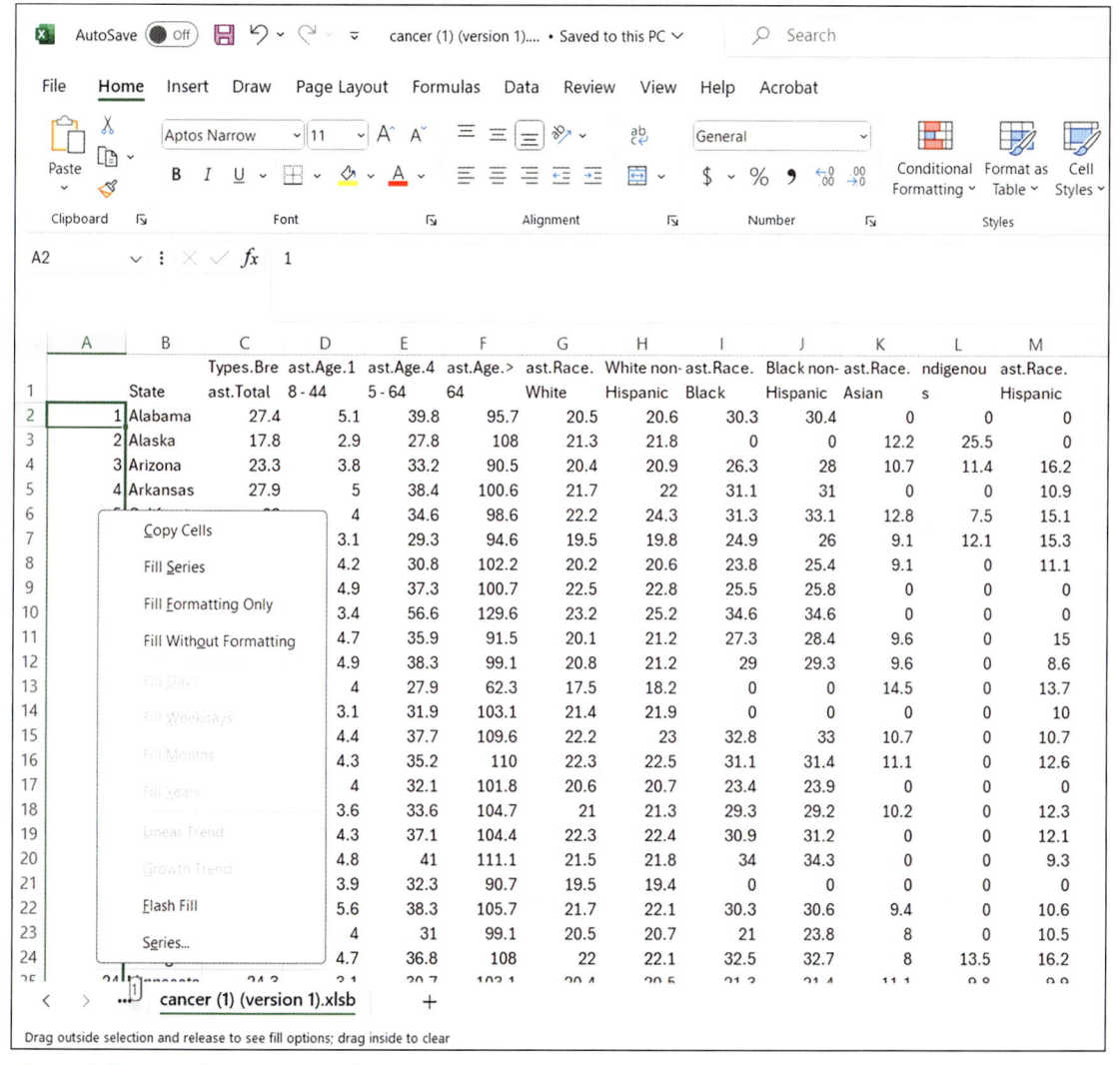

Figure B-13. Autofilling a series of numbers.

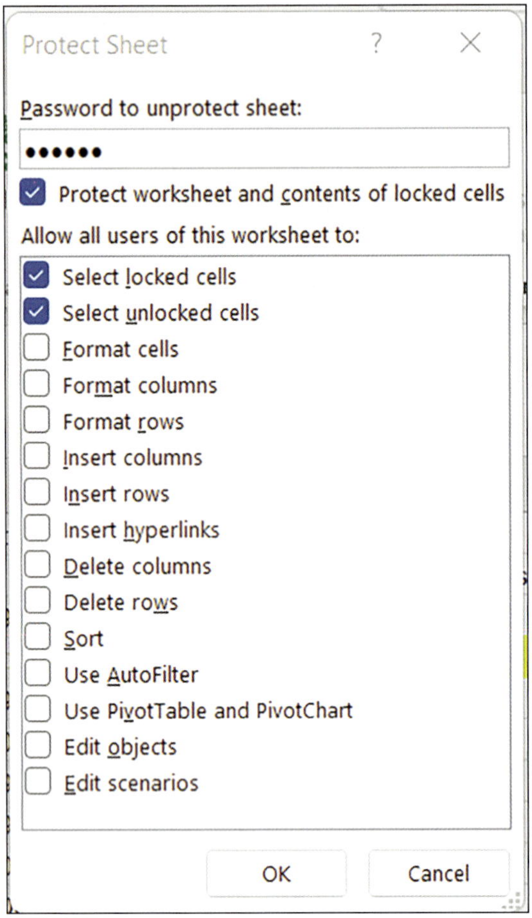

Figure B-14. Protecting sheet feature.

the numbers increase. This formatting allows you to see quickly the states that have low death rates from breast cancer (green) and those that have high death rates (red).

Freezing Rows and Columns

When there are more rows or columns than you can view on a computer screen, it is difficult to know what information is represented. Spreadsheets provide a way to freeze rows, columns, or both. The term "freeze" means you can keep one part of the spreadsheet visible while scrolling to another area on the spreadsheet. Freezing is important for accurate data entry when you get further away from the top column heads or left row names. Freezing the headings on columns is especially helpful to remember the categories as you scroll down a long list of data.

In the cancer death rates spreadsheet, highlight the top row of the cancer worksheet. In the "View" tab, select "Freeze Panes" and freeze the top row. Now, when you scroll down to Wyoming, you can still see the column headers (Fig. B-12).

Using Automatic Data Entry

Sometimes, spreadsheet design requires sequential data such as numbering 1 to 10, days of the week, months of the year, or quarters in the year. Excel includes a feature that allows the user to make a few entries and then have the computer complete the series. The feature can also recognize a series of skipped numbers such as 2, 4, and 6.

To fill cells in a pattern automatically, start typing the first two entries. For instance, if you are numbering a list of rows, start typing 1, then 2, then grab the bottom right corner of the cell with the number 2 using a right mouse click and drag the corner down the column as far as you want to fill. When you release the right mouse click, select "Fill Series" in the menu box that appears. If you have a different pattern, you want to populate, select "Series" and set the rules in the menu box.

Try opening the cancer data set from CORGIS and adding a column to the left of the states. Type a "1" next to "Alabama." Then right click drag the corner of the green box down to "Wyoming" and select "Fill Series" (Fig. B-13). Then try the same thing but instead select "Series" and try adjusting the step value to see how you can fill a series of skipped numbers.

Data Protection and Security

In healthcare, it is especially important to provide data protection and/or security when storing confidential patient data in spreadsheets. Data protection refers to locking cells to prevent

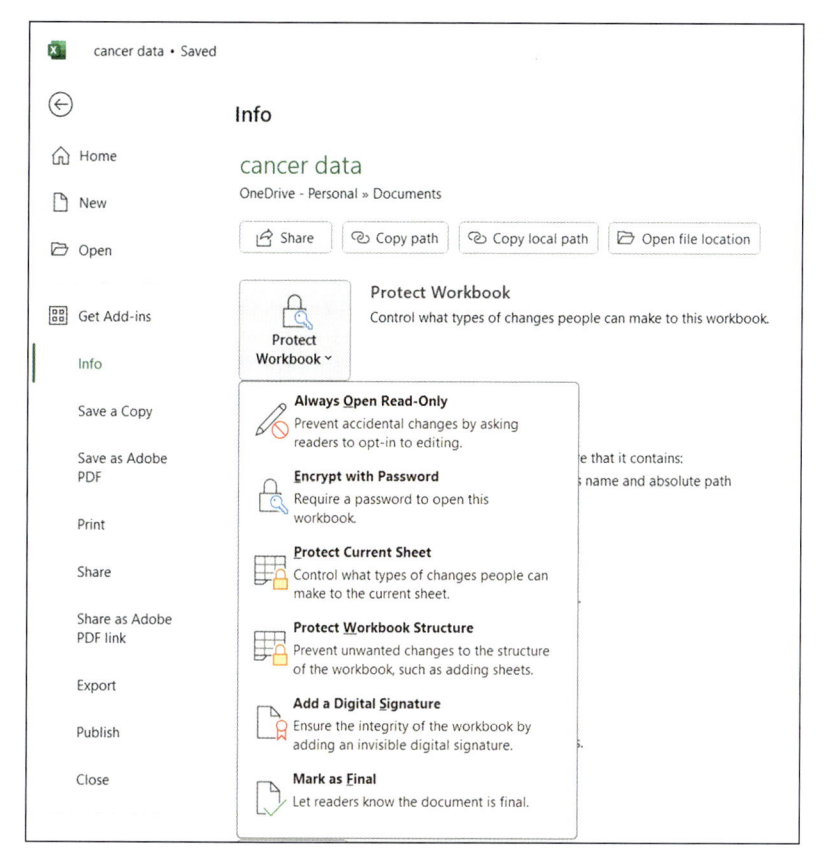

Figure B-15. Encrypting spreadsheet with a password.

users from changing the cell value. This feature is helpful for preventing accidental changes to cell text, numbers, or formulas. To lock cells, go to the "Review" tab menu bar and the "Protect Sheet" button. Choose a password and the features you want to protect (Fig. B-14).

Security means the user must provide a password to view and/or edit the spreadsheet. Security is especially important when using a laptop to work with spreadsheets that contain patient-associated data. To protect an Excel file with a password, go to the "File" tab and then select "Info." Use the "Protect Workbook" button to encrypt with password, or use one of the other security measures available there (Fig. B-15).

Error Messages

When using a spreadsheet software program, if a cell shows an error message such as "#DIV/0," "#NAME?", or "#####Error (#######)," it means data in a cell or formulas are incorrect. This may be due to error with typing or logic or errors associated with omission. It can also occur if your data formatting does not match the data entered. Error messages are like red flags identifying something that needs to be corrected for accurate use of the formula. If you get an error message, you can click on the error to see what type of error it is and find help with fixing it (Fig. B-16).

Creating Charts

Spreadsheet software allows you to create many types of charts. To start chart development, look at the menu bar under the "Insert" tab. From there, you can pick the type of chart to use when presenting data. Practice with the cancer data set. Create a new sheet and copy the data for sex and race for your state into that sheet. To begin the creation of a spreadsheet chart, first identify the cells (in this case, A1:E2) that represent the data. After selecting the appropriate cells, click on the chart tool and select the type of chart that best represents those data. Figure B-17 shows the data in a pie chart.

Excel provides chart suggestions and a preview of how the chart will look before making the final selection. If you do not like the chart, delete it, and begin again. You will not lose your data when you delete the chart. Most spreadsheet software tools provide a way to create and edit the chart title and legends. The chart title is an important part of the chart, so the type of data that are incorporated in the data visualization is clear. Also, be sure to use a legend so readers know exactly what you are presenting in the chart.

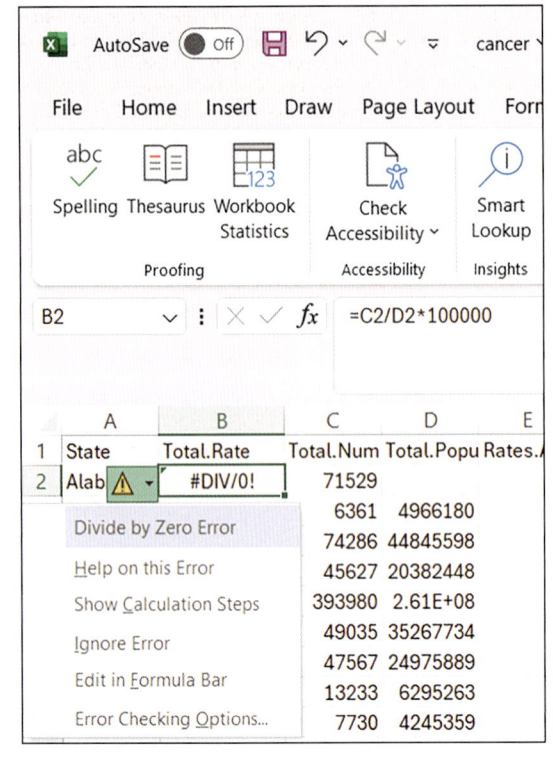

Figure B-16. Error message.

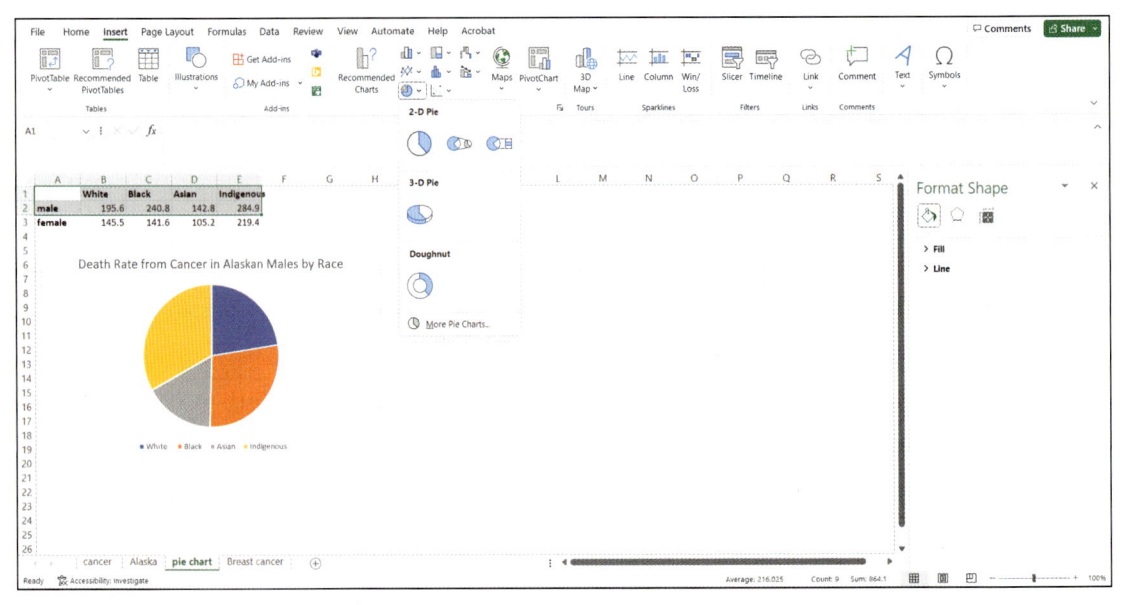

Figure B-17. How to make a pie chart.

You can also modify fonts and colors used in the chart. Once you have clicked on the icon to indicate that you have finished, the chart appears on the spreadsheet. You can always resize, move, or edit a completed chart. To edit the chart, right click the object you want to change to obtain a drop-down menu of choices.

REFERENCES

Kafura, D. (2019, June 27). *Cumulative cancer deaths for the period 2007-2013 reported for each U.S. State.* CORGIS Dataset Project. https://think.cs.vt.edu/corgis/csv/cancer/

Mattessich, R. (n.d.). *Spreadsheet: Its first computerization (1961–1964)*. Retrieved on February 8, 2023 from http://dssresources.com/history/mattessichspreadsheet.htm

Miller, K., Haddad, L., Phillips, K. (2016). Educational strategies for reducing medication errors committed by student nurses: A literature review. *International Journal of Health Sciences Education*, *3*(1). Retrieved from https://dc.etsu.edu/cgi/viewcontent.cgi?article=1012&context=ijhse

Whitcomb, R., Choi, J. M., & Guan, B. (2021, August 31). *AIDS CSV File. 3.0.0.* CORGIS Dataset Project. https://corgis-edu.github.io/corgis/csv/aids/

APPENDIX C

Authoring Scholarly Slide Presentations

Sarah Rusnak and Kristi Miller

You will likely view a slide presentation at some point in your life: a training video with a voice speaking as slides appear with useful information; your instructor presenting a lecture on heart failure to the class; a poster presentation at a research conference on climate change and health outcomes. Sharing knowledge with others is essential in nursing education and practice, and slide presentations are a common way to share knowledge in educational, research, and clinical settings.

As you learn how to create a scholarly presentation, reflect on what makes a scholarly presentation different from one created purely for entertainment. A presentation such as a slideshow of a recent vacation made for your family can include anything you choose, and the format is all up to you. In contrast, a scholarly presentation includes information that is clear, concise, accurate, relevant, objective, interesting, complete, and adapted to the audience and purpose of the presentation. In addition, references should be provided to the audience to support your message. The guidelines suggested in this appendix will help you create a scholarly presentation. Think about the tone, the use of references, and how visuals and imagery can support your presentation goals.

In Appendix D, you will learn the basics of how to write a scholarly paper. This appendix will give you the tools to create an effective visual presentation of that information. It discusses the basics of scholarly presentations including visual design principles, presentation models, how to design slideshows, and tools you can use to make your presentations more effective. There are multiple options when selecting presentation software, including Microsoft PowerPoint and Google Slides. PowerPoint is among the most popular and will be the example used to demonstrate features within this appendix.

As you review this appendix, refer to Box C-1 for common terminology related to presentations and slideshows.

PRESENTATION MODELS

A presentation is a mode of communication used in a wide variety of speaking situations. A lecture is a type of presentation delivered specifically to educate the audience. Lectures are one of the most common ways to deliver medical information with two models of presentation—lecture support and lecture replacement.

Lecture Support Model

The lecture support model guides audiences to follow an oral presentation. This is the type of presentation most often seen in classrooms in which the instructor presents information in conjunction with a slideshow with supporting visuals. The lecture support model is used in face-to-face and online synchronous settings. When supplementing an oral presentation, the slides should help an audience keep track of ideas and illustrate the speaker's points. Slides alone are only an outline of a talk; everything the speaker says should not be included on the slide. Forcing learners to read while you are speaking increases cognitive load and impairs learning. It may even be appropriate to reveal bullet points one at a time and as they

BOX C-1 Scholarly Presentation Terminology

Backward design
Creation principle in which you begin with the end in mind; focus on what the learner needs to know to help determine what information and visuals should be included (i.e., create the conclusion slide first, emphasizing the most important points, and build the presentation around that)

Cognitive load theory
The brain has limited short-term memory and unlimited long-term memory making complex decision making a burden to cognitive load; audio and visual elements of a presentation should work in tandem instead of in opposition to decrease cognitive load of audience

Font
The style of the text characters; presentation font should be chosen with readability in mind; the three types of fonts are serif, sans serif, and script

Lecture
A type of presentation delivered specifically to educate the audience; one of the most common ways to deliver medical information

Lecture replacement model
Presentation that requires text or prerecorded voiceover narration to guide the audience; available on demand since it is prerecorded

Lecture support model
Presentation that guides audiences to follow an oral presentation; most often seen in classrooms in which the instructor presents information in conjunction with a slideshow with supporting visuals; used in face-to-face and online synchronous settings

Multimedia principle
Learning is enhanced when words and graphics are used together rather than words alone; decorative graphics do not enhance learning so it is important to incorporate graphics that serve a specific purpose

Presentation
A mode of communication used in a wide variety of speaking situations; effective way to get across data and knowledge to a group of people

Progressive disclosure
Form of animation on screen in which items are revealed one at a time until all the items on a slide are displayed (e.g., bulleted list appears as one bullet at a time by dropping down from the top or flying in from the side); creates visual interest and can reduce cognitive load

Slide
A single page of a presentation (also called a slideshow) created with software like PowerPoint, Keynote, Google slides, Prezi, or Canva

Slide layout
The arrangement of content on a slide; a template that contains formatting, positioning, and placeholders for the content that appears on a slide; content examples include titles, body text, tables, charts, SmartArt graphics, pictures, clip art, videos, and sounds

Storyboard
A plan for slides and visuals that can organize thoughts; works like an outline that can be easily rearranged in presentation software; assembles ideas into a coherent presentation

Theme
A slide or group of slides that can contain layouts with specified colors, fonts, effects, and background styles

(Continued)

> **BOX C-1** Scholarly Presentation Terminology *(Continued)*
>
> **Transition**
> The way a slide makes an entrance onto the screen (e.g., fade, push, morph); creates visual interest but should not be overused
>
> **Visual literacy**
> The ability to interpret, evaluate, and create images and visual media; skills equip you to understand the components (e.g., context, culture, aesthetic) involved in creation and use of visual materials

are discussed so the viewer will not read ahead and miss important information.

Speaker notes can help a speaker remember information for a given slide. You can print them or use presenter view to see your notes at the bottom of the screen while you are speaking (Fig. C-1). When in presenter view, only the slide is visible to the audience, not the notes. Speaker notes can be used to record narration or when rehearsing the presentation.

Lecture Replacement Model

The lecture replacement model is a slide presentation that requires text or prerecorded narration to guide the audience. You may also see it called voiceover narration when the creators record themselves speaking as they go through the presentation. This method is useful for presenters who have a fear of public speaking. Creating a voiceover presentation is a great way to practice for a live presentation. Instructors often will upload a copy of the classroom slideshow used as lecture support to a learning platform so that students can download and view the slides on their own. Using the lecture replacement model solves the issue of students not understanding the slides without the support of narration.

A major advantage of lecture replacement is that it is available on demand, whenever and wherever the learner wants access. Putting a lecture with voiceover on a website like YouTube allows anyone to watch and comment at any time. In addition, a standalone slideshow, such as an interactive tutorial, can allow for self-guided study. The video can be started, stopped, slowed down or sped up and watched as many times as needed to master the content. Learners with different backgrounds and abilities can study the material as much or as little as is needed to understand it, which helps support equity in the classroom.

Lecture replacement presentations are particularly attractive to patients who need to learn a new skill. A patient learning how to give an insulin injection can access an on-demand video instead of making an expensive and time-consuming visit to the physician's office. Patients can watch the presentation as many times as is needed to master the skill.

Because the learner does not have access to the creator, it is helpful to include explicit learning objectives, and the slides may need to be highly detailed depending on the amount and type of narration provided by the creator. This may be seen as a disadvantage, but a workaround to this is found on sites like YouTube, where viewers can comment and ask questions about videos. The creators can then answer in the comments section.

CREATING A PRESENTATION

Similar to any scholarly document, it is important to have a goal and a plan in mind before beginning to create the presentation. This can be done with backward design. When using the principle of backward design, begin with the end in mind by asking, "What will the learners know or be able to do after this presentation?" If you focus on this, you can determine what information, stories, images, and data you should include to achieve that end (Wiggins & McTighe, 2005). One suggestion to achieve this is writing out the conclusion slide first, emphasizing the most important points and building the presentation around that.

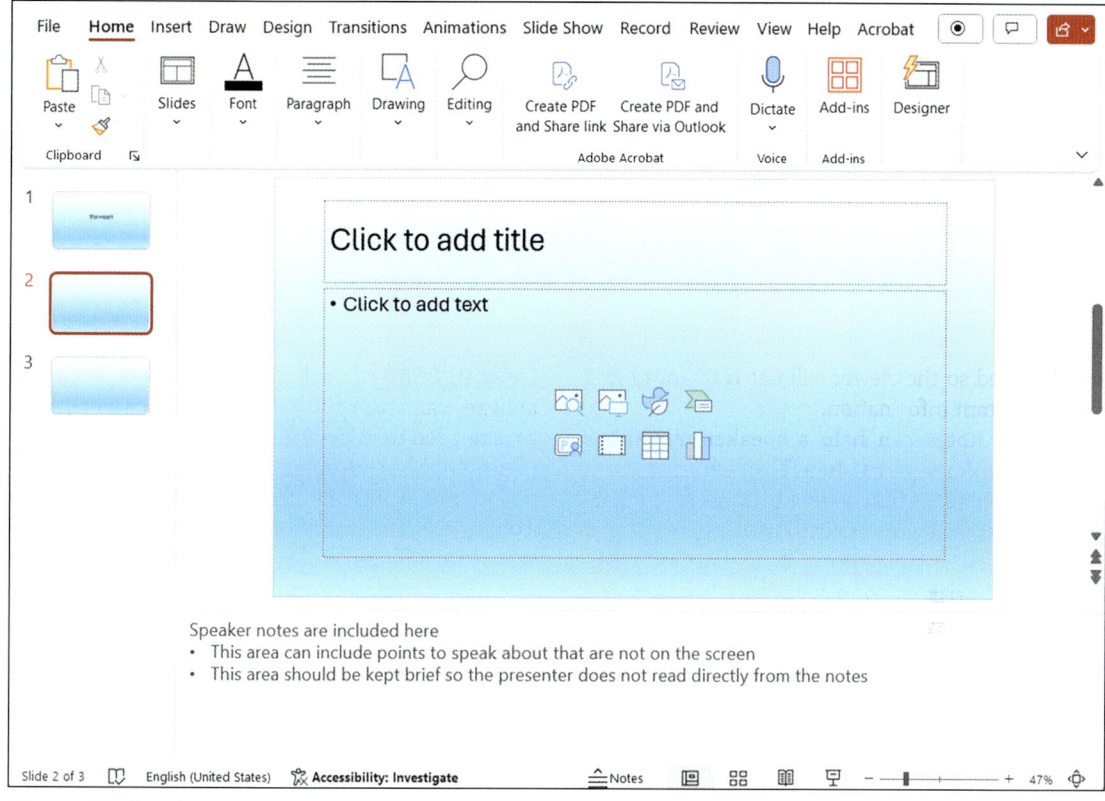

Figure C-1. Speaker notes.

Deciding on a Theme

You can start with a blank presentation or a prepared design using a template or theme. A gallery of themes is included with presentation software and applications. Keep in mind that any graphics or images on your background layer will show on all slides regardless of the layout selected. Although the graphic may be interesting, it may interfere with your message or even cause attention to be deflected from your message. A template is a theme that includes content. For a presentation on climate change, an earth-themed presentation might be appropriate. After opening PowerPoint, select the "New" button along the left side and from there, search the templates for one that is suitable for the topic or design your own (Fig. C-2). You can also create your own custom templates for use in the future or for sharing with others. If you are presenting at a professional conference, ask in advance if there is a template provided by the conference organizers.

When selecting a background for an oral presentation, it is helpful to know the kind of screen that will be in the room and the room lighting. Whether you will present from a high-resolution monitor or from a projector cast onto a screen, high contrast between the background and foreground is important. However, consider using a light background for light rooms and dark background for dark rooms (Prost, n.d.).

Views

Presentation software allows you to look at your slides in many ways, called views. Under the "View" tab, the options are found on the left of the menu bar. You can also toggle between views using the icons on the bottom right of the screen (Fig. C-3). The view that audiences see is the slideshow view, which is only for viewing, not editing.

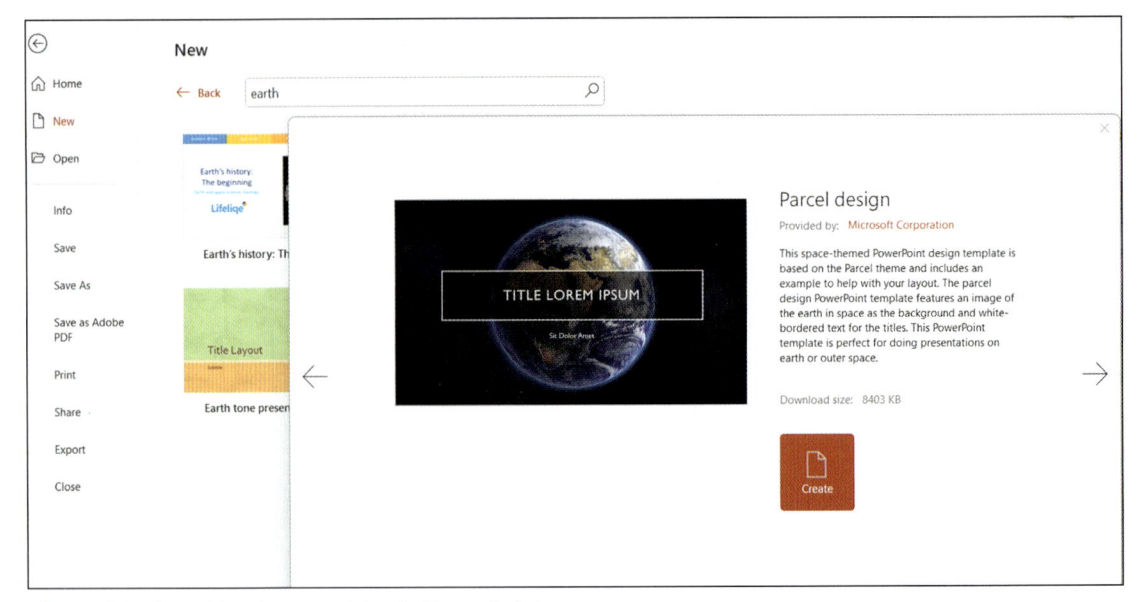

Figure C-2. Searching for templates in PowerPoint.

The normal view is the default creation mode (see Fig. C-1). In normal view, the left side of the screen has a column with thumbnail views of slides, the right has a view of the slide under construction, and the bottom contains any speaker notes you have added.

Slide sorter view (as seen in Fig. C-3) is especially useful when rearranging slides or copying slides from one presentation to another. You can rearrange slides by clicking and dragging slides where you want them. If slides are copied to another presentation, you can select whether they

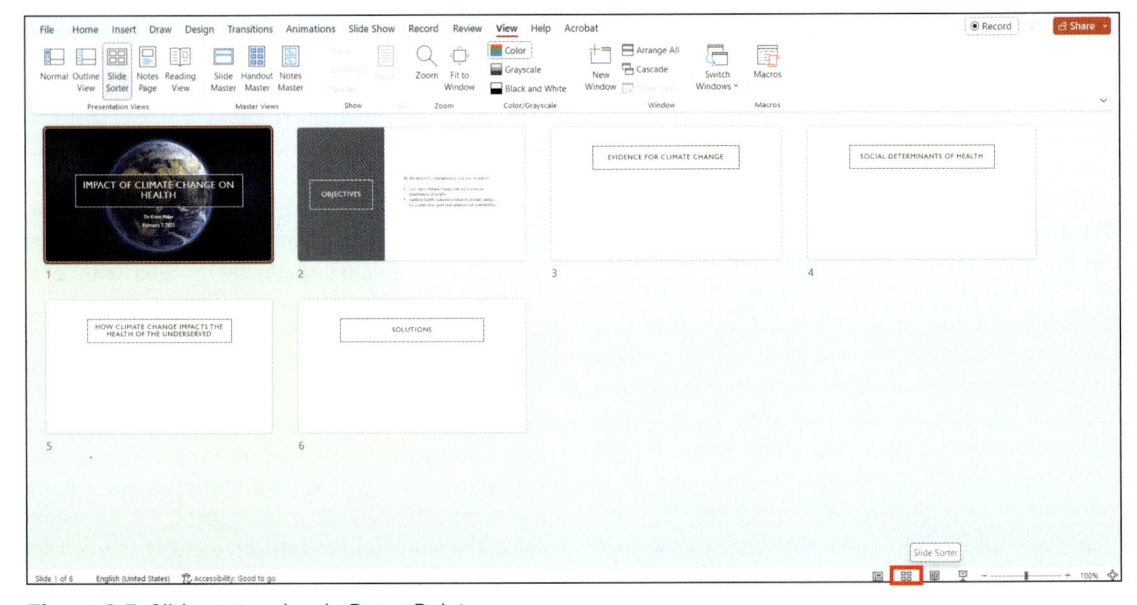

Figure C-3. Slide sorter view in PowerPoint.

take on the style of the new slideshow or retain formatting from the source presentation. Slides can be copied or deleted individually or in selected groups. To select more than one, after clicking on the first one, hold down the "Ctrl" or "Command" key as you select the others. If the slides you wish to select are in order (contiguous), select either the first or the last slide then hold down the "Shift" key as you select the other end of the group.

You can also use the slide sorter view to storyboard the presentation. A storyboard is a plan for visuals that forces you to organize your thoughts and allows you to assemble your ideas into a coherent presentation. As with all projects, planning saves time. With presentation software, you can outline your thoughts using a title and text on a slide. After you complete the first draft, use the slide sorter view to determine if a rearrangement of slides would be helpful. When you have your slides in the correct order, go back to each slide and develop it into a meaningful communication tool. Expect to switch between the slide sorter view and the normal view many times while working on the visuals. Once you have an outline or storyboard, you are ready to begin creating slides.

Collaborating on Slideshow Design

Some slideshow software supports real-time collaboration in which two or more individuals can work on a slideshow at the same time. For example, PowerPoint users can save and share files for collaborative design using OneDrive. You can also share Google Slide files for collaborative work. The cloud computing versions of PowerPoint and Keynote support collaboration. However, the commercial Keynote software allows only the ability to share slides with others as email attachments.

CREATING SLIDES

Electronic presentations, also called slideshows, are created using slides. The word "slide" comes from a time before computers when images were printed on 35 mm slides, inserted into a carousel, and projected onto a screen (Fig. C-4). In the digital age, a slide is a single page of an electronic presentation created with software.

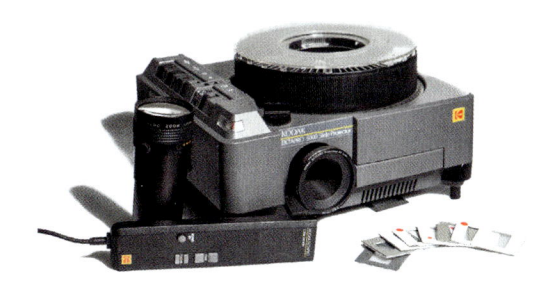

Figure C-4. 35-mm slides in a carousel. (Shutterstock/Joshua Sanderson Media.)

There are multiple steps to slide creation including slide layout, content, special effects, and accessibility. See Table C-1 for a summary of the basic rules for creating slides. Accessibility is covered in the text in Chapters 10 and 14.

The content and design of a presentation depends upon multiple factors:

- What are your goals? Are you informing or attempting to persuade?
- What type of presentation is it—a lecture or a prerecorded video?
- Who is your audience? Are you speaking to nurses, community members, or members of the hospital board?

Keeping these factors in mind is important as you add text content, images, and other features to your presentation.

Slide Layout

The slide layout contains formatting, positioning, and placeholders for the content that appears on a slide. Placeholders are boxes framed with dotted lines on slide layouts that contain titles, body text, tables, charts, SmartArt graphics, pictures, clip art, videos, and sounds (Microsoft, n.d.). The slide layout button is found on the menu bar of the home tab (Fig. C-5). Options for slide layouts include a title slide, title and content, two content, comparison and blank. By default, when you open a new presentation, the title page layout appears as the first slide. The title slide layout has placeholders for a title and a subtitle. Depending on the theme or template you select, the next slide layout

TABLE C-1 Basic Rules for Creating Slides

Text and Fonts	
Fonts	• Choose a sans serif font (e.g., Arial or Helvetica) for projected visuals. • Use no more than three font styles per presentation.
Font size	• Use a font size of 24 or more.
Punctuation	• Be consistent. If using periods to end sentences or bullets, use them for all sentences or bullets.
Colors	
Text and background	• Match slide lighting to presentation setting. Use light colors for light rooms and dark colors for dark rooms. • Use no more than four to six colors per presentation.
Font color	• Use a strong contrast to the background color. Opposite sides of color wheel are ideal.
For emphasis	• Match font color to reactions desired from the audience. Colors convey meaning (e.g., red is intense—use only for emphasis). • Never use color as the sole means of conveying meaning. Patterns, symbols, or text can be added to objects with color to assist viewers with any type of color blindness.
Consistency	• Use the same color, font, symbol, or pattern for the same meaning throughout.
Using Visuals	
Appropriateness	• Use images to enhance the learner's understanding of important information but match the visual literacy of the audience.
Presentation	• Use progressive disclosure for bullet points.

will be chosen for you, but you can change it by selecting the slide layout button.

Text Content

Select a placeholder on a slide to enter text or other objects, such as images, tables, and charts. You can resize, move, delete, or create placeholders as needed. If the default or template font size or color is not appropriate for an individual slide, you can use the font menu under the home tab to change them. Be careful not to introduce too many variations into one presentation.

Choosing fonts for presentation text is an important design choice. Font refers to the style of the text characters. There are three types of fonts: serif, sans serif, and script. Serif fonts like Times New Roman and Garamond have extra tails on the ends of each letter called serifs and are easier to read in print format. These fonts are harder to

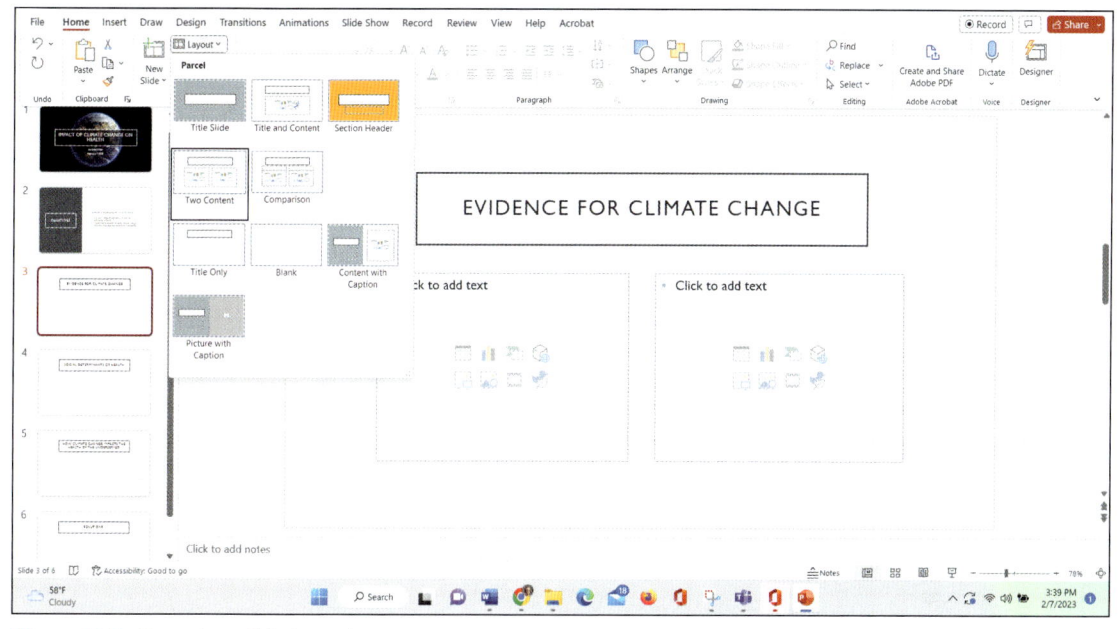

Figure C-5. Choosing slide layout.

read when projected on a screen, so a sans serif font like Arial, Calibri, Helvetica, or Verdana, which are easier to read on a screen, including a projected presentation, are better choices for fonts on slides (Fig. C-6). Though there are many font options available, many are unsuitable for text in a presentation. Choosing a unique font in the hope that it will enliven a presentation can create readability problems.

Fonts should be chosen early in the creation process because changing a font later may alter the layout on some slides due to the difference in size of the text. For example, the default font size in a blank template on PowerPoint is 28, but if too much text is added, the font size decreases to fit it all on the screen (Fig. C-7). If you change the font type later in the process of creating the presentation, you may find that the font sizes vary from slide to slide to accommodate the text.

Sans-serif font: Arial	Generally easier to read on screens and in presentations
Serif font: Times New Roman	Generally easier to read in a print format

Figure C-6. Comparison of sans serif and serif fonts.

In general, text font size should be between 24 and 32 point, though the minimum size needed for readability depends on the size of the screen and the room.

You can add attributes to fonts just as you can in word processing software. Bold or italic text will emphasize a point. Italicizing, however, tends to make text more difficult to read, especially from a distance. If it is used, give the audience more time to read the slide. Use this feature to your advantage when you want the audience to read more slowly. When using font effects, be consistent throughout the presentation: always use the same attribute for the same type of information.

To avoid cognitive overload, limit the text on a slide. When placing text on slides, include only the essential elements of a concept. State ideas as though they were headlines. The audience should grasp the point of the visual text within the first 5 seconds after it appears. Some suggest that a presenter should be quiet for those 5 seconds to allow the audience to grasp the point. The information on a slide can be helpful to the presenter as a guide but should not be used as a teleprompter or a script. In oral and voiceover presentations, do not read the slide to the audience unless for specific emphasis,

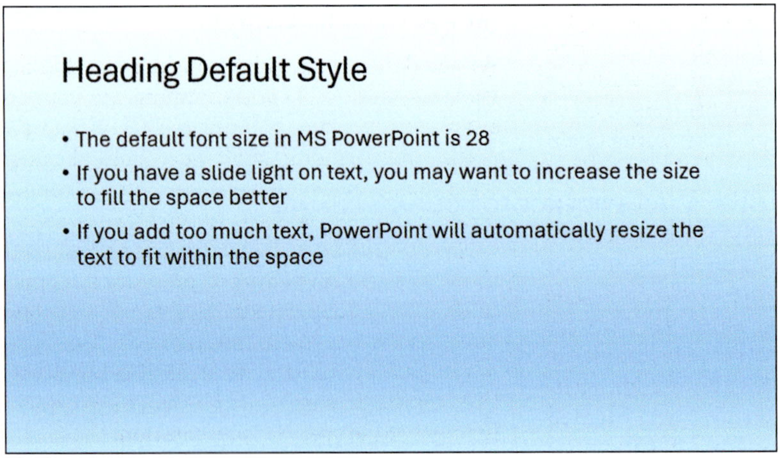

Figure C-7. Default font size **(A)** of a presentation will automatically adjust to accommodate too much text on the screen **(B)**.

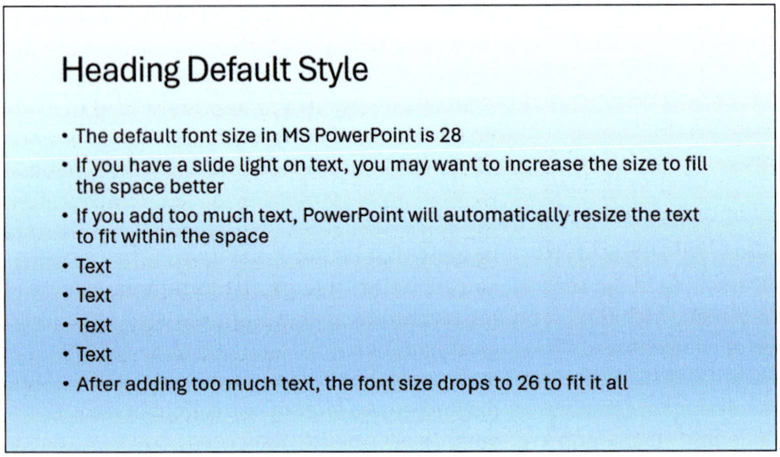

and even then, limit this practice. Audience participants can read faster than a speaker can talk; therefore, their attention can become divided between reading ahead and listening. Visual text serves as a focus to assist the audience in following the presentation, though recall that cognitive load theory shows that learners will have a harder time learning information if what they hear does not match with what they read on the slide.

Visual Design Principles

The images and visual design can make a difference in how ideas are received. The concepts of visual literacy, cognitive load, and Mayer's multimedia principle will help guide the selection of images and graphics for a presentation.

When you use visuals, you need to be aware of the visual literacy of the viewers. Visual literacy is the ability to find, create, and evaluate images and other visual media. Visual literacy skills allow you to understand and analyze the components involved in the creation and use of visual materials (Visual Literacy Standards Task Force, 2022). Culture, which affects visual literacy, can pertain to any part of a learner's background. The ability to interpret the meaning of visual images is an important skill for both the designer and audience (Visual Literacy Standards Task Force, 2022). One audience will view a visual in a different way from another. For example, an image might clearly convey information to a group of healthcare professionals but be confusing to professionals from other disciplines. Consider a presentation on the human heart. A simple stylized graphic of a heart would be appropriate for some audiences (e.g., patients, community members) but an anatomical image would be better suited for medical professionals (Fig. C-8).

According to cognitive load theory, the brain has limited short-term memory and unlimited long-term memory (Sweller, 1988). This means that complex decision making adds to cognitive load. In relation to presentations, it is difficult for the brain to process reading words on a slide while listening to a presenter unless the two are congruent. If a presenter is verbally providing information at the same time as a different written message is displayed visually, the increased cognitive load prevents you from focusing on both, making you miss important parts of both messages. Slide design should have minimal text and appropriate visual images and complement the audio presentation, not conflict with it. This will facilitate learners to process information.

Mayer's multimedia principle brings together the concepts of visual literacy and cognitive load by stating that learning is enhanced when words and graphics are used together rather than words alone (Clark & Mayer, 2016). The type of graphic matters, however, as decorative graphics do not enhance learning. While an aesthetically pleasing design is appealing, it is more important to incorporate graphics that serve a specific purpose. When selecting or creating graphics for your slides, carefully consider the purpose of the image.

Using and Formatting Images

As you design your slides, consider whether a picture, graph, or table will communicate your message better than words. Using images on your slides is easy in presentation software. Right clicking on most images stored on your computer or found on the internet will allow you to copy the image to the clipboard so you can then paste it in a presentation, though some browser-based presentation applications do not support pasting from the clipboard. You can also use the menu bar under the "Insert" tab to add saved images to slides. Remember from the Chapter 10 that copyright must be considered for any images used in a presentation.

Drawing tools and image editing features assist in the slide design process. Slideshow software provides drawing tools that you can use to call out information in images or text or create illustrations. Cropping images allows the designer to cut off the sides of a picture to show a smaller portion of the image. When resizing an image, remember to click on the corner (not a side) to avoid stretching and skewing the image. PowerPoint also makes the placement of images easy. When placing an image on a slide, you can drag it to where you want it placed. As you move into the exact center of the slide, smart guides (dotted red lines) will appear. These guides are in line with the heading or another image, or are in a visually appealing location in another way (Fig. C-9). This helps ensure

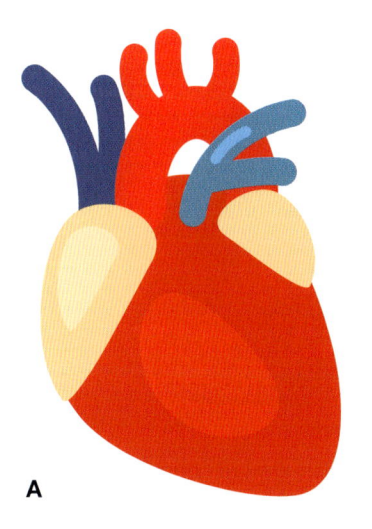

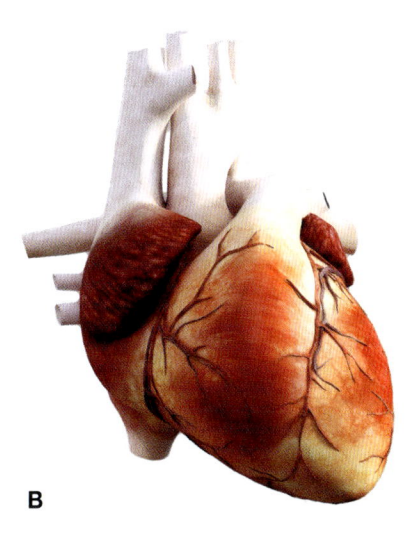

Figure C-8. Using different types of graphics for different audiences. (**A.** Shutterstock/Pogorelova Olga. **B.** Shutterstock/Derya Cakirsoy.)

A

B

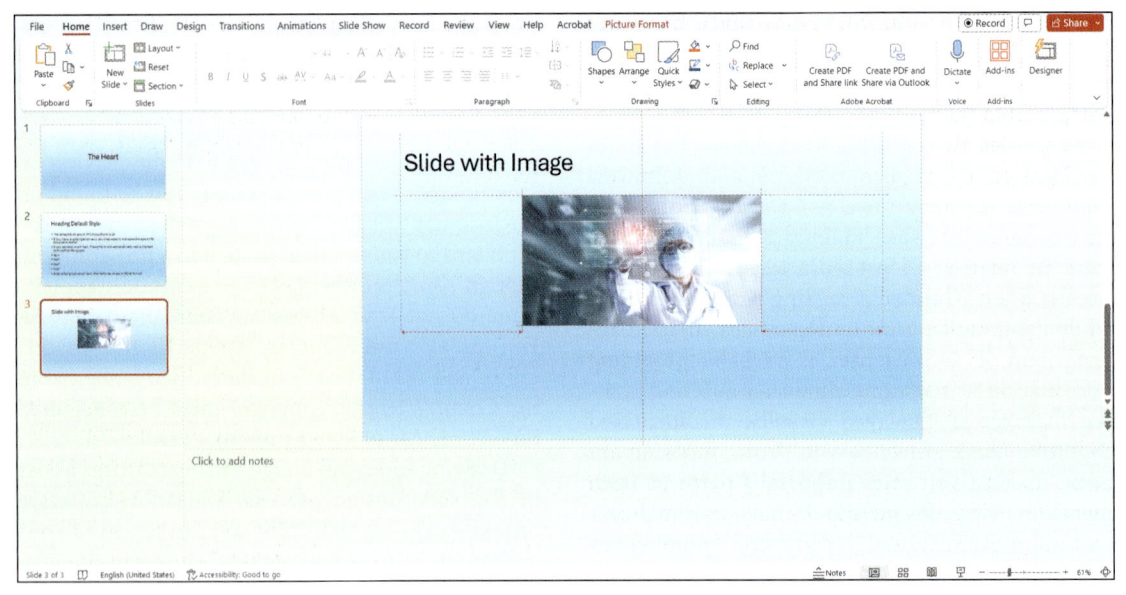

Figure C-9. Using smart guides to help with the placement of an image.

the image placement does not look off, which could be distracting to an audience.

Although it is possible to include detailed pictures, considerations should be made regarding art. First, is the visual pertinent to your message or will it distract from your message? Second, is the image more complicated than necessary to convey the meaning? For example, a presentation that includes an illustration of blood circulation through the heart could be confusing if it were very detailed (Fig. C-10). A simple drawing that depicts only the basic structures make the information easier to understand. A more detailed drawing with many labels may be a good choice for

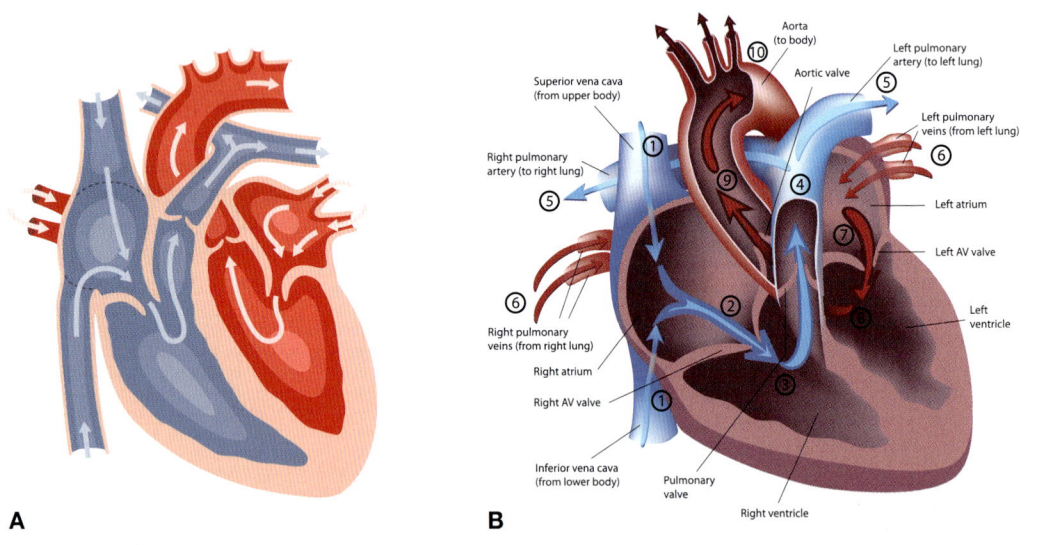

Figure C-10. Less complicated images **(A)** will read better to an audience than a more complicated image **(B)**. (**B.** Shutterstock/Alila Medical Media.)

a printed resource but will be difficult to follow in a projected presentation, especially from a distance. Simple illustrations allow learners to focus on the main points rather than trying to separate them from the details.

Occasionally, an image does not project well. To prevent this from ruining a presentation, check the appearance of the slide in the "Play" or "Show" view before committing to using the visual in the presentation. Generally, if an image looks good in playback mode, it will project well. If possible, check how the image projects using the equipment you will use to make the presentation.

When you add images, remember to add alt text to every image, especially in lecture replacement presentations since learners access these on their own. The point of visuals is to communicate information to the audience, but for people who rely on screen readers, an image has no value. Alt text is used to provide a brief description of the image, which will be read aloud by the screen reader. If you cannot decide how to describe an image to a learner who uses a screen reader, consider whether the image is pertinent to any learner. For help with adding these text descriptions, search for "alt tags" in the search bar of PowerPoint.

Other Features

You can enhance slideshow presentations using special effects such as color, sound, video, animations, and transitions. However, use moderation when adding special effects to a presentation. You want the viewers to pay attention to your message, not the special effect. If you are giving a presentation that uses special effects, test the presentation in the setting where viewers will see it to make sure they can be clearly experienced by the audience.

Color

Color can be used to draw attention to a feature, but should not be the only distinguishing characteristic. Always include additional means of expression so that viewers with limited color vision, or low or no vision, are also able to comprehend the content. This may mean adding a pattern to bars in charts, adding data labels, or adding text descriptions. Note that providing multiple means of comprehension helps all learners. As with fonts, it is important to be consistent in using color and to use no more than four to six different colors. When viewers grasp the implications of a given color, the result is improved comprehension of the meaning of the visuals.

Sound

You can insert sound into all commercial slideshow software and some free versions. Depending on the software, you may be able to insert audio from a file or record narration. To record sound, you need a microphone. External microphones will provide better audio quality than microphones integrated into a laptop or tablet. Record several test clips to find the best option. If you are using PowerPoint, you can record your voice and insert it into your presentation using the audio recording feature under the "Insert" tab (Fig. C-11). In lecture replacement presentations, the audience will then select the microphone icon that appears on each slide to playback the recording.

Video

Video clips are equally easy to insert using the "Video" button under the "Insert" tab (see Fig. C-11). Many applications allow you to embed from a website. If you click the "Video" button in MS PowerPoint, selecting "Online videos" will open a box where you can add a weblink and it will add the video from that source to the slide. You can also use videos from a webcam, most digital cameras, smartphones, and tablet devices. Some slideshow software includes a video editor.

When adding a video to a slideshow, limit the video length to the essential information so it does not lose audience attention. As with sound, before using a video in a presentation, check the equipment in the room where you will present. Make a copy of the presentation without video available and plan for what you will say in case the video portion of the presentation equipment fails on the day of the presentation.

Transitions

A transition is the way a slide makes an entrance onto the screen. Presentation programs have a variety of transitions available. Some cause a slide

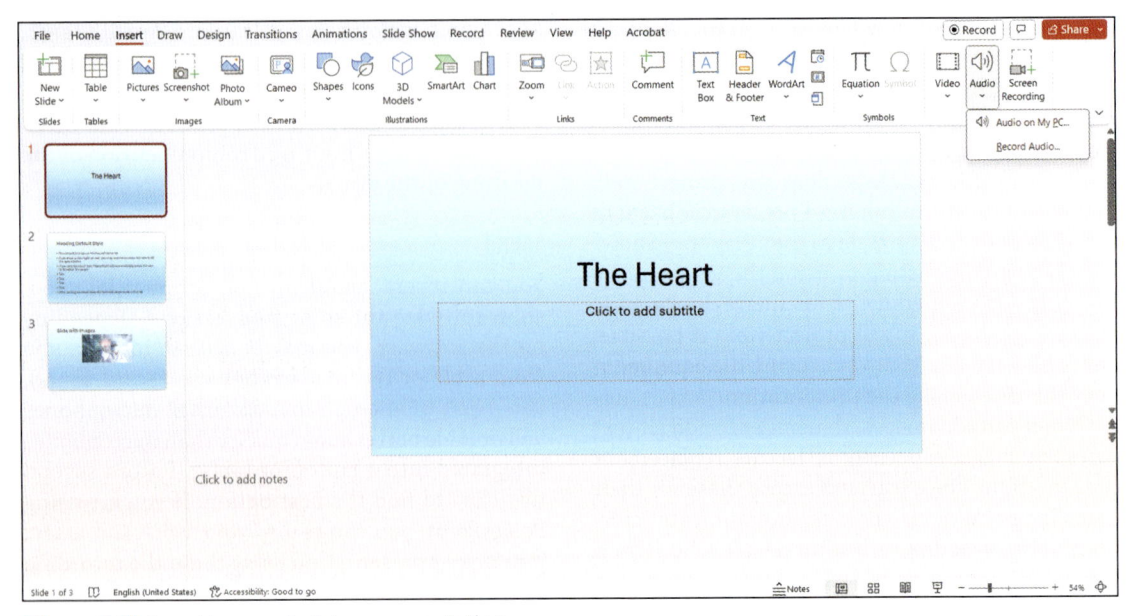

Figure C-11. Inserting media into a presentation.

to fade in, some cause the slide to appear first at the center and then expand, and others cause the slide to sweep across the screen. Transitions can be dramatic, enhance your message, or distract the audience. The best rule is to be consistent and use transitions sparingly. Avoid trying to dazzle the audience with multiple transitions. Transitions can be added and customized under the "Transitions" tab.

Animation

Animation is a tool in some presentation software that makes slide objects move on a slide. When the slide appears on screen, an animation can work to make the slide more dynamic or interesting. Generally, animation takes the form of progressive disclosure in which items are revealed one at a time until all the items are revealed on a slide display. For example, when the items in a bulleted list appear one at a time by dropping down from the top of the screen or flying in from the left or right. During your presentation, you can dim or convert bullets or images already discussed to a different color while the current point takes center stage or makes objects appear or disappear during a presentation. Use of animation can reduce cognitive load for viewers.

To use progressive disclosure as animation, first add all the bullet points or images you want to animate to the slide. Select the first bullet point or image you want to appear. Go to the "Animations" tab and choose a type of reveal (e.g., appear, fade, fly in). Then select the second bullet point or image you want to appear and choose a reveal, and so on. As you add the reveals to individual bullets or images, numbers will appear beside them indicating the order in which they will appear (Fig. C-12). When you play the presentation, the items will be revealed in the order and manner you have chosen.

You can also use animated graphics interchange formats (GIFs, a type of image files from the web that show movement) with many presentation programs. If the animated GIF will be on the screen for a long time, it is a good idea to cover it up after a given time, something you can set to happen automatically. Movement on a screen can become distracting. When using animation, check the animation before your actual presentation to ensure it is functioning the way you want it to.

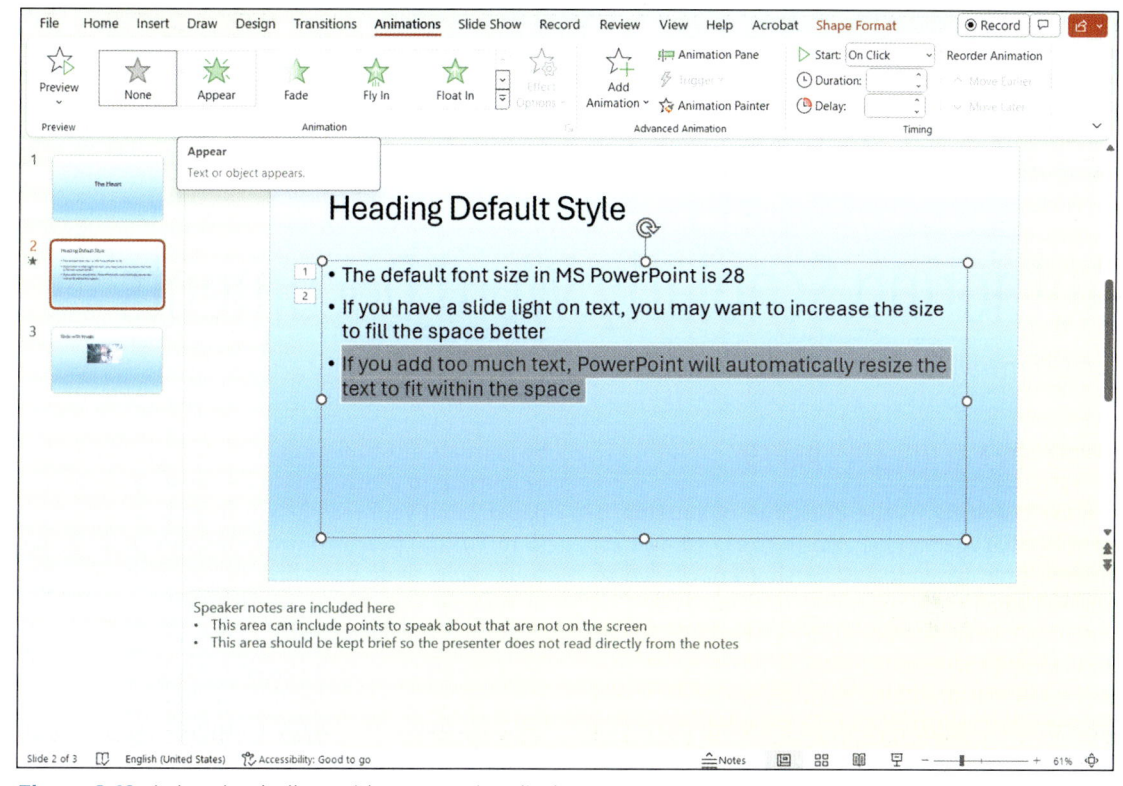

Figure C-12. Animating bullets with progressive disclosure.

REFERENCES

Clark, R. C., & Mayer, R. E. (2016). *E-Learning and the science of instruction: Proven guidelines for consumers and designers of multimedia learning* (4th edn.). Wiley.

Microsoft. (n.d.) *What is a slide layout?* Retrieved February 7, 2023 from https://support.microsoft.com/en-us/office/what-is-a-slide-layout-99da5716-92ee-4b6a-a0b5-bee-a45150f3a

Prost, J. (n.d.). *8 Mistakes made when presenting with PowerPoint and how to correct them.* Retrieved February 8, 2023 from http://www.frippandassociates.com/artprost2_faa.html

Sweller, J. (1988). Cognitive load during problem solving: Effects on learning. *Cognitive Science, 12,* 257–285. http://onlinelibrary.wiley.com/doi/10.1207/s15516709cog1202_4/pdf

Visual Literacy Standards Task Force. (2022). *Companion document to the ACRL framework for information literacy for higher education.* Association of College and Research Libraries, American Library Association. https://www.ala.org/acrl/sites/ala.org.acrl/files/content/standards/Framework_Companion_Visual_Literacy.pdf

Wiggins, G., & McTighe, J. (2005). *Understanding by design* (2nd Expanded edition). Assn. for Supervision & Curriculum Development.

APPENDIX D

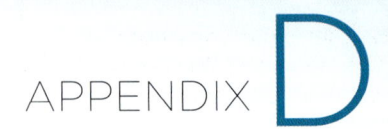

Authoring Scholarly Word Documents

Joni Tornwall and Kristi Miller

WRITING A SCHOLARLY PAPER

Scholarly writing in the discipline of nursing is writing that generates, synthesizes, translates, applies, and disseminates nursing knowledge to improve health and transform healthcare (AACN, 2021). When you set out to write a manuscript for publication, whether the work is conducted while you are in a student or in a professional role, begin with the end in mind. Choose your topic and the main message you want readers to take away from your work and explore your specific topic through a literature review.

After you have a topic, you still need to make many decisions from other authors to writing technique to citation style. Making these decisions before starting to write will make the process easier and more streamlined.

While reading this appendix be sure to review Box D-1, which contains terminology related to scholarly writing and word processing software.

Researching the Paper Topic

Once you choose a topic, start a comprehensive literature review to narrow the paper topic. The paper topic should add to the body of knowledge for nursing. When narrowing down your topic, look for gaps in the literature, meaning topics or areas that are not thoroughly covered by current information in the literature.

Chapter 7 provides detailed guidance for how to use resources such as electronic databases to conduct an initial broad literature search using keywords. In summary, focus on articles published by journals most relevant to your topic of interest or journals in which you would like to publish your paper. Limit your search to include the most recent (5 to 7 years) peer-reviewed literature available on your topic. Only use older literature in the case of seminal work. It is permissible to use sources that are not peer-reviewed or sources found using a general-topic search engine such as Google, but you must do so judiciously and thoroughly evaluate the source for reliability and trustworthiness (Portillo et al., 2021).

Authors

Once you have narrowed down your topic, decide what other authors to include in your writing project. Imagine you wrote an original academic paper on the opioid epidemic for a big project in nursing school and now you want to adapt that paper with a narrower focus for publication. You did all the research and wrote the original paper yourself, but many other people supported your work, including the writing center and your advisor. In addition, you interviewed several people who use drugs and nurses working at a local rehabilitation clinic. How will you decide whom to invite to contribute to the manuscript you will submit for publication? If you ask your advisor and one of the nurses from the clinic, how will you decide in what order to list the names?

Authorship should not be given to someone just because they are a supervisor or advisor. Rather, anyone who has contributed significantly to your journal article should be included as an author. Authors also share responsibility

BOX D-1 Scholarly Manuscript Terminology

Abstract
First part of a scholarly paper that summarizes the information presented in the paper includes a summary of each of the sections in the body of the paper and should contain the most important keywords that help others find the paper in an electronic database

Bibliography
List of all the materials that have been consulted during research, including references that are not cited in the body of the text

Citation
A brief callout to an original source (reference) that appears in the body of the text of a scholarly paper; each in-text citation corresponds to an entry in a reference list at the end of the paper

Header
A section located within the top margin of each page of a document; information in headers could include page numbers and/or article title

Keywords
Words that capture the most important aspects of a paper such as the topic or problem, population, methods or solutions, and findings; they are used in databases to index and retrieve papers

Margins
The white space around the edge of a word processing document; APA style uses 1-inch margins

Page break
A code inserted in a document by the word processor that is used to separate each of the sections; even if additional text or pages are inserted above the page break, everything below it will always start on a new page

Paragraph headings
Topics and subtopics that create organization and flow in a paper together with an outline support usability for all readers by facilitating understanding of a document's hierarchy

Peer-reviewed
A source (such as a journal article) that has been reviewed by experts in the field of the topic prior to publication to assure that the information is valid, applicable, pertinent, and current

Reference
Outside source of information that is used to provide support for writing may include journal articles, books, websites, seminars, etc., listed at the end of a scholarly paper

Seminal work
A literature source that is well known or classic or is the only research on a specific topic; literature source should be current (past 5 to 7 years) but can be older in the case of seminal work

Style
A specific set of rules used to format a paper and cite and credit resources; provides a familiar structure that assists the reader in understanding the information in the text; common styles used in academic and professional writing include American Psychological Association (APA), Modern Language Association (MLA), and American Medical Association (AMA)

(Continued)

> **BOX D-1 Manuscript Terminology** *(Continued)*
>
> **Table of contents**
> A table that includes the main headings used in a paper and the associated page numbers
>
> **Theoretical framework**
> Explanation of previous theories and how they may apply to the study; supports the importance of the thesis statement and shows where it can fill in knowledge or practice gaps
>
> **Thesis statement**
> The main argument of the paper: included in the introduction
>
> **Track changes**
> Feature in Word that keeps track of suggested revisions by all collaborators
>
> **Writing bias**
> Language that others might interpret as favoritism toward or prejudice against people or ideas; examples include terminology used for labels, sex, age, sexual orientation, racial and ethnic identity, and disabilities; avoid writing bias by including characteristics and differences only relevant to your topic

and accountability for the work. A paper is the culmination of designing the study, collecting, and analyzing data and writing the paper. Consider a contributor an author if they have participated in at least two of these steps to publication. You can always list contributors in the acknowledgements section if they do not qualify as authors. If there is more than one author, you will need to decide who will be the corresponding author. This person lists their email address and is responsible for responding to any questions about the article.

If there is more than one author on your manuscript, it is important to determine each author's responsibilities before writing begins. The order in which authors appear on a manuscript matters because it ultimately influences an author's professional reputation. The level of responsibility for each author determines, in part, the order in which the authors are listed on a paper. In nursing, the author listed first is the person who contributed the most to the article (other fields like molecular biology put the most important author last).

The American Psychological Association (APA) organization offers resources for negotiating authorship (2022), and the International Committee of Medical Journal Editors (ICMJE) provides definitions of roles and responsibilities for authors and contributors to journal articles (2022). ICMJE states that all authors must meet all four of the following criteria:

1. Make substantial contributions to all aspects of the work
2. Contribute to writing and revising the work
3. Give final approval for publication
4. Agree to be responsible for the quality of work

Any contributor who is not listed as an author should be mentioned in the acknowledgements section of your paper. These contributors could include anyone that mentored or assisted in the paper or research. If you received help from someone who did not contribute directly to the paper but influenced it in a significant way, include a short statement acknowledging that individual in the paper. In the example, you might mention the names of the people you interviewed after obtaining their permission. Review the journal author guidelines to learn whether and how they use acknowledgement statements.

Outlining the Paper Topic

After you identify and research the topic, create an outline for your paper that includes the main topics. The first topic on your outline should be a description of the problem, question, or situation that gets the reader interested, and the last topic should be an answer to the question, solution to

> **BOX D-2** Sample Outline for Opioid Epidemic Manuscript
>
> General idea: Nursing interventions for supporting people who use drugs during the opioid epidemic
>
> I. Background
>   A. Why is the opioid epidemic a problem?
>   B. What are the traditional ways of dealing with the opioid epidemic?
>   C. What are some nursing interventions for dealing with patients who use drugs?
>   D. Why do we need to change the way we do things?
> II. Methods
>   A. Describe how the literature review was done
>   1. What literature databases were used?
>   2. What search parameters were used?
>   B. Describe interviews
>   1. People who use drugs: how they were found, what questions were asked
>   2. Rehabilitation clinic employees: general description of place and people, what questions were asked
> III. Results
>   A. Compare and contrast what was found in the literature review and provide synthesis or analysis of the articles
>   B. Discuss results from the interviews
> IV. Discussion
>   A. Explain what nursing interventions will work
>   B. Call for advocacy for this issue: provide resources and links
> V. Conclusion

the problem, or explanation of the situation that resolves the issues brought up at the beginning of the paper. All topics in the middle of the outline should be supporting evidence and further elaboration that directly relate to the main topic of the paper. It may be tempting to skip the outline process, but it is an essential step in the process of writing (Johnson & Rulo, 2019). Continuing with the previous example in which you have already written an academic paper on the opioid epidemic, your ideas are already organized. You can still create an outline to organize additional topics and develop more on some of the original topics (Box D-2).

Writing the Manuscript

As you begin to write, your goal is to develop each point on your outline. Do not worry about writing perfect sentences on the first attempt. Simply write down all your thoughts. You do not need to begin with the introduction; in fact, many authors write the introduction after they have written the rest of the paper. Begin with one of the headings you created in your outline and type what you know on that topic, making note of areas that need additional research or information. With word processing software you can write, format, edit, rearrange, and delete sections from your paper with ease.

When writing scholarly manuscripts, expository writing is the primary style used. It informs, explains, or describes, answering the questions, "what," "why," and "how." Other writing techniques include descriptive, narrative, and persuasive. While elements of these will be used within your paper, they will not be the primary technique.

Reducing Writing Bias

Writing bias occurs when an author chooses language others might interpret as favoritism toward or prejudice against people or ideas. General recommendations from experts include focusing on specific characteristics and differences relevant to your topic and choosing and defining sensitive labels (APA Style, 2022c).

An example that might come from research on the opioid epidemic includes the language used to describe the people who use drugs that you interviewed. Words like "addict" or "drug abuser" should not be used due to the stigma associated with those terms (National Institute on Drug Abuse, 2021). Instead, use *"people with substance use disorder."* If terminology is relatively new, you may need to explain why you are using a new term instead of one that has been used for many years. The APA's *Inclusive Language Guide* may be helpful to identify and correct writing bias (APA, 2023).

APA Style

Style refers to a specific set of rules used to format a paper, cite, and credit resources. There are many citation and formatting styles used by scholarly journals. The most common styles used for academic and professional papers include APA, Modern Language Association (MLA), and American Medical Association (AMA). MLA is used in humanities such as English and literature. Physicians writing in the medical field use AMA. APA is the style most used in the social and health sciences, including nursing.

The *Publication Manual of the American Psychological Association* describes APA publication style for authoring scholarly papers, and it serves as a style guide for many nursing programs, journals, and textbooks. It is ideal to obtain a copy of the most current APA *Publication Manual*, but you can also use the official APA website (apastyle.apa.org) as a quick reference. APA provides reliable online tutorials and resources, including the APA Style blog and the Journal Article Reporting Standards (JARS) website. Students may find the *Student Sample* and *Professional Sample* papers especially helpful for formatting papers and understanding the differences between the two types of papers (APA Style, 2022d).

APA style dictates numerous writing techniques, word choices, spellings, and other writing decisions. For example, typically speaking, scientific writing uses the third person point of view, in which the writer does not include themselves within the writing (i.e., does not use "I"). However, when writing in APA style, the first-person point of view can be used (e.g., "I researched …"). Be careful not to write as if the study itself did the research. For example, instead of writing, "the study reported," write "After reading the study, I found…" APA style also encourages using the active voice when writing, instead of passive voice. A sentence is in the active voice when the subject of the sentence performs the action ("I conducted the experiment."). A sentence is in the passive voice when the subject of the sentence is acted on by the verb ("The experiment was conducted."). These are just two examples of writing conventions explained in APA style. The full *Publication Manual* or the APA style website should be consulted when making decisions on writing techniques. Regardless of what style you use, the most important rules to follow are ultimately the ones in the author guidelines for the journal in which you want to publish. Throughout the rest of this chapter, you will find additional tips for APA formatting since this is the style used most often in nursing.

An APA style paper includes four main sections: title page, abstract, body of the paper, and reference list. The body of the paper is the longest section and has multiple subsections within it. It is generally written first, and a reference list is built as the paper is written. The title and abstract are often the final parts created.

Parts of a Paper

This discusses the elements of an effective abstract and introduction as well as the components found in the middle or body of the manuscript. You will learn basic concepts of writing about background information, literature review, methods, and results. Tables and figures will also be discussed. The discussion of the results involves critical thinking and tells the reader how your research adds to current knowledge. It may contain limitations (what you were unable to accomplish and why). An effective conclusion brings everything together and a list of references for all the information cited in your manuscript is included.

Before you read this section, find a published article from a journal that interests you and follow along as you read about the parts. Published articles do not always follow APA style, and sometimes the parts of the paper can be tricky to find, but if you follow along with a published example, it will help familiarize you with the process. As you write your paper, you can use a checklist to be sure you are hitting the main content and formatting points (Table D-1).

Title

The title is a key piece of information that helps the reader find the paper in databases and understand what it is about. The title should be concise and meaningful, and it should contain the most important keywords. For these reasons, it may be best to write the paper before making a final decision on the title. The literature provides mixed recommendations about creating paper titles, but general guidelines are to keep the title around 10 to 12 words, providing just enough essential information to state specifically what the paper is about (Bahadoran et al, 2019).

APA style requires a title page. An APA-formatted title page has a running head (for professional papers), page number, paper title, author name, and institutional affiliation (APA, 2020). Keep in mind, however, that the author guidelines for the journal in which you want to publish may provide different directions.

Abstract and Keywords

The abstract summarizes the information presented in the paper. According to Greer and Wingo (2017), abstracts are "highly strategic mini-stories that create a first impression of a researcher's work and position it effectively to those who matter" (p. 37). The abstract should include a summary of each of the sections in the body of the paper and describe the question or problem; a discussion about potential approaches to resolving the problem or methods to answer the question; the findings or results; and a final response to the question or problem (Bahadoran et al., 2020).

The abstract should contain the most important keywords that help others find the paper in an electronic database. Choose keywords that capture the most important aspects of the paper such as the topic or problem, population, methods or solutions, and findings. Keywords are used in databases to index and retrieve papers when readers search for them. Nurse scholars are highly motivated to help others find and cite their work, and a good title and keywords are essential to that process.

In a word processor when using APA style, center the word "Abstract" in bold font on the first line of the first page. The abstract is a single paragraph, and the first line is not indented (APA Style, n.d.). (All other new paragraphs in the body of the paper are indented.) On the next line following the abstract, indent and italicize the word (with the colon) "Keywords:". The keywords are then listed in lowercase, regular font style, and separated by commas. See the sample papers on the APA Style website for examples (APA Style, 2022d).

Introduction

The body of a paper begins with an introduction and ends with a conclusion. The introduction includes the specific purpose or thesis statement of the paper. The introduction should be clear, concise, and provide a roadmap of how you develop the purpose for the paper. The introduction is an important part of the paper because it is an overview of everything the paper contains. For this reason, it is often written last.

An introduction includes background information on the topic demonstrating why the thesis is important. For a manuscript on nursing interventions for the opioid crisis, you would need to provide evidence that there is a problem and how nurses are uniquely positioned to solve the problem. You may also include a review of the literature which involves critical analysis of research findings on your topic, for example, for evidence-based interventions published in the last 5 years that have reduced death from opioid overdose for people with substance use disorder. Establishing the general and specific context of existing knowledge demonstrates how research builds on that knowledge. You do not have to conduct experimental research to write a manuscript for publication. Many manuscripts are literature reviews conducted by students in an academic setting. When and if you are asked to do a literature review on a topic of interest, keep in mind that you could turn what you learn into a publication.

In a word processor using APA style, you will begin the body of the paper on page 3 with the title of the paper in bold, centered, and in title case. The first paragraph under the title will be

TABLE D-1 Basic Checklist for an APA Paper

Item	Check
Title page is formatted correctly and has an appropriate page header.	
Abstract begins on a separate page with a new header.	
Body of paper starts on a separate page and includes the paper title.	
Spell and grammar checker is used.	
Section headings are formatted for the appropriate heading level.	
All abbreviations used are formatted correctly.	
Acronyms are spelled out the first time they are used.	
In-text citations are near the information they support.	
In-text citations are in parentheses and contain author last names and date (one or two authors, or ", et al." after first author when there are three or more authors).	
Reference list begins on a separate page and is formatted using hanging indent.	
Citations and references match (in text and in reference list) and are formatted according to required style.	
Read each paragraph, preferably aloud to yourself, to verify flow of ideas.	
Ask a secondary reader to review and provide feedback.	
Tables and figures are formatted in APA style and have a number and title.	
All tables and figures are referred to in the body of the paper.	
Select "All Markup" under "Track Changes" to ensure all edits and comments have been deleted before submission.	

the introduction. It does not need a heading of "Introduction" unless the journal requires it. Indent all first lines in each of the body paragraphs, unless APA style requires different formatting (e.g., for a direct quote or heading). Paragraph headings (such as "Theoretical Framework") assist the reader in visualizing and understanding the organization of the paper. When writing the paper, pay attention to paragraph length. If a paragraph is shorter than three sentences or longer than half a page, consider combining or breaking the paragraphs in different places. Grouping text in paragraphs of reasonable length supports readability and comprehension. Each sentence in a paragraph should relate to the topic sentence or theme of the paragraph.

Methods

A methods section tells the reader how to duplicate the study. If you have done a literature review, the methods section will tell the reader what keywords you used, what years you limited your search to, and what databases you searched. You will describe how many articles you found, which ones you decided to use, and the reasoning for why you included them in your study. If you conducted an experimental study, describe your subjects, how they were selected, and if you had to obtain institutional review board (IRB) approval for your research (needed for research studies if there is a potential that subjects might be negatively impacted by the study for protection of human rights). In addition, describe how data was collected, stored, and secured. Any statistics performed on your data will also be described.

Results

The results (also known as findings) section in a research paper describes what you found when you analyzed your data. If you have done a literature review, this is where you will tell the reader how the articles you reviewed support or do not support your thesis statement. For example, if you reviewed the literature looking for evidence-based nursing interventions for people with substance use disorder, you will describe what interventions you found and if they meet the criteria you set up in your methods section. If you have conducted experimental research, you will tell the reader the results of your statistical analysis and if the results support the thesis statement. For example, if you tested the impact of mobile recovery outreach teams on the number of deaths from overdose, this is where you would report your findings.

Discussion

Every manuscript will need a discussion of the findings. This starts by restating the question or idea being explored and then describing how the findings fit in with the research. Was the initial question answered? If not, why not? Was the problem solved or was a new solution found? Think of yourself as a salesperson; this is your final pitch. You need to convince the reader to believe in your statements. In the opioid epidemic example, the initial idea was to find innovative nursing interventions to support those with substance use disorder. The goal is ultimately to prevent people from dying from an overdose. In the discussion, you will need to state how what you found from your search of the literature or your interviews support your ideas.

The discussion should also include any unexpected results, explanations for changes made in the approach, and any limitations to the research. Limitations include things like participants dropping out, a small number of participants, issues with interviews, or study methods. A limitation for the opioid study might be that you were only able to interview two people with substance use disorder and one of them seemed unreliable. Limitations are often outside the researcher's control but acknowledging them is a way to strengthen the argument by identifying the weaknesses before someone else does. Another term sometimes used is delimitations or exclusion criteria. In this example, it would be an explanation of why you included only two people for your interview.

Tables and Figures

Use tables and figures when they present large amounts of information or complex ideas in images better than text. The purpose of tables and figures is to help the reader understand the paper, so use the opportunities that tables and figures offer to present a visualization of data and information that would not otherwise be achievable through text (APA Style, 2019). Always refer to and explain information in tables and figures within the text. Check style and formatting guidelines (especially author guidelines for journal article submissions) for special requirements and example tables and figure captions. The placement and formatting of the tables and figures differ with the type of academic papers, online journal, and print journal.

Author guidelines may specify placing the tables and figures at the end of the manuscript after the reference list or submitting tables and figures as separate files. Note the placement in your manuscript between paragraphs where you want the tables, boxes, or figures to display, but be aware that the publisher may or may not use the suggested placement. If your manuscript is accepted for publication, it is best practice for journals to send a proof of the article showing how it will appear in print for your approval.

If a table or figure was previously published anywhere, such as a journal, textbook, or website, you must obtain the permission from the copyright holder for use in your manuscript. If the figure was originally published in a journal or book, you should contact the publisher, not the author. When the publisher accepts a manuscript for publication, the associated images become the property of the publisher. Some items do not require permission, such as those from government sources (e.g., Centers for Disease Control and Prevention or National Institutes of Health). Look for guidelines for reproduction of any figures or other resources on the pages where they were originally published. In all cases, whether you need to obtain permission for reuse or not, you must cite the source of the figure and include any necessary permission information.

Conclusion

The conclusion provides a visual signal to the reader that the paper is ending. It is a summary of the important points of the paper, but it does more than simply restating everything that was said. It is the final opportunity to show the reader the practical implications of the findings and how the work fits into the bigger picture of all other literature on the topic. A conclusion can also contain recommendations for future research or what the next steps are to find a solution to the problem. For the paper on the opioid epidemic, you might state that your next steps will be to interview more people with substance use disorder or to test one of the interventions in an outpatient clinic. A conclusion should deliver a strong impact with a small number of words. Most conclusions are just a few sentences to a couple of paragraphs long.

References

Citation of research sources provide evidence to the reader that you have based your assertions on scientific or scholarly evidence and the work of scholars that have gone before you. Citations give credit to the scholars who generated the evidence, and it also helps the reader find the original source for the evidence you are citing. Your readers will want to know what evidence on which you based your assertion, and they may want to find the original source to explore on their own whether the evidence is sound and generated by rigorous research and scholarly expertise.

A reference is an outside source of information used to provide support for writing. A citation is a brief callout to a reference that appears in the body of the text of a scholarly paper. In APA style, this is done with the author's last name and year inside parentheses. Other styles, like AMA, use superscript numbers in the paper that correspond to a numbered reference list at the end of the paper. The reference list appears immediately after the conclusion and contains all the sources cited in the text. All in-text citations must appear in the reference list, and all references in the reference list must be cited somewhere in the paper (APA Style, 2022e). Do not include references that you did not cite in your paper unless an instructor or editor directs you to do so. Of note, a reference list is not the same thing as a bibliography. A bibliography includes all the materials that have been consulted during your research, including references that are not cited in the body of the text. A bibliography is sometimes required in student work but not always in scholarly publications.

In a word processor when using APA style, the section name "References" should be in bold separate from the body of the paper using a page break. APA style requires using a special kind of indentation called a hanging indent for each reference. Hanging indent means the first line of the reference is not indented but all the subsequent lines are. To format the reference list in Microsoft Word, go to the "Home" tab and expand the "Paragraph" section in the menu bar (Fig. D-1). Then select "hanging indent" under the special drop-down. Do not simulate the appearance of hanging indent using the space or tab key because doing so will cause problems with the appearance of your document when opened in other file formats, on other computers, or in other applications.

In today's information-rich environment, there are a wide variety of information (e.g., books, journals, web documents, conference presentations, video, emails) and a growing number of ways to transmit information (e.g., print, audio, video, electronic files). There are specific rules for formatting various types of references, and APA documentation covers almost every possible type and format for communication. Even those that are not covered follow a specific convention with four elements aimed at identifying the original source: author, date, title, and source (APA Style, 2022b). Using a consistent style to format citations, and references create a common framework among scholars for understanding types of sources and where to find them. Although it is tempting to copy and paste preformatted citations and references from other sources (or to use reference manager applications or online citation generators), this strategy often produces errors in APA format for new writers. It is better to develop skills in creating APA-style citations and references first. The APA style website and the APA *Publication Manual* cover citations and the reference list in extensive detail. Once you are able to easily spot errors and problems in reference list formatting, then you can explore digital options for speeding up the work of creating citations and references.

WORD PROCESSING FEATURES

To work efficiently and focus on writing, use a word processing tool to write your paper. If a commercial word processing application is not available to you, use one of the free cloud computing apps. Microsoft Word is a popular word processing

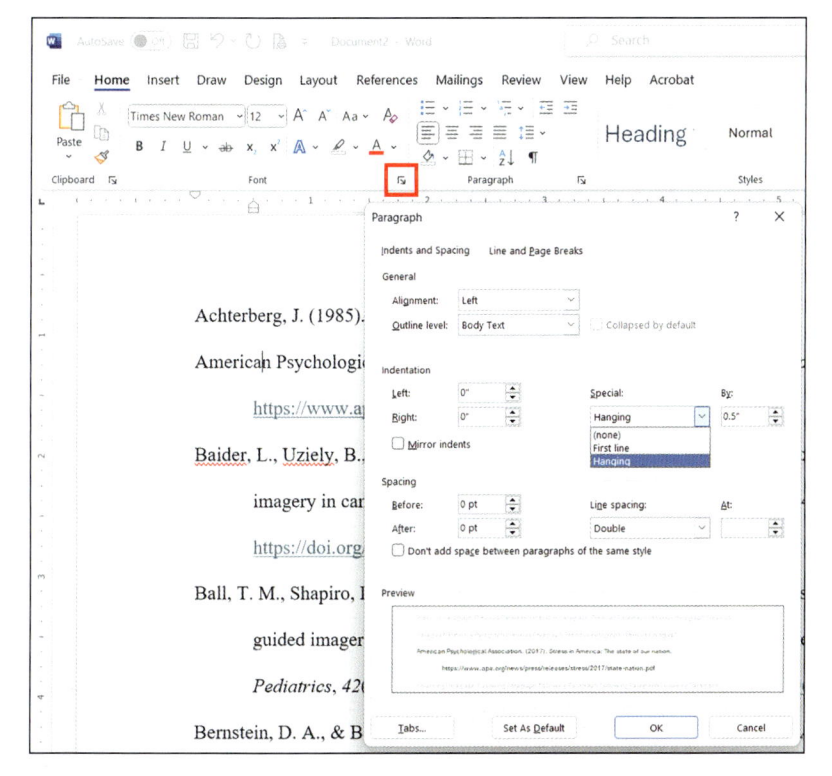

Figure D-1. Adding a hanging indent.

application among nurse scholars and will be used for the examples in this chapter.

Foundational word processing skills are essential for nurses who want to communicate their work to colleagues and stakeholders and produce scholarly writing in the most efficient and effective manner. Word processing applications have many features and tools to support successful writing. Some features you might find helpful are described in the following sections, but information and tutorials about other features can be found online.

To familiarize yourself with the features in Word, open a blank document and create a sample manuscript with a mock title, an outline with several headings, and some text. You can copy and paste text from anywhere into this sample document just to try out the features. You could also download one of the sample papers from the APA Style website to experiment with (APA Style, 2022d). Keep your document open so you can continue adding mock content and trying out the features discussed below.

As you work through this section, you may have additional questions about the tools and features in the specific word processing application you are using. The availability, location, and function of specific features vary in each application and tend to change over time as improvements are made to the application. There are two good sources for help with almost any word processor, regardless of operating system, application, and feature:

1. Look for the "Help" option in your word processor and search for the feature of interest. (In Word, the "Help" tab opens a menu bar.)
2. Search for help online using search terms that include the name of your word processing application and the feature you want to explore.

Formatting a Document

When using APA style in a word processing program, there are several general requirements for formatting that you should adhere to. APA requires a document to be double-spaced, have 1-inch margins, and use a legible font such as size 12 Times New Roman or size 11 Calibri. The font and spacing can be easily adjusted in the menu bar of the "Home" tab (Fig. D-2). However, there are often multiple ways to set the format in Word. For example, to adjust the margins, you can go to the "Layout" tab and select "Margins" from the menu bar (Fig. D-3). You can also type "margins" in the search bar at the top of the screen, which will also take you to a drop-down menu. Finally, if you have the ruler showing in your document, you can drag the margin markers to the left or right to adjust

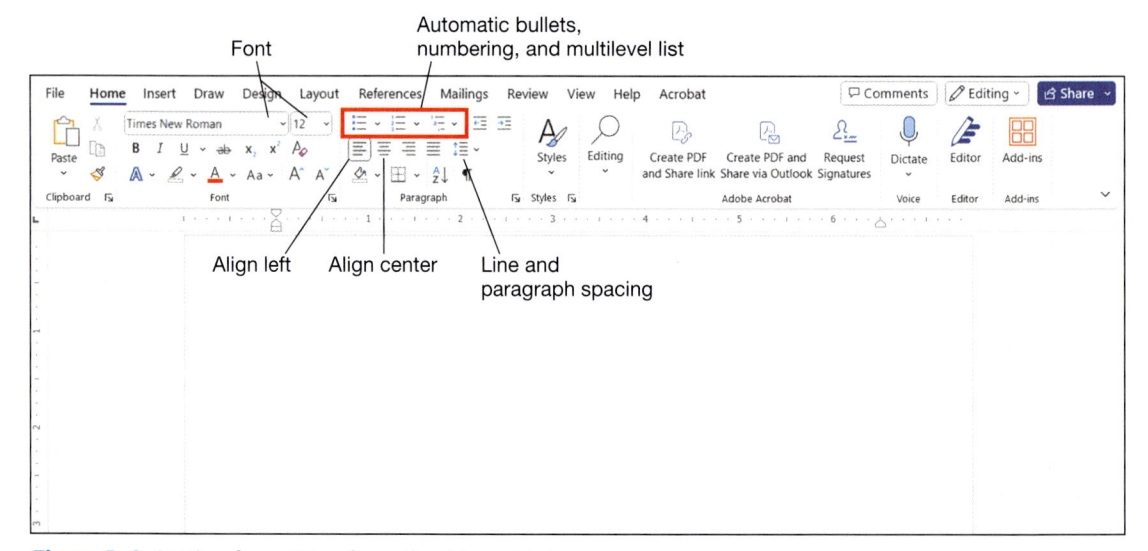

Figure D-2. Setting formatting from the "Home" tab.

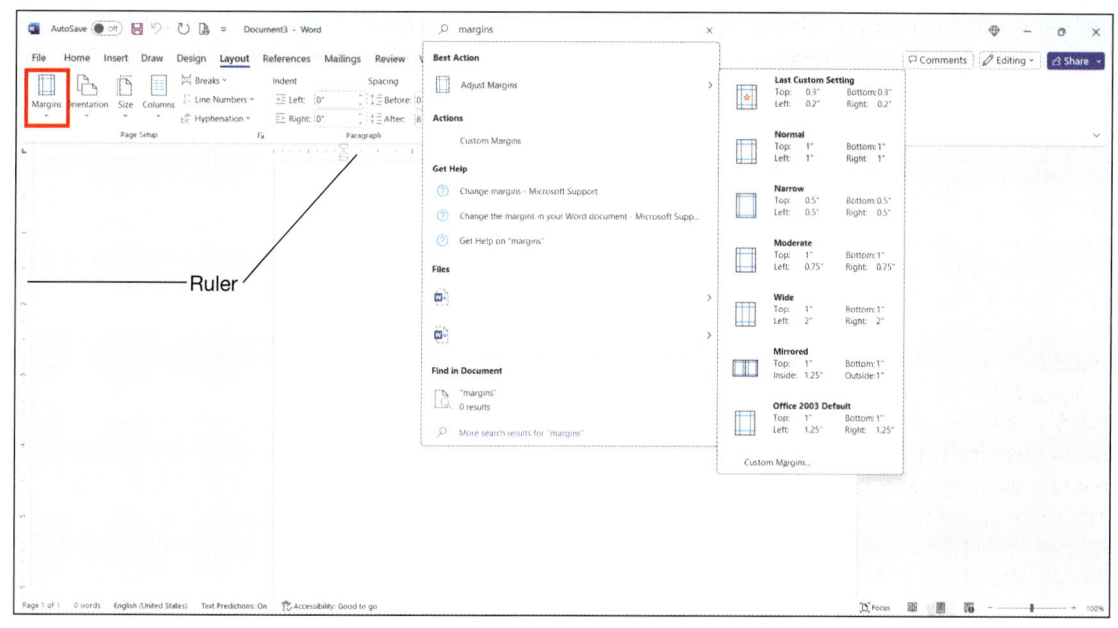

Figure D-3. Multiple ways to adjust margins in Word.

them manually. Word is a good option as a word processor because it is user-friendly, allowing you to access functions in multiple ways.

For the body of the paper, each regular paragraph should be indented 0.5 inch from the left margin. If this is not already set as a default, you can adjust the tab in the "Paragraph" menu shown in Fig D-1. Do not use the space bar to mimic an indent because it will result in formatting and printing irregularities. The title and certain headings will be centered on the page, but the body of the paper should be aligned to the left margin (this is called "left-justified" or "align left") (see Fig. D-2). The right margin will be uneven (i.e., text on the right side of the paper will appear "ragged" rather than evenly aligned along the right margin).

For additional help with APA formatting style, use an APA template in Word. Select the "New" icon on the left side, which shows a menu of template options. Type "APA" in the search bar and you can create your document using this template or experiment within it to get used to the APA style (Fig. D-4). You can also refer to the sample papers on the APA website (APA Style, 2022d).

Paragraph Headings

In addition to creating organization and flow in a paper, creating an outline allows you to identify paragraph headings, which are topics and subtopics discussed in the paper. You can create a thorough outline, and then match your paper to that hierarchy, but you may also identify paragraph headings as you write the text, and then add those to your outline. Headings help the reader anticipate the topic of discussion in the section, and they support usability for all readers by facilitating understanding of a document's hierarchy (APA Style, 2022a). Use of paragraph heading styles also makes your document more accessible to readers who use a screen reader. Word also uses paragraph headings to generate a table of contents, which you may or may not need for your paper.

The ""Styles" tool is used to format each paragraph heading to represent the appropriate level in the document hierarchy. You can use existing heading styles available in Word, which you view by expanding the box in the "Styles" area of the "Home" tab (Fig. D-5). If none of the existing styles work for your needs, you can customize or create new styles. Table D-2 shows examples of heading

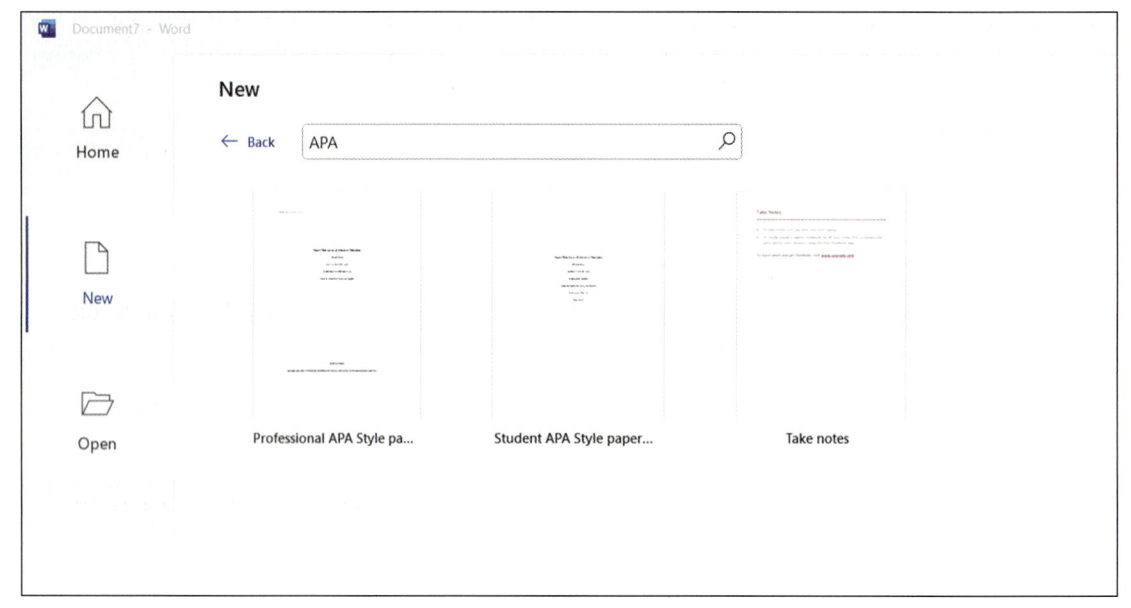

Figure D-4. Finding an APA template in Word.

styles from APA. In the sample document you have opened, create a new heading style to match one of these headings. Expand the "Styles" section in the menu bar with the icon, and then in the menu that comes up, select the "add style" button (Fig. D-6). Give the style a name in the top box, set the style elements (font, alignment, etc.), and select "New documents based on this template" at the bottom to save the style for future documents. This process takes only a few minutes and can save a great deal of time in formatting current and future APA style papers.

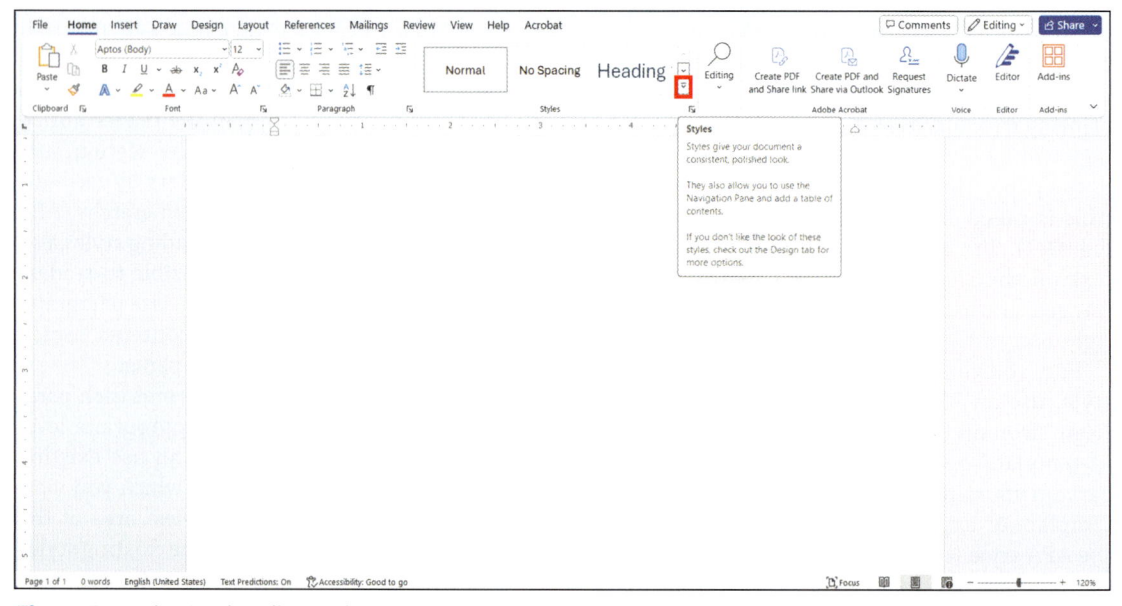

Figure D-5. Viewing heading styles.

TABLE D-2 Formatting APA Headings

Heading Level	APA Formatting
1 (and paper title)	**Title Case, Centered, Bold**
2	**Title Case, Flush Left, Bold**
3	***Title Case, Flush Left, Bold, Italic***
4	**Title Case, Indented, Bold, Ends with a Period.** Paragraph text begins on the same line.
5	***Title Case, Indented, Bold, Italic, Ends with a Period.*** Paragraph text begins on the same line.

Data from American Psychological Association. (2020). *Publication manual of the American Psychological Association* (7th ed.).

Now that you have set paragraph heading styles, Word can automatically generate a table of contents with page numbers. Type "Table of Contents" in the search bar at the top of Word for additional assistance.

Headers

A page header is a separate section located in the top margin of each page of the document (whereas a footer is located at the bottom). Depending on the audience for the paper (e.g., instructor, workplace supervisor, journal editor), a page header may or may not be needed. Typically, APA-style professional papers have a running head and student papers do not (Adams, 2020). In APA style, the running head is an abbreviated paper title of no more than 50 characters appearing in all capital letters. Always check with your instructor or review the journal submission guidelines for paper formatting requirements.

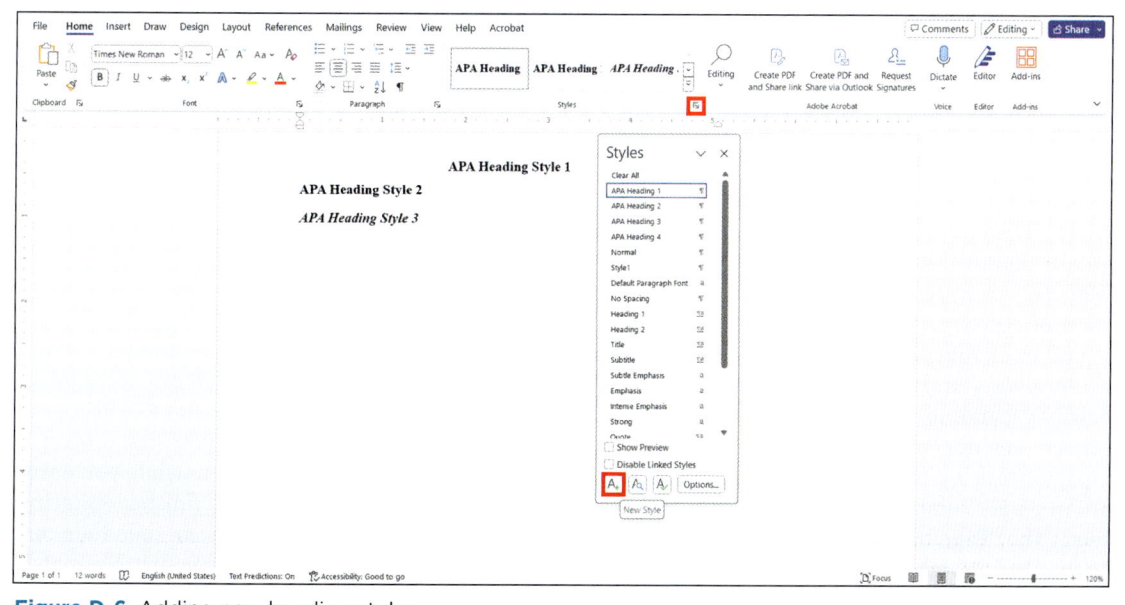

Figure D-6. Adding new heading styles.

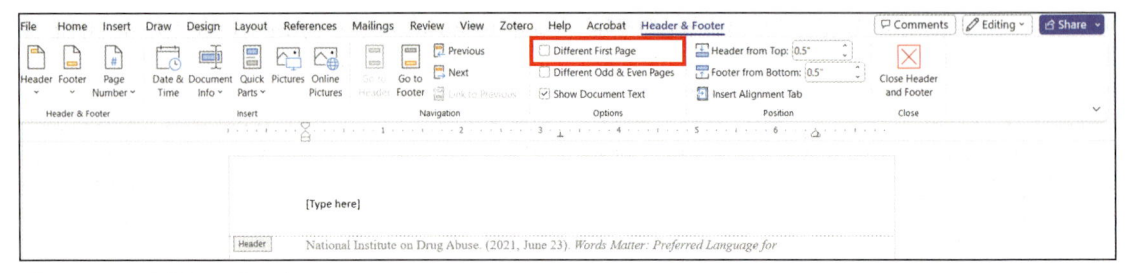

Figure D-7. Editing a header.

In addition to a running head, APA style calls for page numbers on all pages, including the first (title) page. If you are required to have a different first page for your document that does not include a running head or page numbers, in Word there is a checkbox for "Different first page" in the "Header & Footer" menu bar (Fig. D-7).

You may find that the "Header & Footer" tab is not visible in your Word document. To access that tab, either double click in the header area, or go to the "Insert" tab to the "Header." From there, you can select a preformatted header, or select "Edit header" to create your own. Format the header so that the running head is flush left and the page number is flush right on the same line. Once the header is created, double click on the main (body) part of the document to close the header editor and continue as usual with document editing.

Page Breaks

A page break separates a new section on a separate page by forcing the end of one page and starting any additional text on the next. For example, if you want your reference list to start on a new page, you can add a page break following the end of the body of the paper. Page breaks should be used instead of tapping the "Return" or "Enter" key many times to force the start of a new page. The page break allows you to add to or subtract from the body of the paper while always starting your reference list on a new page; adding the lines with the "Return" or "Enter" key does not. When using Word, insert a page break by tapping "Ctrl" (or "Command" on an Apple computer) + "Enter". You can also select the "Page break" button in the menu bar of the "Insert" tab.

Automatic Numbering

Word processors have automatic bullet and number features that allow you to generate a numbered or bulleted list quickly. Like most word processor features, you can apply the feature before or after you enter the text. If you type the number 1, a period, and a space and then enter text, most word processors assume by default that you are creating a numbered list and will automatically enter the number 2, a period, and space on the next line when you press the "Enter" key. To stop automatic numbering, select the text and use the automatic numbering tool from the "Home" tab menu bar (see Fig. D-2) to choose the format you need. To create a hierarchal multilevel list, use that button from the "Home" tab menu bar. You can change the format to multilevel lists before or after you enter any numbers and text. These guidelines also apply to bulleted lists. Automatic numbering saves time and effort in creating a properly formatted numbered list. It is valuable when reordering items in the list because the numbers change automatically, so they remain in sequence. As useful as the automatic bullet and number features are in word processors, it is important to check instructor, journal, and APA guidelines for lists of all kinds to be sure yours are formatted correctly.

Tables

Use the table tool in your word processor to create tables. From the "Insert" tab, you can add a table. Once you have added a table, a new tab will appear called "Table Design". When you first create a table, be sure to show all borders while you enter the table data. When you have finished entering content into the table cells, you can then hide certain borders as needed to make your table match

APA style. In Word, the "Borders" tool in the "Table Design" tab allows you to show or hide borders as well as make some table borders heavier or lighter, depending on the table style you want to achieve (Fig. D-8A). Online resources that demonstrate APA-style table setup are available from many different sources including Microsoft Support and the APA Style website. Alternately, use the table already set up in the Professional Sample paper on the APA Style website (APA Style, 2022d).

If a long table spans across two or more pages, repeat the header rows on each page, which makes it easier for the reader to follow from page to page. Highlight the top row and right click, then select "Table Properties". From this box, you can select "Repeat as header row at the top of each page" (Fig. D-8B).

Figures

Figures are visual representations of data in the form of images, charts, graphs, or any other type of illustrations that help communicate essential information in your paper. Figures differ from tables primarily in that tables display information in rows and columns, whereas figures are based more often on graphics or images. Graphs usually display quantitative data in a visually appealing and understandable format. Diagrams are typically simplified representations of a process or structure. Drawings and images show information using pictures and photographs.

Videos or hyperlinks to videos, as well as other objects, can also be inserted in documents, but you will need to be judicious about how your audience will view your document (online or in print), whether they will have a connection to the internet to view the media, and how it will be displayed to the reader. Videos and interactive objects may not be acceptable as an element in a student paper or a journal article submission. Check with your instructor or journal editor before embedding or hyperlinking to media in your paper.

To display a figure in a document, use the "Insert" menu or drag and drop the graph, chart, diagram, or image into place. Use the formatting tools in the word processor to resize and position the image appropriately in the document. Image formatting tools included in word processors allow you to position the figure to the left or right of your text, or you can wrap text around the image. When working with multiple images, you can align them, layer them, rotate them, and choose from many other options. However, review APA style or check with your instructor or journal submission guidelines for specific requirements for figures.

Spelling and Grammar Check

Word processing programs have built-in spelling and grammar check features that automatically check for errors and make suggestions for replacements. The spelling and grammar check functions are active by default in word processors and can be accessed under the "Review" tab by selecting the "Spelling and Grammar" button in the menu bar. A squiggly red underline is a signal to alert writers about a misspelled word. To make a spelling correction, click on the word to view replacement suggestions (Fig. D-9A). Right-clicking on a misspelled word brings up additional features such as a read aloud option and definitions for the replacements (Fig. D-9B). Spelling and grammar checkers are quite effective but will occasionally miss correctly spelled words that are used incorrectly in the text or they may make suggestions that are not improvements or corrections. Use these tools to support accuracy in your paper but consider each suggestion before accepting it. If in doubt, use online resources such as *Merriam-Webster Collegiate Dictionary* to double check spelling, abbreviation, and hyphenation. Always proofread all documents created in word processors to ensure accurate spelling and appropriate word usage.

Find and Replace

Find and replace is a useful tool available in most word processors (and in many other applications) for locating and editing text. The "Find" feature is accessible in the "Home" tab by selecting "Editing" in the menu bar or by pressing the "Ctrl" (or "Command" on Apple computers) key + F at the same time (Fig. D-10A). It will locate every instance of a set of characters that you type into the find box. The "Find and Replace" feature can replace one set of characters with another. Select "Replace" from the drop-down menu beside the

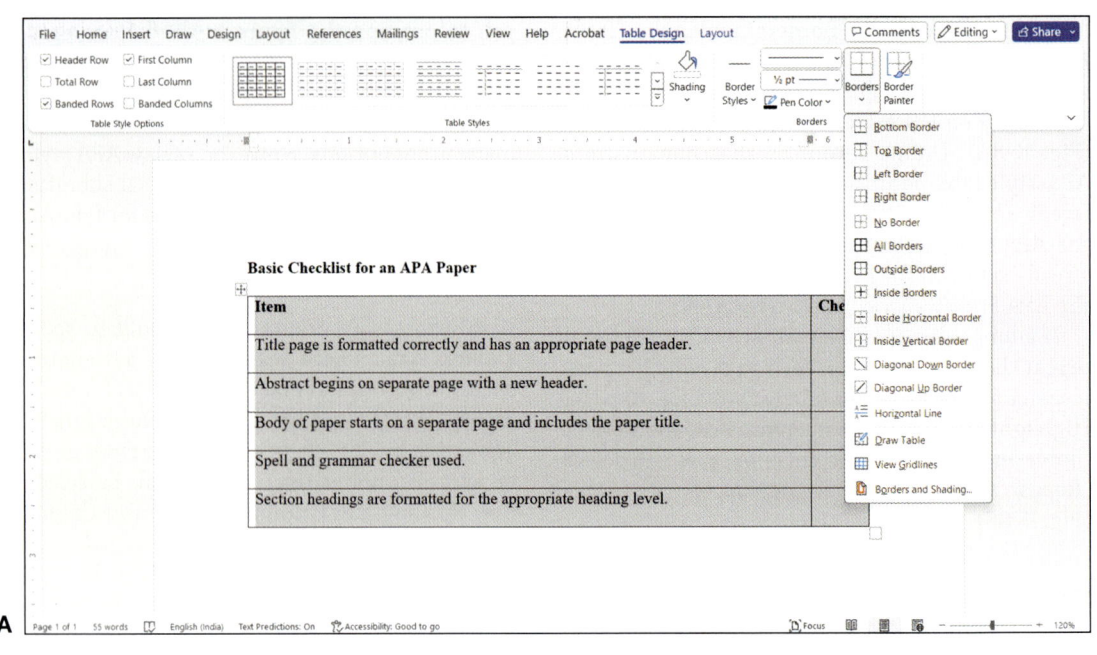

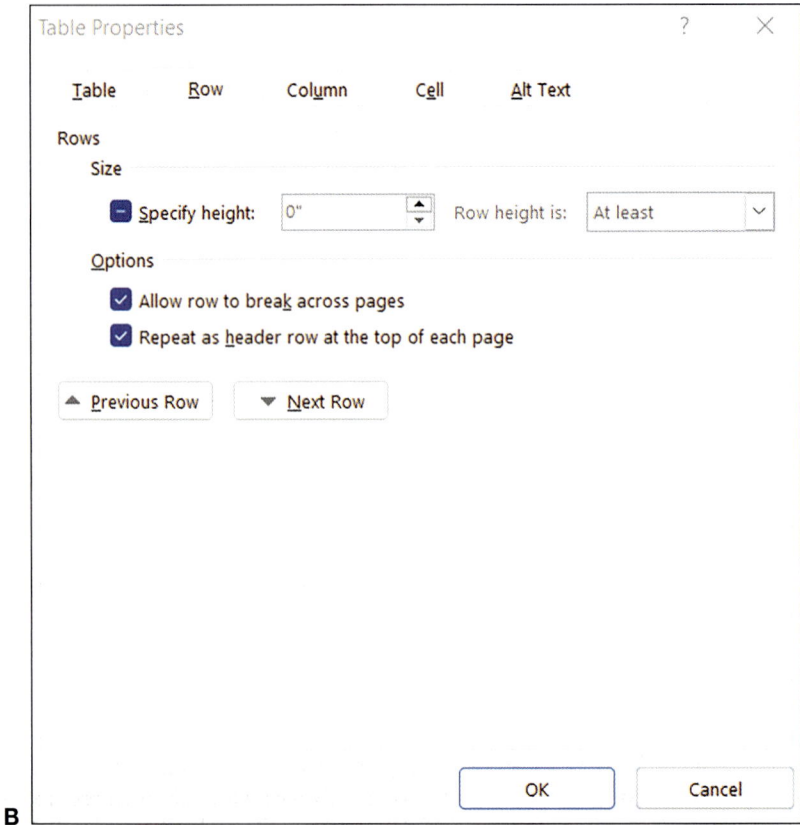

Figure D-8. Formatting a table. **A.** Changing the borders. **B.** Table properties.

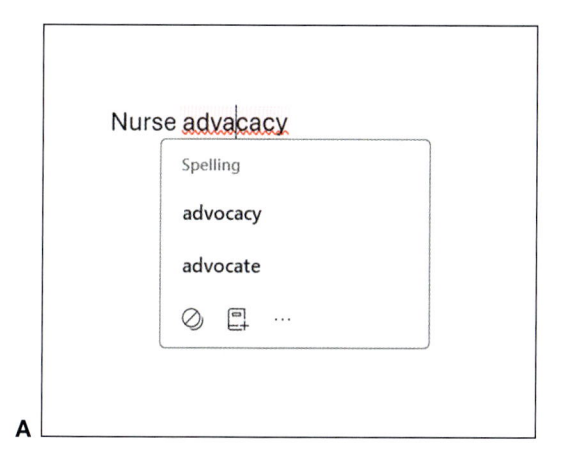

Figure D-9. Viewing spell-check options with a normal mouse click **(A)** versus a right mouse click **(B)**.

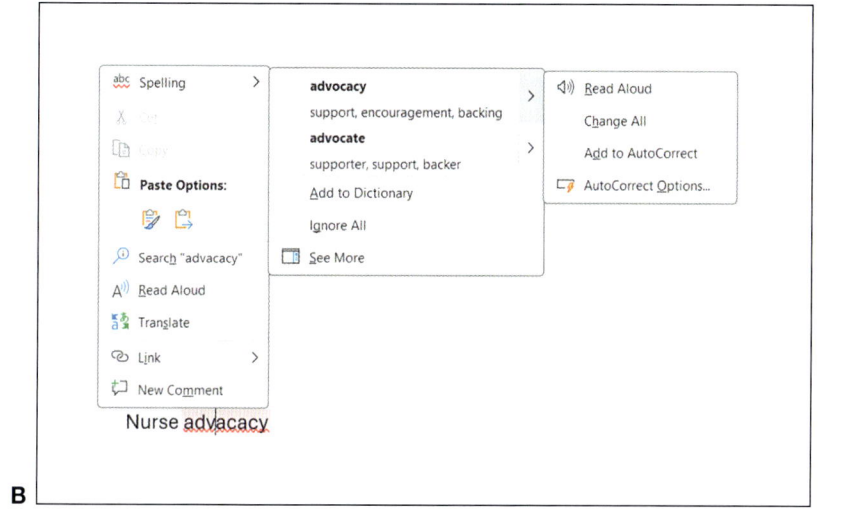

A

B

"Find" box. For example, if you want to replace every instance of the word "nurse" in your document with "registered nurse", type those into the "Find" and "Replace" fields (Fig. D-10B). Then you can make the desired change in your document quickly and without risk of overlooking any instance.

Track Changes Tool

When you need to collaborate with others on a document, the review features in word processors that track changes and allow commenting and feedback are exceptionally useful. In collaborative authoring projects, it is almost essential for all authors to see proposed changes while maintaining the ability to see the original document.

The "Track Changes" feature in Word keeps track of suggested revisions by all collaborators if they are all using Word. (Before you begin a collaborative writing project, agree on one word processing application so that your group can take advantage of this important word processing feature.) When the track changes feature is active, edits and comments display in text of a different color for each author or contributor, and comments display in the right margin of the document.

Access the "Track Changes" tools under the "Review" tab and in the "Tracking" area of the menu bar. From there you can turn tracking on or off, change the look of the tracked changes and switch between different views of an edited document. "All Markup" displays all edits in detail and can become difficult to read after several iterations

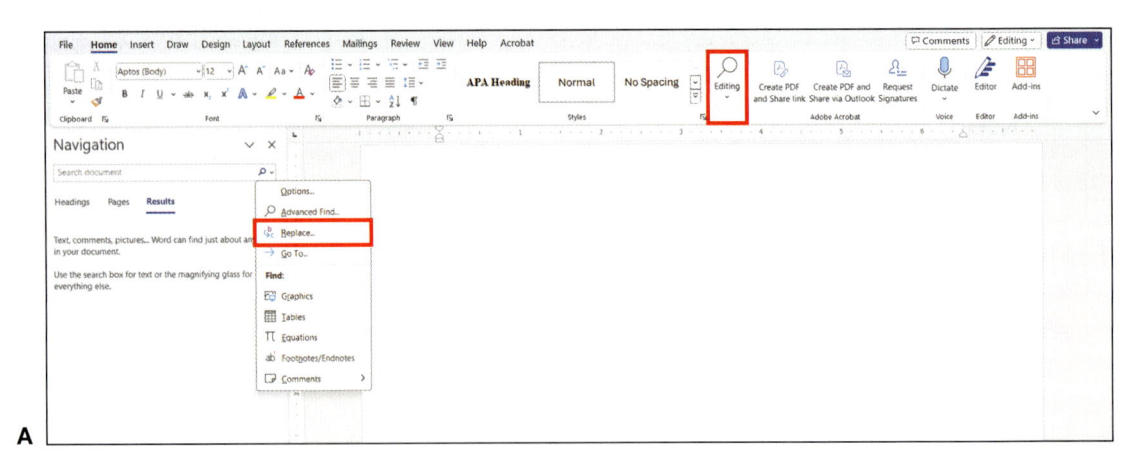

Figure D-10. Accessing the "Find" feature **(A)** and the "Find and Replace" feature **(B)**.

of the document. At that point, the author can switch between "All Markup" and "Simple Markup" as needed for readability. To view a current copy of the document with no editing or markup, select the "No Markup" view. The original view is also preserved among the available views. As editing on the document progresses, individual edits can be accepted or rejected one by one, in individual paper sections, or throughout the entire document.

Cloud word processing applications allow authors to edit a single document, usually synchronously, without needing to email a document file back and forth. Storing your collaborative document online where all authors can access and edit it makes collaborative authorship quite feasible. It is important to know what the effect of simultaneous editing will be in your chosen word processing application. That is, if two people edit a document at the same time (i.e., synchronously), will the word processing program save the changes both people make? This is important to know ahead of time because two or more people may edit a document at the same time during an online meeting of the authors. Be sure you understand how your cloud application behaves on collaborative documents before important edits are lost.

Be careful as you prepare your paper for submission to an instructor or a journal to save a separate copy of the document, accept or reject all edits, delete all comments, and stop tracking changes. The document should be completely free of any remaining markup before sharing with any reader who is not an author or contributor and especially before submission to an instructor or a journal.

Accessibility

Ensuring accessibility of your scholarly documents, whether they appear in print or online, is essential. Checking for accessibility in Word and other prominent word processing applications has become much easier over time. The feature that checks for accessibility will automatically review

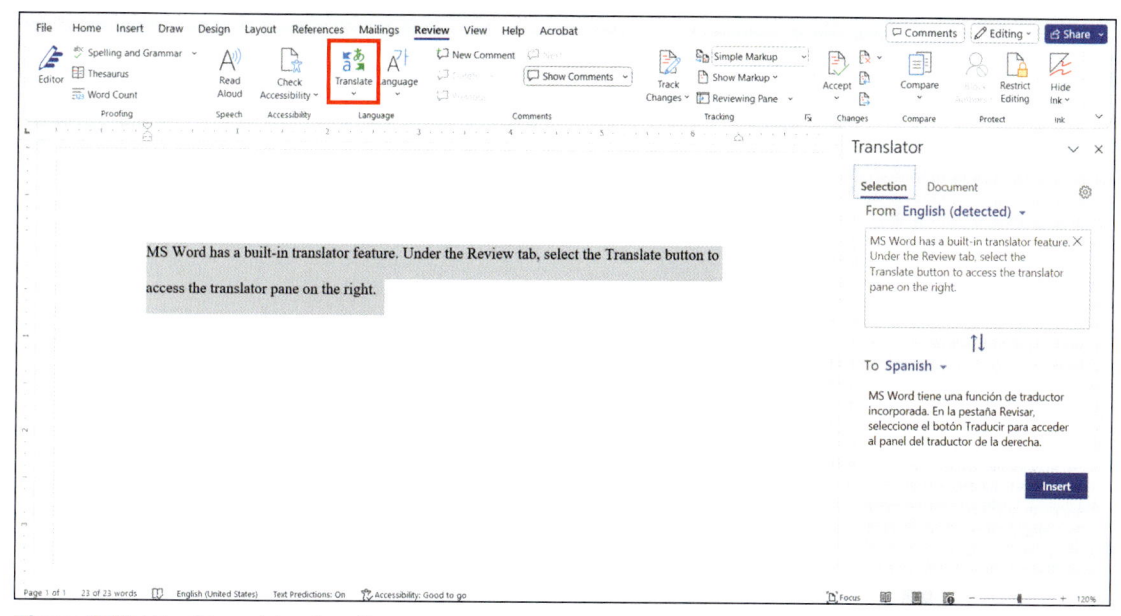

Figure D-11. Word translator function.

the headings, fonts, hyperlinks, color contrast, and readability by a screen reader and provide a report on your document listing potential problems. For example, the accessibility checker may suggest that you include alt text explanations for images or graphics in your document. Tables may trigger warnings in the accessibility checker, but keeping your tables as simple as possible (using table headers and avoiding nested tables, for example) can improve accessibility. The checker also checks for meaningful use of color and sufficient contrast in the document to assist readers with low vision or color blindness. The accessibility checker looks for built-in headings and styles that are in a logical, hierarchical order because screen readers use them to navigate through a document. Try the "Immersive Reader" feature in MS Word to hear how your document will sound if you read aloud with a screen reader. The "Check Accessibility" menu is under the "Review" tab or you can type "accessibility" into the search bar.

Language Translation

Given today's global culture, there are times you might need to translate text into a different language. Some word processors, including Word, have a built-in translator feature. Under the "Review" tab, select the "Translate" button to access the translator pane on the right (Fig. D-11). A variety of language translators are also available online, such as Google Translate and Yandex. The quality of computer translators varies, so use them carefully. When translating a document into another language, such as a manuscript you are preparing for publication, be sure to have a native speaker of the language assist you in producing an accurate and meaningful translation.

Word processors also make it possible to write characters in another language, such as letters with accents or umlauts. Single instances of these letters can be added by selecting "Symbol" in the menu bar under the "Insert" tab. You can change the keyboard language to type in languages that use special letter characters and diacritics. If you need to write in a language other than the default on your computer, use the "Help" feature.

REFERENCES

Adams, A. (2020, January 17). *Running head or no running head? For student papers, APA Style says bye, bye, bye* [blog post]. American Psychological Association. https://apastyle.apa.org/blog/running-head

American Association of Colleges of Nursing (AACN) (2021). *The essentials: Core competencies for professional nursing* education [PDF]. AACN. https://www.aacnnursing.org/Portals/42/AcademicNursing/pdf/Essentials-2021.pdf

American Psychological Association (APA). (2020). *Publication manual of the American Psychological Association* (7th ed.). https://doi.org/10.1037/0000165-000

American Psychological Association (APA). (2022). *Tips for determining authorship credit* [webpage] https://www.apa.org/science/leadership/students/authorship-paper.

American Psychological Association (APA). (2023). *Inclusive language guide* (2nd ed.). https://www.apa.org/about/apa/equity-diversity-inclusion/language-guidelines.pdf

APA Style. (n.d.). *Abstract and keywords guide* [web document] https://apastyle.apa.org/instructional-aids/abstract-keywords-guide.pdf.

APA Style. (2019, September). *Tables and figures* [webpage] https://apastyle.apa.org/style-grammar-guidelines/tables-figures.

APA Style. (2022a, June). *Accessible headings* [website] https://apastyle.apa.org/style-grammar-guidelines/paper-format/accessibility/headings.

APA Style. (2022b, July). *Basic principles of reference list entries* [website] https://apastyle.apa.org/style-grammar-guidelines/references/basic-principles.

APA Style. (2022c, July). *General principles for reducing bias* [webpage] https://apastyle.apa.org/style-grammar-guidelines/bias-free-language/general-principles.

APA Style. (2022d, July). *Sample papers* [webpage] https://apastyle.apa.org/style-grammar-guidelines/paper-format/sample-papers.

APA Style. (2022e, July). *Works included in a reference list* [webpage] https://apastyle.apa.org/style-grammar-guidelines/references/works-included.

Bahadoran, Z., Mirmiran, P., Kashfi, K., & Ghasemi, A. (2019). The principles of biomedical scientific writing: Title. *International Journal of Endocrinology and Metabolism, 17*(4), e98326. https://doi.org/10.5812/ijem.98326

Bahadoran, Z., Mirmiran, P., Kashfi, K., & Ghasemi, A. (2020). The principles of biomedical scientific writing: Abstract and keywords. *International Journal of Endocrinology and Metabolism, 18*(1), e100159. https://doi-org.proxy.lib.ohio-state.edu/10.5812/ijem.100159

Greer, J. L., & Wingo, N. P. (2017). My research article was accepted for publication! *American Nurse Today, 12*(1), 37–39. Retrieved from https://www.americannursetoday.com/wp-content/uploads/2016/12/ant1-Abstracts-1213.pdf

International Committee of Medical Journal Editors (ICMJE). (2022). *Roles and responsibilities of authors, contributors, reviewers, editors, publishers, and owners* [webpage]. https://www.icmje.org/recommendations/browse/roles-and-responsibilities/

Johnson, J. E., & Rulo, K. (2019). Problem in the profession: How and why writing skills in nursing must be improved. *Journal of Professional Nursing, 35*(1), 57–64. https://doi.org/10.1016/j.profnurs.2018.05.005

National Institute on Drug Abuse. (2021, June 23). *Words matter: Preferred language for talking about addiction.* https://nida.nih.gov/research-topics/addiction-science/words-matter-preferred-language-talking-about-addiction

Portillo, I. A., Johnson, C. V., & Johnson, S. Y. (2021). Quality evaluation of consumer health information websites found on Google using DISCERN, CRAAP, and HONcode. *Medical Reference Services Quaterly, 40*(4), 396–407. https://doi.org/10.1080/02763869.2021.1987799

Glossary

5G: fifth-generation technology standard for broadband cellular networks

academic paper: a paper written for an instructor or professor in an educational setting

accessibility: the design of a resource, such as a website, that allows individuals with disabilities to access the resource; the resource design should allow for use of screen readers for persons with limited eyesight, as well as alt tags for images and close captioning for videos for those who are hearing disabled

actionability: ability of people to identify what actions can be taken based on the information presented in material

adware: software that includes pop-up advertisements; paying to register the software installation may remove these ads

aggregate data: data from more than one source and grouped for comparison

algorithm: a set of well-defined instructions to solve a particular problem

alt tag: a text alternative for a graphic because screen readers cannot "read" a graphic; the tag should provide either textual information used by a screen reader in place of the illustration or a link to a site that explains the illustration in text

alternative text (alt text): text that describes an image or table and the information it conveys so that people with vision impairments can engage with the material

application programming interface (API): enables the real-time connection of phones, computers, and other technologies; examples include Google Maps, PayPal, E-commerce, and Travel Booking

applications (apps): various types of computer programs designed to assist the user to accomplish tasks, such as office software and web browsers

artificial intelligence (AI): ability of a machine to imitate human behaviors, like understanding their surroundings, reasoning, and problem-solving

assessment: systematic strategy for gathering data and measuring learning outcomes achieved by learners because of instruction

asynchronous telehealth: term describing store-and-forward transmission of medical images and/or data because the data transfer takes place over time, and typically in separate time frames; the transmission typically does not take place simultaneously

audit trail: a chronologic record detailing electronic transactions that is commonly used with clinical information systems to monitor appropriate access of information

authentication: the process of verification of a person's identity

author guidelines: guidelines provided by a journal or other publication for author submitted manuscripts; contain detailed instructions for formatting, citations, references, figures, and tables

automatic logout: built-in safety feature for clinical information systems in which the information system (e.g., electronic medical record) automatically logs the user out after a designated period; used to preserve data confidentiality and unauthorized access

backdoor: undocumented way of gaining access to a computer system or encrypted data that bypasses the system's customary security mechanisms; a potential security risk

backup: a duplicate copy of a digital file

bandwidth: the rate of digital communication for data transmission

bar chart: chart generally associated with comparisons of amounts in which data is displayed horizontally in bars

barcode medication administration (BCMA): point-of-care application for validation of medication administration that supports real-time recording of medications given to patients; uses electronic medication administration record and barcode scanning to verify patient identity and ensures the patient receives the right medication, in the right dose, via the right route at the right time (commonly known as "The Five Rights")

beaming: allows for wireless, very short-ranged, transmission of information to other beam-enabled devices with the same operating system using infrared, Bluetooth, or near field communication (on Android devices); AirDrop emulates beaming with Apple devices for file sharing

benchmarking: a process for comparing or evaluating something against a standard; healthcare organizations use benchmarking to compare their performance using metrics or data from national and international databases

best-of-breed approach: choosing systems that best meet the needs of services or departments from different vendors to obtain the best offering for each application area, but requires building an integrated interface

bibliographic database: indexes of published literature, often limited to a particular area such as health sciences, business, history, government, law, and ethics; contains citations for indexed items, often with abstracts and sometimes with full-text

bibliographic record: a short description of an item indexed in a database or library catalog consisting of searchable fields such as author, title, journal name, subject, etc; also known simply as a record

big bang conversion: used when switching from one computer system to another; the entire institution implements the system at the same time

big data: massive collections of complex and diverse data that cannot be analyzed or explored without the use of additional technology

biometrics: a secure method of authentication that uses physiologic characteristics such as iris scan, fingerprint, or a voiceprint that is presumably unique to the person

blog: an online web log or discussion about thoughts or topics of interest written in informal style

Bloom's Taxonomy of Learning: delineates progressively complex domains of learning to include knowledge, comprehension, application, analysis, synthesis, and evaluation; was later modified to make "creating" rather than "evaluating" the highest level of learning

Bluetooth: allows for a wireless, short-ranged (32 feet), low-powered radio frequency connection to other Bluetooth-enabled devices

Boolean connectors: a form of algebra in which matches are either true or false used in database searching to find keywords in database records; three concepts make up Boolean logic: "AND" finds records with all words, "OR" finds records with one or more words, and "NOT" finds records without words

botnet: a malware threat using a group of computers connected to the Internet that, unbeknownst to their owners, have software installed on their computers to forward items such as spam or viruses to other computers

Braille reader: a screen reader for people with visual impairments that can send information to a Braille reader placed near or under the keyboard; users then use their fingers to "read" the information

broadband: a high-capacity transmission technique; how much data the connection can transmit at once, the size, or bandwidth, determines the speed of the network connection

bugs: computer system errors and issues

business continuity plan: the term used by information technology (IT) for disaster recovery; some resources differentiate "business continuity" and "disaster recovery," indicating that "business continuity" refers to how to continue IT services in the case of a disruption and "disaster recovery" refers to the recovery of IT services after a disaster

cell phone: a shortwave wireless communication phone that has a connection to a transmitter to receive calls over a wide geographic area; requires a paid subscription to the transmission service provider

central processing unit (CPU): the part of the computer that processes and executes inputs from hardware and software; CPU speed is an important element to consider when purchasing a computer

certified EHR technology (CEHRT): a health IT product that has met or surpassed testing on specific standards and criteria set by Centers for Medicare & Medicaid Services (CMS) and a component of CMS Promoting Interoperability Program

change control: a systematic approach to managing all changes made to a product or system

chaos theory: a theory that deals with the differences in outcomes depending on conditions at the starting point; often associated with the "butterfly effect"

chat: interactive messaging on an online platform that involves two or more individuals; users type their conversation and tap the "enter" key to send the message and then others respond

Chromebook: like a laptop, but with limited functionality; can only be used when connected to the Internet; less expensive and lower maintenance than laptops but have fewer features

civility: formal politeness and courtesy in behavior or speech

click fraud: a person or bot pretends to be a legitimate user on a web page, clicking on an ad, a button, or some other type of hyperlink to trick a service into thinking a real user is interacting with the page

client: a computer needing access to services

Clinical Care Classification (CCC) System: standardized coded terminology for nursing care

clinical decision support system (CDSS): a computer application that uses a complex system of rules to analyze data and presents information to support the decision-making process of the knowledge worker

closed caption: a textual representation of video narration

cloud computing: use of remote computers for applications and file storage

code: describes text written by a computer programmer using a programming language; e.g., C, C#, C++, Java, Linux, Perl, and PHP

code of ethics: statements of the professionals' values and beliefs that are based on ethical principles

Code of Ethics for Nurses: created by the American Nurses Association (ANA), addresses issues that concern acting on behalf of the patient's interests, privacy, and confidentiality; in relation to nursing informatics, it provides general statements that could be useful when addressing conflicts or dilemmas in interactions with others resulting from the creation of, access to, and/or disposition of electronic health information data

cognitive science: the study of the human mind and intelligence and how information can be applied; it is interdisciplinary, including philosophy, psychology, artificial intelligence, neuroscience, linguistics, and anthropology, and is a part of social informatics

collective intelligence: intelligence that emerges from group collaboration

column chart: chart commonly used to compare data over time or show comparisons among two or more sets of data; data is usually presented vertically

computer: an electronic device that manipulates information (data) based on a program, software, or instructions; can store, retrieve, and process data

computer literacy: the ability to perform various tasks with a computer efficiently

computer programming: the process of writing instructions for computing devices and systems, also known as coding; a program is made up of computer code

computer virus: a malware program from the Internet designed to execute and replicate itself without the user's knowledge

computerized provider order entry (CPOE): the process of providers entering and sending treatment instructions (e.g., medication, laboratory, and radiology orders) via a computer application rather than paper, fax, or telephone

confidentiality: authorized care providers maintaining all personal health information as secret, except to other care providers who need access to that information and to others that the patient has consented to allow access

consumer informatics: a field of study related to healthcare information that is accessible to consumers in a useful, understandable manner

cost-benefit analysis: an examination of the difference between the projected revenues and expenses; an analysis assigns a monetary value to health outcomes and calculates the net benefit (benefit minus cost)

continuous data: a type of structured or quantitative data that is measured on a scale or continuum, meaning it can be divided into smaller parts and have any numeric value; height and weight are examples

cultural competence: the ability of all health organizations and providers to recognize the cultural beliefs, values, attitudes, traditions, language preferences, and health practices of diverse and vulnerable populations and to apply that knowledge to produce a positive health outcome

culture of safety (just culture): the combination of attitudes and behaviors toward patient safety that are conveyed when walking into a health facility

cyberchondria: people who become distressed and frightened after repeated and excessive web searches for health information and is a play on "hypochondria," an illness anxiety disorder

cyber criminal: individual or teams of people who use technology to commit malicious activities on digital systems or networks with the intention of stealing sensitive company information or personal data and generating profit

dashboard: a user-friendly way to deliver business intelligence and data analytics; delivers real-time information on key performance indicators to drive decision-making in healthcare

data: discrete, objective facts that have not been interpreted

data breach: stealing information; after breaking in to an unauthorized system (called a "security breach"), a cybercriminal getting away with unauthorized information

data encryption: encoding information that requires a password for files to be viewed by authorized individuals; method of protecting vulnerable data from cyber criminals

Data, Information, Knowledge, and Wisdom (DIKW) Model: facilitates the management and communication of nursing information within the field of healthcare with a focus on nursing actions and interventions; provides a nursing perspective, clarifies nursing values and beliefs, produces new knowledge, and develops standardized nursing terminology for use in electronic records

data mining: the process of finding anomalies, patterns, and correlations within large data sets to predict outcomes, then using this information to increase revenues, cut costs, improve customer relationships, reduce risks, and more

data scraping: a technique in which a computer program extracts data from output generated from another program that is often malicious; commonly manifest as web scraping, the process of using an application to extract valuable information from a website

data security: includes three aspects: ensuring the accuracy of the data, protecting the data from unauthorized eyes, and dealing with internal or external loss or damage to the data; responsibility of the computer user

data warehouse: a centralized repository for all the healthcare information retrieved from multiple sources like electronic health records (EHR), electronic medical records (EMR), enterprise resource planning systems (ERP), radiology and lab databases, or wearables

database: software that is a collection of related objects, such as tables, forms, queries, and reports

database model: the way data are organized in a database; includes flat, hierarchical, network, relational, and object-oriented models

database management system (DBMS): a software application that provides tools for creating a database, entering data, and retrieving, manipulating, and reporting information contained within the data

debugging: process of correcting computer system errors

demographics: the social characteristics and statistics of a human population including the size, age structures, and economics

descriptive data analysis: a meaningful summary or description of data points shown in a constructive way such that patterns might emerge that fulfill every condition of the data; one of the most important steps for conducting statistical data analysis

digital subscriber line (DSL): a home network that connects a router to the Internet; uses a regular phone line

discovery search: a type of digital search that simultaneously pulls results from the library catalog (including physical references) and a selection of library databases; also called a federated search

discrete data: a type of structured or quantitative data that involves only integers (i.e., it cannot be subdivided into parts; the number of people in a study is an example

disinformation: an intentional version of misinformation that includes misleading or biased information, manipulated narratives or facts, and propaganda

distributed denial of service (DDoS): when a botnet owner (or herder) directs all the computers in its botnet to send requests to the same site at the same time, overwhelming the website and preventing legitimate access

domain name: a string of text that maps to a numeric IP address, used to access a website from client software; the text that a user types into a browser window to reach a particular website (e.g., "google.com")

drive-by-download: the unintentional download of malicious code onto a computer or mobile device that exposes users to different types of threats; may happen when visiting a website, opening an e-mail attachment or clicking a link, or clicking on a deceptive pop-up window

electronic health record (EHR): an electronic record of a patient's health history, established by President George W. Bush in 2004; one's health information is available from any location where there is Internet access and a health information exchange

electronic medical record (EMR): an electronic record of health-related information on an individual that can be created, gathered, managed, and consulted by healthcare providers; the institution or provider that creates EMRs owns and manages them, and they are accessible to consumers; not a true electronic health record because outside agencies cannot interface with them

e-intensive care: a form of telemedicine designed to enhance the delivery of intensive patient care; achieved with tele-intensive care units or robotics

enterprise system integration: the process of connecting existing systems/applications to share and communicate information; enables data to flow between systems with ease, simplifying IT processes

ethernet: a system for connecting multiple computer systems to form a local area network, with protocols to control the passing of information and to avoid simultaneous transmission by two or more systems

evidence-based practice (EBP): a cyclical process of moving knowledge from original research into patient care

extranet: an extension of an intranet with added security features, providing accessibility to the intranet to a specific group of outsiders

factual database: contain point-of-need information that may include reference books such as dictionaries and encyclopedias, drug and laboratory manuals, and statistics and data sets; e.g., Nursing Reference Center

fake news: a news article that is intentionally and verifiably false

field: a column in a database table; the smallest structure in a database; a single element of a database record, such as title, that is searchable through the database interface

firewall: a computer network system that blocks incoming and outgoing data using a set of rules

fishbone diagram: a diagram that places the problem at one end of the chart with the many suspected causes branching out; also referred to as a cause-and-effect or Ishikawa diagram

flash drive: a data storage device that connects to a computer using a universal serial bus (USB)

flash memory: computer memory that it is nonvolatile, meaning that the applications and data will not disappear after the loss of battery power

flat database: all of the data are located in one table, such as a spreadsheet, worksheet, or an address book; very simple to construct and use but have limitations when it comes to tracking items that belong in a record when there are more than one of the same item

Flesch Reading Ease: measures how easy it is to read text from a formula using the average sentence length and the average number of syllables per word; the recommended score for patient education resources is between 60 and 70

Flesch-Kincaid Grade Level: calculates a U.S. school grade level with a formula that uses the average number of words per sentence and the average number of syllables per word; the recommended level for patient education resources is 6

flowchart: a chart of the sequence of movements or actions of people or things involved in an activity

focus group: a data collection tool with the characteristics of an interview but in a larger group, usually 6-12 subjects

folksonomy: word descriptor tags used for content and often achieved by group consensus

foundational interoperability: the transmission and reception of information so that it is useful, but with no need for interpretation; these systems can send and receive useable data from different systems

freeware: an application the programmer has decided to make freely available to anyone who wishes to use it, but is protected by copyright

full-text collection: a collection of documents in which the complete text of each referenced document is available for online viewing, printing, or downloading; images are often included, such as graphs, maps, photos, and diagrams; JSTOR, ProQuest Central, and Directory of Open Access Journals (DOAJ) are examples

general systems theory: a method of thinking about complex structures such as an information system or an organization

graphical user interface (GUI): the point and click interface used on computers today

hacked: when unauthorized access to data in a system is gained through use of another computer or technology by hackers

hacker: a person or group skilled in information technology who use technical knowledge to achieve a goal or overcome an obstacle, within a computerized system by non-standard means; can have good or bad/criminal intentions

hard disk drives (HDDs): a storage drive for a computer that contains moving parts; a motor-driven spindle that holds one or more flat, circular disks coated with a thin layer of magnetic material and can hold 500GB-1TB of data

hardwired: computers wired together or wired to something that physically exists, usually done using ethernet

hashtag: the pound sign (#) that identifies the keyword or topic of a social media post

health information exchange (HIE): allows doctors, nurses, pharmacists, other health care providers and patients to appropriately access and securely share a patient's vital medical information electronically thereby improving the speed, quality, safety, and cost of patient care; facilitated by the Office of the National Coordinator for Health Information Technology (ONC)

healthcare information technology (HIT): information technology used specifically for healthcare; involves the processing, storage, and exchange of health information in an electronic environment

Health Insurance Portability and Accountability Act (HIPAA): a law passed in 1996 that protects the privacy and security of health information and provides patients the right to see their own healthcare records

health literacy: the ability to obtain and understand health information for decision-making; includes the capacity to understand instructions on prescription drug bottles, appointment slips, medical education brochures, doctor's directions, consent forms, and the ability to negotiate complex healthcare systems

health numeracy: the ability to interpret and act on numerical information to make effective health decisions

health portal (patient portal): a secure way for patients to access the electronic health record information

healthcare data analytics (business intelligence): using applications and tools to analyze data integrated from financial, patient, and quality data; crucial to inform decisions, identify opportunities for improvement, and improve outcomes

healthcare informatics: a discipline specializing in the management of healthcare information with computer technology

hierarchical database: an early database model with tables organized in the shape of an inverted tree, like an organizational chart; often called a tree structure, records are linked to a base, or root, but through successive layers

high reliability organizations (HROs): organizations that have fewer than normal accidents; when faced with unexpected situations, they follow five principles of "mindfulness" that prevent error: preoccupation with failure, reluctance to simplify, sensitivity to operations, commitment to resilience, and deference to expertise; examples include aviation and nuclear power

HIPAA Privacy Rule: requires that an individual provide signed authorization to a covered entity before the entity may use or disclose certain protected health information

hoax: a message warning the recipients of a non-existent computer virus threat; usually a chain e-mail that tells the recipients to forward it to everyone they know, but can also be in the form of a pop-up window

holoportation: allows 3D models of healthcare providers to be reconstructed, compressed, and transmitted live and in real time; users can see, hear, and interact with remote participants in 3D as if they are actually present in the same physical space

hotspot: a Wi-Fi-enabled area that allows Wi-Fi-enabled mobile devices to connect to the Internet; many hotspots use encryption for security reasons and require an access code or a fee for use

hypertext transfer protocol (HTTP): transmission protocol used by the browser on the client computer to request a file from the server; server has special software for using the protocol to receive the message, find the file, and send it back to the requesting computer

hypothesis: a proposed explanation made based on limited evidence as a starting point for further investigation

impact factor (IF): a calculated index that reflects the yearly mean number of citations of articles published in the last two years in a given journal; journals with higher IF values carry more prestige in their respective fields; frequently used as a measure of the relative importance of a journal within its field; frequently used by universities and funding bodies to decide on promotion and research proposals

infodemic: large amounts of conflicting information being shared by numerous types of media; often used in conjunction with the COVID-19 pandemic

informatics: application of information technology to the arts and sciences

informatics nurse (IN): a nurse who enters the nursing informatics field because of interest or experience; work to optimize information management and communication to improve the health of individuals, families, populations, and communities

informatics nurse specialist: a nurse with either a graduate education degree in nursing informatics or a field relating to informatics who has successfully passed an American Nurses Credentialing Center (ANCC) specialty certification exam

information: data that have context, that is, some type of interpretation or structure

information disorder: the sharing or developing of false information with or without the intent of harm that is categorized as misinformation, disinformation, or fake news

information governance: the management of information at an organization

information literacy: the ability to know when one needs information and how to locate, evaluate, and effectively use it

information technology (IT): use of electronic systems like computers or telecommunications for storing, retrieving, and sending information

information technology skills: the ability to use computers, computer software, and peripherals to access electronic information efficiently

instructional design: use of models to define activities that will guide the development of educational interventions; example includes Analyze, Design, Develop, Implement and Evaluate (ADDIE) model

intangible assets: values that are not easily calculated or in which the results cannot be directly attributed to the investment; examples include improved decision-making, communication, and user satisfaction

integrated interface approach: selection of a collection of systems that are already interfaced but that may not all be the best choice for each application

interface: the search screen for a database; multiple databases from a single vendor may share the same or similar interface

interface terminology: terminology that allows the exchange of computer clinical information with the user

Internet: a global computer network providing a variety of information and communication facilities, consisting of interconnected networks using standardized communication protocols

Internet of Medical Things (IoMT): the network of Internet-connected medical devices, hardware infrastructure, and software applications used to connect healthcare information technology; allows wireless and remote devices to securely communicate over the Internet to allow rapid and flexible analysis of medical data; sometimes referred to as Internet of Things (IoT) in healthcare

Internet service provider (ISP): an organization that provides access to and use of the Internet

Internet telephone: computer software and hardware that can perform functions usually associated with a telephone

interoperability: ability of two or more systems to pass information between them and to use the exchanged information; means that healthcare information systems can transmit and receive information within and across organizational boundaries to provide the delivery of optimum healthcare to individuals and communities

invisible web (deep web): sites not reachable by traditional search tools

interview: a data collection method that involves a formal meeting between two individuals in which the interviewer asks the interviewee questions to gather information

intranet: a private network within an organization that allows users of an organization to share information, including features similar to the Internet, such as e-mail, mailing lists, and user groups

Iowa Implementation Framework (IIF): includes 81 implementation strategies for evidence-based practice (EBP) and new technology with suggested timing of four implementation phases; based on the Iowa EBP process model

IP address: an identifier of four sets of numbers separated by periods or dots, making it possible for each computer on the Internet to be electronically located; abbreviation for internet protocol address

journal article: a manuscript that has been published in a journal

journal manuscript: a paper written for journal readers

keylogger: a software program that tracks all keystrokes made by a user; can be used to trace and steal passwords and bank account numbers

knowledge: the combination of things learned and skills developed over time

Lewin's Field Theory: a theory identified by Kurt Lewin that provides a guide for helping individuals achieve a positive decision related to an innovation change

Likert scale: a way to collect ordinal data using a 5-7-point linear scale; a continuum from strongly agree to strongly disagree is an example

limiter (filter): a way to select specific attributes (such as peer-reviewed journal or a publication date range) that must be present in records brought up in a database search; limiters and filters appear on both the initial search interface and on pages for search results in most databases

line chart: a chart that uses lines to connect data; category data are displayed on the horizontal axis and the data values displayed on the vertical axis; one type communicates changes in elapsed time and one type shows data trends

listserv: an e-mail discussion list that has participants who discuss various aspects of a topic

literacy assessment tools: tools that are used to determine a person's ability to read, understand, and utilize written information; can then be used for education, research, training, or program planning purposes

local area network (LAN): a network confined to a small area such as a building or groups of buildings

login: a name that you enter into a device to be able to use the systems and applications that the device can access; most systems rely on a login name and a password for authentication

mainframe computer: a large, high-speed computer that supports many workstations or peripheral computers

malware: all forms of computer software designed by criminals to damage or disrupt a computer system; often used to generate a profit

mapping: a form of matching concepts with similar meaning from one standardized terminology to another

meaningful use: the use of aggregated data from electronic health records (EHRs) for decision-making to improve healthcare delivery; was originally part of Centers for Medicare & Medicaid Services (CMS) efforts to improve interoperability of EHRs but has been replaced with certified EHR technology; term still used to refer to the ability of an organization to meet a set of reporting requirements

medical device: a device intended by the manufacturer to be used, alone or in combination, for a medical purpose; could be any instrument, apparatus, implement, machine, appliance, implant, reagent for in vitro use, software, material or other similar or related item

medical error: the failure of a planned action to be completed as intended or the use of a wrong plan to achieve an aim; a preventable adverse effect of care, whether it is evident or harmful to the patient

medical subject headings (MeSH): the controlled vocabulary of terms used to index materials in PubMed and MEDLINE databases; differs from many other subject heading lists because the basis is a hierarchal structure

medication error: an error of commission or omission during any part of the medication process beginning when a clinician prescribes a medication and ending when the patient takes the medication

medjacking: the practice of hacking a medical device with the intent to harm or threaten a patient

meta-analysis: research on previous research; systematic reviews

metadata: data that describes other data; in library databases metadata is used to create bibliographic records, or descriptions of items indexed in the database

microblogs: very brief web journaling; text-based communication tools include Twitter, text messaging, and chat

minimum data set: a list of categories of data, each of which has an agreed definition as to what it includes; they specify the type of data that will meet the essential needs of data users for a specific purpose, such as billing

misinformation: false or inaccurate information

mobile device: a device small enough to hold and operate in the hand with a flat screen interface that may or may not be touchscreen along with a keyboard or physical buttons; many can connect to the internet and with other devices such as headsets via Wi-Fi, Bluetooth, and cellular networks; smartphones, tablets, and personal digital assistants (PDA) are examples

mobile healthcare technology (mHealth): the use of mobile devices, such as mobile phones and patient monitoring devices, in medicine; encompasses everything from healthcare apps to electronic healthcare records (EHRs) to home healthcare

mobile medical application (app): a software application designed to operate on a mobile platform that is intended as an accessory to a regulated medical device or to transform a mobile platform into a regulated medical device

mobile medical device: a medical device that can send or receive information wirelessly via Wi-Fi, Bluetooth, or cellular networks; insulin pumps, pulse oximeters, smart card readers for identification, and medication bar code readers are examples

mobile network: a communication network where the link to and from end nodes is wireless

model for improvement: based on the plan-do-study-act cycle but adds three questions: What are you trying to accomplish? How will you know that a change is an improvement? What change can you make that will result in an improvement?

modem: a device that transmits digital information

motherboard: primary circuit board holding the hardware in place providing a connection between hardware components and devices

nanotechnology: science, engineering, and technology conducted at the nanoscale, which is about 1 to 100 nm; the study and application of extremely small things and can be used across all science fields, including chemistry, biology, physics, materials science, and engineering

National Database of Nursing Quality Indicators (NDNQI): a national database to which hospitals submit nursing-sensitive data about structure, process, and outcomes of nursing care; the database aggregates the data quarterly and returns reports to participating hospitals

National Patient Safety Goals (NPSG): a quality and patient safety improvement program established by The Joint Commission in 2003 to help accredited organizations address specific areas of concern related to patient safety

Natural Language Processing (NLP): the branch of computer science, specifically the branch of artificial intelligence, concerned with giving computers the ability to understand text and spoken words in much the same way human beings can

natural language searches: searching with the natural spoken phrasing rather than focusing on specific key terms

near field communication (NFC): a way for devices to communicate; a subset of radio-frequency identification (RFID) designed to be a secure form of data exchange; a device can be both an NFC reader and an NFC tag allowing devices to communicate peer-to-peer

needs assessment: an initial step of the systems life cycle used to identify the requirements for system performance; comparable to a brainstorming session

netiquette: the correct or acceptable way of communicating on the internet

network: a connection of two or more computers that allows the computers to communicate

network authentication: a standard for work and home computer networks that requires a user to enter an authentication code to use a secure WiFi network

network model: a database model with tables organized in the shape of an inverted tree, but in which the trees can share branches; like the hierarchical database model but with shared components; because of the data structure, this model is complex and inflexible

NANDA International (NANDA-I): an organization that exists to develop, refine, and promote terminology that accurately reflects nurses' clinical judgments; created a standardized language used in nursing care; began as North American Nursing Diagnosis Association, but was changed to NANDA International to reflect global membership

nodes: tiny routers with a few wireless cards and antennas that pick-up signals sent by a user and transmit them to the central server or rebroadcast them to another node

nominal data: a type of unstructured data used for labeling variables that have no specific order; race and gender are examples

data normalization: a process that uses rules in relational databases to organize, aggregate, and display data; each table represents a category of data, and each field should be unique to the database

non-relational databases (NoSQL): database type used to analyze unstructured data, which is qualitative in nature

nursing informatics: subspecialty of nursing that focuses on managing information pertaining to nursing; nursing specialty that transforms data into information and uses technology to improve patient outcomes

Nursing Interventions Classification (NIC): standardized terminology to describe nursing interventions; often used with NANDA-I and Nursing Outcomes Classification (NOC)

Nursing Management Minimal Data Set (NMMDS): designed to capture data useful to nurse managers, administrators, and healthcare executives; complements the Nursing Minimum Data Set (NMDS)

Nursing Minimum Data Set (NMDS): list of categories of data with a definition of what is included; categories specify the type of data that meets the essential needs of users for a specific purpose, such as billing

Nursing Outcomes Classification (NOC): standardized terminology to describe nursing outcomes; often used with NANDA-I and Nursing Interventions Classification (NIC)

nursing knowledge: a component of nursing informatics theory; information known to nursing practice which defines the profession

nursing research: a systematic process of inquiry that involves collecting, documenting, analyzing, and reporting data to contribute to nursing knowledge; the scientific foundation for practice

object-oriented model: a database model that combines database functions with object programming languages to make a more powerful tool with better management of complex data relationships; better suited to applications with complex relationships between data such as hospital patient record systems

observation: a method of data collection that enables you to directly visualize how people are behaving

open access: free and open online access to academic information such as publications and data; journals that publish peer-reviewed articles with no user fees and that may have limited copyright/licensing restrictions to allow anyone with an Internet connection to download, copy, and distribute the articles

Open Systems Interconnection (OSI) model: a conceptual model created by the International Organization for Standardization (ISO); a universal language for computer networking that supports interoperability; allows health information exchanges to communicate using standard protocols; provides a way for different computer systems to communicate with each other

open-source software: software that has copyright protection but with source code available to anyone who wants it

operating system (OS): coordinates input from the keyboard, mouse, and touchpad with output on the screen; heeds commands to save or retrieve files, transmits commands to printers and other peripheral devices, and provides access to applications

ordinal data: a type of unstructured data that can be placed in order; year and satisfaction ratings are examples

organizational health literacy (OHL): the degree to which organizations equitably enable individuals to find, understand, and use information and services to inform health-related decisions and actions for themselves and others

organizational interoperability: facilitates the secure, seamless, and timely use of data both within and between organizations; includes governance, policy, social, legal, and organizational considerations of entities and individuals that enable shared consent, trust, and integrated end-user processes and workflows

parallel conversion: information system transition that requires the operation and support of the new and the old computer system simultaneously for a period

parameter query: queries that require the user to enter a constraint to define data output; only records that match that parameter are returned

password manager: a software program that helps create, store, and encrypt passwords

Perioperative Nursing Data Set (PNDS): standardized language used to support perioperative nursing practice

personal health literacy: the degree to which individuals are able to find, understand, and use information and services to inform health-related decisions and actions for themselves and others

personal health record (PHR): a record of health information owned by the individual; may be maintained using computer document or a paper record

pharming: a web scam in which an attacker infiltrates a domain name server and changes the routing for addresses to get personal information from an individual

phased conversion: a computer system implementation strategy used to bring up a new system gradually in a controlled environment; done incrementally with several alternative approaches

phishing: a web scam in which an individual receives an email message with a hyperlink that directs the person to confirm an account or enter personal information in an attempt to get personal information from the individual

picture archiving and communication system (PACS): medical imaging technology that provides storage and easy access to images, or non-image data scanned as a PDF, from multiple different machine types; images are transmitted digitally via PACS, eliminating the need to manually file, retrieve, or transport physical images; universal format for PACS is Digital Imaging and Communications in Medicine (DICOM)

pie chart: chart that communicates the proportion of various items in relation to the whole (classified as area charts); "part-to-whole" charts designed to show percentages, not amounts, and use only one data series

pilot conversion: a computer system implementation strategy done to "test the waters" to see what issues might occur when making a transition to a new computer information system; this approach enables the testing of a system on a smaller scale

plagiarism: using someone else's work as your own; two common types include copying the exact text written by others without citing the source and reordering the words of a source text without citing the source

plain old telephone service (POTS): devices can be connected to the internet using a dial-up modem through a regular telephone line; used in some rural areas

plan-do-study-act (PDSA) cycle: a four-stage problem-solving model used for quality improvement

poll: simple way to record an opinion or collect votes quickly; typically limited to one question with no demographic or other details collected

portable monitoring devices: healthcare monitoring devices not connected to plugs; include an input device and various types of peripheral monitoring equipment; many of the input devices use a touch screen with text and audio to ask assessment questions about the patient's health

primary data: generated by the researcher from surveys, interviews, and experiments that were designed for answering a specific research question

privacy: the right of patients to control what happens to their personal health information

Privacy Rights Clearinghouse: organization that maintains an online record of all types of security breaches

process improvement: the application of actions taken to identify, analyze, and improve existing processes within an organization to meet requirements for quality, customer satisfaction, and financial goals

professional networking: a subset of social media by which interactions focus on business themes

project management: uses knowledge, skills, tools, and techniques applied to projects to deliver a successful project result

project scope: all the elements that are entailed in a project, as in, the boundaries of a project

protected health information (PHI): any information about health status, provision of health care, or payment for health care that is created or collected by a Covered Entity, and can be linked to a specific individual; The HIPAA privacy rule provides federal protection for PHI

protocol: a system of rules required for data transfer

public domain software: software with no copyright restrictions that can be used in any way the user desires, including making changes

push notification: a message that is received on a mobile device, such as alerts for elevated lab values, poor air quality, or notification of an upcoming appointment; can be set up through patient care management software or other applications

qualitative: non-numerical data (and methods to collect it) that allows freedom for varied or unexpected answers; sources include interviews, focus groups, documents, personal accounts or papers, cultural records, or observation; in qualitative studies, the researcher may conduct interviews or focus groups to collect data that is not available in existing documents or records

Quality and Safety Education for Nurses (QSEN): initiative aimed at improving nurses' education to deliver safe and quality care and now incorporated into the AACN essentials of nursing; focused on six competencies of nursing, including patient-centered care, teamwork and collaboration, evidence-based practice, quality improvement, safety, and informatics

quality improvement (QI): a process to improve outcomes by the introduction of change, repeat measurement, and comparison of outcomes over time

quality measures: tools that help measure or quantify healthcare processes, outcomes, patient perceptions, and organizational structure/systems that are associated with the ability to provide high-quality health care or that relate to one or more quality goals for health care

quantitative: numerical data (and methods to collect it) that lends itself to numerical analysis and can test causal relationships among variables; data collection forms include experiments, questionnaires, surveys, and database reports

QWERTY keyboard: a keyboard layout common to the PC and typewriter that comprises the first six letters on the top row of letters; data using a QWERTY keyboard is available on all smartphones and tablets

random-access memory (RAM): one of three types of built-in memory for mobile devices; stores all the add-on applications and data files and requires a small amount of continuous battery power; this memory is volatile and all data stored in RAM are lost with the depletion of battery life

randomized controlled trial (RCT): prospective studies that measure the effectiveness of a new intervention or treatment by randomly assigning participants to either the intervention or the comparator group; randomization reduces bias and provides rigorous tool to examine cause-effect relationships between an intervention and outcome

ransomware: malicious software that blocks access of victims to their computers without paying a ransom; ransomware has attacked healthcare information systems worldwide

readability: the ease with which a reader can successfully decipher, process, and make meaning of text; typographical features of the text are critical: letter shape, size, and spacing all meaningfully impact fluency and comprehension

read-only memory (ROM): one of three types of built-in memory for mobile devices, it stores the operating and standard applications such as contacts, calendar, and notes

record: a row in a database table; all the information about a single "member" of a table

reference manager: software that allows for the collection and organization of citations from search findings; commonly include ability to store digital copies of full-text articles, cite sources, and automatically generate a formatted reference list with word processing software

reference terminology model: a set of terms based on evidence-based research; potential uses include facilitating the documentation of nursing problems (diagnosis) and actions (interventions) in electronic information systems

Regional Extension Centers (RECs): center with trained staff members to assist healthcare providers in understanding and implementing electronic health record adoption; educational components include vendor selection, workflow analysis necessary to decide on a vendor, and meaningful use requirements; component of the Health Information Technology Extension Program;

regression testing: testing application functionality in computer systems using a set of situations, commonly called scenarios or test scripts, to test application functionality

relational database: a flexible database model which uses two or more tables connected by identical information in key fields in each table; allows data in a record from one table to be matched to any piece or pieces of data in records in another table

remote patient monitoring: ability to monitor certain aspects of a patient's health (e.g., weight, blood pressure, blood sugar levels, oxygenation levels) from their own home; lets providers manage acute and chronic conditions and it cuts down on patients' travel costs and infection risk

request for information (RFI): a document sent to vendors with a summary of information requested; information from return of the RFI is used to determine which vendors should be considered in the development of a new computer system

request for proposal (RFP): a detailed document sent to potential vendors asking for information on how their product will meet the users' needs

return on investment (ROI): the cost savings that are realized because of an investment

risk assessment: assessment that helps an organization ensure it is compliant with administrative, physical, and technical safeguards required by the Health Insurance Portability and Accountability Act (HIPAA); helps reveal areas where an organization's protected health information could be at risk; HIPAA Security Rule requires that covered entities and business associates conduct a risk assessment of their healthcare organization

robotics: the use of robots; used in a variety of healthcare settings

Rogers' Diffusion of Innovations Theory: theory that examines the pattern of acceptance that innovations follow as they spread across the population; process of decision-making that occurs in individuals when deciding whether to adopt an innovation

root cause analysis (RCA): method used for the systematic analysis of the factors that contribute to medical error; guides implementation of interventions that will decrease the likelihood of similar events happening in the future; required by The Joint Commission for major safety events and sentinel events

router: a device that connects multiple devices to the same network; has one or two antennas (which may be internal) to transmit the Wi-Fi signal

satellite: Internet access provided through communication satellites

scholarly nursing journal: contains articles about studies and research conducted by those with expertise in nursing with the goal of increasing nursing knowledge; articles are rigorously peer reviewed prior to publication

scholarly writing: in the nursing discipline, writing related to generation, synthesis, translation, application, and dissemination of nursing knowledge to improve health and transform healthcare

scope creep: unanticipated growth of the project that can result in cost overruns

screen reader: computer accessibility feature with speech recognition for those with limited eyesight; can translate text to speech; some readers can send information to a Braille reader

search engine: a program that searches for and identifies items in a database that correspond to keywords or characters specified by the user; used especially for finding particular sites on the World Wide Web

secondary data: using existing data generated by large government institutions, healthcare facilities, and other organizations as part of organizational record keeping; data is extracted and used for other purposes

security breach: incident that results in unauthorized access to computer data, applications, networks, or devices; typically occurs when an intruder is able to bypass security mechanisms

self-plagiarism: when authors publish work that they published previously and present it as new work

semantic interoperability: information transmitted is understandable; at its highest level, the interpretation and action on messages exchanged by two computers occurs without human intervention; effectiveness depends on the interaction between algorithms (rules), the data used in the message, and the terminology used to designate that data

seminal work: work frequently cited by others or that influences the opinions of others

sentinel event: a patient safety event that results in death, permanent harm, or severe temporary harm; the most serious type of medical error

server: a computer that provides information or services to other computers on a network

shareware: software that the developers encourage users to give copies of to friends and colleagues to try out for a trial period; protected by copyright

skills assessment: assessment to identify the level of skill of users who will use an electronic system and identify those who need additional training

single sign-on: one login/password for authentication that allows user to access multiple clinical applications; efficient but if compromised, risks all linked applications and services

smart infusion pumps: enable the automatic delivery of intravenous (IV) fluids and medications within the bounds of preset parameters (e.g., drug concentration and dose); uses dose error reduction systems, drug libraries, preset limits, and alerts for infusion rates outside of acceptable boundaries to reduce medication error

smartphone: cell phones with Internet connectivity

social bookmarking: saves bookmarks to the cloud where they are available on an individual's computers and devices with an Internet connection

social determinants of health (SDoH): nonmedical factors that influence a person's health outcomes

social engineering: tricking victims into downloading and installing malware by clicking on link or viewing a file

social informatics: a good design is based on an understanding of how people work and the context of the work, not just technologic considerations

social media: allows people to share stories, pictures, videos, and thoughts with others online using the Internet

social networking: the use of websites that serve to connect millions of users worldwide

sociotechnical theory: focuses on the impact of technology's implementation on an organization

software: the part of a computer that is not physical; includes data, programs, applications, and protocols

software piracy: using a copyrighted program without following the rules for use

solid-state drive (SSD): a memory chip using integrated circuits instead of a rotating disk (no moving parts); nonvolatile, meaning it does not require power to retain data; the most common storage drive in use

spam: unsolicited, usually commercial messages (e.g., emails, text messages, or Internet postings) sent to numerous recipients or posted in a large number of places

speech-recognition software: software with the ability to translate spoken word into text; type of biometric used for security by creating voiceprints with two authentication factors: what is said and the way that it is said

spyware: tracks web surfing to tailor advertisements to the user, often appearing like legitimate adware; can monitor keystrokes and transmit it to a third party and scan hard drives, read cookies, and change default home pages on web browsers

stacked bar chart: a bar chart that is a "part-to-whole" chart that measures in percentage and compare differences in groups of clustered data; each data set uses the previous data set as its baseline

standardized nursing terminology (SNT): uses words or multiword expressions to describe symptoms, diagnoses, diseases, treatments, and outcomes that are consistent (or standard) across an organization or across the entire nursing discipline; supports interoperability of electronic health records for use by nurses for seamless health information exchange

standards: an agreement to use a given protocol, term, or other criterion formally approved by a nationally or internationally recognized professional trade association or governmental body

statistical analysis: the process of analyzing a collection of data in order to identify trends and patterns

stop words: words that a search engine generally does not search for unless they are a part of a phrase enclosed with quotes (e.g., articles and prepositions)

storage drive: stores the operating system, applications, and data files like documents and images; computers need at least one storage drive to function

store and forward (S&F): a digital camera, scanner, or other technology (e.g, x-ray machine) generates electronic images that are sent electronically to a specialist for interpretation later

strategic planning: creating a roadmap that guides an institution to meet its mission, directs decision-making practices over a 3- or 5- to 10-year period, guides the acquisition of resources and budget priorities, and serves as a living and breathing document that allows for flexibility

structural interoperability: defines the format of data exchanged between systems; begins the process of transforming data into information by adding meaning and purpose to the information; data exchanged between information systems allow for interpretation at the data field level; also known as syntactic or technical interoperability

structured data: data that is quantitative in nature, involving numbers and letters that are organized and factual; can be analyzed in tables like spreadsheets

structured query language (SQL): coding that is used for querying in many databases; an American National Standards Institute (ANSI) standard computer language for retrieving and updating data in a database

subject headings: a standardized term used to index or catalog reference materials; each library chooses a standard subject authority or thesaurus for all of its cataloging

supercomputer: a large and powerful mainframe computer capable of processing data measured in petabytes (a million gigabytes)

super user: an individual identified to assist in the computer system building and testing; clinical nurses and staff who are recruited from each of the areas where the system will be deployed

survey: a method of data collection that uses a questionnaire to gather data from a set of respondents

synchronization (sync): technology that allows users to share files between devices through a cloud sharing application where changes are copied back and forth

synchronous telehealth: healthcare provided by a provider to a patient in real time, often using a camera and specialized monitoring devices such as blood pressure, pulse rate, heart rhythm, and pulse oximetry

systematic review: a research process designed to carefully review and analyze the results of multiple, similar research studies; reduces bias inherent in individual research studies

systems lifecycle: the process that begins with the conception of a computer system until the system is implemented; a systematic approach for designing, developing, implementing, and maintaining information systems

tablet: a compact and portable computer that does not require a keyboard or mouse to receive or transmit information

tacit knowledge: knowledge that is difficult to share with others in written or verbal formats

tangible assets: values that can be clearly measured, calculated, and quantified with numerical data; examples include length of stay, medication costs, number of unnecessary medications or tests, and charges per admission

Technology Informatics Guiding Educational Reform (TIGER): initiative aimed at providing the global health workforce with innovative informatics tools and resources and to integrate informatics into healthcare education, certification, practice, and research through an equitable, inclusive, interdisciplinary, and intergenerational approach

telehealth: health services delivered using electronic technology to patients at a distance; extends beyond the delivery of clinical services

telehomecare: the monitoring and delivery of healthcare in the patient's home rather than the provider's work setting; benefits include allowing the patient the comforts of his or her own home, improving quality of life, and avoiding time-consuming costly visits to office appointments or hospital admissions

telemedicine: the electronic exchange of health information between two sites using telecommunication tools

telemental health: use of telehealth to deliver psychiatric healthcare

telenursing: using telecommunications technology (telehealth) to provide home nursing care

telepresence: the use of technology to provide the appearance of a person's presence, although he or she is located at a remote site

teletrauma: used to obtain second opinions and advice from trauma care experts; used by rural hospitals and clinics and parts of the world torn by violence and war

The Joint Commission (TJC): a U.S. non-profit organization that strives to ensure quality healthcare for patients, prevent harm, and improve patient advocacy; accredits more than 22,000 healthcare organizations and programs that comply with TJC standards

throughput: the movement or flow of patients through the hospital system

topology: how nodes in a computer network are arranged; bus, ring, star, and mesh are examples

Trojan horse: type of malware that appears to be a legitimate program (e.g., a game), but places malicious software on a computer or creates a backdoor when the program runs

trolls: people who post or make inflammatory, insincere, digressive, extraneous, or off-topic messages online to obscure and drown out opposing views and evidence-based content

truncation: a technique that broadens your Internet or database search to include various word endings and spellings; for example, enter the root of a word and put the truncation symbol at the end (e.g., child*) and the database will return results that include any ending of that root word (e.g., child, childs, children, childrens, childhood); truncation symbols may vary by database

two-factor authentication (2FA): requires additional personal information (beyond standard login/password authentication) for account access to prevent unauthorized users from hacking an account

understandability: ability of people from different backgrounds with different levels of health literacy to understand the materials and extract important messages

Unified Medical Language System (UMLS): integrates and distributes standard terminology, classification and coding standards, and resources to promote interoperable health information exchange, including electronic health records; designed by the National Library of Medicine

universal design for learning (UDL): a teaching approach that accommodates the needs and abilities of all learners and eliminates unnecessary hurdles in the learning process

universal patient identifier (UPI): a single identification number that links each patient with his or her individual health record; also known as a unique patient identifier

universal resource locator (URL): a complete web address used to find a particular web page; assigned to all web documents; contain descriptors, domain name (unique name that identifies a website), and may include a folder name, a file name, or both

universal serial bus (USB) port: a port installed on a computer that allows a device with a USB connection to be plugged in and accessed on the computer

unstructured data: data that is qualitative in nature that does not have a predefined structure; subjective data can be categorized depending on its characteristics and traits (e.g., social media posts, emails, text files, videos, images, audio, and sensor data); makes up more than 80% of data; stored in raw form and analyzed using non-relational databases since traditional methods and tools cannot be used

usability: ability of people with different backgrounds and abilities to use a website or other material; websites should meet certain criteria to make them useable for their audience (e.g., considering location of drop-down menus, amount of information on the screen, font size, number and detail of instructions for finding things, and navigation issues); websites need to be compliant with the American Disability Act usability principles

user interface (UI): the space where interactions between humans and healthcare information technology (HIT) occur; goal of the interaction is to allow effective operation and control of HIT from the human end while HIT simultaneously feeds back information that aids the decision-making process

video conference: a meeting participants join from various physical locations using video and audio technology to display participant presence and multimedia content

virtual private network (VPN): an intranet with an extra layer of security that operates as an extranet; allows an organization to communicate confidentially by transmitting files using an encrypted tunnel blocking the view by others

visible web (surface web): sites reachable by traditional search engines

Voiceover Internet Protocol (VoIP): terminology for telephony products that allows a telephone call to be made from anywhere in the world with voice and video by using the Internet, bypassing the phone company

warez: illegal and pirated software used by botnets

wearable: smart device worn on the body used to obtain, analyze, and track patient data

web browser (browser): a tool enabling users to retrieve and display files from the Internet

webcast: a one-way electronic presentation, usually with video, to an audience who may be present either in a room or in a different geographical location

webinar: a live seminar over the Internet where users must log in to a website address to view; audience members can ask questions during the presentation and the speaker can ask for feedback

website: a set of related web pages located under a single domain name, typically produced by a single person or organization

white hat hackers: people who have the skills to be cybercriminals but are ethically opposed to security abuse; often work for organizations by looking for security weaknesses

wide area network (WAN): a network that encompasses a large geographical area; might be two or more local area networks

Wi-Fi protected access (WPA): a security standard for computing devices equipped with wireless internet connections; developed by the Wi-Fi Alliance to provide more sophisticated data encryption and better user authentication than wired equivalent privacy (WEP), the original Wi-Fi security standard

wiki: a piece of server software that allows users to freely create and edit content on a web page using any web browser; allows for collaborative knowledge sharing

wildcard: a searching method substituting a symbol for one letter of a word useful for terms spelled in different ways but with the same meaning; for example, typing wom!n or colo?r will return search results with woman and women or color and colour; wildcard symbols may vary by database or search engine

wireless (Wi-Fi): a network connection in which a device does not need to be hard wired to the Internet but connects to it using a modem and router that emits a signal through an antenna

wisdom: a component of nursing informatics theory that is achieved through evaluating knowledge with reflection

workflow: the sequence of steps that need to be completed from the beginning to the end of a process

workstation: a desktop computer in a network with many others; more powerful than a personal computer due to the connection with the mainframe

world wide web (the web): an information system enabling documents and other web resources to be accessed over the Internet; documents and downloadable media are made available to the network through web servers and can be accessed by programs such as web browsers

worm: a small piece of malware that uses security holes and computer networks to replicate itself

Index

Note: Page numbers followed by "*f*" indicate figures, "*t*" indicate tables, and "*b*" indicate boxes.

A

AAACN. *See* American Academy of Ambulatory Care Nursing (AAACN)
ABI/INFORM (ProQuest), 145
Abstracts, 200
Academic paper, 207
Academic writing, 207–208
Accessibility
   Alt text, 210–211
   checking, 210
   color perception, 211
   instructional design features, 209
   slides, 210
   questions about, 210*b*
Accuracy of data, 325
Actionability, health literacy, 302
Active learning techniques, 203
ADA. *See* American Disabilities Act (ADA)
ADDIE instructional design model, 201, 201*f*
Adult Literacy and Life Skills (ALL) survey, 297
Advanced Encryption Standard (AES), 52
Advanced search, 147, 154
Advancing Research and Clinical practice through close Collaboration (ARCC), 137, 139*f*
Adverse drug event (ADE), 335
Adware software, 69–70
Affordable Care Act (ACA), 11
Affordable Connectivity Program, 65, 125
Agency for Healthcare Research and Quality (AHRQ), 152, 185, 186*f*, 237, 294, 338

Aggregate data, 182
AHIMA. *See* American Health Information Management Association (AHIMA)
AI. *See* Artificial intelligence (AI)
Algorithms, 66
AliveCor heart smartphone, 119, 119*f*
Alliance for Nursing Informatics (ANI), 13
All patient-refined Diagnosis-Related Groups (APR-DRGs), 264
Alternative payment models (APMs), 236–237
Alt tags, 304
Alt text, 210–211
American Academy of Ambulatory Care Nursing (AAACN), 116
American Academy of Nursing (AAN), 294
American Association of Colleges of Nursing (AACN), 14–15, 15*b*, 31, 73, 294
American Association of Critical-Care Nurses, 200
American Disabilities Act (ADA), 209
American Health Information Management Association (AHIMA), 12, 183
American Health Quality Association (AHQA), 238
American Medical Informatics Association (AMIA), 12–13, 222
American Nurses Association (ANA) Code of Ethics, 7, 7*b*, 17, 17*b*, 45, 73, 199, 279
American Nurses Credentialing Center (ANCC), 32

American Nursing Informatics Association (ANIA), 13
American Recovery and Reinvestment Act, 273
American Telehealth Association (ATA), 116
AMIA. *See* American Medical Informatics Association (AMIA)
ANA. *See* American Nurses Association (ANA)
ANA Code of Ethics. *See* American Nurses Association (ANA) Code of Ethics
ANCC. *See* American Nurses Credentialing Center (ANCC)
Anecdata, 171
ANI. *See* Alliance for Nursing Informatics (ANI)
ANIA. *See* American Nursing Informatics Association (ANIA)
Antivirus software, 72
APMs. *See* Alternative payment models (APMs)
Apple Macintosh computer, 48
Apple macOS, 48
Application programming interfaces (APIs), 257
Application software, 53
ARCC. *See* Advancing Research and Clinical practice through close Collaboration (ARCC)
Artificial intelligence (AI), 107, 190–192
Association of Colleges and Research Libraries (ACRL), 294
Association of periOperative Registered Nurses (AORN), 282

441

Index

Asynchronous telehealth, 115, 115f
ATA. *See* American Telehealth Association (ATA)
Audit trail, 325
Authentication
   login name and passwords, 317
   two-factor authentication, 317–318
Author guidelines, data publishing, 208
Automated dispensing cabinet (ADC), 349
Automatic Data Processing (ADP), 67–68
Automatic logout, authentication, 318–319
Automatic pill dispensers and reminders, 119

B
Backdoor, 69
Backup, 50
Bandwidth, 63
Bar charts, 188–189, 188f
Barcode medication administration (BCMA), 349–350
Beaming, 97, 97f
Benchmarking, 184, 235–236
Best-of-breed approach, 226
Best-of-breed approach, to vendor selection, 226
Biased survey questions, 168b
Bibliographic databases, 140, 142–145
   Cumulative Index to Nursing and Allied Health Literature (CINAHL), 142
   evidence-based practice databases, 144
   Nursing & Allied Health Premium, 143–144
Bibliographic records, 141
Big bang conversion, healthcare information technology, 228
Big data, 181–184
   asthma patient care, 184
   characteristics, 182
   chronic obstructive pulmonary disease (COPD) patient care, 184
   information privacy, 183–184
   management, 182–183
   software and applications, 191
Billing terminology standardization
   Healthcare Common Procedure Coding System (HCPCS), 264

International Classification of Disease (ICD), 264
Medicare Severity Diagnosis-Related Groups (MS-DRGs), 264
Outcome and Assessment Information Set (OASIS), 264–265
Patient Protection and Affordable Care Act (ACA), 264
Biometric two-factor authentication (2fA), 318, 318f
Blogs, 75
Blood pressure cuff, 98f
Bloom's Taxonomy of Learning, 201–202, 203f
Bluetooth, 96, 96f
Boolean connectors, 146
Botnets, 69
Braille reader, 304
British Computer Society (BCS) Nursing Specialist Group, 13
Broadband connection, 63
Bugs, 49
Business continuity plan, 233–234, 234b

C
California Consumer Privacy Act (CCPA), 184
California Medication Error Reduction Plan framework, 342
Cardiac rhythm devices, 119
CareDo robot and system, 122–123
CARES Act. *See* Coronavirus Aid, Relief, and Economic Security (CARES) Act
CCHP. *See* Center for Connected Health Policy (CCHP)
CCPA. *See* California Consumer Privacy Act (CCPA)
CDSS. *See* Clinical decision support system (CDSS)
CEHRT. *See* Certified electronic health record technology (CEHRT)
Cell phone, 91
CEN. *See* Comité Européen de Normalisation (CEN)
Center for Connected Health Policy (CCHP), 127
Centers for Disease Control and Prevention (CDC), 117, 152, 257
Centers for Medicare & Medicaid Services (CMS), 124, 152, 185, 236–237, 255–256, 274

Medicare Promoting Interoperability Program, 255–256
Merit-Based Incentive Payment System (MIPS), 256, 256f
Central processing unit (CPU), 46
Certified EHR technology (CEHRT), 255
Certified electronic health records (CEHRs), 274
Certified electronic health record technology (CEHRT), 230
Certified Professional in Healthcare Quality (CPHQ) certification, 238
Certified Professional in Patient Safety (CPPS), 356
Certified Quality Improvement Associate (CQIA) certification, 238
Change adopters, Rogers's theory, 27
Change/control management
   business continuity plan, 233–234, 234b
   unintended consequences, 232–233
Change theories, informatics, 27–29
   Lewin's field theory, 28–29, 29f
   Rogers's diffusion of innovations theory, 27–28, 28f
Chaos theory, 30–31
Charts
   bar, 188–189, 188f
   column, 188, 188f
   line, 189
   pie, 188, 188f
Chat, 79
ChatGPT, 192
Chief nursing informatics officer, 224
Chrome OS, 48
Chronic Disease Indicator (CDI), 184
Chronic illness management, telehealth, 123–124
CINAHL. *See* Cumulative Index to Nursing and Allied Health Literature (CINAHL)
Civility, 74, 74t
Classic search algorithms, 66
Click fraud, 69
Client-server network, 61
Clinical analyst, 224
Clinical Care Classification (CCC) system, 282
Clinical decision support system (CDSS), 192, 348–349

Index   **443**

Clinical informatics
  directors and manager, 224
  specialist, 223
Clinical information system (CIS), 103, 228
Clinical reasoning, 192
Cloud computing, 50, 52*f*
  advantages, 53
  benefits, 50–51
  cloud storage and encryption, 52
  file sharing, 52–53
  limitations, 53
Cloud office suite software, 78
CMS. *See* Centers for Medicare & Medicaid Services (CMS)
Code, 48
Codes of ethics, 15
Cognitive science, 31
Collective intelligence, 79
Column charts, 188, 188*f*
Comité Européen de Normalisation (CEN), 263
Commercial software, 54
Communication systems, 232
Compact disks (CDs), 50
Competencies
  informatics education, 31–32
  informatics nurses, 33*b*
  information literacy standards, 294, 295*b*
  nursing informatics, 13–15
Computer
  cloud computing, 50, 52*f*
  components, 45–46, 46*f*
  data storage, 49–50, 49*f*
  ethical considerations, 45
  hardware, 45–46
  operating system (OS), 47–49
  software applications, 53–55
  types, 46–47, 46*f*
    mainframes, 47
    mobile devices, 47
    personal computers, 47
    server, 46–47
Computerized provider order entry (CPOE), 26, 229, 348
Computer literacy, 6
Computer malware
  adware software, 69–70
  botnet, 69
  computer virus, 67
  drive-by-download, 67
  hoaxes, 70
  pharming, 68

  phishing, 67–68
  ransomware, 68–69
  social engineering, 67
  spyware, 70
  Trojan horse program, 69
  worms, 69
Computer network, 82
  architecture, 60–61
  connections, 60–64, 63*t*
  internet, 64–66
  nodes, 60
  protocols, 60
  security issues, 66–72
  types, 61, 62*t*
Computer programming (coding), 48–49
Computer Stored Ambulatory Record (COSTAR), 273
Computer virus, 67
Confidentiality, 314
  authentication, 317–318, 318*f*
  automatic logout, 318–319
  healthcare records, 316
  single sign-on (SSO), 319
Confusing answer scale options, 168*b*
Consumer informatics, 305
Consumer-mediated exchange, health information, 277
Content sharing, 77
Continuous data, 181
Controlling phase, project management, 244
Coronavirus Aid, Relief, and Economic Security (CARES) Act, 126
Cost-benefit analysis, 241
Country-specific top-level domain (TLD), 66
CPOE. *See* Computerized provider order entry (CPOE)
CRAAP test. *See* Currency, Relevance, Authority, Accuracy and Purpose (CRAAP) test
Cultural competence, 302, 303*f*
Culture of safety
  high reliability organizations (HROs), 351–352
  measurement
    surveys for healthcare organizations, 353
    surveys for schools of nursing, 353–354
    patient safety organizations, 354–356
  root cause analysis (RCA), 352
  tenets, 351, 352*b*

Cumulative Index to Nursing and Allied Health Literature (CINAHL), 142, 144*f*, 147, 147*f*, 154–156, 155*f*
Currency, Relevance, Authority, Accuracy and Purpose (CRAAP) test, 307, 308*t*
Current procedural terminology (CPT) codes, 264
Cyber attacks, mobile devices, 106
Cyberchondria, 307
Cyber criminals, 67

D

Dashboards, 183, 183*f*
Data, 24, 163
  analysis
    artificial intelligence (AI), 191–192
    clinical decision support system (CDSS), 192
    data standards, 184–185
    data types, 180–184, 180*f*
    electronic health records (EHRs), 180
    health information technology (HIT), 191
    in nursing, 179–180, 179*f*
    tools, 186–191, 193
  big data, 181–184
  breach, 326
  encryption, 52, 72, 328
  lakes, 191
  loss, 326, 328
  mining, 170, 191
  presentation, 201–205, 202*f*
  scraping, 170–171
  structured, 181
  types, 180*f*
  unstructured, 181
  warehouse, 172
Database management system (DBMS), 172
Databases, 140–145
  ABI/INFORM (ProQuest), 145
  bibliographic, 140, 142–145
  database management system (DBMS), 172
  design, 173–174
  digital, 171
  Education Resources Information Center (ERIC), 145
  Embase (Elsevier), 145
  factual, 140
  full-text collection, 140
  LexisNexis, 145

Databases *(Continued)*
  metadata and records, 141
  models, 172–173
    flat database, 173
    hierarchical database, 173
    network model, 173
    relational database, 173
  Physician Data Query (PDQ), 145
  plagiarism, 141–142
  PsycINFO, 145
  reference managers, 141
  software, 174
  visible web (surface web), 145
Data collection
  databases
    database management system (DBMS), 172
    design, 173–174
    digital, 171
    models, 172–173
    software, 174
  demographic data, 165
  ethical considerations, 166
  guidelines, 163–166
  tools
    data mining, 170
    data scraping, 170–171
    experimentation, 170
    focus groups, 169–170
    interviews, 169
    observations, 169
    polls, 166–167
    primary data, 170
    records and documents, 170
    secondary data, 170
    surveys, 167–169
Data dissemination
  American Nurses Association (ANA), 199
  assessment and evaluation, 207
  clinical practice guidelines, 199
  data presentation
    access sharing, 204
    active learning, 203
    fonts and colors, 205
    images, 204
    instructional design, 201, 201*f*
    learning objectives, 201–203, 202*f*
    oral presentation, 203
    questioning, 203–204
    software, 200–201
    special effects, 204
    venue selection, 200
  data publishing
    academic writing, 207–208

journal selection, 208–209
scholarly writing, 207–208
poster presentations, 205–207
universal design for learning (UDL), 209–213
Data, information, knowledge, and wisdom (DIKW) model, 24–25
Data security
  breaches, 326–328
    prevalence, 326, 327*f*
    prevention, 327–328
  data accuracy protection, 325
  data loss, 326
  unauthorized external data access, 325–326
  unauthorized internal data access, 325
Data storage, 49–50, 49*f*
  compact disks (CDs), 50
  data backup, 50
  flash drive, 50
  floppy disks, 50
  hard drive, 49–50
  secure digital (SD) cards, 50
  solid-state drive (SSD), 50
DBMS. *See* Database management system (DBMS)
DCI score. *See* Digital civility index (DCI) score
Debugging process, 49
Decision making stages, Rogers's theory, 28
Deep learning, 190
Demographic data, 165
Descriptive data analysis, 187
Digital civility index (DCI) score, 74
Digital databases, 171
Digital Imaging and Communications in Medicine (DICOM) organization, 262–263
Digital Millennium Copyright Act of 1998, 100
Digital rights management (DRM), 100
Digital subscriber line (DSL), 62
Digital video disks (DVDs), 50
DIKW model. *See* Data, information, knowledge, and wisdom (DIKW) model
Directed exchange, health information exchange, 277
Disaster healthcare, 124–125
Discovery search, 140
Discrete data, 181
Disinformation, 81
Disk operating system (DOS), 48

Distributed denial of service (DDoS), 69
Domain name system, 6566
DOS. *See* Disk operating system (DOS)
Dose error reduction systems (DERSs), 350
Double-barreled questions, 168*b*
Double negatives, 168*b*
Drive-by-download, 67
DRM. *See* Digital rights management (DRM)
DSL. *See* Digital subscriber line (DSL)
Dull-text collection, database, 140

E
eBook, 99–100
EBP. *See* Evidence-based practice (EBP)
Eclipsys, 45
Education Resources Information Center (ERIC), 145
EHRs. *See* Electronic health records (EHRs)
e-intensive care units
  robotics, 122–123
  tele-intensive care units, 120, 122
Electronic health records (EHRs), 103, 103*f*, 178, 273, 276–277
  benefits, 275*b*
  certification, 230
  complaints about, 278
  data analysis, 180
  design problems, 278–279
  vs. electronic health record (EHR), 276*t*
  Electronic Medical Records Adoption Model (EMRAM), 230
  ethical considerations, 284
  implementation manager, 225
  medical errors, 336
  modern adoption, 274, 274*f*
  nursing advocacy, 279–280
  nursing research, 279
  solutions, 279
  standardized nursing terminology (SNT)
    ANA-recognized, 281*b*
    implementation barriers, 284
    interface terminologies, 281–283
    minimum data set, 281
    Nursing Information and Data Set Evaluation Center (NIDSEC), 283
    patient care, 280–281

reference terminologies, 283
super users, 229–230
task force, 230
Electronic laboratory reporting (ELR) services, 265
Electronic medical record (EMR), 275–276
Electronic Medical Records Adoption Model (EMRAM), 230, 231t
Electronic patient records
   benefits, 275b
   conceptual organization, 276f
   transition to, 273–274
   types
      electronic health record (EHR), 276–277
      electronic medical record (EMR), 275–276
      personal health records (PHRs), 277
Electronic posters, 205
Electronic protected health information (ePHI), 273
ELR services. *See* Electronic laboratory reporting (ELR) services
Emergency Care Research Institute (ECRI), 354–355
Empowerment, healthcare consumers
   consumer informatics, 305
   information literacy
      advocacy for internet access, 306
      healthcare misinformation clarifying, 307–308
      internet resources, 306–307
      legislative developments, 305
EMR. *See* Electronic medical record (EMR)
EMRAM. *See* Electronic Medical Records Adoption Model (EMRAM)
Encryption
   ransomware, 68
   software, 72
Enhanced Nurse Licensure Compact (eNLC), 127
eNLC. *See* Enhanced Nurse Licensure Compact (eNLC)
Enterprise system integration, 228
e-paper, 47
e-reader, 47
e-textiles, 118
Ethernet, 61
Ethical considerations
   computer concepts, 45
   patient safety, 351

professional behavior, 73
professional growth, 35
European Federation for Medical Informatics (EFMI), 12
European Union's General Data Privacy Regulation (GDPR), 184
Evidence-based practice (EBP)
   cyclical nature, 137–138
   databases, 144
   implementation strategies, 226f
Execution phase, project management, 242–244
   design and testing, 243
   implementation, 244
   preparing end users, 243–244
   workflow redesign, 243
Experimentation, data collection, 170
Extranet, 61

F
Facebook, 76
Factual databases, 140
Failure Modes and Effects Analysis (FMEA), 356
Fake news, 81
Fast Healthcare Interoperability Resources (FHIR), 261
Federal Communications Commission's (FCC) Lifeline program, 306
Federal Health Information Technology (IT) Strategic Plan, 5f
Federal laws, 11
Federation of State Medical Boards (FSMB), 127
Firewalls, 71, 325
Fitbit, 119
Fitness app, 102f
Fitness trackers track metrics, 47
5G, 64, 96
Flash drive, 50
Flash memory, 91
Flat database, 173
Flesch–Kincaid Grade Level test, 301, 301f
Flesch Reading Ease, 301, 301f
Floppy disks, 50
Focus groups, data collection, 169–170
Folksonomies, 79
Foundational interoperability, 253
Free cloud office applications, 54–55
Freeware, 54

G
GDPR. *See* European Union's General Data Privacy Regulation (GDPR)
General systems theory, 29–30, 30f
Glucose monitor, 98f
Graphical user interface (GUI), 48, 48f
Group discussion forums, 79
GUI. *See* Graphical user interface (GUI)

H
Hacked, 67
Hacker, 67
Hard disk drives (HDDs), 49–50
Hard drive, 49–50
Hardwired, 61
Hashtag, 78
HCAHPS survey. *See* Hospital Consumer Assessment of Healthcare Providers and Systems (HCAHPS) survey
HCPCS. *See* Healthcare Common Procedure Coding System (HCPCS)
Healthcare Common Procedure Coding System (HCPCS), 264
Healthcare data analytics, 182
Healthcare informatics, 6
   federal standards, 11
   professional organizations, 11–13
Healthcare Information and Management Systems Society (HIMSS), 12, 31, 222, 294
Healthcare information technology (HIT), 6, 222, 333
   conversion methods, 227f
   informatics nurse (IN) responsibilities
      change/control management, 232–234
      Iowa Implementation Framework (IIF), 225, 226f
      system development, 230, 232
      system implementation, 225–229
      system optimization and utilization, 229–230
      systems life cycle, 225, 226f
   medication error prevention
      automated dispensing cabinet (ADC), 349
      barcode medication administration (BCMA), 349–350
      clinical decision support system (CDSS), 348–349

Index

Healthcare information technology (HIT) *(Continued)*
  computerized provider order entry (CPOE), 348
  smart infusion pumps, 350, 350*f*
Healthcare records
  electronic records, 273–274
  history and trends
    paper records, 272–273
    Swedish medical record, 272, 272*f*
Healthcare-related software, 53–54
Health Evaluation through Logical Processing (HELP), 273
Health information exchange (HIE), 253, 274, 277
Health information technology (HIT), 191, 274
  adoption dashboards, 257
Health Information Technology for Economic and Clinical Health (HITECH) Act, 11, 222, 241, 273, 321
Health Insurance Portability and Accountability Act (HIPAA), 79, 187, 273, 316
  limitations, 324–325
  sample authorization form, 319, 320*f*
  universal patient identifier (UPI), 321
  violations
    individual, 322*b*–323*b*
    organizational, 322*b*
    penalties, 323–324, 324*t*
    types, 321
Health level seven (HL7) standards, 261, 265
Health literacy, 293
  actionability, 302
  assessment, 299
  cultural competence, 302
  ethical considerations, 299
  factors affecting, 298
  health literacy movement, 296–297
  Healthy People 2030 objectives, 296, 297*b*
  and numeracy surveys, 297–298
  online resources, 300*b*
  oral communication, 300
  personal health literacy, 296
  skills needed, 296*b*
  understandability, 302
  web design
    accessibility, 302–304
    usability, 304
  written communication, 300–302
Health Literacy Precautions Toolkit, 299
Health numeracy, 297
Health on the Net (HON) Foundation, 307
Healthy People 2030, 296
Hierarchical database, 173
High reliability organizations (HROs), 351
HIMSS. *See* Healthcare Information and Management Systems Society (HIMSS)
HIPAA. *See* Health Insurance Portability and Accountability Act (HIPAA)
HITECH Act. *See* Health Information Technology for Economic and Clinical Health (HITECH) Act
Hoaxes, 70
Holoportation, 114
Home healthcare devices, 124*b*
Hospital Consumer Assessment of Healthcare Providers and Systems (HCAHPS) survey, 167, 185, 237
Hospital Quality Alliance (HQA), 237
Hotspot, 92
HQA. *See* Hospital Quality Alliance (HQA)
Human resource management system (HRMS), 239
Hypertext transfer protocol (HTTP), 66
Hypothesis, 164

I

ICD. *See* International Classification of Disease (ICD)
Identity Theft Resource Center (ITRC), 326
Image-based platforms, 77
Image sharing, 77
IMIA. *See* International Medical Informatics Association (IMIA)
Impact factor (IF), 150, 208–209
IN. *See* Informatics nurse (IN)
Incident reporting system (IRS), 340
Inclusive instruction, 211–212
Individual Health Insurance Portability and Accountability Act (HIPAA) violations, 322*b*–323*b*
Infodemic of information, 81
Informatics, 5*f*
  social, 26
  healthcare informatics, 6
  informatics nurse (IN), 7–10
  nursing informatics, 6–7, 7*f*
  theories supporting, 24–31, 25*t*
    change theories, 27–29
    chaos theory, 30–31
    cognitive science, 31
    data, information, knowledge, and wisdom (DIKW) model, 24–25
    general systems theory, 29–30, 30*f*
    Lewin's field theory, 28–29, 29*f*
    Rogers's diffusion of innovations theory, 27–28, 28*f*
    social informatics, 26
    sociotechnical theory, 26
Informatics nurse (IN)
  bedside experience, 31
  benefits, 10
  certification, 32, 34
  education
    continuing education, 35
    programs, 32
    standards and competencies, 31–32
  job titles, 223–225
  leadership, 245
  professional practice areas, 8
  project management, 240–245
  quality improvement (QI)
    benchmarking, 235–236
    Centers for Medicare & Medicaid Services (CMS), 236–237
    certification, 238
    The Joint Commission (TJC), 237
    models, 235
    National Quality Forum (NQF), 236
    and staffing, 238–239
    tools, 238
  roles and responsibilities, 36, 37*t*–38*t*
  specialists, 223, 225*b*
  specialty components and relationships, 7–8, 8*f*
  system responsibilities
    change/control management, 232–234
    Iowa Implementation Framework (IIF), 225, 226*f*
    system development, 230, 232

Index

system implementation, 225–229
system optimization and utilization, 229–230
systems life cycle, 225, 226f
systems life cycle, 225
Informatics nurse specialist (INS), 35–36, 37t–38t
Information, 24
  governance, 183
  privacy, 183–184
Information disorder, 81
Information finding
  library resources and services, 139–140
  literature search, 154–157
  nursing knowledge, 137–139
    evidence-based practice (EBP), 137–138
    PICOT Question, 138–139
  sources, 150–154
  research databases, 140–145
  search interface, 145–149
Information literacy, 6
  competency standards, 294, 295t
  in healthcare, 293–294
  health literacy, 293
  nursing organizations promoting, 294
Information technology (IT), 6
  healthcare. See Healthcare information technology (HIT),
  skills, 293
Initiating phase, project management, 240–241
  project goals, 241
  project scope, 241
INS. See Informatics nurse specialist (INS)
Institute for Healthcare Improvement (IHI), 294, 342
Institute for Safe Medication Practices (ISMP), 341, 341f
Institute of Medicine (IoM), 273
Institutional review board (IRB), 170
Insulin pump, 98f
Intangible assets, 241
Integrated interface approach, 226
Interface terminologies, 281–283
  Clinical Care Classification (CCC) system, 282
  International Classification for Nursing Practice (ICNP), 283
  North American Nursing Diagnosis Association (NANDA) International, 282
  Nursing Interventions Classification (NIC), 282
  Nursing Outcomes Classification (NOC), 282
  Omaha System, 282–283
  Perioperative Nursing Data Set (PNDS), 282
International Classification for Nursing Practice (ICNP), 283
International Classification of Disease (ICD), 261–262
International Classification of Functioning, Disability, and Health (ICF), 262
International Council of Nurses (ICN) Code of Ethics, 17–18
International Electrotechnical Commission (IEC), 261
International Health Terminology Standards Development Organization, 263
International Medical Informatics Association (IMIA), 12
International Standards Organizations (ISO), 260–261
  Comité Européen de Normalisation (CEN), 263
  Digital Imaging and Communications in Medicine (DICOM) organization, 262–263
  health level seven (HL7) standards, 261
  International Classification of Disease (ICD), 261–262
  International Classification of Functioning, Disability, and Health (ICF), 262
  International Electrotechnical Commission (IEC), 261
  SNOMED International, 263
Internet, 82
  domain name system, 65–66
  initial development, 64
  internet of medical things (IoMT), 64
  IP addresses, 65
  search engines, 66
  social determinant of health (SDoH), 64–65
  universal resource locator (URL), 65
  web browser, 66
Internet Corporation for Assigned Names and Numbers (ICANN), 65–66
Internet of medical things (IoMT), 64, 92
Internet service provider (ISP), 62
Internet telephone, 100
Interoperability, 228
  billing terminology standardization
    Healthcare Common Procedure Coding System (HCPCS), 264
    International Classification of Disease (ICD), 264
    Medicare Severity Diagnosis-Related Groups (MS-DRGs), 264
    Outcome and Assessment Information Set (OASIS), 264–265
    Patient Protection and Affordable Care Act (ACA), 264
  Comité Européen de Normalisation (CEN), 263
  Digital Imaging and Communications in Medicine (DICOM) organization, 262–263
  electronic laboratory reporting (ELR) services, 265
  ethical considerations, 259
  foundational, 253
  global data infrastructure, 265
  health information exchange (HIE), 253
  health level seven (HL7) standards, 261
  International Classification of Disease (ICD), 261–262
  International Classification of Functioning, Disability, and Health (ICF), 262
  International Electrotechnical Commission (IEC), 261
  International Health Terminology Standards Development Organization, 263
  international standards development, 263
  International Standards Organizations (ISO), 260–261
  levels, 253–254
  organizational, 254
  semantic, 253–254
  standards, 252, 254, 255b
  structural, 253
  U.S. efforts for promoting
    Centers for Disease Control and Prevention (CDC), 257

448 Index

Interoperability *(Continued)*
    Centers for Medicare & Medicaid Services (CMS), 255–256
    Office of the National Coordinator for Health Information Technology, 256–257
    Unified Medical Language System (UMLS), 257, 259
Interviews, data collection, 169
Intranet, 61
Invisible web (deep web), 145
IoMT. *See* Internet of medical things (IoMT)
Iowa Implementation Framework (IIF), 225, 226*f*
IP addresses, 65
ISO. *See* International Standards Organizations (ISO)

J
Journal article, 208
Journal editors, 208
Journal manuscripts, 208
Just Culture Assessment Tool (JCAT), 353
Just Culture Assessment Tool for Nursing Education (JCAT-NE), 353–354

K
Keylogger software, 69
Keylogger Trojan, 69
Knowledge, 24–25

L
Leadership, 245
Leading questions, 168*b*
Lesbian, gay, bisexual, transgender, questioning/queer, intersex, and asexual/agender (LGBTQIA), 164
Lewin's field theory, 28–29, 29*f*
    moving stage, 29, 29*f*
    refreezing stage, 29, 29*f*
    unfreezing stage, 28–29, 29*f*
LexisNexis, 145
Library resources and services, 139–140
Likert scale, 181
Limiters (filters), 141
Line charts, 189, 189*f*
LinkedIn, 76–77
Linux, 48
Liquid crystal display (LCD), 91
listserv, 79

Literacy assessment tools, 299
Literature search
    best evidence search, 154–157
    critical appraisal, 157
Loaded questions, 168*b*
Local area network (LAN), 61
Lock screen ransomware, 68
Logical Observation Identifiers Names and Codes (LOINC), 263, 283
Login name and passwords, authentication, 317

M
Machine learning, 190
Mail servers, 46
Mainframe computer, 47
Meaningful use, 255
Measures Management System (MMS), 236
Medical device, 97, 97*b*
Medical errors
    causes
        electronic health record (EHR), 336
        incivility, 336
        nursing behavior, 335–336
    counting, 337
    financial cost, 336–337
    measurement, 341–342
    prevention
        root cause analysis (RCA), 343–345, 346*f*, 347–348
        systems approach, 342–343
    Swiss cheese model, 343*f*
    types, 334*b*
    voluntary error reporting (VER), 337–338, 339*b*, 340–341
Medical subject headings (MeSH), 148
Medicare Promoting Interoperability Program, 255–256
Medicare Severity Diagnosis-Related Groups (MS-DRGs), 264
Medication error, 335
    health information technology (HIT)
        automated dispensing cabinet (ADC), 349
        barcode medication administration (BCMA), 349–350
        clinical decision support system (CDSS), 348–349
        computerized provider order entry (CPOE), 348
        smart infusion pumps, 350, 350*f*

    reporting, 341
Medjacking, 67
MEDLINE, 142
Merit-Based Incentive Payment System (MIPS), 236–237, 256, 256*f*
Meta-analyses, 154
Metadata, 141
Microblogs, 78
Microsoft Windows OS, 48
Minimum data set, 281
MIPS. *See* Merit-Based Incentive Payment System (MIPS)
Misinformation, 83
    combating, 82
    detection, 81–82
MMS. *See* Measures Management System (MMS)
Mobile devices, 47
    bluetooth, 96, 96*f*
    clinical practice, 103–104, 108–109
    cyber attacks, 106
    data transfer functions, 92
    internet of medical things (IoMT), 92
    near-field communication (NFC), 96–97, 97*f*
    networks, 96
    nursing research, 104
    self-monitoring, 119
    smartphones, 91
    synchronization (sync), 92
    tablet devices, 91
    wireless (WiFi) networking, 92, 93*t*–95*t*, 96
Mobile healthcare technology (mHealth)
    advantages and disadvantages, 104–105, 109
    artificial intelligence (AI), 107
    barcode medication administration (BCMA), 99, 99*f*
    eBook, 99–100
    ethical considerations, 108
    internet telephone, 100
    mobile devices, 90–97
    mobile medical devices, 97–98, 97*b*
    nanotechnology, 107–108
    smartwatches, 98–99
    software categories and examples, 101–103, 102*b*
    speech recognition software, 106–107
    video conferencing, 100–101
    wearables, 98, 99*f*

Mobile medical application, 101, 102b
Mobile medical devices, 97–98, 97b, 98f
Model for Improvement, 235
Modem, 62
Motherboard, 46
Motivational interviewing (MI) technique, 308–309

N
NANDA-I. *See* North American Nursing Diagnosis Association International (NANDA-I)
Nanotechnology, 107–108
National Academy of Medicine (NAM), 355
National Aeronautics and Space Administration (NASA), 114
National Coordinating Council for Medication Error Reporting and Prevention (NCC MERP), 341
National Council of State Boards of Nursing (NCSBN), 73, 79, 127
National Database of Nursing Quality Indicators (NDNQI), 237
National Electronic Disease Surveillance System (NEDSS), 257
National Healthcare Quality and Disparities Report (NHQDR), 340
National Informatics Agenda for Nursing Education and Practice, 7
National Institute of Nursing Research (NINR), 180
National Institutes of Health (NIH), 152, 300
National League for Nurses (NLN), 7, 31, 79, 294
National Patient Safety Goals (NPSGs), 355
National Pressure Injury Advisory Panel (NPIAP), 254
National Pressure Ulcer Advisory Panel (NPUAP), 254
National Quality Forum (NQF), 236
Natural disasters, 124–125
Natural language processing (NLP), 190
Natural language searches, 146
NCSBN. *See* National Council of State Boards of Nursing (NCSBN)
NDNQI. *See* National Database of Nursing Quality Indicators (NDNQI)

Near-field communication (NFC), 96–97, 97f
NEDSS. *See* National Electronic Disease Surveillance System (NEDSS)
Needs assessment, 242
Netiquette, 74–75
Network authentication, 63
Network connection
 speed, 63–64
 wireless connections, 62–63
Network model, 173
Network of Patient Safety Databases (NPSD), 340
Network security issues, 82–83
 breaches
  prevalence, 70–71
  protecting against, 71–72
 computer malware, 67–70
 cyber criminals, 67
Neuromuscular blocking agents (NMBAs), 349
NI. *See* Nursing informatics (NI)
NIC. *See* Nursing Interventions Classification (NIC)
NINR. *See* National Institute of Nursing Research (NINR)
Nodes, 60
Nominal data, 181
Nonrelational databases (NoSQL), 189
North American Nursing Diagnosis Association International (NANDA-I), 282
North American Treaty Organization (NATO), 124
North Carolina Nurses Association (NCNA), 200
NoSQL databases, 191
NPIAP. *See* National Pressure Injury Advisory Panel (NPIAP)
NQF. *See* National Quality Forum (NQF)
Nurse educators, 224
Nurse Licensure Compact (NLC), 127
Nursing & Allied Health Premium, 143–144
Nursing informatics (NI)
 American Nurses Association (ANA), 24
 benefits, 10
 competencies, 13–15, 14b
 continuum, 25–26
 data, 24
 definition, 6
 and ethics, 15–18
 frame-work model, 6, 7f

information, 24
 job responsibilities, 224f
 job titles, 223f
 knowledge, 24–25
 organizations, 13
 patient safety
  certification, 356
  culture, 350–356
  ethical considerations, 351
  measurement strategies, 337–342
  medical errors. *See* Medical errors
  program goals, 7
  recommendations, 7
 as specialty, 35–36
 specialty components and relationships, 7–8, 8f
 wisdom, 25, 26f
Nursing Informatics Workforce Survey, 222
Nursing Information and Data Set Evaluation Center (NIDSEC), 283
Nursing Interventions Classification (NIC), 282
Nursing knowledge
 library databases, 143t
 sources, 150–154
  government and not-for-profit specialty organization, 152
  laws, rules and regulations, 153
  levels of evidence, 154, 154b
  magazines, 152
  newsletters, 152
  newspaper and website articles, 152
  online evidence-based resources, 153, 153t
  online journals, 150–151
  open-access journals, 151–152
  professional nursing organization information, 152–153
  scholarly nursing journals, 150
Nursing Management Minimum Data Set (NMMDS), 281
Nursing Minimum Data Set (NMDS), 281
Nursing Outcomes Classification (NOC), 282

O
OASIS. *See* Outcome and Assessment Information Set (OASIS)
Object-oriented model, 173

Index

OBQI. *See* Outcome-Based Quality Improvement (OBQI)
Observations, data collection, 169
Office of the National Coordinator for Health Information Technology, 11, 256–257
OJIN. *See* Online Journal of Issues in Nursing (OJIN)
Omaha System, 282–283
ONC-Coordinated Federal Health Information Technology Strategic Plan, 11
One-time passcode (OTP), 318
Online communication, 83
   civility, 74
   group discussion forums, 79
   netiquette, 74–75
   professional behavior, 73
   social bookmarking, 78–79
Online evidence-based resources, 153, 153*t*
Online Journal of Issues in Nursing (OJIN), 151
Online journals, 150–151
Open-access journals, 151–152
Open medical record system (OpenMRS), 280
OpenNotes project, 280
Open-source software, 54
Operating system (OS)
   commercial software, 54
   computer programming (coding), 48–49
   examples, 47–48
   freeware, 54
   graphical user interface (GUI), 48
Oral communication, 300
Oral data presentation, 203
Ordinal data, 181
Organizational Health Insurance Portability and Accountability Act (HIPAA) violations, 322*b*
Organizational health literacy (OHL), 296
Organizational interoperability, 254
Outcome and Assessment Information Set (OASIS), 264–265
Outcome-Based Quality Improvement (OBQI), 264
Overly broad answer scale, 168*b*

P

PACS. *See* Picture archiving and communication system (PACS)
Paper records, 272–273
Parallel conversion, 227
Parameter query, 173
Password manager, 105*b*
Patient classification systems, 239
Patient Education Materials Assessment Tool (PEMAT), 302
Patient privacy and confidentiality data security
   breaches, 326–328
   data accuracy protection, 325
   data loss, 326
   risk assessment, 327
   unauthorized external data access, 325–326
   unauthorized internal data access, 325
   ensuring, 315–316
   ethical considerations, 315
   Health Insurance Portability and Accountability Act (HIPAA), 319–325
   regulation, 316
Patient Protection and Accountable Care Act (PPACA), 222, 264
Patient safety
   certification, 356
   culture, 350–356
   ethical considerations, 351
   measurement strategies, 337–342
   medical errors. *See* Medical errors
Patient Safety and Quality Improvement Act (PSQIA), 337
Patient safety organizations (PSOs), 338, 354–356
Patient satisfaction survey, 167
Patient Tracker program, 103
PDQ. *See* Physician Data Query (PDQ)
PDSA cycle. *See* Plan-do-study-act (PDSA) cycle
Peer-to-peer (P2P) architecture, 61
Perioperative Nursing Data Set (PNDS), 282
Personal computers, 47
Personal digital assistant (PDA) concept, 91
Personal health literacy, 296
Personal health records (PHRs), 277
Pharming, 68
Phased conversion, 228
PHIN. *See* Public Health Information Network (PHIN)
Phishing, 67–68
Physician Data Query (PDQ), 145
PICOT question, 138–139, 154
Picture archiving and communication system (PACS), 229
Pilot conversion, healthcare information technology, 228
Plagiarism, 141–142
Plain old telephone service (POTS), 62
Plan-do-study-act (PDSA) cycle, 235, 236*f*
PMBOK Guide. *See* Project Management Body of Knowledge (PMBOK) Guide
Polls, data collection, 166–167
Polydimethylsiloxane (PDMS) dermal patch, 118
Portable monitoring devices, 118
Positive patient identifier (PPID) system, 229
Poster handouts, 206–207
Poster presentations
   accent colors, 206
   design guidelines, 206, 206*b*
   electronic posters, 205
   handouts, 206–207
   print posters, 205
Predictive analytics, 191
Prescription software, 53
Primary data, 170
Print posters, 205
Print servers, 46
Privacy, 315
Privacy Rights Clearinghouse, 316
Process improvement, 240
Professional informatics organization, 35
Professional networking, 75
Professional nursing organization information, 152–153
Program for the International Assessment of Adult Competencies (PIAAC) survey, 297
Project ECHO, 117
Project goals, 241
Project management
   closing phase, 244–245
   controlling phase, 244
   execution phase, 242–244
      design and testing, 243
      implementation, 244
      preparing end users, 243–244
      workflow redesign, 243
   initiating phase, 240–241
      project goals, 241
      project scope, 241
   leadership, 245
   planning phase

Index

financial considerations, 241–242
project requirements, 242
process improvement, 240
steps involved, 240, 240f
Project Management Body of Knowledge (PMBOK) Guide, 240
Project requirements, 242
Project scope, 241
Protected health information (PHI), 316
Psion Organiser, 91
PsycARTICLES, 145
PsycINFO, 145
Public domain software, 55
Public Health Information Network (PHIN), 257
PubMed, 142–143
Pulse oximeter, 98f

Q

QI. See Quality improvement (QI)
QSEN initiative. See Quality and Safety Education for Nurses (QSEN) initiative
Qualitative data, 165
Quality and Safety Education for Nurses (QSEN) initiative, 14, 352
Quality improvement (QI)
 benchmarking
  Centers for Medicare & Medicaid Services (CMS), 236–237
  The Joint Commission (TJC), 237
  National Quality Forum (NQF), 236
  quality measures, 235
 certification, 238
 models for, 235
 and staffing, 238–239
  human resource management system (HRMS), 239
  patient classification systems, 239
 tools for, 238
Quality improvement organizations (QIOs), 238
Quality measures, 235
Quality Payment Program, 236–237
Quantitative data, 165, 181
Queries, 173
Query-based exchange, health information, 277
QWERTY keyboard, 91, 92f

R

Random access memory (RAM), 46, 91
Ransomware, 68–69
Readability of Mayo Clinic Web Page on Heart Failure, 301b
Read-only memory (ROM), 91
Reddit, 78
Reference managers, 141
Reference terminologies, 283
Reference terminology model, 260
Regional extension center (REC), 279
Registered nurse (RN), 222
Regression testing, 243
Reimbursement, telehealth, 126–127
Relational database, 173
Remote patient monitoring, 115, 116f
Request for information (RFI), 242
Request for proposal (RFP), 242
ResearchGate, 77
Return on investment (ROI), 241
RFI. See Request for information (RFI)
RFP. See Request for proposal (RFP)
Risk assessment, 327
Robotics, 115–116
 telepresence, 122–123, 122f
 and virtual reality, 115
Rogers's diffusion of innovations theory, 27–28, 28f
 change adopters, 27
 decision making stages, 28
Root cause analysis (RCA), 343–345, 346f, 347–348
Router, 62
R programming, 191

S

Safe networking, 80–81
Safety Attitudes Questionnaire (SAQ), 353–354
Satellite connections, 62
Scholarly nursing journals, 150
Scholarly writing, 207–208
School of Nursing Culture of Safety Survey (SON-COSS), 354
Schwirian's model of informatics, 6, 7f
Screen reader, 304
Search engines, 66
Search interface
 advantages, 148–149
 Boolean connectors, 146
 medical subject headings (MeSH), 148
 natural language searches, 146
 stop words, 146
 subject headings, 148
 truncation and wildcards, 147
Secondary data, 170
Second-level domain (2LD), 61
Secure digital (SD) cards, 50
Security breach, 321
Self-plagiarism, 142
Semantic interoperability, 253–254
Seminal work, 157
Sentinel event, 334–335
Servers, 46
Sexual orientation, gender identity, and variations in sex characteristics (SOGISC), 165
Shareware, 54
Sigma Theta Tau International (STTI)-sponsored journals, 153
Single server, 46
Single sign-on (SSO), 319
Situation, background, assessment, recommendation (SBAR) technique, 356
Skills assessment, 244
Smart clothing, 118
Smart infusion pumps, 350, 350f
SMART learning objectives. See Specific, measurable, actionable or achievable, reasonable or relevant, and time-bound (SMART) learning objectives
Smartphones, 47, 91, 105
Smart thermometer, 114f
Smartwatches, 98–99
SNOMED International, 263
SNT. See Standardized nursing terminology (SNT)
Social bookmarking, 78–79
Social determinants of health (SDoH), 64–65, 271, 298
Social engineering, 67
Social informatics, 26
Social media, 83
 guidelines, 79–80, 80t
 image-based platforms, 77
 microblogs, 78
 popular social networks, 75, 76f
 professional networking, 75
 safe networking, 80–81
 social networking sites, 75–77, 77t
 video-sharing and streaming platforms, 77–78
Social networking sites, 75–77, 77t
Social Security number (SSN), 321
Sociotechnical theory, 26

Software, 46
  commercial software, 54
  freeware, 54
  open-source software, 54
  shareware, 54
SOGISC. *See* Sexual orientation, gender identity, and variations in sex characteristics (SOGISC)
Solid-state drive (SSD), 50
Space Technology Applied to Rural Papago Advanced Health Care (STARPAHC) program, 114
Spam, 69
Sparklines, 189, 189*f*
Specific, measurable, achievable, relevant, and time-bound (SMART) learning objectives, 201, 202*f*, 241
Speech recognition software, 106–107
Spreadsheet, 171
Spyware, 70
SQL. *See* Structured query language (SQL)
Stacked bar chart, 188–189
Standalone personal health records, 277
Standardized nursing terminology (SNT)
  ANA-recognized, 281*b*
  implementation barriers, 284
  interface terminologies, 281–283
  minimum data set, 281
  Nursing Information and Data Set Evaluation Center (NIDSEC), 283
  patient care, 280–281
  reference terminologies, 283
Stanford History Education Group (SHEG), 82
STARPAHC program. *See* Space Technology Applied to Rural Papago Advanced Health Care (STARPAHC) program
Stop words, 146
Storage drive, 46
Store-and-forward (S&F) technology, 115
Strategic planning, 245
Structural interoperability, 253
Structured data, 181
Structured query language (SQL), 173, 181
Subject headings, 148
Subreddits, 78
Supercomputer, 47

Super user, 34
Survey of Patient Safety (SOPS), 353
Swedish medical record, 272*f*
Swiss cheese model, medical errors, 343*f*
Synchronization (sync), 92
Synchronous telehealth, 115, 115*f*
Systematized Nomenclature of Medicine-Clinical Terminology (SNOMED CT), 263, 283, 285
System implementation
  big-bang conversion, 228
  interoperability and system integration, 228–229
  parallel conversion, 227
  phased conversion, 228
  pilot conversion, 228
  system selection, 225–227
Systems development
  change/control management, 232–234
  communication systems, 232
  user interface (UI), 232
Systems life cycle, 225, 226*f*

T
Tablet devices, 47, 91
Tangible assets, 241
"Teach-back" technique, 300
Technology Informatics Guiding Education Reform (TIGER) initiative, 13–14, 14*b*, 294
Telehealth
  asynchronous, 115, 115*f*
  chronic illness management, 123–124
  disaster healthcare, 124–125
  and education, 117
  e-intensive care units, 120–123
  issues, 129
    fraud, 127–128
    high-speed internet access, 125–126
    regulation, 127
    reimbursement, 126–127
  portable monitoring devices, 118–119
  primary care, 120
  remote patient monitoring, 115, 116*f*
  robotics, 115–116
  self-monitoring, 119
  standards, 116–117
  store-and-forward (S&F) technology, 115
  synchronous, 115, 115*f*

  telehomecare, 118
  telemedicine, 114
  telemental health, 120
  telenursing, 116
  teletrauma, 123
  types, 115–116, 115*f*
Telehomecare, 118
Tele-intensive care units, 120, 122
Telemedicine, 53, 114
Telemental health, 120
Telenursing, 116, 129
Telepresence, 115–116
Teletrauma, 123
Tethered personal health records, 277
Text Readability Analyzer (TRAY) tool, 301
The Joint Commission (TJC), 237, 334, 345
Third-level domain (3LD), 61
TIGER initiative. *See* Technology Informatics Guiding Education Reform (TIGER) initiative
TikTok, 78
TJC, 355
Top-level domain (TLD), 66
Topology, 61, 61*f*
Trojan horse program, 69
Trolls, 81
Truncation, 147
Two-factor authentication (2*f*A), 317–318, 318*f*

U
UDL. *See* Universal design for learning (UDL)
UMLS. *See* Unified Medical Language System (UMLS)
Unauthorized internal data access, 325
Unbalanced answer scale options, 168*b*
Understandability, health literacy, 302
Unified Medical Language System (UMLS), 257, 259, 259*b*, 283
Universal design for learning (UDL), 209–212
  accessibility
    alternative text, 210–211
    checks, 210
    closed captions, 209
    color perception, 211
    design, 210
    online instruction, 209
    inclusive instruction, 211–212
    usability, 211
Universal patient identifier (UPI), 321

Universal resource locator (URL), 65, 65f
Universal serial bus (USB) port, 50
Unstructured data, 181, 189–190
U.S. Census Bureau, 185
U.S. Department of Health and Human Services (USDHHS), 117
U.S. Department of Justice (USDOJ), 127–128
User interface (UI), 232
U.S. Government, 185

V
Video conferencing, 100–101, 116
Video-sharing platforms, 77–78
Virtual private network (VPN), 71
Virtual servers, 46
Visible web (surface web), 145

Voice over Internet Protocol (VoIP), 100
Voluntary error reporting (VER), 337–338, 340–341

W
WAN. *See* Wide area network (WAN)
Warez, 69
Wearables, 98, 99f
Wearable technology, 47
Web Accessibility in Mind (WebAIM)., 211–212
Web browser, 66
Webcast, 101
Webinar, 101
Web servers, 46
White hat hackers, 325
Wide area network (WAN), 61
Wikipedia, 79
Wildcards, 147

Wireless (WiFi) connections, 61–63, 92, 93t–95t, 96
Wireless (WiFi)-protected access (WPA), 63
Wisdom, 25, 26f
Workflow, 241
Workplace
  civility, 74, 74t
  incivility, 336
Workstation, 47
World Wide Web, 64
Worm, online security, 69
Written communication, 300–302

Y
YouTube, 77–78

Z
Zotero, 141